PREHOSPITAL CARE ADMINISTRATION

·

ISSUES

·

READINGS

·

CASES

PREHOSPITAL CARE ADMINISTRATION

•

ISSUES

•

READINGS

•

CASES

Joseph J. Fitch, PhD

Acquisitions Editor: Rina Steinhauer
Editorial Assistant: Melissa Blair

Printed in the United States of America.

Library of Congress Cataloging-in-Publication Data
Prehospital care administration : issues, readings, cases / Joseph J.
  Fitch, [editor].
      p.   cm.
  Collection of previously published and original articles.
  Includes bibliographical references and index.
  ISBN 0-8151-3391-X (softcover)
  1. Emergency medical services—Administration. 2. Emergency medical
services—United States—Administration.   I. Fitch, Joseph J.
  [DNLM: 1. Emergency Medical Services—organization &
administration—collected works.   WX 215 P9229 1995]
  RA645.5.P72 1995
  362. 1'8'068—dc20
  DNLM/DLC
  for Library of Congress   94-49606
                                       CIP

ISBN: 0-8151-3391-X
Book Code: 25879
Jems Product Code: JP0203

Jems Communications
A division of Mosby-Year Book, Inc.
P.O. Box 2789
Carlsbad, California 92018
(619) 431-9797

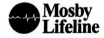

Dedicated to Publishing Excellence

Mosby-Year Book, Inc.
11830 Westline Industrial Drive
St. Louis, Missouri 63146

Publishing coordination and book production by
Laing Communications Inc., Redmond, Washington, and Edmonton, Alberta

Design and Production: Sandra J. Harner
Editorial Coordination/Copyediting: Susan B. Bureau

Contents

Preface

Many people contribute to the birth of a book—friends, clients, colleagues. This is particularly true with the collection of articles in *Prehospital Care Administration: Issues, Readings, Cases.*

The impetus for this book came from the frequent requests for reprints of articles published in the *Journal of Emergency Medical Services* (*JEMS*). The book was also envisioned as a companion reading and case book for the college text *EMS Management: Beyond the Street.* Our goal was to put together, in a single volume, a ready reference that both EMS leaders and students would want on their bookshelves.

As Development Editor Rick Minerd and I began the process of sorting through more than a thousand articles in the *JEMS* library, it became obvious that exciting things were occurring within EMS about which no one had written. As a result, a number of talented EMS leaders were asked to submit original articles addressing specific topics.

In addition, we felt that articles appearing in other journals and magazines were excellent and should be included. We are appreciative of the authors and publishers who were willing to share their knowledge and manuscripts. A list of these publications is included in the Acknowledgments section.

As you read this book, remember that we are all learning. Please provide feedback and let us know about articles you would recommend for inclusion in future editions. Write Rick Minerd or me at the Kansas City offices of Fitch & Associates, Inc., P.O. Box 170, Platte City, Mo. 64079-0179, or call us at (816) 431-2600.

—Jay Fitch

Publication Acknowledgments

WHILE THE COLLECTION OF ARTICLES from *JEMS* was the focal point in our search for significant management material, chapters and articles from a number of other books and publications were also used. These previously published contributions are mentioned in the source information at the end of each article, but we would like to especially acknowledge the following publishers and publications.

Ambulance Industry Journal
American Ambulance Association
3800 Auburn Boulevard, Suite C
Sacramento, Calif. 95821-2102

Annals of Emergency Medicine
American College of Emergency
　Physicians
P.O. Box 619911
Dallas, Tex. 75261-9911

Emergency
Hare Publications
6300 Yarrow Drive
Carlsbad, Calif. 92009

EMS Insider
Jems Communications
P.O. Box 2789
Carlsbad, Calif. 92018

Fire Chief
35 East Wacker Drive, Suite 700
Chicago, Ill. 60601-2198

*Journal of Emergency Medical
　Services*
Jems Communications
P.O. Box 2789
Carlsbad, Calif. 92018

Management Focus
Fitch & Associates, Inc.
303 Marshall Road
Platte City, Mo. 64079

Prehospital and Disaster Medicine
Jems Communications
1 University Avenue, Room 434
Madison, Wisc. 53705

the Research Evaluation
Scott Bourn Associates, Inc.
557 Burbank Street, Unit B
Broomfield, Colo. 80020

And excerpts from the books:

*Infection Control for Prehospital
Care Providers*, 2nd ed. Reprinted
with permission from Mercy
Ambulance, Grand Rapids, Mich.
Copyright © 1993.

*The New Owner: Making the
Transition from Employee to
Employer.* Reprinted with permission
from Business One Irwin,
Homewood, Ill. Copyright © 1993.

Introduction

It's important to make certain that our efforts are directed at the decisive core of the problem, and not on distracting issues. The more complex the difficulties we face, the more important it becomes to bear this in mind, for it is human nature to try to evade what we cannot cope with.

—Bernard Baruch

ONE OF MY IDIOSYNCRASIES is being an avid *Star Trek—the Next Generation* fan. On the show, the characters frequently refer to observing the "prime directive." Star Trek's prime directive is to seek new life forms without interfering or otherwise compromising the newly discovered culture and way of life. Those in charge of EMS systems also have a prime directive.

The prime directive for EMS leaders is to develop and sustain sophisticated, future-oriented EMS systems that are clinically efficacious, operationally efficient, and—at the same time—cost effective. That, as Bernard Baruch would put it, "is at the core of the problems we face."

Many distractions can steer us away from our EMS prime directive. People can present puzzling problems—and when they do, the EMS leader must focus on the prime directive. When we become complacent with the operational status quo, we must concentrate even harder on the prime directive. When we become jaded about current clinical care, we must redouble our efforts to achieve the prime directive. And regardless of how politically powerful or powerless we become—as EMS leaders, we must constantly focus on the prime directive.

The unique difficulties in, and opportunities for, achieving the EMS leadership prime directive are outlined in the articles and cases presented in the five parts of this book. Human resources topics are presented in Part One. Parts Two, Three, and Four deal with evolving operations, financial issues, and managing in the changing clinical and technological environment, respectively. Part Five presents issues and options in system design and the political process. This last part concludes with a section outlining visions of the future from several different perspectives.

Each article in this book is introduced with a brief synopsis describing its relevance to EMS leaders.

Even though Bernard Baruch believed it is human nature for us to evade what we cannot cope with, I believe it is our calling as EMS leaders to steadfastly move toward the future. Many talented authors throughout this book have provided information and differing perspectives to—as Enterprise Captain Jean-Luc Picard would say—"make it so!"

—Jay Fitch

Part One

Understanding Cultural and Human Resources

A house divided against itself cannot stand. . . . Our cause must be entrusted to and conducted by its own undoubted friends—whose hands are free, whose hearts are in the work—who do care for the result.

—Abraham Lincoln

Lincoln's comments have particular meaning for those who lead EMS systems today, even though he lived almost 140 years ago. EMS leaders have to recognize the value and dignity of others if they are to unite the house and help others keep their hearts in the work.

Lincoln fully understood the importance of leadership, motivation, and ethics. Recruitment and retention of troops throughout the Civil War were major issues for this president. He built strong alliances during his presidency and gained the trust and respect of his subordinates. Known as the Great Emancipator, Lincoln knew how to accommodate cultural differences. Finally, through his own life and the lives of those he touched, he was familiar with the toll that stress can take.

It is often said that EMS is a "people business." However, human resources issues are not always given high priority. To achieve success, EMS leaders must shift their focus from effect to cause, from treatment to prevention, from responding to an issue to anticipating the issue. Experience consulting with hundreds of organizations has underscored, for me, the importance of understanding and optimizing human resources on a proactive basis. The authors contributing to this section bring this concept to life.

—Jay Fitch

Leadership, Motivation, and Ethics in EMS

It All Starts With Leadership

Jay Fitch, PhD

The function of leadership either propels EMS systems and their people into the future or condemns them to constantly relearn the lessons of the past. In this original article, the author describes 10 common characteristics found in some of the most effective leaders in the EMS profession.

LEADERSHIP IS OFTEN a very personal topic that defies adequate description. What is it? How does it happen? What are the characteristics and attitudes of effective leaders? One example from early in my own EMS experience comes to mind.

It had been a long, hot summer. I was 24 years old and the new director of St. Louis's troubled EMS system. Response times were long, equipment was poor, and an invisible color line divided the city. Our staff had its own racial tensions as well. The majority of the staff was not excited about the rapid implementation of change.

Suddenly, the radio crackled loudly as a unit staffed by two black crew members put out a distress call. Several inebriated family members had verbally abused the crew while they "packaged" the elderly white patient for transport. The verbal taunts had quickly progressed into a shoving match. By the time another supervisor and I arrived to rescue the crew with the help of several police officers, the crew's resolve to transport the patient had diminished considerably.

"Do you want to get a white crew to take the patient in?" the staff member quietly asked me. I instinctively responded, "If he doesn't want you—he doesn't want *any* of us. So go ahead and take care of your patient. If he gives you any more guff, let him die where he lies."

Popular leadership and management texts might describe this incident in terms of my leadership role. Was I an agent of change? A visionary? Intuitive? Peter Drucker's distinction between *effective* and *efficient* is relevant. Getting an all-white crew to make the assignment would have been an efficient response, "doing things right" as Drucker puts it. But clearly, "doing the right thing" had a more effective impact on the crew members and on the system as a whole. The tension within our organization seemed to subside a bit as staff heard about the incident. It became a statement that we were all on the same team.

EMS leadership is about creating teams of people committed to both doing things right and doing the right thing.

10 Key Leadership Characteristics

In my 25 years in EMS, I have had the opportunity to work with and observe a variety of leaders, chiefs, and managers. The great leaders of our profession share 10 common attitudes and characteristics. They are

- The ability to integrate vision and strategy
- Proving that performance is primary
- Expectations that stretch rather than directives that compress
- Ensuring optimal service through development of team members
- Clear, no-nonsense accountability for results
- Intuitive communication abilities
- Building on team members' strengths rather than dwelling on their weaknesses
- Passion for change
- Uncompromising ethical behavior, in the broadest sense
- *Lots* of hard work

Consistently applied, these attitudes, concepts, and characteristics can transform both the EMS organization and its members. A more detailed exploration of the 10 characteristics follows.

The Ability to Integrate Vision and Strategy

Leadership textbooks describe the need for leaders to be visionaries, but few explain what that means in the context of the workday world. Being an EMS visionary is having the ability to see the possible *and* move the organization toward it. This requires thinking around the corner—or outside the box—and developing strategies that empower individuals to accomplish the vision.

To fulfill the dual leadership role of having one's head in the clouds (vision) and feet on the ground (solid strategy), the leader must use both a telescope and a microscope. The telescope is used to understand the big picture and ensure perspective. The microscope is used to keep a microscopic command of critical details, which is necessary for implementing strategy.

The ability to integrate these two distinct parts of the leadership role is a crucial step. Integration is defined as bringing the parts together as a whole. In the context of leadership, integration also involves linking each individual's vision and goals to the mission and strategies of the organization. This multilevel integration is the method great EMS leaders use to link vision and strategy.

Proving that Performance Is Primary

Good leaders consistently deal with performance and *only* performance. They avoid getting caught up in egos, personalities, preferences,

EMS leadership is about creating teams of people committed to both doing things right and doing the right thing.

Good leaders stretch their employees, but they never expect more than employees are capable of performing.

turf battles, and the like. In short, good leaders focus on fulfilling commitments rather than targets and intentions.

Response times illustrate this point. In the past 10 years, the standards for response times have become increasingly specific. Response time performance, which used to be shrouded in the generalities of averages, is now typically measured on a definitive basis. For example, the acceptable urban response time is generally considered to be four minutes with 90-percent compliance for fire department first responder units, and eight minutes with 90-percent compliance for transporting ALS units, as measured from call receipt. There can be little confusion about the system's actual performance when it's measured so objectively.

The same is true for measuring the performance of other aspects of the EMS program and its personnel. When there are no objective benchmarks, the measurement tools become subjective and far less fair. Developing standards and consistently relying on objective performance indicators rather than being unduly influenced by personalities, preferences, and egos is a characteristic of a true EMS leader.

Expectations that Stretch Rather Than Directives that Compress

Current management literature underscores the fact that managers can't *give* motivation. Instead, EMS leaders create an environment in which *self*-motivation can occur. A sure way to do this is to create expectations that expand roles and invite contributions.

Most employees want to participate and will initially make efforts to do so. If an EMS leader recognizes the employee for the contribution and simply comments that it's an interesting idea rather than telling the employee why the idea won't work or that it has already been suggested, then the leader has begun the process of creating expectations that stretch workers.

Good leaders stretch their employees, but they never expect more than employees are capable of performing. However, they often do expect more than employees believe they can accomplish. This approach is key for developing confidence and helping workers feel empowered.

Creating expectations that lift and stretch employees rather than directives that compress them has several specific advantages for EMS organizations. Team members feel they are listened to and involved, they make an emotional investment in their plan, and they work harder to fulfill new expectations.

Ensuring Optimal Service Through Development of Team Members

One strength of the EMS profession is that it is highly focused on the needs of patients and customers. Future-oriented leaders are also aware of the needs within their organizations. They treat employees as one of the most important consumer groups that the organization serves.

Organizations cannot achieve greatness unless people throughout the organization are constantly growing. Growing individuals seek better ways of doing things both professionally and personally. Providing growth opportunities can be likened to the biblical story of sowing seeds. Some seeds will fall on the rocks and will not grow. Others will begin to grow but will be taken over by weeds. Still others will grow and return a full yield. While not every person will grow at the same rate, EMS leaders should encourage all members of their organizations to develop the full range of their talents.

To avoid the "arrested development syndrome," in which workers get limited satisfaction from caring for patients and almost no satisfaction from being a member of their EMS organization, leaders must encourage individual growth. Only growing, learning, motivated individuals can provide optimal service.

Clear, No-Nonsense Accountability for Results

Good EMS leaders set high expectations through mutually agreed-upon performance objectives and hold each individual accountable for his personal results. The individual's results are building blocks for the organization's mission, goals, key result areas, and action plans. This approach provides a way to move from generalities to tough-minded specifics throughout the organization.

Leaders work with each employee to develop performance standards based on results. True accountability means holding someone responsible for achieving results in all key jobs. To ensure success, the EMS leader must break down the responsibilities to *measurable* components and require clear and concise progress reports.

Effective leaders reward performance in a variety of ways. They dismantle rigid compensation systems that reward mediocrity and instead employ policies that ensure all team members are rewarded generously for measurable contributions to fulfilling customers' needs and the organization's mission.

Intuitive Communication Abilities

The Latin root of communicate means "to make common." Communication skills are at the core of the EMS leader's job. The effectiveness of leaders is measured in their face-to-face communication skills and their interpersonal insights and actions.

Being a great communicator involves using intuitive communication. Leaders must share their vulnerability, send a signal of approachability, and constantly practice positive listening. Vulnerability in professional relationships can be defined as openness to experiences and the absence of defensive, petty, or suspicious behavior. Approachability means reaching out to become interested in others. Through openness, we let ourselves out and the other person in.

We all think we know how to listen, but too often managers participate in simultaneous one-way communication rather than in active listening to the other person. We must become alert enough to find the

> **Leaders work with each employee to develop performance standards based on results.**

Clear, objective, and consistent affirmation of strengths—not frivolous undeserved praise—is the most powerful tool the EMS leader has.

positive in what other people are saying and reinforce it rather than judge the content or the context.

In other words, share, care, and dare to be intuitively in touch. Cultivate a curious and zestful interest in the uniqueness of your team members. Ask—and really listen. Focus on their strengths and link them to your organization's vision, mission, and goals to dissolve their defenses.

Building on Team Members' Strengths Rather Than Dwelling on Their Weaknesses

True EMS leaders recognize that they, like all people, have weaknesses. Their primary concern, however, is strengths. They know that strengths—not weaknesses—will make their organizations thrive.

Overemphasizing weaknesses shackles employees with miserable self-images. Finding strengths and using them in a meaningful way sets employees free. Clear, objective, and consistent affirmation of strengths—not frivolous undeserved praise—is the most powerful tool the EMS leader has. People have a great need to have their strengths properly and fully used. Tapping into this motivational source provides tremendous implications for morale and performance.

Passion for Change

Great EMS leaders truly love what they do. They have a passion for their job and see it as a "calling" to make a difference. They understand that this means constantly changing perspectives, work methods, techniques, and a whole host of other items. Understanding the constancy of change serves as an internal guidance system allowing leaders to point the way and to radiate energy that both empowers and sustains the team. EMS leaders who work in this state of mind use every thought, word, and action to enhance people and reassure them rather than diminish them or play upon their fears.

EMS leaders are fortunate. In almost all respects, ours is a noble profession. Many opportunities exist for blending personal and professional pathways. Typically, those with a passion for their leadership responsibilities keep it alive by growing and expanding their own dreams. As individual leaders grow, their image and reality of "the possible" also grow. In inspiring success and moving to a new level of performance, leaders facilitate change through the reinvention and transformation of team members and the organization.

Uncompromising Ethical Behavior, in the Broadest Sense

Personal and professional ethics and principles are inextricably intertwined. Those who believe that they can be separated are simply deceiving themselves. Leadership expert Steven Covey describes principles as being "like a compass, always pointing the right way." As long as you know which way true north is, you won't get lost or confused by conflicting paths. "At the root of societal declines," said Covey, "are foolish practices that represent violations of correct principles."

The philosophy of the organization must make it absolutely clear that integrity is the beginning and end of all policies, procedures, practices, programs, and people in the organization.

Lots of Hard Work

No one who has advanced in the EMS profession will tell you it's an easy road. It takes commitment, conviction, and hard work.

Philip D. Reed, former chairman of General Electric, observed that those who get the most out of life are those who "do whatever they do, all out. Whether it be work or play, dull or exciting, little or big, they give the matter their undivided attention and try to do their best. Without being stuffy about it, they have made a habit of being satisfied with only their utmost effort."

Remember, it is your attitude—not your aptitude—that determines your ultimate altitude in EMS.

One Final Thought

Leadership in EMS comes in many shapes, sizes, and sources. Sometimes it comes from where you least expect it. Never forget to show appreciation for others' hard work.

I began this article by sharing an incident that occurred when I worked in St. Louis. One of my leadership mentors in that community was a 43-year-old woman who had worked her way up from nurse's aide to deputy health commissioner. Florence Hill was an elegant, quiet leader who could also be quite intimidating when she drew herself up to her full height of six feet. She was a kind, gentle soul who saved my "political bacon" on more than one occasion my first year on the job.

She stood with me, often putting her 25 years of experience in the system in jeopardy, to fight for the resources necessary to improve care and reduce response times from 16 minutes down to four. She gently "suggested" improvements in my place while reinforcing my dignity and worth.

She died suddenly, and I never was able to share my appreciation. Don't let that happen to you. Find a way to say thank you each day to both those who help shape and those who follow your leadership.

References

Batten, J. D. *Tough-Minded Leadership*. New York: Amacom, 1989.
Covey, S. R. *Principle Centered Leadership*. New York: Fireside/Simon & Schuster, 1992.
Drucker, P. R. *Management Tasks, Responsibilities, Practices*. New York: Harper & Row, 1974.
Tomasko, R. M. *Rethinking the Corporation*. New York: Amacom, 1993.

Source
Original article.

Carrots to Kudos: Motivating EMS Providers

John M. Norris,
MPA, NREMT-P

Motivating staff is one of the most complex challenges any EMS manager faces. In this article, John Norris describes a number of nuts and bolts models that have been proven to motivate EMS providers.

JOHN SMITH AND MARY JONES are paramedics in a large metropolitan fire department. John's biannual performance rating is consistently the highest on his shift, and he gets along well with his supervisors and peers. He regularly attends extracurricular educational functions and earned a bachelor's degree in emergency health services management while employed full-time. He attends monthly staff meetings while off duty and regularly submits suggestions and plans for improving his division to his supervisor.

Mary's performance is the opposite of John's. Her performance ratings are generally low, and she attends only the required educational functions. She has problems dealing with peers and was recently transferred to another shift because of personality conflicts. She often speaks about the poor morale of personnel in the emergency medical services division and expresses her desire to transfer to another division.

Why do some employees, such as John, consistently work to their potential while others, such as Mary, do not? This is a problem faced by numerous managers whose responsibility it is to motivate their employees.

Fortunately, there are specific methods that can be used to motivate low-performing personnel to the point that, in many cases, their productivity increases to peak levels. But EMS responders who are promoted to mid-management positions often don't know about these methods. These newly promoted managers and supervisors have been taught how to manage an airway or accident scene, but not how to manage people!

The Persuasion Model

Mike Warren, a paramedic, has been late for work three times in the past month, one time arriving five minutes late with his shirt unbuttoned and without any shoes or socks on his feet. His ratio of successful IV attempts has dropped significantly, and his partner has complained that Warren has become incapable of making routine decisions. The paramedic supervisor recently held a meeting with Warren and determined that he suffers from a lack of motivation, which has resulted in the loss of his "can-do" attitude.

At some point in their careers, EMS providers may suffer from a lack of motivation. This condition is not necessarily irreversible; a manager well versed in motivational techniques can often help providers regain their professional drive. While conventional wisdom might advocate the use of monetary incentives for such low-performing providers, non-monetary incentives can work just as well. As Thomas Peters, in his book *In Search of Excellence*, says:

> All of us are self-centered, suckers for a bit of praise, and generally like to think of ourselves as winners. But the fact of the matter is that our talents are distributed normally—none of us is really as good as he or she would like to think, but rubbing our noses daily in that reality doesn't do us a bit of good. The systems in the excellent companies are not only designed to produce lots of winners, they are constructed to celebrate the winning once it occurs. Their systems make extraordinary use of non-monetary incentives.

A manager can use two specific techniques to help restore employees' motivation: Help them develop a "can-do" attitude, and convince them that hard work will be rewarded.

An EMS provider can lack a "can-do" attitude for a variety of reasons. He may have experienced a recent performance setback that others are unaware of, such as being unable to locate a trapped person or experiencing a conflict with a nurse or physician who may have criticized his competency. Or his attitude may have developed after being repeatedly told by his supervisor that he is incompetent. Whatever the reason for an employee's lack of confidence, the manager can improve it by

- Giving positive feedback at every opportunity, followed by any gentle negative feedback that may need to be given, so that the provider's self-esteem is gradually improved
- Establishing a trial period with the provider for measuring his performance and effort—during this period, the manager will provide regular and direct performance feedback in a personal and supportive manner
- Not ignoring any disappointments the provider may experience—errors can be interpreted as indicators of progress; learning often does not take place until mistakes are made

A manager can attempt to reward employees by using the existing formal awards available within the system. Another option is to develop other, more imaginative ways of rewarding good performers. An example of this type of reward might be providing the responder with interesting assignments and challenging tasks, such as allowing him to participate in a new equipment study, sending him on trips to inspect new vehicles, or asking him to contribute to important research or committees.

Another example would be to manipulate rules and regulations so that providers are able to interpret them in a more favorable way. Compensatory time off or time off with permission is often a coveted reward.

A third example of imaginative rewards would be to allow the provider more opportunities to work unsupervised. The use of praise, recognition, awards, and symbols of accomplishment, such as certificates, badges, and medals, can also be effective. One other type of reward to compensate good performers is to allow them increased access to higher man-

A manager can use two specific techniques to help restore employees' motivation: Help them develop a "can-do" attitude, and convince them that hard work will be rewarded.

agement. An invitation to participate in a senior-level staff meeting, for example, or to meet with the boss might be suitable. When granting rewards, however, keep in mind that different people may have different values. The manager should therefore be sensitive to the awards that his workers value the most.

Unlike Warren's case, there may be occasions when a provider is putting out significant effort but is still not performing adequately. To address this problem, the manager should try to remove the impediments to good performance and help the employee understand what is expected of him.

When impediments to good performance exist that are beyond the provider's control (e.g., poor equipment, inadequate budgetary resources, or insufficient training), he will begin to show signs of frustration. The manager must be aware of these signs and remove the impediments as soon as possible. If an employee's performance is blocked for an extended period of time, he will be very difficult to motivate. Some common signs of frustration include the following:

- The provider deals with peers and the public aggressively.
- The provider shows anger in dealing with inanimate objects, such as a stretcher or tool.
- The provider repeatedly uses an incorrect procedure to accomplish a basic task, such as assembling a scoop stretcher.
- The provider often appears to be inattentive, and he daydreams.
- The provider is unrealistically negative.
- The provider seems to have given up.

When impediments are identified and removed, the manager can then help the provider understand what is expected of him. This can often be done during a counseling session using management by objectives (MBO), a management method in which management and the employee mutually establish the employee's goals.

Another method is to provide the employee with an action plan, a written statement that is very specific. Avoid statements such as, "Do the best you can," and include statements such as, "You need to improve your IV ratio from one out of three to two out of three." The plan should deal with performance rather than effort, and it should be developed with the provider's input.

Fostering Motivation Through Persuasion

Is the provider trying hard enough?

Yes	No
Help him develop a "can-do" attitude.	Remove impediments to good performance.
Convince him that hard work will be rewarded.	Develop goals or action plans with the provider.
Be fair with punishments and rewards.	

The Productivity Gainsharing Model

Productivity gainsharing is designed to motivate providers by allowing them to become directly involved in decisions regarding how their work can be improved. It achieves this by allowing for job rotation, open communication, and performance feedback.

Job Rotation

At specific time periods, the provider rotates to a different location. The purpose of the rotation is not to relieve boredom; rather, it is to teach each person how the other positions function. For example, the types of patients and methods of treatment in a small residential district may be vastly different from those in a large industrial area. This type of rotation also helps reduce burnout by relieving providers of the pressure associated with a district that has a high call volume. Similarly, providers who move from a slow district to a busier one are given the opportunity to increase the number of incidents they see. They are thus able to practice their skills more often.

Providers can also be rotated to positions other than those within fire and ambulance stations. A provider could, for example, be rotated into an administrative position or be assigned to ride along with his battalion chief. Other job rotation options for smaller EMS organizations might include assignment to an emergency department or to a teaching facility as an assistant. The options are limited only by the resources available and the manager's imagination.

Open Communication

An open network of communication is essential in productivity gainsharing; it is important for providers to voice their concerns and to see that their concerns are acted on. In Ohio, for example, one successful manager spends two hours a day just talking with employees! They discuss job-related problems and any other matters that may be on an employee's mind. And in Baltimore County, Md., all EMS providers are invited to attend EMS staff meetings. The minutes from these meetings and other management-level meetings are published and sent to each station weekly. In addition, a portion of the semiannual continuing education curriculum is devoted to "gripe sessions," in which providers are encouraged to voice their concerns and recommendations. The input is recorded and acted on by the system's managers.

Performance Feedback

As in the persuasion model, performance feedback is an essential element in letting the providers know how their job performance is measuring up to their own goals and those of the department. The provider needs to be told what is going right or wrong and why. This feedback should be provided often and regularly. Strengths and weaknesses should be discussed, and a plan for improvement in the coming months should be developed.

The Job-Enrichment Model

Job enrichment is not a one-time solution to motivation problems but a continual function of management. It provides an opportunity for increasing an employee's psychological growth by using motivators rather than hygiene factors. Hygiene factors relate to lower-level needs, such as hunger, thirst, security, and safety. Motivators, on the other hand, relate to higher-level needs, such as self-actualization, self-esteem, and a sense of belonging. The use of motivators often results in long-term motivational gains that cannot be achieved with hygiene factors alone.

Motivators Versus Hygiene Factors	
Motivators	*Hygiene Factors*
Achievement	Company policy and administration
Recognition of achievement	
The work itself	Supervision
Increased responsibility	Interpersonal relationships
Job-related growth	Working conditions
Advancement	Salary
	Status
	Security

In a job-enrichment study conducted by IBM Corp., one group of employees had their jobs enriched by various motivators while the members of the control group continued to perform their jobs in the traditional way. No hygiene changes were made other than instituting normal pay raises for both groups.

At the beginning of the six-month study period, the performances of the enriched group declined slightly, probably due to some uncertainty about the newly acquired responsibilities instituted as a motivator. After the first quarter, however, this decline was followed by a significant increase in performance for the remainder of the study, and after six months, members of the enriched group were found to be outperforming the control group. In addition, they showed increased admiration for their jobs, had a lower absenteeism rate, and had a much higher rate of promotion.

At the conclusion of the study, both groups were asked 16 questions designed to assess motivation levels; the answers were scaled from one to five, with a maximum possible score of 80 points. Results of the study indicated that members of the enriched group began to feel much more positive about their jobs, while the control group did not demonstrate any significant change.

There are seven steps that managers should take in effecting job enrichment among their providers:

- Approach the job with the conviction that it can be changed. Many managers believe that if a job has been around for a long time, it can no longer be significantly changed.
- Brainstorm a list of changes with employees without regard to how practical they are.
- Screen the list, and remove items that involve hygiene changes rather than motivators.

- Remove generalities from the list, such as "give them more responsibility."
- When beginning job enrichment, set up a control group so that results can be measured.
- Be prepared for a drop in performance for the first few weeks. Achievement levels may not increase until providers become comfortable with their newly assigned duties.
- Expect some hostility or anxiety from first-line supervisors about the changes being made; they may view the providers' new duties as a threat to their own job security or as a loss of control over their subordinates.

The Separation Model

Occasionally, a manager will try every possible alternative to motivate a marginal provider but will not succeed. Since marginal providers can drag down the performance of others, action must be taken to determine whether the provider should be kept or whether the process of separation should be started. Knowing that poor performance may result in termination can work as a motivational tool for employees. Good management, which may include terminating a provider, can motivate others toward good performance.

Individual Approaches

Other approaches to motivation have been designed to satisfy providers' needs in unique ways. One involves adapting the workweek so that providers can determine the format of their schedules. For example, formats may include 10 hours a day for four days each week or two 10-hour days followed by two 14-hour nights. This approach obviously requires much planning, coordination, and agreement with the administration and thus may not be acceptable in some jurisdictions.

Baltimore County offers educational leave and "exchange time," in which personnel are allowed to exchange time with others as long as they have corresponding certification levels. If the exchange is done to allow one provider to attend school, the substituting provider is awarded compensatory time off so that the provider attending school does not have to pay back the time.

Quality circles also seem to be gaining nationwide acceptance. A quality circle is a group of providers who meet regularly to discuss problems and recommend solutions. EMS providers experience problems every day, so it makes sense that they would have ideas their supervisors might overlook. Employees who participate in quality circles begin to feel more a part of their organization, and they take more pride in and are more committed to the solutions they have helped develop.

Non-monetary incentives, such as those mentioned in the persuasion model, should be used often. As Peters says, "Managers should be

Source

Reprinted with permission from JEMS, *February 1992. John Norris is a fire captain and a nationally registered paramedic with the Baltimore County Fire Department. He has an under-graduate degree from the University of Maryland in emergency health services management and a graduate degree in public administration from the University of Baltimore.*

constantly looking for methods and reasons to provide incentives and positive feedback." A decal on an ambulance for each "saved" cardiac arrest, annual awards ceremonies, and certificates for outstanding service, perfect attendance, and extracurricular activities are a few examples of non-monetary incentives.

In spite of the many theories of motivation and the numerous approaches taken by managers, problems will continue to persist in motivating EMS providers. Any solution applied to a group of providers will satisfy some problems but not others, as each provider is a unique individual who responds to stimuli in various ways. Members of management should not expect quick solutions. Instead, they must take the time to properly diagnose each problem before pursuing a course of action. Thus, managers can aim to initiate or improve a process that has often been ignored in EMS.

References

Drazan, F. "By Ridding Your Business of a Poor Employee, You May Be Able to Improve the Performance of the Rest of the Staff in the Process." *American Printer* 202 (1988): 134.

Hatcher, L., T. L. Ross, and R. A. Ross. "Gainsharing: Living Up to its Name." *Personnel Administrator* 32 (1987): 155.

Herzberg, F. "One More Time: How Do You Motivate Employees?" *Harvard Business Review* (January-February 1968).

Moberg, J. D. *Interactive Cases in Organizational Behavior.* Glenview, Ill.: Scott, Foreman & Co., 1988.

Peters, T. J., and R. H. Waterman. *In Search of Excellence.* New York: Harper & Row, 1982.

THE STAFF MEMBER left the meeting in a huff. The supervisor's insides were churning. Emotions ran high, and no one knew why.

Is this a familiar scenario? Unfortunately, frustration and conflict in EMS organizations are as prevalent as the common cold. They can also be as contagious; attitudes can quickly spread throughout the organization. Supervisors and workers need to learn how to reduce the risk of exposure and how to care for afflicted individuals. Doing so can improve the health of the entire organization.

Sources of Conflict

Interpersonal conflict within most EMS agencies can be attributed to one of three primary sources: abilities, role perception, and motivation. When viewpoints in these areas differ, frustration builds and conflict becomes more likely.

An individual's job-related abilities and skills are the main areas in which EMS conflicts arise. Every employee needs manual, intellectual, and social abilities to survive on the job, but many new EMS staff members are underprepared. And, while most individuals' skills develop over time, some employees never progress beyond their entry-level point. For others, only the ego grows. This can become an early source of frustration for co-workers and the agency's leadership.

Role perception refers to one's view of what he is supposed to do to be successful in the organization. That view is shaped by the expectations and behavior of supervisors and peers. Role perception can be a subtle yet important cause of conflict. For example, EMS agencies often offer entry-level employees opportunities for fast promotion, challenging work with significant early responsibility, and a professional work environment. Yet despite these benefits, there is high turnover among new staff; some estimate that 30 to 40 percent leave the field within three years. Some of the turnover is traceable to attractive alternative job offers. Some, however, is traceable to the new staff members' perception of their roles.

Long before EMTs are hired, they receive an impression of their new roles. College faculty members tell EMT students there is greater prestige in being a paramedic than an EMT. Recruiters devote their time to courting students who may have paramedic training potential. Supervisors and physicians make clear the superior nature of paramedics' abilities and give the impression that EMTs are simply low-level assistants. Students are further introduced to the paramedic mystique through insti-

Dealing With EMS Frustration and Conflict

Jay Fitch, PhD

Harry Truman once said, "Leadership is the ability to get people to do what they don't want to do, and like it." That doesn't happen automatically; conflict sometimes occurs along the way. This article explores the sources of conflict, the situations in which conflict is likely to occur, and how you can reduce the risk of conflict that can create a dysfunctional organization.

Empowerment can be summarized simply: Always treat others with respect, and whenever possible, give them the opportunity to be involved in decisions that affect them.

tutional mechanisms, such as specialized ALS quality review sessions to which EMTs are not invited.

Thus, before their first day on the job, new employees have developed certain perceptions. And new information concerning appropriate attitudes, beliefs, and behaviors are received over time. This information is frequently personalized by employees; if the EMT does not rapidly progress to being a medic, the message received is that he is not successful.

If abilities and skills represent what the EMT or medic can do and role perception represents what the medic is supposed to do, motivation represents what the medic will do. Motivation is the force that energizes, directs, and sustains a person's behavior.

The current buzzword for motivation is empowerment. There is no right way to encourage motivation in an EMS organization. Supervisors don't motivate; staff members choose whether to be motivated. However, the supervisors' actions and behaviors are imitated by staff. Consequently, supervisors often influence the choices made by employees. Empowerment describes an environment in which there is a higher likelihood that an employee will remain energized and committed over time. It can be summarized simply: Always treat others with respect, and whenever possible, give them the opportunity to be involved in decisions that affect them.

Understanding the three sources of conflict—when staff members are unable to perform (skills and abilities); when expectations are unclear (role perceptions); and when staff members are unwilling to perform (motivation)—is the first step toward controlling it. In addition, EMS leaders need to know when conflict is likely to occur and how it can be managed.

When Conflict Occurs

A group of EMS supervisors was recently asked when conflict occurred in their respective organizations. The five most frequent instances they reported were

- Dealing with routine employment matters, such as attendance, completing paperwork, and checking vehicles
- Conducting clinical reviews/quality assurance activities
- Handling coaching sessions and annual performance appraisals
- Working in small groups
- Dealing with their own supervisors

Dealing with routine employment matters can be perplexing. Attendance problems can be a mix of role perception and motivation. Employees learn it is acceptable to be a little late for work or to call in sick when they really aren't by watching others do it without any adverse consequences. Supervisors often don't like to deal with these issues because they think they are nit-picking. However, with this approach, supervisors often set up conflict by ignoring some infractions and not ignoring others. Employees perceive inequitable treatment and become angry that they're being picked on, rather than focusing on the behavior that caused the problem.

Quality assurance/improvement issues can be rooted in any of the three causes of conflict: skills, perception (expectations), or motivation. Supervisors must answer two questions before dealing with any QA or QI situation: "Did this problem occur because the person did not have the necessary skills or ability?" and "Was the person's behavior in the situation the norm despite policies and protocols, or did he simply decide not to do the right thing?"

For example, if the person was never trained in a new procedure, such as the appropriate method of decontaminating a unit after exposure to an infectious disease, the conflict experience is related to skills. However, if the person has been trained but observes that other, more senior staff (including supervisors) rarely follow the procedure, the conflict may center in role perception. If the person has been trained and knows (based on experience) that it is common practice to follow the vehicle cleaning procedure—but instead decides to watch television—motivation may be the issue.

Supervisors describe providing feedback in coaching sessions and annual performance appraisals as periods when they experience frustration and conflict. Conflict frequently occurs in this situation because the feedback given is non-specific or has not been provided in a timely fashion. This frustrates both employee and supervisor. The sooner someone receives the feedback, the easier it is to act on it. When teaching someone to drive an ambulance, for example, a person wouldn't wait until the next day to tell the student the hazards of entering an exit ramp. The teacher would want the student to know the error being made before colliding head-on with oncoming traffic.

The other key issue in these sessions is to be sure the feedback being provided is specific and non-evaluative. Feedback should be based on measurable performance criteria. For example, sitting down with the employee to review a bar graph comparing the service's desired out-of-chute times, the service's actual out-of-chute times, and the individual employee's performance during the previous month is far more useful to the employee than saying, "You've been slow getting out the door lately, and you need to do better."

Working in groups also was described as being frustrating and producing conflict. While the result may be a better work product, working in groups often takes longer than doing it alone. Ensuring that the group has the expertise, organizational power, required information, and ownership of both the problem and outcome is the best way to avoid frustration. Some conflict within the group can be useful; healthy discussion of differing opinions can help illustrate the issues and move the group toward consensus.

Communicating with top management often frustrates supervisors and causes conflict. Not understanding the preferred communication style

Quality assurance/ improvement issues can be rooted in any of the three causes of conflict: skills, perception (expectations), or motivation.

and not recognizing time pressures are some underlying causes of tension. For example, knowing whether the supervisor is a "reader" or "listener" may reduce tension and improve communication. Readers like to see reports on projects or problems before discussing them. If the supervisor is a reader, offer a written outline or description of the problem or project. If the supervisor is a listener, don't send a memo. Go in and talk about it first, and then follow up with a written report.

Knowing the flow of the supervisor's day and his time limitations can be helpful in choosing the best time for interaction. Trying to get the supervisor's full attention immediately prior to an important meeting will be frustrating for all. Carefully selecting the method and time for communicating can improve the outcome.

Reducing the Risk

Regardless of the source of frustration and the situation in which the conflict occurs, strategies can be employed to reduce the risk of conflict. They include improving communication, maintaining relationships, and using a defined conflict-resolution mechanism.

Improving communication and, more specifically, listening are the most frequently identified skills for reducing frustration and conflict. Many people have had public speaking classes in high school or college, but few in EMS have had specialized training in listening. In fact, most learn how not to listen before entering kindergarten. Ask any parent who's tried to put a preschooler to bed to confirm this. Poor listening has a profound effect on frustration and conflict from any of the three sources. Communicating assertively without guilt or anxiety can help get things done in the best possible way.

What are the barriers to effective listening? Sperry Corp. (now called Unisys) conducted extensive research on listening during the past decade and came up with these barriers: daydreaming, listening primarily for facts instead of ideas and central themes, judging, and becoming personally antagonized by emotion-laden words.

What are some of the components of effective listening? As with all aspects of good communication, body language is important. Making eye contact is a good start. Smile appropriately. If facial muscles become tense or you impatiently begin to make a counter argument, you are engaging in evaluative rather than non-evaluative listening.

One of the most effective tools in listening is reflecting back the content of the other person's statement. The idea is to convey the other's meaning without being obvious. This can be accomplished with phrases such as "What I'm hearing you say is . . ." or "I understand you're saying. . . ." This type of paraphrasing lets someone correct his or her comments and reshape what's been said or heard without escalating a conflict.

Communication is a fundamental component of EMS work, yet we often fail to communicate effectively when dealing with one another. Managing communication is an important component in reducing conflict.

Another mechanism for reducing conflict is preventive maintenance of relationships. Maintaining human relationships requires as much attention as technical issues do because emotions condition and color the way people handle information. If the relationship has been well maintained, it can mean the difference between flying with a tail wind and flying into a head wind. Discussions about EMS procedures tend to involve issues of power and turf. Having a positive relationship is especially important when trying to resolve these types of conflicts.

Relationship maintenance does not imply that intimate knowledge of each staff member is necessary, but a working knowledge of the employee's off-duty interests is helpful. Furthermore, spending time with a staff member can guide the supervisor in how the member processes information and help the supervisor establish a positive basis for communication. President Coolidge said that nothing in the world can take the place of persistence. Neither talent nor genius can replace it. The same is true in maintaining positive work relationships.

Conflict resolution is a process of negotiation. Despite using excellent planning, approach, and follow-through, conflict sometimes cannot be avoided. Anticipating problems and how to resolve them improves the effectiveness of the EMS leader. Positively resolving a conflict involves finding alternatives that all parties believe are equitable. Negotiation can be boiled down to four key points:

- People—separate the people and personalities from the problem
- Interests—focus on interests, not positions
- Options—generate a variety of options before deciding what to do
- Criteria—insist that results be based on objective criteria

To effectively deal with conflict, a recognized mechanism for resolving disputes may be needed. When asked to mediate between individuals, a five-point approach may be helpful for supervisors. Ask each party to

- Write down his views of the situation and the factors driving it
- Note the factors each believes might be the basis for the resolution, as well as acceptable behavior or alternative solutions to the situation
- Meet and trade lists, comparing and contrasting one another's assessment of the situation and proposed solutions
- Negotiate acceptable behavior that can improve the situation and ask people to agree on checkpoints to assess their progress
- Spell out the desired behavior from your perspective as a supervisor

Source

Reprinted with permission from Emergency, *May 1993.*

There is no simple way to resolve frustration and conflict in an EMS organization. Some believe both are as inevitable as getting a cold. If that's true, understand the underlying reasons you are getting sick (the sources of conflict). Know when you're most likely to come down with the cold (when conflict is likely to occur). Finally, know how to keep the common cold from becoming something more serious by implementing strategies to reduce the risk and manage the problem.

Repairing Middle Management "Brown-Out"

Cathy E. Vacirca

Every leader on a middle management team experiences some flickering light bulbs. In this original article, author Cathy Vacirca outlines a number of specific steps the EMS leader can take to prevent the light from going out, or from becoming so dim that it can't be followed.

MIDDLE MANAGEMENT IS A GREAT place to be, especially in prehospital medicine. Think about it—many of us now in management began as EMTs or paramedics. During our time in the field, nearly every conversation with fellow workers included discussions about management and how we could "do it better." Supervisors and mid-level managers have numerous opportunities to effect change in EMS organizations, as well as provide for overall system improvements.

Being chosen for a supervisory position is a vote of confidence in your ability to tackle new responsibilities. Others believe that your decisions and actions will be guided by reason and ethics. You are valued for your ideas—not just your EMS skills. What could be better than a job that offers daily challenges and the personal satisfaction that comes with making a real difference in the lives of so many people? Well, consider the following scenario.

You are the senior operations supervisor at Helping Hand Ambulance Service. As you listen to the alarm go off Tuesday morning, a voice inside your head says, "Just call in sick. They can manage without you for one day." It feels like there is a great weight on your body and mind. Facing the dispatcher's complaints, the boss's demands, vehicle problems, staff disputes, and customer dissatisfaction without any help or support seems like more than you can handle today. A "mental health" break would certainly be in order, even though you just came back from vacation last week.

What happened? When did the patient's family members or, for that matter, your fellow workers become the enemy? How did the exciting opportunities of this job become overwhelming burdens? The answers to these questions are complex and numerous; however, the scenario described is not so unique. Many EMS supervisory and mid-level management personnel leave or go back to their medic positions because they cannot find a way to deal with middle management "brown-out." When these talented individuals are lost, EMS organizations sacrifice a key link in their operational structure. The ultimate costs can be substantial. Sometimes they cannot even be measured.

How can this distressing situation be prevented? How can those affected refocus on the important issues and regain the perspective and self-confidence needed to do their jobs effectively? There are practical, positive, alternative responses to the negative environments that perpetuate middle management brown-out.

Coping With Frustration, Stress, and Change

We are all faced with a series of great opportunities brilliantly disguised as impossible situations.

—C. R. Swindoll

Frustration and stress are not owned by middle management, although sometimes it may appear that way. Numerous roadblocks can stand in the way of achieving success. You often feel like you're spinning your wheels. In addition to the daily pressures described in the scenario, specific causes of stress can include having to make tough decisions, dealing with complex or difficult interpersonal relationships, and coping with rapid technological changes.

Responsibility overload can also become an issue if the parameters of your position are not clearly defined, or if non-management tasks are not effectively delegated. One of the complaints most often heard from mid-level managers is that their responsibility and accountability far exceed the amount of authority or control vested in their positions.

The physiological and psychological effects of prolonged stressful circumstances can be devastating, both to the individual and the organization. Antagonism, apathy, lowered self-esteem, increased absenteeism, and high rates of turnover can all be indicators of problems.

How do we begin to approach this dilemma? Implementing some or all of the following ideas will enable individuals to reduce daily frustrations and ward off the symptoms of brown-out.

Identify the Source of Your Stress/Frustration

Determine the sources of stress that you have control over (some you do not), and examine positive courses of action that will reduce or eliminate them from your work activities. Also, take a hard look at how appropriate your reactions are to stressful situations. You may be a major cause of your own stress.

Define the Responsibilities and Authority of Your Position

Discuss your interpretation of your responsibilities and authority with your superior. When your approach is one of concern for the overall success of the organization, and specifically your part in that success, most top-level managers will appreciate your initiative and gladly engage in such a discussion. The more clearly you understand what is expected of you, the better you can set priorities for yourself and your subordinates.

Learn to Manage Your Time Effectively

Learning to better manage your time will be to your benefit both on the job and in your personal life. Many resources are available to assist you with this. *The One Minute Manager* and *If You Haven't Got the Time to Do It Right, When Will You Find the Time to Do It Over?* are two good books. Both are also available on cassette.

Review Your Development

Objectively review your development as a manager and what you brought to the job. In many instances, just working to your maximum capability is not enough. Accomplishments that are visible and demonstrate increased operational efficiency and effectiveness are often necessary to "justify your existence." By developing or working on projects that are relevant to organizational needs, you can sharpen your management skills while at the same time cultivate the relationships and support that every manager needs to be successful.

Understand Your Own Motivations

What personal and professional achievements or goals are important to you? Do you need to be the star, or does being a team player serve as your primary incentive for work? Is it high salary or respect and appreciation that give you satisfaction? Consider these motivations in relation to your position and the goals and objectives of the organization. Perhaps they are not in alignment. If so, face the decisions that must be made. It may be difficult, but if the decisions are made with the best interests of all parties in mind, the respect of fellow workers—and your own self-respect—will be retained.

Individuals, as well as organizations, need to experience and react to change in order to thrive. Throughout the lives of organizations, there are periods of crisis, growth, and stability. Individuals experience similar evolutions. It can be frightening when the crisis stage hits and there is no plan to seize the opportunities presented by that crisis. Making the change from medic to manager can have a significant impact on who you are, both in fact and in perception. The expectations others in the organization have about your performance or allegiance can cause difficulties if you have not realistically examined your capabilities and intentions.

Change, however, might also be seen as a wonderful thing. It can provide the opportunity for improvement that draws most people to EMS management positions. It is a chance to shape events rather than being shaped by them. Support and participation are keys to the successful implementation of change. It should begin with you. Making a personal decision to be flexible in the face of change is critical. Holding steadfastly to operations or procedures merely because they have become habit, without being willing or able to evaluate the benefits of change, will not serve you or the organization in the long run. In creating a positive, involving change environment, managers will sometimes have to fight inertia and convince a workforce that may not see the advantages of exceeding the currently accepted norm. Many will not see the potential individual benefits that will be theirs, but the battle is worth fighting on all fronts. When waged with sincerity and commitment, pockets of support and even widespread enthusiasm can be the result.

The idea of synergy is one that extols the virtues of teamwork and declares that the whole can be greater than the sum of its parts. In other

> **Individuals, as well as organizations, need to experience and react to change in order to thrive.**

Listening actively, encouraging feedback, and responding in a timely and appropriate manner are as important as getting your point across.

words, if all members of the organization share common goals, objectives, and planned courses of action, they can achieve more than if they each had their own agenda and proceeded independently toward change. Mid-level managers can initiate and foster the concepts of teamwork and synergy in many areas of operations. These concepts are visible, relevant, and self-perpetuating.

Listening, Learning, and Sorting Out the Options

I'd rather know some of the questions than all of the answers.
—James Thurber

Occasionally, it is a good practice to take stock, revisit the skills that make good managers, and see how we measure up. What does this have to do with brown-out? Sharpening these skills can serve to expand your current viewpoints and enable you to see new ways to handle responsibilities more efficiently and effectively. This will give you the opportunity to get past the daily grind and focus on real needs and organizational issues. Similarly, it offers a way to gain new perspectives. The more clearly you are able to address what you *have* to do, the sooner you will be able to accomplish what you *want* to do. Communication, decision making, and the role of continuing education should figure prominently in this skill assessment.

Communication

Consider the familiar story of the tree falling in a forest. If no one hears it, does it make a sound? Communication is not one-sided. If no one is listening and there is no exchange of ideas, does communication really happen? Listening actively, encouraging feedback, and responding in a timely and appropriate manner are as important as getting your point across. Being a successful communicator involves understanding that there are inherent problems in the communication process. One primary consideration is that "senders" and "receivers" are individuals and have different perceptions and interpretations of the words, phrases, and non-verbal signals projected. Practicing the techniques of two-sided communication will allow a better understanding of the receiver's frame of reference.

Think about your superiors. They rely on you for a great deal of information on a variety of management issues. Identify how and when they need certain data and keep them informed. Solicit clarifications if requests for information are unclear. Provide progress reports on projects or changes in operational procedures. Call attention to potential problems before they become major disasters. Give positive feedback; be appreciative of support or confidence in your capabilities. The result of such actions can only serve to enhance your position and your ability to effect change.

Your new management position within the organization can sometimes inhibit communication. Subordinates may not feel comfortable discussing ideas or improvements because historically this type of exchange has not been taken seriously or has been ignored. Remember that words and actions need to be consistent. If the goal is to create an environment where open communication is an essential part of organizational growth, the first step is to design and identify the manner in which such exchange takes place. The next crucial step is to ensure that the communication system developed is respected by all involved. Saying to employees, "We want your ideas and suggestions," only to have them sit in a drawer is of little benefit. What you do can often speak louder than what you say.

Much of the success and satisfaction in life is achieved through communication with others. Max DePree, a noted author of leadership texts, stated, "The first responsibility of a leader is to define reality. The last is to say thank you. . . ." There are two communication truths expressed here. First, all employees will be more competent and more enthusiastic if the importance of their work has been communicated to them. Second, and perhaps more significant, simple and sincere recognition of that work is one of the best "bonuses" any of us can ever get. Be a communication leader.

Decision Making

When viewing the essentials of good decision making, several fundamental steps apply universally. Using a solid decision-making process can reduce brown-out.

Identify the problem. Get to the heart of the matter. Understand the type of problem to be addressed. For example, is the problem part of a larger, more complex issue that will require a series of decisions? Know that there is always a connection between decisions and the resulting consequences. Study the scope of the problem—recognize who and what in the organization will be touched by the decision.

Gather data and consider alternatives. Maximize your access to information. Avoid relying solely on information from others. Realize that there are always options; you may just need to activate some creative thinking to see them. Also appreciate that some of the "costs" and "benefits" you may attach to a decision may be intangible but very real all the same.

Make the decision. Indecision and procrastination can be detrimental to any manager and organization. When making the decision, remember that the thought process does not necessarily need to include a recalculation of the national debt. Some problems actually have simple, clear solutions. As a "B.C." comic strip explains, "The secret of perpetual motion . . . a slinky on an escalator."

Communicate and implement the decision. This may require an incremental approach to afford time for developing support for the decision and implementing subsequent changes in operations. Occasionally, during the implementation phase, it becomes evident that a poor decision has been made. If that is the case, cease action and re-evaluate the problem, the alternatives, and the method of implementation. Being committed to a bad decision can only compound the original problem, and even create others.

In sum, decisions should be purpose-driven and meaningful, provide practical benefit to the organization, and have a workable implementation plan. When considering alternatives, favor proactive, positive approaches. Know that reasonable people will often disagree on solutions. Do not be discouraged; use logic and communication skills to make the best decision possible.

Continuing Education

Continuing education is often considered a luxury, something we do when the time and money are available. The fact of the matter is that it doesn't always take a great deal of time or money to reap the benefits of continued learning. First, forget algebra, English, world history, or whatever it was about your last stint with formal education that brought you to your knees. You are a different person now. You can participate by pursuing knowledge in your areas of interest. The key is taking the initiative, being involved because you have a desire to be better at what you do and who you are.

There are many sources of continued learning. With technological advances, learning today is not limited to traditional forms. The use of audio- and videotapes or computer-aided instruction can provide learning within student-defined time frames. Reading, of course, is still a tried and true option. There are also numerous seminars and adult or college classes available. The advantage to this source of learning is that it encourages interaction among participants. Opportunities abound to speak with and pose queries to experts in your field of interest. Seminars often provide a non-competitive environment to converse with peers and share different approaches to common problems.

Continuing education is one of the best ways to attack brown-out. Management and leadership styles are always evolving. Different styles affect motivation and performance. Staying current with new studies or ideas in these areas can help make you a more effective manager. Every now and then among the new ideas you discover, there will be one that you have already put into practice. What a confirmation of your competence and creativity! The overall result of continuing education is an awareness that there is always a way to "make it better." Additionally, the greater the variety of experience and learning you bring to the job, the more satisfaction you will be able to derive from it.

Empowering Yourself and Reviving the EMS Spirit

The highest reward for man's toil is not what he gets for it, but what he becomes by it.
—Ralph Waldo Emerson

Many of us in middle management become tangled in the web of position, power, and politics. The more entangled we become, the further from reality are the notions of freedom and autonomy in our daily work life. It has been said that empowerment (which has become a buzzword of the 1990s) can only exist in a supportive environment. Perhaps that is true in part; however, is it not also true that we are ultimately responsible for enabling or empowering ourselves to meet life's challenges? We are always capable of putting our own signature on our work, and the better our performance in meeting the challenges of the workplace, the greater our satisfaction. The key here is knowing that you can make a difference just by motivating yourself. Practice the following ideas to impact your daily work life.

Mentor: You can help create your own support network; you can be your own best teacher.

Openness to change: Seize the opportunities.

Translate: Interpret organizational goals and turn them into positive actions.

Inspiration: Seek out new experiences and acquaintances that will serve to inspire you.

Value: Although kudos may not always come your way, do not underestimate the value of your work.

Achievements: Celebrate them!

Trust: Be comfortable in your own skin; trust your instincts.

Empower: Enable yourself to be better; empowering others can often be the result.

Sometimes the nurturing elements of prehospital medicine leave us when we get behind a desk. The sad result is that we not only neglect our co-workers, but we fail to nurture ourselves. That desk can be a symbol of success, or an obstacle to it. Each of us needs to understand that simple fact. Taking time to achieve a balance in life, planning for yourself, and finding ways to enjoy the moment can be very worthwhile. Taking another look at the overall mission of EMS, and choosing proactive approaches to your tasks and responsibilities can do much to keep the brown-out situation from developing. Although frustration may always be present on some level, it is within our power to make the choices that will help us to maintain a positive outlook and renew our sense of purpose.

Source

Original article. Cathy E. Vacirca, MPH, is a department director at McCabe Ambulance in Bayonne, N.J., and the director of the McCabe Training Institute. She has been an EMT instructor since 1978 and has earned her master's in public health.

References

Costley, D. L., and R. Todd. *Human Relations in Organizations*. 4th ed. New York: West Publishing Co., 1991.

Daft, R. *Organization Theory and Design*. New York: West Publishing Co., 1989.

Fitch, J., et al. *EMS Management: Beyond the Street*, 2nd ed. Carlsbad, Calif.: Jems Communications, Inc., 1993.

Johnson, S., MD. *Yes or No; The Guide to Better Decisions*. New York: Harper Publishers, 1991.

Newkirck, W., MD, and R. Linden. *Managing Emergency Medical Services, Principles and Practices*. Englewood Cliffs, N.J.: Prentice Hall Publishing, 1984.

Stoner, J., and R. Freeman. *Management*. 4th ed. Englewood Cliffs, N.J.: Prentice Hall Publishing, 1989.

Ethics in EMS: Making Choices You and Your Patients Can Live With

Jeffrey Salomone, BS, REMT-P

EMS staff members face ethical conflicts every day. Thousands of choices are made, and in most cases they are the right choices. But by what standards do staff members make these ethical choices? Belief in a value system is just one of the areas highlighted by Jeffrey Salomone in this article.

- WHEN, IF EVER, should an EMT refuse to carry out a physician's orders?
- When, if ever, should an EMT lie to patients or their families about their conditions or treatment?
- When, if ever, should an EMT initiate lifesaving therapy against patients' or their families' desires?
- When, if ever, should an EMT violate a law to treat a patient?
- When, if ever, should an EMT refuse to treat a patient?
- When, if ever, should an EMT jeopardize patient care to keep his job?

These questions represent just a few of the many situations in which an EMT may face a moral dilemma while providing emergency care. EMTs are frequently confronted with situations involving such issues as confidentiality, informed consent, patients' rights, and truth telling. Yet all too often, EMTs are confused about how to approach these issues and how to justify their decisions.

It would be impossible to cover all the possible situations requiring ethical decisions by EMTs or to provide a list of actions that would be universally accepted as ethical. Instead, the purpose of this article is to provide a better understanding of the often neglected—yet very important—ethical issues involved in prehospital medicine. Because the current ethical training of EMTs is deficient, more attention must be focused on providing EMTs with the tools to make informed, intelligent decisions that will stand up under the scrutiny of their peers and medical colleagues.

According to medical ethicist Vincent Barry, ethics involves "the study of what constitutes good and bad human conduct, including related actions and values." Ethicists concern themselves with questions of good versus bad and right versus wrong. They are also interested in how personal values affect decision making, and they address questions of moral responsibility, attempting to define acts that one is obligated to perform. Ethicists do not see their role as prescribing to society what actions are moral or immoral. Instead, most believe their function is to ensure that all points of view are considered while pointing out inconsistencies or weaknesses in people's justifications of their acts. In short, ethicists attempt to frame and pose the moral questions that society as a whole must consider.

As a branch of philosophy, ethics has long been a subject of debate, dating back at least to the ancient Greek philosopher Aristotle. In more recent times, ethics has assumed a more practical nature. The development of medical ethics (also known as biomedical ethics or bioethics) is one example of applied ethics, in which philosophical concepts and theories are used to assess actual moral dilemmas within the health-care setting.

The union of morality and medical care dates back to the fifth century B.C. One of the most well-known documents discussing the ethical behavior of the physician is the Hippocratic Oath. Hippocrates has long served the medical profession as an ethical role model who in many ways is still revered today.

In the past two decades, medical ethics has become a subject of widespread study and debate in the United States. Many health professionals no longer consider it sufficient to perform acts that fall within accepted legal and professional boundaries; actions must also be morally acceptable. Additionally, some healthcare professionals have found in bioethics the necessary guidance for situations in which their moral convictions conflict with legal or professional obligations. The medical and nursing professions are addressing ethical issues with more frequency and intensity than ever before.

Barry has identified four reasons for this increased interest in bioethics, and most have some relevance to EMS: advances in medical science; consumer rights; medical malpractice; and the Nuremberg trials of Nazi war criminals.

Technological advances during the past three decades have presented healthcare workers with situations few would have imagined 50 years ago. CPR and prehospital advanced life support improve the chance of recovery for many victims who would have previously been classified as "dead on arrival." But this benefit also poses serious questions for EMTs: If resuscitated, what will the victim's quality of life be? Can we afford to provide ALS care to all communities and, if not, how do we fairly allocate these resources?

Increased medical knowledge has served as a catalyst for the development of new medical specialties, including EMS. With the increased size of the healthcare team, questions now surface as to who should serve as the team leader and how conflicts among team members should be resolved. Must the EMT always follow the doctor's orders?

The concept of patients' rights grew out of the civil rights movement of the 1960s. The stage was set for discussions about informed consent and the rights of those mentally or physically incompetent to consent.

While most states have laws defining informed consent, patients do have rights that have been defined and clarified through malpractice litigation. Almost without exception, EMTs must abide by the principle of nonmaleficence ("do no further harm") while caring for patients. In fact, failing to follow by this principle may lead to a judgment against the EMT.

The Nuremberg trials concluded that a person cannot be excused for immoral actions simply because he was following orders. The "Bormann defense," named after a Nazi official, is frequently offered by those in the

> Many health professionals no longer consider it sufficient to perform acts that fall within accepted legal and professional boundaries; actions must also be morally acceptable.

health professions when confronted with the choice of losing their jobs or following a supervisor's dubious instructions.

A Lack of Ethical Training

EMTs are often unprepared to face moral dilemmas for several reasons. Using Barry's term, they face "healthcare's moral quandary" due to the lack of a clearly defined and universally accepted moral standard, controversies regarding rights and responsibilities, and a vague understanding of moral accountability. But unlike many physicians and nurses, the quandary EMTs face is compounded by the emergent nature of their business, limited training, and a shortage of experienced colleagues.

Healthcare workers have failed to adopt a moral standard to serve as a guide when confronting ethical matters. The result is chaos. Professionals are forced to choose between their personal ethics and those of their patients, employers, or colleagues. Conflicts arise when healthcare workers attempt to reconcile personal responsibilities with the rights advanced by different members of society.

Barry sees moral accountability as "blaming or praising someone for an action." When the rights and responsibilities of various members of society conflict, it becomes impossible to determine who should be held accountable for a specific action. Furthermore, because medical care is performed by a team of health professionals, many may share in the praise or blame for an action. Ethicists often attribute moral accountability by defining the circumstances in which healthcare workers are ordinarily excused from accountability—if none of these excusable circumstances exists, one ought to be accountable for his actions. While the Bormann defense is not considered sufficient grounds to excuse people from being held accountable for their actions, Barry identified four situations that may protect people from being held accountable.

- Excusable ignorance of consequences. A reasonable person would not have foreseen the consequences of a particular action. Example: A patient suffers a life-threatening side effect after an EMT injects a drug the medical community believes to be safe.
- Constraints. One is forced to perform an unethical act against his wishes. Example: An EMT is prevented by law enforcement personnel from initiating resuscitation on a shooting victim.
- Uncontrollable circumstances. Circumstances are truly beyond the person's control. Example: A patient dies from injuries received in a motor vehicle accident that occurs while being transported in an ambulance, and the accident is not the fault of the EMT.
- Lack of alternatives. An individual lacks either the ability or the opportunity to do the right act. Example: An EMT can-

not obtain informed consent from a patient because of the patient's neurological condition.

Other factors may affect one's ability to act ethically. EMTs and others working in emergent situations are frequently called on to make split-second decisions regarding life and death. Delaying treatment to assess the ethical issues often results in an increased risk of injury or death. EMTs frequently lack experienced colleagues to turn to when dealing with ethical issues. A physician can consult a peer who has decades of experience practicing medicine, but the majority of EMTs have fewer than 10 years of experience in the field. Few EMTs have completed a bachelor's degree, compared with many nurses and virtually all physicians. A college education can provide the skills necessary to critically analyze issues and arguments and increase problem-solving abilities. At a time when more and more nursing programs, medical schools, and residencies are providing ethical training to their students, most EMTs receive little more than a brief discussion of the EMT Oath or the EMT Code of Ethics. These documents, like most other medical oaths and codes of ethics, prove to be of little practical assistance in guiding ethical decisions in the field. Despite these factors, EMTs are often expected to make prudent, moral decisions in situations in which time is of the essence.

How Values Affect Opinions

Anyone who answers ethical questions should be aware of how personal values affect opinions. But from where do people derive their values? Barry argues that the four main sources of values are experience, culture, science, and religion. Our life experiences can greatly influence our values. For example, an EMT who has a comatose family member under constant nursing care as a result of "successful" CPR most likely has different opinions regarding CPR than an EMT whose family member was resuscitated and returned to a productive life. Understanding one's biases is the first step toward ethical behavior, but values cannot serve as the only guide for ethical action.

Like other healthcare professionals confronted with ethical dilemmas, the EMT may seek guidance from two additional sources: the law, and professional oaths and codes. Rarely will either provide the guidance necessary to act morally. In recent years, the medical profession has become the target of increased litigation, and many EMTs are concerned about protecting themselves from medical malpractice actions. This increased awareness has provoked many to turn to the law when looking for answers to moral questions. After all, many people equate acting legally with acting morally—but is this necessarily the case?

In theory, laws should reflect the values and priorities of society and therefore should constitute socially acceptable standards. But laws cannot be expected to address the countless and often complex situations that might arise in the practice of medical care.

Box 1.1

Code of Ethics for Emergency Medical Technicians

Professional status as an emergency medical technician is maintained and enriched by the willingness of the individual practitioner to accept and fulfill obligations to society, other medical professionals, and the profession of emergency medical technician. As an emergency medical technician, I solemnly pledge myself to the following code of ethics:

- The fundamental responsibility of the emergency medical technician is to conserve life, to alleviate suffering, and to promote health.
- The emergency medical technician provides services based on human need, with respect for human dignity, unrestricted by considerations of nationality, race, creed, color, or status.
- The emergency medical technician does not use professional knowledge and skill in any enterprise detrimental to the public good.
- The emergency medical technician respects and holds in confidence all information of a confidential nature obtained in the course of professional work unless required by law to divulge such information.
- The emergency medical technician as a citizen understands and upholds the laws and performs the duties of citizenship; as a professional person, the emergency medical technician has a particular responsibility to work with other citizens and health professionals in promoting efforts to meet the health needs of the public.
- The emergency medical technician maintains professional competence and demonstrates concern for the competence of other members of the medical profession.
- The emergency medical technician assumes responsibility in defining and up-

A law might prohibit EMTs from performing a specific lifesaving procedure, but if they have been properly trained and have received a physician's order, it could be argued that it would be immoral to withhold the therapy. Here, a legal obligation to refrain from an action is conflicting with a moral obligation to perform that action. Such dilemmas frequently occur when an EMT has training from a related health field (respiratory therapy or nursing) or when EMTs are undergoing further training to advance their skill level (i.e., to paramedic) yet do not have licensure to function in that new capacity.

Conversely, one could easily imagine a situation in which no specific law exists but a moral obligation does. Unless a state requires an off-duty EMT to stop at all accident scenes and render emergency care, no legal duty to act exists. Yet one could argue that the EMT has a moral obligation to provide treatment. Thus, a legal standard often provides insufficient assistance when faced with an ethical question.

Some believe professional oaths and codes are useful sources of moral direction. While these documents are often designed for that purpose, they contain weaknesses as well. The Code of Ethics for Emergency Medical Technicians and the EMT Oath (Boxes 1.1 and 1.2) are both based on the Hippocratic Oath, which was written more than 2,000 years ago. Obviously, issues such as organ transplantation, human experimentation, and patients' rights are not addressed.

The EMT Oath and the Code of Ethics for EMTs are both brief documents, and any attempt to codify all proper ethical behavior within a few sentences simply fails. Like the Hippocratic Oath, few important ethical issues are addressed. The authors' efforts to produce an all-inclusive guide for behavior results in vague statements that lack adequate definition and leave much to individual interpretation. A reader of the Code of Ethics will find obscure phrases such as "respect for human dignity" and "dignity of the profession." And what are "dependent and independent emergency functions"? Most would agree that EMTs should refuse to "participate in unethical procedures" and commit themselves to "expose incompetence or unethical conduct," yet the reader is left without a clear definition of what procedures and conduct are unethical.

Finally, the EMT who seeks advice from the EMT

Oath and Code of Ethics will find no guidance for settling disputes when his values differ from those expressed in these documents. The EMT may, in fact, be more confused when confronting conflicting statements within the Code of Ethics itself. For instance, the Code asserts that the EMT's "fundamental responsibility" is "to conserve life [and] to alleviate suffering." But what is an EMT to do when, as with certain cancer patients, efforts aimed at alleviating suffering (e.g., narcotic pain medications) may not necessarily conserve life and could in all likelihood hasten death?

Because of the shortcomings of laws and professional codes in guiding moral decisions, bioethicists have turned to ethical theories. Many different philosophers have developed ethical theories. However, only three of the most well known will be addressed here: utilitarianism, Kant's categorical imperative, and natural law.

In utilitarianism, an act is ethical if it produces the largest possible ratio of good to evil. Put simply, one should provide the greatest good to the greatest number. Triage is a medical application of utilitarianism. During mass casualty incidents, EMTs commonly accept the idea that care should be delivered to the greatest number. In doing so, a person with a potentially survivable injury but requiring extensive intervention and a drain of manpower may not receive treatment so many others with less severe injuries may be saved.

Immanuel Kant argues that one is acting ethically only when acting from a sense of duty. His concept of categorical imperative states that one should act the same way in all similar situations. If an action is not universal, it must be rejected as unethical. An EMT would therefore be obliged to render lifesaving therapy out of respect for human life.

The Roman Catholic Church promotes a system of natural law ethics in which moral decisions can be reached through the God-given ability of reason. Good or moral actions derive from good intentions and produce good results. In this ethical system, actions that produce both good and bad effects may involve the principle of double effect. The following is an example of this principle, applied to the prehospital setting. An EMT is called on to treat a critically injured, pregnant victim of a motor vehicle accident. Application and inflation of a pneumatic antishock garment may jeopardize the viability of the fetus, yet the mother and the

Box 1.1 (cont.)

holding standards of professional practice and education.
- The emergency medical technician assumes responsibility for individual professional actions and judgment, both in dependent and independent emergency functions, and knows and upholds the laws that affect the practice of the emergency medical technician.
- The emergency medical technician has the responsibility to participate in the study of and action on matters of legislature affecting emergency medical technicians and emergency service to the public.
- The emergency medical technician adheres to standards of personal ethics that reflect credit upon the profession.
- The emergency medical technician may contribute to research in relation to a commercial product or service but does not lend professional status to advertising, promotion, or sales.
- The emergency medical technician, or groups of emergency medical technicians, who advertise professional services, do so in conformity with the dignity of the profession.
- The emergency medical technician has an obligation to protect the public by not delegating to a person less qualified in any service that requires the professional competence of an emergency medical technician.
- The emergency medical technician works harmoniously with, and sustains confidence in, emergency medical technician associates, the nurse, the physician, and other members of the health team.
- The emergency medical technician refuses to participate in unethical procedures and assumes the responsibility to expose incompetence or unethical conduct in others to the appropriate authority.

This Code of Ethics was drafted and adopted by the National Association of Emergency Medical Technicians in 1978.

Box 1.2

The EMT Oath

Be it pledged as an emergency medical technician, I will honor the physical and judicial laws of God and man. I will follow the regimen which, according to my ability and judgment, I consider for the benefit of patients, and abstain from whatever is deleterious and mischievous, nor shall I suggest any such counsel. Into whatever homes I enter, I will go into them for the benefit of only the sick and injured, never revealing what I see or hear in the lives of men unless required by law.

I shall also share my medical knowledge with those who may benefit from what I have learned. I will serve unselfishly and continuously in order to help make a better world for all mankind.

While I continue to keep this oath unviolated, may it be granted to me to enjoy life, and the practice of the art, respected by all men, in all times. Should I trespass or violate this oath, may the reverse be my lot. So help me God.

This EMT Oath was drafted and adopted by the National Association of Emergency Medical Technicians in 1978.

fetus will probably die if the treatment is not performed. The therapy would be moral even if it resulted in fetal death because four crucial elements would be satisfied: First, applying the device is morally neutral; second, a fetal death would not save the mother; third, the intent is to save the mother and hopefully also the fetus; and last, saving the mother's life is at least equivalent to loss of the fetus.

In addition to ethical theories, bioethicists also use the principles of autonomy, beneficence, nonmaleficence, and justice when examining moral questions.

Autonomy is a person's capability to make his own decisions. Unless one is incapable of exercising this right, as in the case of minors, the mentally ill, or comatose patients, most ethicists argue that humans should be permitted to act autonomously. Two fundamental patient rights, the right to informed consent and the right to refuse treatment, arise from the principle of autonomy.

Beneficence has evolved out of the Christian tradition that advocates performing actions to aid other people either by preventing harm or by promoting good. An EMT may think that he is doing good by initiating resuscitative measures and laboring to save a life, but the patient, if he could express his feelings, might feel that death is welcome because of the great pain or disability he must face.

Nonmaleficence is commonly associated with the Hippocratic tradition in medicine, which advocates not causing further harm. Yet an EMT may need to inflict pain while starting an IV to administer a lifesaving drug or while manipulating a fractured extremity to improve circulation.

The principle of justice involves "giving each his right or due." In a mass casualty situation in which victims exceed supplies and personnel, each patient cannot receive an equal share, and treatment must be distributed based on individual need.

While all of these ethical theories have weaknesses, they can provide important assistance in decision making, especially by providing ethical alternatives and a "defensible standard" for debating the following case studies.

Improper Physician Orders

A paramedic and his partner are attempting resuscitative efforts on a middle-aged female victim of an apparent heart attack. After the paramedics report to the base station physician that the patient's heart is now showing a slow idioventricular complex on the cardiac monitor, the physician orders 50 mg lidocaine to be administered intravenously. Realizing that the drug is inappropriate in this case and that it may prevent a successful outcome of the resuscitation, are the paramedics obligated to administer the medication?

This case raises the issue of whether an EMT is always required to follow the medical control physician's orders. By ignoring the physician's order, the paramedics would be preventing further harm to the patient (nonmaleficence). This action, however, could set a dangerous precedent after which paramedics might begin to routinely deviate from the base station physician's orders.

Such an outcome, while possible, seems quite remote. A utilitarian would argue that ignoring a physician's order when it jeopardizes a patient's life will in the long run produce a greater ratio of good over evil. Could the paramedic be held accountable for the death if he administered the drug and then claimed he did so because he was simply following orders? Certainly. Blindly carrying out orders when aware of the negative consequences amounts to nothing more than the Bormann defense.

Patients' Rights

An EMT is called to the local bus station to examine a bus driver who complains of chest pain and associated symptoms that suggest an acute heart attack. After a few minutes on oxygen, the patient states that his chest pain seems to have subsided. The EMT recommends that he be transported to the local emergency department for a cardiac evaluation, but the patient refuses treatment. Instead, he tells the EMT he wants to drive his fully loaded bus back to his hometown and that he will consult his family physician the following day. Furthermore, he asks the EMT not to tell his supervisor about the incident.

This situation poses several ethical dilemmas. First, the patient appears to be a competent, autonomous adult and has the right to refuse treatment. Others might argue that his potentially serious condition may be clouding his thinking and that he should be forced to seek a medical evaluation. The EMT must also consider the safety of the bus passengers. Should he breach the patient's confidentiality and report his concerns to the driver's supervisor?

Kant would have advocated taking some action to protect the lives of the passengers, as well as that of the bus driver. Similarly, utilitarians might recommend that the EMT breach the patient's confidentiality to maximize good. The benefit of protecting the passengers may well justify jeopardizing the patient's privacy.

Confidentiality

While caring for a victim of an automobile accident, an EMT is told by the patient that he was drinking quite heavily before the accident. The driver of the other vehicle apparently died instantly. As the EMT is preparing to transport the patient to the hospital, a law enforcement officer asks if the EMT has any reason to believe that the patient was driving under the influence of alcohol. What should his response to the officer be?

In most if not all states, it is unclear if an EMT is bound by the same legal obligations as a physician to protect his patient's confidentiality. Although the legal duty is vague, many ethicists believe that all healthcare professionals have a moral obligation to protect the confidentiality of their patients. Most states, however, clearly define some circumstances in which the healthcare professional has a legal duty to breach confidentiality, such as in cases of suspected child abuse. One may approach this case by deciding if a larger social good would be served by exposing the patient's admission of alcohol use. While this may lead to a conviction and remove a single criminal from the streets, the long-term effect of this action on the patient/helper relationship deserves serious consideration. Future patients may withhold information from EMTs and other health professionals if they fear that statements offered in confidence would be disclosed to others, especially when illegal acts are involved.

To Code or Not to Code

An EMT has responded to an elderly victim of cardiac arrest. The firefighters state that they would have initiated CPR, but the wife requested that they withhold any treatment. The wife claims that both she and her husband are in their 80s, and it was her husband's wish that "no heroic measures" be used to prolong his life. The patient's medical history includes only mild hypertension and no history of terminal illness. Neither the wife nor the husband have signed living wills. Is CPR indicated?

This situation raises many complex ethical issues. Once again, there is conflict between the patient's reported wish to refuse lifesaving care (autonomy) and the rescuer's belief that continued life is better than death. Some ethicists would focus on the quality of life. In most studies, less than 25 percent of those cardiac arrest patients undergoing resuscitation in the field are ever discharged from the hospital, and about one-half of the survivors suffer permanent brain damage.

The principle of double effect comes into play also. Does the good effect (continued life) outweigh the bad effect (brain damage)? When the risk for brain recovery versus injury are approximately equal, natural law would argue for resuscitation. However, when the risk of brain injury and permanent disability greatly exceeds the hope for recovery, proponents of natural law might opt for allowing nature to take its course and refrain from resuscitation.

The cost of resuscitation and subsequent hospitalization should also be considered, as the family could find itself under a severe financial burden if the patient survives only to be in a comatose condition requiring long-term nursing care. Also, the patient's life expectancy at the time of the cardiac arrest might be a factor in this decision.

Human Experimentation

The employees of a local EMS service have been informed that they will be assisting the medical center in conducting research on an experimental drug for patients with multitraumatic injuries. The preliminary laboratory studies on animals suggest that the drug may be effective. On odd-numbered days, all multitrauma patients will receive the drug, while on even-numbered days, no drug therapy will be administered. Should the EMT be concerned that he is acting as an agent of the researcher, yet no mention has been made of obtaining informed consent from the patients?

Even if written consent was obtained from the patients, some ethicists would claim that such consent may not be truly valid. Because of the duress of the illness or injury, patients may not fully comprehend the consequences of their agreement to participate in the research. Altered levels of consciousness may also render them incompetent in giving informed consent. For the unconscious patient, the law "implies" consent for emergency medical therapy. Without sufficient moral justification, some researchers have interpreted this implied consent to include not only consent for treatment, but also for participation in emergency medical research.

The EMT who is troubled by the lack of informed consent may find himself in an untenable situation in which he must choose between keeping his job by following his medical director's orders and refusing to assist in the research. Those EMTs who did participate would remain morally accountable along with the researchers for any adverse reactions to the experimental treatment.

The moral dilemmas faced by EMTs are complicated by conflicting rights and responsibilities, a poorly defined concept of moral accountability, limited ethical training, and the emergent nature of the industry. As humans, many of our values are subject to bias and may cloud our ethical decision making. The law and professional oaths or codes alone are insufficient tools to help in making such ethical choices. Theories and principles, although somewhat flawed, can supply us with a rational, justifiable framework on which to develop our personal moral standards.

There are no protocols for all of the possible ethical dilemmas EMTs face. Perhaps, though, by stimulating the discussion of ethical issues among EMS personnel, we can spark the interest of not only the EMTs in the field today, but also those who will teach the EMTs of tomorrow.

Source

Reprinted with permission from JEMS, *May 1989. At the time of original publication, Jeff Salomone, NREMT-P, taught extensively on EMS topics and had been involved in prehospital emergency care for more than 10 years.*

References

Arras, J., and R. Hunt. *Ethical Issues in Modern Medicine.* 2nd ed. Palo Alto, Calif.: Mayfield Publishing, 1983.

Barry, V. *Aspects of Healthcare.* Belmont, Calif.: Wadsworth Publishing, 1982.

Beauchamp, T. L., and J. F. Childress. *Principles of Biomedical Ethics.* 2nd ed. New York: Oxford University Press, 1983.

Lloyd, G. *Hippocratic Writings.* New York: Penguin Books, 1983.

Recruitment and Retention

Hiring Top-Notch Employees: Unmasking the Best Applicant

Gail Hallas, PhD

As the available labor pool contracts in a post-baby boom era, recruitment and retention become increasingly important. Hiring top-notch employees requires both skill and practice. Author Gail Hallas provides 12 helpful hints on how to unmask the best candidate.

INTERVIEWING A JOB APPLICANT is like watching *The Wizard of Oz*. It's impressive. It's convincing. And you get fooled if you don't look behind the curtain.

EMS providers know that operational survival depends on the ability to hire top-notch employees. But the truth is, when job applicants start lining up, most providers don't quite know what to do. So they talk too much, ask illegal questions, and don't listen. And when they finally select someone for the job, the odds are that many will make a mistake.

Less than 12 percent of EMS providers have any previous formal training on how to effectively hire people, and only 17 percent receive formal training once they're on the job. The lucky ones learn by trial and error after years of making costly mistakes, but most never learn. Consequently, the industry is riddled with low productivity and high turnover costs. These problems may be alleviated, however, by initially hiring the right person for the job.

There are three main skills to master for interviewing job candidates:

- Regulating what you do and don't say
- Asking the right types of questions
- Listening well

Once you master these skills, you'll spend less time later cleaning up messes that result from poor choices now. It's well worth the effort to become an expert at interviewing applicants, because hiring the wrong person is wretched and costly—not only for you and the person you hired, but for the rest of your employees, for the physicians and facility administrators with whom you work, and, most of all, for the patients you serve. Aside from the emotional drain on everyone, the cost of turnover can choke the life out of your budget.

Becoming expert at the three hiring skills is merely a matter of following a structured agenda during the interview. What's more, with the right frame of mind, you'll discover that interviewing applicants can be rewarding and fun. Clearly, however, the biggest problem for most interviewers is trying to overcome two very normal, very human psychological forces that not only hinder wise hiring decisions but affect all human interaction.

The first force is called the primacy effect, or the tendency to give credibility to whatever the applicant says and does at the beginning of an interview. Interviewers, hoping to zip through the whole hiring mess and get down to business, tend to listen for good news from the applicant—reasons to hire him—rather than the more effective method of looking for reasons not to hire him. Then, when the manager's good-news appetite is satisfied, he makes up his mind. His thinking goes on hold, and subsequent messages from the applicant, good or bad, are disregarded. The primacy effect is a big part of the reason that the majority of all hiring decisions turn out to be mistakes.

The second psychological force that causes hiring mistakes is the recency effect, or the tendency to remember only recent information. The recency effect comes into play after interviewing several people in a relatively short period of time. As information from applicants is stored in the interviewer's brain, things start running together and becoming jumbled. For example, the interviewer forgets what people said and what they looked like. A sense of frustration and urgency ultimately prompts a snap judgment based on input that he remembers—or input from the most recent applicant interviewed. Managers tend to hire the last person interviewed more often than anyone else.

The good news is that the primacy and recency effects can be curbed, and interviews can become more organized. The following is a list of 12 guidelines that will help keep interviewers on track and unmask the winning applicants from the rest of the group.

Welcome Applicants Up Front

Greet job candidates in the reception area or outer office rather than from behind your desk. This maneuver helps the applicant relax and allows his true personality to come through.

Interview Privately

Interview applicants in a quiet place where you won't be interrupted. If you can keep the rest of the staff from disturbing you, your office is probably the best location. If you can't find a private area, find a place that is removed from foot traffic. Instruct the person who answers the phone to hold your calls.

Spell Out Details of the Interview

Tell the applicant exactly how you intend to structure the interview and how long it will take. This way, the applicant knows exactly what to expect, and you establish a feeling of trust. The person will likely shed remaining defenses at this point.

Lean on a Clipboard

There are two advantages to this. First, it reminds you to write. By documenting ongoing impressions about each applicant, you're more likely to overcome the primacy and recency effects. Using a clipboard also prevents the applicant from reading your notes, which makes you less inhibited about documenting any thoughts you may have.

Change the Subject if the Applicant Looks Stressed

If this happens, stop that specific line of questioning, and go to something else. Make note of the troublesome topic, however, to put it into context with the rest of the interview. It may be significant, or it may mean nothing at all.

Monitor What You Do and Don't Say During the Interview

Let the applicant talk 90 percent of the time. This is the hardest part for most interviewers, but one technique is to stick a note on your clipboard with the word *listen* written on it.

When you do talk, be precise about job responsibilities and what you expect of your staff. Studies show that most problems with new employees stem from the fact that they don't know what is expected of them.

Legally, there are some things you can't say during an interview. In fact, not knowing what your parameters are when conducting interviews and during the candidate-selection process can prove costly.

Federal law prohibits employers from discriminating against people because of sex, age, race, national origin, or religion. Effective July 26, 1992, the Americans with Disabilities Act prohibits employer discrimination in hiring, firing, promoting, awarding benefits to, and managing employees and applicants with disabilities. Because of ongoing legislative changes, it's wise to remain up-to-date on federal and state laws that protect people who fall into these categories.

Ask Open-Ended Questions

Avoid asking questions that require only yes or no answers. Instead, use statements that start with, "Tell me about . . . ," "Describe . . . ," "What kind of . . . ," and "Give me an example of . . . ." Choose four or five questions, and use the same ones with all applicants for that job so that the competition is measurable and fair. There are no right or wrong answers to these questions, only appropriate or inappropriate responses. Later, tally the scores based on whether the answers are suitable to your needs.

Tune in for Lies

Body language changes when people lie. Their eyes tend to shift, and their voices drop. If you're suspicious, ask the applicant to explain further. Most people will stumble on details about events they're making up.

Ask About Pet Peeves and Pastimes

It's important to listen carefully here, as the applicant's answers will draw a picture of his strengths and weaknesses. With encouragement,

What Not to Say During an Interview

To prevent legal vulnerability during interviews, remember that legal issues usually hinge on whether the questions you ask have any bearing on the applicant's qualifications or ability to perform the job. The following are examples of what you can and cannot say during an interview.

DON'T ASK . . .	INSTEAD, ASK . . .
About the applicant's national origin, parentage, ancestry, naturalization, or the status of parents, spouse, or children.	If the applicant is a U.S. citizen or a resident alien with the right to work in the United States.
About the applicant's religion, church, synagogue, parish, or the religious holidays he observes.	If the applicant foresees any scheduling problems since the company operates seven days a week, 24 hours a day, and needs people to work those times.
About the applicant's native language or the language spoken at home. Also, don't ask how the applicant learned to read, write, or speak a foreign language.	What languages the applicant is fluent in (but only if knowledge of a foreign language is needed for the job).
About marital status, number of dependents, children's or spouse's occupation, maiden name or whether the applicant has changed his or her name.	If the applicant has ever worked for the company under a different name.
Whether a woman wants her name preceded by Miss, Mrs., or Ms.	How she would like to be addressed.
About applicant's age or date of birth, or the ages of his children.	If the applicant is older than 18.

If you wonder whether an interview question is legal, ask yourself, "Does this question have any bearing on qualifications or abilities to perform this job?" It's a safe bet that if your answer is yes, the question is legal. If your answer is no, don't ask.

most people will talk about themselves. Hence, you can establish whether the person is goal-oriented, hostile or friendly, enthusiastic, energetic, and so forth. You'll learn critical information for your immediate hiring decision as well as information for the future should you decide to hire the applicant.

Use Hypothetical Problem Situations

Hypothetical problem situations (HPS) are 50- to 100-word prepared statements of real-life work situations that the person you hire is likely to face. The purpose of the HPS is to reveal how the applicant sizes up a situation and makes decisions. Read at least one statement to the applicant and then ask, "How would you respond to this situation?"

A quick way to get ideas for your hypothetical problem situations is to ask a few tenured employees to write down problems they've encountered with co-workers, patients, physicians, and outside agencies. With a little editing, you'll end up with an excellent resource file of HPS for future use.

During applicant responses, watch for clues as to how the applicant processes information, makes judgments, incorporates leadership style, shows ability to delegate, indicates attitude problems or prejudices, and other important traits. This is a valuable technique for predicting future performance.

Think of Resumes as Rubbish

Unfortunately, some applicants are just plain talented at fabricating impressive references and bureaucratic rhetoric for their resumes—neither of which qualifies them for the job. Personnel selections that rely primarily on resumes and overlook the applicant's personality are destined to fail. High turnover rates are usually the result of personality flaws or conflicts, not the inability of employees to do the job. Turnover may occasionally appear to be due to inability because an employee does not produce, but a lack of productivity usually stems from a lack of motivation, a poor attitude, and an unwillingness to learn.

Fortunately, these are all characteristics that can be recognized during the interview. The "80/20 rule" covers it well: 80 percent of management's personnel problems come from 20 percent of the employees. If you trust hunches and weigh personality over resumes, you'll likely weed out that mind-maddening 20 percent before they're ever hired.

Stick to the Interview Format

Tell the applicant when 10 minutes remain in the interview. Use the remaining time to elicit questions or to let the applicant say anything not yet covered. Then, at the precise time you said the interview would end, stand, shake the person's hand, and make it clear that the interview is over. Walk the applicant back to where the initial greeting took place. At that point, smile and say three things:

- "Thank you for your interest in the position."
- "Someone will call you in about a week" (or whatever time frame you choose).
- "Please don't call me before that time is up."

Then return to your office and write down any last-minute impressions you may have. With the applicant gone, you'll think of details that escaped you before. To lessen the recency effect, don't schedule another interview for at least two hours.

Let's face it. Hiring top-notch employees can be risky business. But it can be done if you follow these 12 guidelines to peek past deceptive drapes. To blindly assume that an enchanting applicant represents the ideal employee is to click your heels three times and wish you were back in Kansas.

Source

Reprinted with permission from JEMS, *February 1992. At the time of original publication, Gail Hallas, PhD, was a management consultant, writer, and speaker on medical-legal, personnel, and stress management topics.*

Discovering Professional-ism in EMS

John M. Becknell

Helping staff members become professionals is one of the most important responsibilities of EMS leaders. John Becknell shares a method for defining and discovering professionalism.

ON AN UNUSUALLY WARM DAY last spring, a paramedic I know took off his shirt to sun himself in a chair while awaiting calls in the fire department driveway. The warm sun felt great until the ambulance service director drove by, observed his shirtless behavior, and stopped to decry it as "acting in an unprofessional manner."

Hearing the phrase "acting in an unprofessional manner" led me to reflect on the topic of professionalism in EMS. It's something you hear much about these days. Somewhere between attending EMT school and learning IV therapy, you may start to ask, "Just what is professionalism?" Many people hear the word and think of doctors, lawyers, teachers, and highly paid athletes. You may want a professional to paint your car instead of letting the local high school shop class do it. Or you may think of professionalism in terms of receiving payment for something. (The oldest profession is reputed to be prostitution!)

Most of us might agree that the shirtless medic was not acting professionally. We might look at a list of behavioral standards and divide the list into professional and nonprofessional categories. But a concrete, black-and-white definition of professionalism is elusive. In asking various people how they would define it, I've discovered that professionalism is a concept that can be very personal and subjective.

Defining Professionalism

Some background on the word may shed light on the topic. In a religious sense, professional relates to the practice of taking vows, with motivation coming from within the individual. Along with the profession comes a specific code of conduct. The calling, the profession, the conduct—all are related.

In a secular sense, the word is applied to a calling to or training in a vocation to which one has become committed. The professional has more than a job—he has a special calling and thus willingly subscribes to the concept of personal conduct and ethics that go along with his profession.

In the early twentieth century, there was a marked rise in the teaching of professionalism—that is, in the number of professional schools that included special training and preparation for the practice of a profession. In the 1950s, a musician friend of mine attended Eastman Conservatory of Music, a school for musicians in Rochester, N.Y. He reports that Eastman was as busy teaching the concept of professionalism as it was teaching music itself. The school taught ethics, dress, and social behavior. There was a very specific idea of what professional musicians should look like, how they should act, and what they should be able to do. Another friend just out of medical school stated—tongue-in-cheek—that 50 percent of medical school was learning not medicine, but how to act like a doctor!

If paramedics are to be considered professionals, then they should be expected to follow the standard of ethical conduct that applies to medical work. The trouble is, many in EMS are not taught professionalism.

I learned my definition of EMS professionalism by watching others. Early on, paramedics had to beat the "ambulance driver" syndrome. Largely, that meant "be credible, act educated, and instill confidence." However, I still believe that the bulk of what most paramedics know about professionalism is "caught," not taught.

Professionalism and Management

In the real world of EMS, the people who teach and talk most about professionalism are EMS managers. Management experts tell us that managers set the tone for an organization. Managers recognize that professional conduct is not always an automatic for street paramedics. Unfortunately, managers themselves are often at a loss for a clear concept of professionalism and thus are reduced to defining it in terms of their specific agendas.

Concerned with organizational image, quality assurance, industry innovations, growth, bottom lines, and career ladders, managers are the ones assigned to see that an organization looks good and prospers.

Thus, when managers tell EMS workers to "act professional out there," they mean in a way that relates to the specifics of their organizational goals. And these goals and agendas can change.

Because of unclear expectations for street paramedics, managers often try to instill their concepts of professionalism through policy making. A policy that states, "Paramedics shall not take off shirts while on duty," only covers shirts and suggests that a policy must eventually be made to cover every other detail. Obviously, the shirtless medic needed a better understanding of his specific manager's concept of professionalism—of how that concept related to the organizational image.

Furthermore, teaching through policy is often negative and can cause more confusion than constructive edification. I have a positive feeling toward the idea of improving my professional image. I have a very negative feeling toward a policy that defines my image strictly in terms of rules and regulations.

Managers must honestly ask themselves if they see the people who work for them as professionals. Those who already see their employees as professionals will find ways to enhance professionalism through respectful listening, sharing of ideas, and an absence of the charge "act like a professional," which implies that the person is not a professional.

Professionalism on the Streets

If TV police shows were written by people in the police business, the managers might have written *ADAM 12*, and the street cops might

> If paramedics are to be considered professionals, then they should be expected to follow the standard of ethical conduct that applies to medical work.

The very nature of taking care of the sick and injured outside the hospital setting suggests that no matter what is taught as professionalism, the streets will always be a classroom of contradictions.

have written *Hill Street Blues*. Whatever the ideal concept of professionalism, life on the streets presents paradoxes that defy our ideals. The very nature of taking care of the sick and injured outside the hospital setting suggests that no matter what is taught as professionalism, the streets will always be a classroom of contradictions.

Not long ago, while kneeling next to the angulated legs and ankles of a cement mason who had fallen two floors to the ground, I was faced with a professional dilemma. A crowd of construction workers and volunteer firefighters stood in a semicircle and protested as we began the painful process of easing off the man's boots to assess and tend to his injuries. The sharp broken end of the tibia scraped against the rough leather, and the man screamed with pain. Someone in the crowd called out, "You guys don't know what the hell you're doing!"

The bystanders hated to see the man suffer, and they saw us as adding to his pain. But the best thing for the man was a thorough assessment of distal circulation and bleeding control. While we wanted to instill confidence and trust in the patient and represent ourselves as quality EMS professionals, our image in the eyes of the volunteers and bystanders was that of insensitive "ambulance drivers." It would have been easy to leave the boot in place and please the crowd. The public relations and marketing value may have been better for our company. But the professional thing to do that day was not the most popular. Thus, the patient care priority at times seems at cross-purposes with the professional image.

Living in the tight space of an ambulance cab or in musty quarters at odd times of the day and night understandably can make EMS professionals feel rather unprofessional. The "easy life" of just sitting around and waiting is often a very trying life. Under media lights, it is natural to think of oneself as a professional, but the real work of EMS includes scraping bugs off the light bar and putting up with the unique habits of the people you must work with so closely. The image of the professional as a starched, uniformed medic in a shiny rig is only part of the picture. Professionalism is elusive for the street paramedic because of the stark contrast between waiting for calls and caring for people in extreme need.

When I experience a number of tragic calls in a short space of time, I am affected. As tempers run short, run forms get sloppy and thoughts travel to things other than professionalism. Herein lies another paradox. Thinking back over all the EMS workers I've known, the ones I look up to are not always the best dressed or the ones with the winning charm. The irony of professionalism is that some of the best EMS people are those with the ability to blend human compassion with an uncanny street sense that allows them to filter out distractions and respond like heroes in a Robert Ludlum thriller.

How do we define this sort of professionalism? It's a quality that comes only from the hard education of experience. It is not laid down in a guide book.

A Personal Discovery

Whether others see me as a professional is not something over which I have exclusive control. And because management may change its agendas, I do not want to be dependent on its circumstantial definitions. I need an understanding of professionalism that honestly embraces the basics and will give mileage no matter where I take my medic work. So over the years I've had to develop my own understanding of how I see myself in the job I do. That image—the inner discovery of what being a professional means to me—has led me to the formulation of a model that is of concrete use in my daily work.

This personal model suggests four areas of focus that assist me in sorting out what is important in EMS. While the areas obviously overlap, I have suggested them in the order of my perception of their importance.

Value Yourself and What You Do

If anything can be learned from modern psychology, it is the importance of self-esteem. Viewing yourself as a professional requires that you believe in your own worth and in the worth of your work. Often this means going back to the beginning of your career and rediscovering why you are in EMS instead of the insurance or computer business. Is the daily job of caring for the sick and injured worth the time you invest? The common laborer says, "Tell me exactly what I have to do to earn my wage." The professional says, "I desire to do this work because the work itself has value to me."

Others will respect you only as much as you respect yourself. Sometimes paramedics think that the long line of people waiting to get into the field must diminish the importance of what they do as individuals. Not so. If you believe in your choice of EMS as an occupation and see its real value, you will respect yourself as a professional.

Seek the Best for Those You Help

Beyond the basic company policy is the belief that you must always seek the best for those you are called on to help. For me, this means that my skills need to be sharp and my knowledge fresh. It means that I have to be honest enough to admit when I can improve in an area. Simply looking good is not enough.

Most of us in EMS are great at looking good. But the real proof is in the care we are able to give. When I have to make a decision about a specific action or behavior, I need not await a management policy. The patient's best interest directs and sometimes limits my action. Doing the best for the patient demands that my response times are not jeopardized by personal comfort or interest, but rather served by an honest drive to fulfill my duty to those who need me.

Learn and Grow

Nothing in life is static. Everything is in a process of either growing

Source

Reprinted with permission from JEMS, *December 1987. John Becknell, EMT-P, is a writer, consultant, and lecturer with over 18 years of experience as an EMS provider. He is a frequent contributor to* JEMS *and has recently published his first book,* Medic Life: Creating Success in EMS.

or dying. I believe this to be true of professionalism. Most EMS workers are either excited and growing in the field, or they're figuring out a way to change careers. If a healthy personal professionalism is to be maintained, growth is imperative.

For me, growth has not meant studying more advanced emergency care—it has meant reflecting on what it means to do this work. What does EMS teach me about modern medicine? What does it teach about death and the art of living? In growing in this field, I have discovered that EMS involves so much more than fast emergency care. It is a world of relationships with partners and a world of insight into the private lives and homes of the people I care for. EMS is an ongoing lesson in the value of life in an unpredictable world.

How you grow in your profession will depend on who you are and what you see, but the first step is to believe that you can learn and grow.

Maintain a Good Image

My father will be happy to know that I at last realize that how I appear to others is indeed important. How I appear to myself is vital to my performance; if I feel good about how I look, I feel better about what I do. This does not mean I copy some unrealistic military image of a paramedic. Yet my image in an emergency situation is vital to the task of establishing credibility within a few short seconds. Gaining the respect and trust of those around me in chaotic situations is a must if I am to continue in EMS. Also, my ability to help people in emergency situations indeed depends on the survival of the organization I represent, thus demanding attention to how I represent that organization.

Professionalism and Integration

We live in an odd world. Sometimes we get the idea that our careers and professions are all there is. But long before the call to EMS, we are all called as human beings. And long after the retirement plaque hangs dusty on the wall, we will still be human.

I believe the ultimate challenge of professionalism is to integrate into the career experience our total world view. EMS provides a wonderful opportunity to develop a concept of professionalism that carries over to just about everything we do. Sure, it's a job, and I look forward to my days off. But it's the sort of work that helps me know how to spend those non-working hours. Maybe the profession of EMS is one of life's great callings.

Before You Quit, Read This: A Personal Perspective on Motivation for Street Paramedics

John M. Becknell

Motivation and satisfaction throughout your career are not automatic. A number of factors can cause you to believe you have no options other than quitting. John Becknell describes how to balance expectations and reality to achieve long-term career success.

LAST YEAR ON A RAINY April night, my partner Tim and I had just cleared the hospital after unloading two patients from a successful trauma call. With our adrenaline spent, we cruised through the wet night toward a coverage point and began to talk. Our conversation drifted from the patients to the run and, finally, to our futures in the emergency business.

"I've really been giving serious thought to quitting," Tom said. "I used to be so pumped about being a medic, but recently I've been thinking about what a dead-end job this is. I'm not motivated anymore. On most shifts, I barely check out the rig. Like everyone says, there doesn't seem to be any future for paramedics."

As we pulled into an empty parking lot and watched a busy intersection, Tim continued. "But there's another side of me that really likes this job. I feel good about what I'm doing when I can use my skills on a good trauma call. I really like the freedom of being out and talking to my partners on nights like this. But everyone keeps talking about going back to school and changing careers. It's frustrating not knowing what to do."

Tim's confession started me wondering whether a street medic can retain his motivation for a long and satisfying career. Tim's frustration suggested that although he did not really want to go into real estate or work toward his MBA, something was driving him in that direction. Forced to reflect on my own experience and on numerous conversations I've had with street medics over the years, I discovered there are some good answers to the questions about career motivation and satisfaction in EMS.

High Expectations

It's no secret to career-conscious baby boomers that we need to feel positive about our work to do a good job. At the beginning of EMS careers, motivation comes fairly easily. New medics are overflowing with vigor. They are the ones who shine the rig, check out the drug box, and spend hours crafting beautiful and complete run reports. When management asks for a volunteer to do a special project, odds are the candidate will be a new guy.

But that new energy doesn't seem to last long. For most street medics, early motivation evaporates within a few years. There are exceptions— the medics who enter EMS with designs on management are able to remain motivated because their sights are set on pin-striped suits and a desk— but they are in the minority. Most medics who stay on the street are looking for some continuation or renewal of their early enthusiasm for street work.

This loss of motivation is nothing new. Managers continually discuss the lack of motivation they observe in experienced field paramedics. They bemoan sloppy run forms and the absence of professional attitudes. In search of answers, the experts blame stress and job burnout. Journal articles, conference speakers, and front-office discussions attribute the turnover and loss of motivation to the witnessing of too much blood and death and the need to talk about it. But from my own experience and that of the many medics I've talked with around the country, stress and burnout do not fully account for the lack of motivation and the desire to leave EMS.

So why do so many lose their spark and think seriously about leaving the field? The answer seems to lie in the very nature of the career.

Imagination and Reality

Careers, like vacations, new cars, and sex, are often a lot different in reality than in our imaginations. People are attracted to the emergency field by the promise of excitement, freedom, high visibility, and the opportunity to make a difference in the world. During paramedic training, one's thoughts often dwell on these desires, and the medic imagines how satisfying it will be when he is finally certified and out on his own. But graduation and reality unveil a very different experience.

Anyone who has spent much time in an ambulance knows that the thrills are there but that they are short-lived and quite different from what may have been anticipated. The canceled calls and nursing home runs, the countless hours on the road subsisting on fast food, the energy expended trying to convince an ED doc that you know how to recognize a PVC—all contribute to a sense of frustration. For every call that leaves you pumped and satisfied with your work, there are a hundred others that inspire only tedium. Somehow, in all of your training and preparation, you never imagined how draining the endless waiting could be.

After a few cardiac arrests, deliveries, suicides, and highway grinders, the thrill of being a medic is not as intense. And herein lies the one reality lesson street medics discover more acutely than most people: Excitement is relative. An international airline pilot recently complained to me that motivation based on excitement is one of the biggest problems in his profession. He added that many pilots think they'll be more motivated if they can fly bigger and faster planes only to discover that the guys flying the 747s have also lost the thrill.

High Responsibility and Low Control

As excitement fades into routine, paramedics begin to discover another aspect of EMS work that saps motivation. The medic is responsible for performing with high-level professionalism but has very little control and only casual influence over the setting. Not long ago, I sat in a run review session and listened to a medical director admonish a young paramedic for failing to score an IV and respond quickly enough to an elderly woman suffering from a leaking "triple A." I could hear the anger building in the young medic's voice as he tried to explain how a snarling dog and an equally snarling husband had made his job next to impossible. The woman died, and the QA-minded doc wanted to be sure the medic felt his responsibility.

This lack of control in life-and-death situations often results in a feeling of helplessness that destroys any sense of satisfaction. Medics get into this work in part to make a difference in crisis situations, but far too often that is impossible. The responsibility, however, doesn't stop.

Yet oddly, even in the face of this imbalance, most medics like street work for what it is—pulling odd hours, getting close to partners, living on the edge, and occasionally making a difference in someone's crisis. They appreciate the flexible schedules, the freedom of rig work, and the opportunity to pursue other interests in addition to their medical work.

Society's Demand on Careers

So why is it so difficult for paramedics to remain content in their work? Part of the answer lies in our success-oriented society, which does not allow people to settle for mere satisfaction in their work. Instead, we are constantly driven to move on to bigger and better things.

At a party last fall, I counted how many people questioned me about my career. The gist of the questioning was if and how I was getting ahead. By evening's end, I was overwhelmed with the sense that the only way to be considered successful in today's world is to make more money and move up. The same pressure is often felt in EMS circles. In ambulance quarters, at conferences, and in publications, there is a heavy push to be something more than a street medic.

But becoming a mover and a shaker is not necessarily what the street medic wants. A medic friend from Ohio told of how he enjoyed his medic work but felt the pressure to move up so acutely that he finished his business degree, quit his medic job, and took on a junior executive position with banker's hours and more money. Two years later, he privately laments about how much he misses EMS work.

I have observed firsthand how difficult it is for medics to admit that they like street work and want to remain on the streets despite the calling to consult, manage, or change careers. The motivation toward excellence and longevity in prehospital work may indeed be hampered by the climate of our high-pressure society.

Staying or Leaving

In view of all the things that cause us to lose motivation and want to leave EMS, is it possible to make a sound career evaluation and rediscover motivation? The answer is yes, but only after asking tough questions and taking control of our own career satisfaction.

Throughout any career, human nature causes us to doubt our own work and whether we should seek something new. These occasional doubts are simply part of the life cycle. But in a medic career, the doubts seem to be more than occasional. I've often heard comments like, "I've

Satisfaction in your career comes from taking charge of your own happiness.

got to get a real job." Indeed, many people in EMS move on. Yet a lot of us, like Tim, linger. My own experience was one of vacillation between staying and quitting until I eventually learned how to deal with the doubts effectively.

Admitting to myself that staying in EMS is OK was the first step toward dealing with the doubts. Coming to such a decision freed me from the notion imposed by society that EMS is not a career anyone stays with.

One of the happiest men I know is approaching 60 and has worked as a clerk in the same family-owned hardware store for most of his life. Everyone who knows Claude thinks he's bright enough to have been something other than a clerk, but Claude simply smiles and says that as a young man, he found something he liked and "just stuck with it." Giving yourself permission to do what you like is the first part of developing a fulfilling work life.

Second—and most important—is conducting personal reviews. During my tenure in EMS, I have frequently reviewed why I got into the emergency business and why I enjoy the work. I have found that I like the personal value I receive from going on calls, as well as the freedom my "down time" affords me. The odd scheduling and having weekdays off have helped me construct a unique lifestyle, and the special relationships I share with partners have been very satisfying. I have also found that there is a lot of nonsense and frustration in EMS, but I realize that this is the case in every field. In short, my reviews confirmed that I was doing something I truly enjoyed.

As I went through this review process, I discovered that I had clarified my reasons for staying in street work. This sense of purpose is central to motivation. It provides the power within ourselves to do our job well and feel some satisfaction.

On the other hand, you may discover through your review and evaluation that you do not enjoy your work and see no purpose in it. Such a finding should be a signal to move on. At the very least, the review process can help you prepare to change careers with confidence and clarity.

Personal Responsibility

Simply knowing why you started in paramedic work and deciding to stay will not guarantee total job satisfaction. Satisfaction in your career comes from taking charge of your own happiness. In any area of life, be it careers, marriage, where we live, or personal achievements, human nature compels us to blame something or someone else for our lack of happiness. This passing of the buck seems especially prevalent in EMS careers.

Modern self-help psychology books continually espouse the notion that we alone are responsible for our personal happiness. Often, it is our attitude that prohibits us from finding satisfaction in our work. It is a myth of the modern work world that we have to find the perfect job to be happy.

There will always be rotten nursing home transfers, rigs that overheat, and managers who won't listen. These problems simply come with the territory. Do not allow them to destroy your satisfaction in your work. Finding fulfillment is possible if you accept that you hold the cards to your career attitude.

Being Your Own Advocate

For reasons yet unexplained, our society has not seen fit to reward me for being a paramedic. In truth, I'm just one of hundreds of city employees who does his job and goes home at the end of his shift. I'm not paid a lot of money for being an "emergency worker," and I'm certainly not overloaded with power and prestige.

Thus, many of us conclude that being a medic is no big deal and accept society's lack of accolades as an appropriate appraisal of our profession.

Medics are often guilty of underestimating the worth of their work. With the goal of not being considered "siren heads" by our peers, we have adopted an attitude that suggests being a medic is nothing to be proud of. But if we don't admire and believe in what we do, how can we expect anyone else (including management) to see value in our work?

A few years ago, while I was evaluating whether to quit EMS, my youngest son asked if he could have an old *JEMS* calendar he had found in a pile of magazines. I gave him the calendar, smiling at the "action hero" pictures. Later that night, he called me into his room. He had taped the photos up on the wall and wanted me to explain them. After a while, he looked up and said, "Is that what you really do, Dad?" Suddenly, for the first time in my career, I saw my work through the eyes of someone else. I was proud to be working on the streets and doing something that indeed was more than a tactic to get ahead. Paramedic work makes a lot of sense when seen through new eyes for what it really is.

Downside-Up Management

In the corporate world, people begin at entry-level positions and hope to work their way up the ladder. The possibility of moving up is often a motivating force. But EMS isn't like the corporate world. Most medics are not in the business because they hope to move up but rather because they like street work and are good at it. Good street medics often do not become managers since their interests lie with the rigs, not the front office.

In many EMS organizations, an adversarial relationship exists between bosses and workers, with management viewed as the upper rung of the ladder while street medics remain on the lower rungs. For the most part, EMS management has not had time to mature as rapidly as the medics being managed, leading some street medics to blame their frustrations on management.

> Most medics are not in the business because they hope to move up but rather because they like street work and are good at it.

Source

Reprinted with permission from JEMS, *August 1989.*

Because the paramedic profession is still young, EMS managers have much to learn about managing the seasoned street medic. But in the meantime, street medics can empower themselves, stimulate their personal motivation, and help their managers by practicing downside-up management. This concept requires street medics to see themselves as street professionals and experts and to assist the EMS manager in understanding how to better manage the organization.

Contrary to a reactive, complaint-oriented attitude toward management, this concept conveys a positive reminder: "I am a professional, and here is how management can help me do what I do best." Because the medic believes in himself, he is uniquely qualified to assist management in knowing how to better the service. After all, the real product of EMS is on the street, not in the front office.

Practicing downside-up management requires us to be willing to tackle problems side by side with management rather than assuming an "us versus them" stance.

Motivation and career satisfaction are not automatic. They have to be desired and worked on, but the rewards can be great. Career experts tell us that we can expect to change careers at least three times in our lives. Some of us will continue to lift stretchers, while others may find the next career to be better. But if I've learned anything on my shifts, it's that the time to start enjoying life is now. Time is the one resource that no amount of money, applause, or power can replace. More than any other profession, our work teaches us that the time we have is truly a gift. Perhaps with a closer look, Tim and other medics will discover that grumbling about quitting is not the only option at hand.

DESPITE RECENT ATTENTION paid to volunteer organizations, most notably through former President Bush's Points of Light program, such organizations still experience great difficulties in recruiting new members. And unless social and economic climates change drastically, those difficulties are not likely to go away any time soon.

Increasing demands for people's time and the growth in the number of families in which both partners work have made recruitment of volunteers a major concern for administrators of volunteer ambulance and rescue squads. But just as tough is the retention of established volunteers. To appreciate the size of the problem, compare the time it takes to recruit and train any new employee (a minimum of 150 hours) to the fact that the average length of productive service for an EMT volunteer is approximately six years. For many volunteer programs, the two never even out.

Recruiting and retaining volunteers involves much more than simply "roping them in" and hoping they'll stay. Other factors, such as orientation, training, and individual provider growth, also play a part. These elements must be worked into an ongoing, proactive personnel policy that does more than just exist for an agency. The leadership must be committed to a continual process of ensuring that the volunteers fully understand what they are being asked to do and the commitment that it will take.

It All Starts With a Plan

To attract the best people, the leadership of the EMS organization must develop a cohesive and comprehensive recruitment plan. Since such a plan must have grass roots support among other members of the organization, all personnel should be involved in its formation and execution.

Getting volunteers to work on your ambulance requires a personal touch. Indeed, one-on-one contact made by enthusiastic members of the agency is the most effective tool in obtaining new members.

It's important to remember to keep an open mind when recruiting people to join your agency. Yes, patient care practitioners are essential to maintaining an ambulance service, but do not overlook the fact that many other skills are also needed. There are individuals in your community who can be assets to your organization even if they don't have the inclination to provide direct patient care. A comprehensive cadre of backup personnel who can carry out administrative duties, for example, can be an invaluable addition to your resource pool.

So exactly how do you go about recruiting new EMS volunteers?

Here to Stay? Recruiting EMS Volunteers

John Morrissey, NREMT-P

Volunteers make up one of the most unique groups in EMS. In this article, John Morrissey asks volunteers, "Are you here to stay?" He also outlines some techniques for recruiting and retaining these valuable individuals.

People want to join a successful organization, and successful recruitment is one of the results of a good PR program.

One way is to conduct promotional events in your community. Sponsoring events in a local shopping mall that have specific themes relating to family, home, or health is an excellent way to promote your agency and look for new members. Exercise centers and allied healthcare meetings can also offer valuable recruitment opportunities.

Using slide shows, videos, or overhead presentations to pitch your volunteer agency during these events can pique people's interest and draw them in. As you develop your recruitment strategy, however, avoid sensationalizing EMS; instead, show a true picture of your agency in terms of the types of work involved and the commitment necessary to be an effective member. Be honest about the requirements. It does no good to sweet talk someone into joining; new members brought in that way will probably leave quickly because the time commitments or requirements were misrepresented. And high turnover of new volunteers makes your agency lose credibility.

Business cards listing the names and phone numbers of key contact people should be printed and handed out to prospective volunteers whenever possible. They are easy to carry, and the person is left with something tangible in his hand—not just an impression.

Another useful recruitment tool is a brochure describing the role of your agency and its importance to the community. The brochure should be professionally produced and should reflect your agency's current activities.

Your agency can also sponsor CPR and first-aid programs. These are invaluable public relations opportunities and demonstrate in a tangible way the role of your agency's members and their impact on the community.

Provide schedules of ongoing entry-level training programs to the agency membership and community media. The media—whether television, radio, or newspaper—can help publicize your EMS agency. To capitalize on such publicity, a public relations officer should be designated. The PR officer will manage the type of message communicated to the public and will make regular contacts with the local media to promote the agency.

Events worthy of media attention include the arrival of a new vehicle, a sizable donation by a corporate benefactor, agency social events and awards, election of officers, a personnel recruitment drive, or calls in which the agency saved a person's life. People want to join a successful organization, and successful recruitment is one of the results of a good PR program.

Allowing prospective members to ride along on a shift can also get people interested in joining an agency and get them involved quickly. Observation either in the field or in the dispatch office is a great way to get people hooked on joining EMS. This also provides prospective members an opportunity to find their niche in the organization and get a feel for what is expected of them as members of the agency. A word of caution, however: Control the observation experience, and limit how long it lasts. Don't allow anyone to become a "terminal observer."

Also, instruct the crews to avoid inappropriate initiation rituals. EMS personnel sometimes give new members meaningless tasks as a form of hazing, but this should be avoided if you want the recruit to stay.

A strong orientation program should include descriptions of the roles of new members as well as personnel manuals. In addition, introductions to the membership and crews with whom the new recruits will work is a necessity. A bulletin board with the new members' photos, special interests, and qualifications will make the new members feel like part of the operation. The presence of such a board also sends a message of caring.

Examine the dynamics of your organization. "Good ol' boy" networks or cliques must be dismantled; new members will be sensitive and will shy away from situations that will require them to prove themselves. Existing members should be well-trained, disciplined role models who arrive on time, complete tasks quickly, and are friendly. Vehicles, buildings, and equipment should be neat, clean, and ready for use.

Finally, initiate a buddy system by assigning a key contact person to help the new recruit through the process of becoming an active and productive member.

> It is counterproductive for an agency to recruit a great number of new members if no one stays long term.

Now You've Got 'em, How Do You Keep 'em?

Retention is an often overlooked—but essential—part of the recruitment process. Obviously, it is counterproductive for an agency to recruit a great number of new members if no one stays long term (i.e., more than 10 years), but some agencies do little or nothing to retain their personnel.

Effective retention of volunteers can be achieved by establishing a number of guidelines in the recruitment and retention plan.

First, assigning new members responsibility for certain tasks as soon as possible will give them a vested interest in the organization and its success. However, it is important not to push people beyond their capabilities too quickly; many new and talented providers are pushed too quickly into a role and become intimidated by the responsibility it demands. This is often a direct result of being moved into solo leadership positions too soon. Nevertheless, new—and existing—members should be encouraged to continually upgrade their skills.

Second, dealing with problems promptly and consistently will show new recruits that agency leadership is responsive and cares about working conditions. As with any conflict, good avenues of communication among all parties involved are extremely important. Problem solving is easy when communication is effective; when communication fails, small problems become huge, and large problems become unmanageable.

Third, communication should not just come down from the top but should also move upward. For example, when a volunteer leaves,

Source

Reprinted with permission from JEMS, *February 1993. John Morrissey, NREMT-P, is a senior emergency medical representative for the Syracuse area office of the New York State Department of Health. He has been involved in various volunteer and paid prehospital activities since 1975.*

management should conduct an exit interview to get the volunteer's perspective on various situations and to be clear about the reasons for the departure. This information is invaluable to an agency's ongoing efforts to retain members.

Fourth, leadership should be dynamic. Rotating the leadership brings fresh perspectives to an agency's agenda and prevents dynasties or empire-building. Bylaws should be established that limit the length of time leaders can serve. These rules communicate to members that there is a career ladder within the organization, with opportunities for clinical growth (e.g., becoming an EMT or paramedic) or managerial growth (e.g., becoming a supervisor).

Finally, acknowledging EMS volunteers' accomplishments is a positive gesture that acts as a powerful retention tool. Recognizing members for hours or years of service, outstanding patient care, a particularly well-executed program, or upgrading of credentials sends a strong message of thanks for a job well done. Publicizing these events in the local paper can't hurt either. Remember, there's no such thing as too much recognition; often, there is not enough.

Conclusion

Recruiting and retaining volunteer members of an EMS organization is not easy. A proactive recruitment and retention program, however, is a sure-fire way to maintain strength and remain on the cutting edge of EMS into the next century.

Reference

Bargue, S. *New York State Department of Health EMS Program, 1986 EMT Study.* Albany, N.Y.: New York State Department of Health, 1986.

Working With Employees and Employee Organizations

Trauma and Triumphs in Transforming a Third Service

S. W. Cartwright

Calgary, Alberta, was witness to the tremendous forces at work when an EMS organization desires change. Director S. W. Cartwright provides an insider's perspective on the change process.

SINCE ITS INCEPTION, Calgary, Alberta, EMS has experienced continual change and improvement. This constant change has occasionally produced an unstable environment, due mainly to fear and mistrust between management and labor. In addition, the unions have changed executive board members almost every year since 1984 and changed names twice in the same period.

Even so, this article is a success story. It shows that interested and motivated people can deal with and master change, and at the same time develop an approach to prehospital care that is patient-oriented, success-seeking, and intent on improvement. The following is a short-hand account of the seminal events that have molded and formed the prehospital care program in Calgary.

Located in western Canada, the city of Calgary has been involved in emergency medical services since 1971, when EMS was based in the fire department. Over time, relationships within the fire department deteriorated, and prehospital workers complained about inequity and bias. A 1982 report revealed these serious conflicts: managerial bias; significant cultural differences between firefighters and paramedics; confused lines of authority; lack of medical accountability and audit; skills atrophy and inadequate medical training; promotional discrepancies; pay inequities; and biased budgets with emphasis on fire suppression.

The city council approved a new emergency medical services department under separate management from the fire department. Total physical separation, although approved in 1984, was postponed for economic reasons, and currently only the EMS headquarters (ironically, a former fire station) exists as a totally separate facility.

Management and Systems

EMS management in Calgary has always encouraged directness,

Issues were never ignored or hidden, and the "truth" invariably figured in discussions. This direct approach led to confrontations and grievances, but the issues were always on the table.

clarity, and a lean approach to organization. Issues were never ignored or hidden, and the "truth" invariably figured in discussions. This direct approach led to confrontations and grievances, but the issues were always on the table.

Requests for increased resources followed careful analysis and statistical information that demonstrated the need, alternative solutions, and recommended actions. This lean approach led to many criticisms from staff who compared EMS with the less-than-lean fire department.

Medical Control

No EMS or prehospital care program can exist and evolve without enlightened medical control and physician interest. Fortunately, in Calgary the emergency physician group, encompassing six hospitals and three medical jurisdictions, is remarkably well founded and concerted in its approach. The physicians' uniform view of prehospital care is important when EMS deals with the Medical Control Board. The six physicians have a consistent approach to prehospital care, quality assurance, training and educational needs, and the importance of a sound and well-run EMS. When issues arise, the emergency physician group supports the ALS service in Calgary.

Management/Labor Relations

Relationships between labor and management have fluctuated over the years from very friendly to definitely hostile. This has primarily been due to the atmosphere of change and improvement; labor contract negotiations that sometimes treated symptoms rather than the real issues; major issue resolution; and changes in union executive personnel. A gradual change from what was perceived as autocratic management to the present participative/democratic form of management has both helped and hindered management/labor relations. Mutual involvement invariably smoothes the way in problem solving, but is hindered by slowness and the perception that management's lack of speed is a signal of reluctance. At present however, relationships have improved to an all-time high since the strikes of 1991-92.

A few examples illustrate the different matters dealt with in management/labor meetings. The early union executive proposal was a policy that mirrored the historical fire department model—promoting people on seniority only and requiring no performance or ability measurement. EMS management envisioned another approach. The negotiations lasted for weeks, with two major problems: The positions were poles apart, and EMS management felt that the classic compromise would result in a less than acceptable promotion policy.

Management eventually convinced the union that a merit-based promotion policy was the solution. Although an agreement was finally reached, full acceptance wasn't achieved for years. Another agreement was recently reached to provide seniority pay after seven and 10 years.

"Taints" have been another area of conflict. The term describes employees who hold jobs as EMT-As but are qualified as paramedics (EMT-Ps). The expression came from "he t'ain't one thing or the other."

Paramedics applied for the lower-paid technician jobs because of the attraction to Calgary EMS, i.e., pay, benefits, training, etc. This, coupled with a generally slow economy, made Calgary a very attractive employment focus. Eventually all EMT-A jobs were held by qualified EMT-Ps, and criticisms grew against EMS for using "cheap labor." EMT-P staff members asked to practice their skills, even though they were employed as EMT-As. This was granted based on sound legal advice.

Department statistics showed an approximate 60/40 split of EMT-Ps to EMT-As (based on hired position), while the real ratio was nearer 96/4. It was finally agreed to pay personnel at their qualification level—not the position held or applied for. This was a major victory for the union, although the issue is still hotly debated today.

These are just two of many issues that have created labor/management conflicts over the years.

The 1988 Winter Olympic Games

Significant challenge, change, and maturity came to Calgary EMS with the 1988 Winter Olympic Games. Calgary EMS was able to prepare, stage, and manage an event of great proportions. The Games were staffed solely by Calgary EMS. Equipment was provided for the event by mothballing everything that was usually replaced on a regular basis. In this way, fully equipped ambulances were activated to create a separate EMS fleet dedicated to the Olympic Games. The existing Calgary EMS fleet met the needs of the city's citizens and visitors to the Olympics. Personnel were scheduled on their off-duty days to staff Olympic venues. Vacations were not taken and training/personnel development was suspended.

The department's ability to work together toward common goals improved management/labor relations. The overall sense of accomplishment following these exciting times carries over to this day.

Value for Money Audit—1987 to 1992

The process of examination and justification is recommended only for the most resourceful, mature, and professional EMS groups. It is a difficult task because it requires a close scrutiny of operations and produces many crises and confrontations along the way.

Calgary EMS conducts value for money audits routinely in two to three departments per year. Because there are 22 separate departments, a department can expect to be audited every seven to 10 years. The process flows from the audit committee to a city council committee, which in turn appoints an audit task force. The EMS consultant selected by the task force to assist with the audit was Fitch & Associates of Kansas City, Mo.

The value for money audit process follows a predictable pathway

> The department's ability to work together toward common goals improved management/labor relations.

of research and analysis, draft reports for departmental comment and response, final report to the audit task force and subsequent approval by the city council. The audited department usually implements the final recommendations. However, in this case Fitch & Associates assisted in the implementation.

The final report produced 42 separate recommendations, with the implementation taking place over a three-year period. Including the initial stages, the audit took four years. This reflects the complexity and size of the audit and its outcomes.

The recommendations were grouped into three categories—clinical, operational, and human resources. The following briefly outlines the major recommendations contained in the audit.

Clinical Recommendations

The following clinical changes were recommended.

- Improve medical protocols for paramedics and technicians
- Add required medical protocols
- Separate medical/administration protocols
- Establish a comprehensive quality assurance program
- Link training to quality assurance
- Ensure continuing medical supervision
- Treat quality problems as medical issues
- Establish a medical control board responsible to the city council
- Establish patient care as the paramount reason for existence

Many of the clinical recommendations were enhancements rather than new ventures. The importance of the changes, however, was clear and had a lasting impact: The process established the relationship between the medical community and the prehospital providers.

Operational Recommendations

Operational recommendations included the following.

- Confirm ALS versus BLS
- Establish industrywide compliance standards for all responses
- Develop quality assurance for communications data
- Assume responsibility for ambulance dispatch
- Move ambulance dispatch to EMS headquarters
- Establish citywide and zone response time standards
- Set and enforce dispatch standards
- Match shifts to demand (flexible deployment)
- Equalize coverage by day/hours
- Institute centralized crew relief
- Eliminate midshift briefings

- Maintain fire department first responder role
- Establish an ambulance post location study
- Institute medically oriented dispatch
- Staff dispatch with best paramedics
- Improve fleet utilization, monitor costs

These recommendations virtually turned Calgary EMS on its head. The changes and impacts on personnel were both profound and difficult to deal with. However, the recommendations were implemented on the basis of *cost avoidance* rather than *cost savings*. This allowed the staff to participate from a secure position, rather than in fear of cutbacks.

Human Resources Recommendations

Changes in this difficult area were the most demanding and significant because they were changes in approach, philosophy, and style. The many changes in management initially resulted in increased mistrust between management and labor. Recommended changes included the following.

- Relieve superintendents of non-managerial duties
- Establish a relief superintendent position
- Ensure replacement staff members are qualified
- Maximize career opportunities
- Revitalize the staff development division
- Give middle management specialized training
- Establish field training officers
- Rename operational staff (crew chief, crew member)
- Rotate station assignments
- Revise the organization structure
- Appoint an assistant to the medical director
- Assign dispatch to manager of operations
- Utilize participation of field staff in decision making
- Change management style from autocratic to participative/democratic

These changes were difficult to accept and implement. Acceptance really only came after the city council endorsed and approved the recommendations. The lack of trust between management and labor was difficult to overcome. However, the department's implementation plan was validated by more than 80 percent of the EMS staff. Very few of the meetings held were paid meetings. This illustrates the staff's interest and commitment.

The value for money audit process was a traumatic and insightful journey. The Calgary EMS staff was forced to look very closely at the service, examine its purpose and goals, and consider the outcomes. More importantly, approach, philosophy, and values were dispassionately reviewed and flaws and shortcomings exposed. Defensive posturing did nothing to alter the validity of the recommendations. It was tough to admit that good intentions are not enough or that believing strongly in some-

If EMS in Calgary is to remain at the top, change will always be present.

thing does not make it so. While Calgary EMS workers worked hard, believed in their role, and always sought to improve, the department came up short when measured against industry standards.

Crisis number one was realizing that improvements were necessary. Crisis number two came when the changes and impacts were discussed with staff. Nobody likes change. It was daunting to accept radical change that affected all and required everyone's hard work for implementation. Morale plummets when an extreme effort is needed to overturn a lot of what you have worked hard to put in place.

The process took four years. If EMS in Calgary is to remain at the top, change will always be present. Many aspects of the value for money audit are not measurable. Intangible benefits flow from the process itself—from the debate, analysis, and consensus. Some of these benefits were an increase in knowledge, improved personal relations, and general improvements in mutual esteem. In addition, since the value for money audit was instituted, Calgary EMS has increased productivity by more than 30 percent and avoided expenditures in excess of $4 million. Not bad for a municipal-based third service.

Labor Dispute 1991-1992

This major work disruption lasted from December 1991 to January 1992. The contract negotiations between Calgary and CUPE Local 3421 had been going on for months, the bargaining unit had been without a contract for approximately a year, and significant issues had not been resolved. The most difficult issue was pay, specifically pay equity with firefighters. Since ambulance service began in Calgary in 1971, comparisons between firefighter and paramedic pay had been made and never successfully dealt with. This issue was the main reason for the work stoppage. The union claimed a promise to "work toward and achieve parity with firefighters" had been reneged on time and again. The union slogan was "Fairness—it's not too much to ask."

The strike occurred in two phases—a 10-day work stoppage prior to Christmas 1991 after which a settlement was signed, and a three-day stoppage in early January 1992 when the city council refused to ratify the settlement negotiators agreed to. The additional three-day strike produced a better settlement than the one turned down by the city council.

Labor disputes are enormously disruptive and emotional. The striking workers were deeply hurt by the need to strike. The dichotomy of wanting to work and needing to deal with "the issue" created an extreme effect on field staff. However, votes throughout the dispute always carried large majorities. The workers were both united and resolved.

Calgary EMS management was equally torn between its public duty to the city and its recognition of the fundamental correctness of the union position. Yet the management team and other staff continued to maintain ALS ambulance service. "Doctor" cars were also used, employing an emergency physician and a management driver. They responded to lower priority calls and eventually to all calls, as the demand overwhelmed the plan to limit doctors to house calls. Volunteers from local emergency nursing staffs also rode on ALS ambulances. The workload during the strike actually increased in spite of public pleas to call only in real emergencies. The management staff worked 16-hour shifts with eight-hour breaks. The breaks eroded over time, and 20-hour shifts were not uncommon. Performance standards were impacted, with a one-minute average increase in response times. However, there were no critical incidents and no complaints. One medic delivered four babies during the dispute!

The strike also had great political impact . The need for politicians to send a fiscal message to the public collided with the merits of the union position. This explains the initial refusal by the city council to ratify the agreement.

The positive outcomes of the strike included

- Union justification, as wage parity is now a reality
- Management satisfaction in successfully handling a major service delivery crisis
- Growth of management/labor respect
- Confirmation that sound planning and preparation do work
- Consolidation of the principles of compromise and cooperation
- Reduction in management/labor friction
- Increased confidence in management's paramedic skills after years away from the street

The strike's negative outcomes were fewer, yet still significant.

- Principles can and will be compromised if the issue is important enough.
- Behavior deteriorates as a labor dispute progresses.
- Professionalism is damaged when such conflicts occur.

While recrimination was absent at the end of the strike, a patient abandonment complaint was filed by the Medical Control Board to the prehospital care professional association. This complaint is still pending.

Calgary EMS/Fire Department Relations—Post-Strike

The 1991-92 strike created a serious dispute with the Calgary Fire Department. During the strike, firefighters were disturbed by media comments made by paramedics that besmirched their professionalism. The firefighters took great exception to the fact that a strike occurred at all; they maintained that true professionals would have continued to serve the public. The paramedics pointed out that this was a "holier than thou" attitude from firefighters unable to strike due to legislation.

Firefighters also claimed that paramedics accused them of being overpaid and underworked through comparisons of call volumes and pay

A strategic planning process has been established to deal with issues before they become problems.

rates. Because paramedics require a two-year full-time diploma before they can practice, firefighters inferred this meant that they were ignorant or uneducated. While no evidence was produced to support these allegations, it resulted in serious disharmony.

The primary paramedic strike spokesperson was singled out for negative attention. Firefighters refused to work with him at his home station. The paramedic was supported by Calgary EMS, and he ultimately prevailed. As a result, this paramedic's stock increased overall, ironically including those in the fire department.

During this period of severe friction, the paramedics continued to do their work, walking away from conflict and steadfastly refusing to get involved with the media. This professionalism produced a sense of gratitude and admiration from most sources.

The maturity and professionalism that emanated from the staff of Calgary EMS bode well for the future. A strategic planning process has been established to deal with issues before they become problems.

Change—Trauma and Triumphs

EMS Consultant Jay Fitch once characterized the prehospital care business as riding up a downward escalator: If you stand still, you go backwards; if you work hard, you manage to stand still; and if you work real hard, you can make progress and improve your position. This means that hard work and change are inevitable unless you want to regress.

Although all these changes created clear benefits, the shift made by EMS management requires further discussion. What started off as an autocratic management style, necessary because of a lack of expertise and ability at that time, has evolved into a management team that is now a facilitative rather than a directing force. It doesn't mean that decisions and direction are not taken or given, but that an enlightened view of management now exists.

Calgary EMS is organized in a traditional hierarchical pyramid structure. In practice, however, the organization operates as a reversed pyramid. Imagine at any time between 13 and 17 ALS ambulances are on duty providing prehospital care. They cannot be supervised or directed in the traditional manner. The units operate autonomously, controlled only by protocols and radio waves. This control ensures proper deployment and security and the application of medical input as dictated by circumstances. The work performed requires knowledge, skill, and judgment in an unsupervised environment. As a result, the field staff are well trained and equipped and given the support necessary to do a good job. Through the application and scrutiny of performance standards and various quality assurance programs, individual and collective performance levels are monitored. Remedial actions are constructive and not punitive. The field staff are both trusted and appreciated. Management's major role is to facilitate, monitor, and assist its staff to be the best they can be.

Change has affected all departments involved in the delivery of prehospital care in Calgary. The medical community has been affected in a vicarious manner, while the fire department has been impressed by the extent and complexity of change over the years. The ability to ride the wave and deal with the crises as they unfolded is a tribute to the staff of the Calgary EMS department. The department is as good as the people it employs, who in turn decide how good they want to be. They have, not always willingly or with good grace, decided they want to be pretty good.

Finally, the people most affected by all the trauma, tribulations, and triumphs of transformation are the patients. They have reaped the rewards of hard work, training, and dedication. The result has been measurable increases in patient care levels, greatly improved patient outcomes, and response time compliance comparable with any EMS service in North America. This was and remains the reason for EMS Calgary's existence; the department hopes never to lose this sense of direction and focus. In the meantime, it awaits and "dreads" the next series of changes. This is a process one does not get used to—ever.

Source

Original article. S. W. Cartwright is the director of the Calgary EMS Department.

Discipline With Due Process

James O. Page

Jim Page's article on discipline describes the principle of due process as a guide to forming policies. He takes neither the employee's nor the employer's position, but rather points out how case law has shaped the scope and limitations of disciplinary actions.

EACH OF THE SEVERAL DEFINITIONS of the word *discipline* portrays the concept in a different way. For example, Webster's *New World Dictionary* defines discipline as "training that develops self-control, character, or orderliness and efficiency." But Webster's also defines discipline as "strict control to enforce obedience" and "treatment that corrects or punishes."

It should be apparent that the first definition, which implies a positive, non-punitive effort to create desired attitudes and behaviors through training, preceptorship, motivation, and personal example, is the preferable approach to discipline. But when that approach fails, it may be necessary to employ a negative, punitive approach.

Throughout the EMS field, many systems have recently imposed requirements for quality assurance programs, presumably to ensure that the quality of emergency medical care consistently meets minimum standards. While there have been elaborate designs developed for QA programs, almost all of them seem to avoid a critical issue—how to correct the behavior and performance of an individual when the QA process reveals deficits in these areas. Most QA proposals simply advise that, when errors are detected, the employer or regulator should "take appropriate corrective action."

But just what is meant by "appropriate corrective action"? Does such action refer to a concentrated period of training that attempts to improve the self-control, character, orderliness, or efficiency of the individual? Or does it mean imposing strict control on individuals to enforce obedience? Is corrective action treatment that corrects or punishes using methods such as suspension of employment or certification, revocation of certification, and/or discharge from employment?

Whenever the punitive approach is selected, it sets the stage for a collision between the authority of the employer or regulatory agency and the constitutional rights of the individual who is to be disciplined. In most states, regulations have been developed to guide and control the process, but frequently, these are poorly written or confusing. Furthermore, EMS agencies, medical-control hospitals, and medical directors tend to apply these regulations inconsistently and, in some cases, without apparent regard for the certificate holder's right to due process.

What Is Due Process?

The Fourteenth Amendment to the U.S. Constitution prohibits any state or local government from depriving any person of life, liberty, or property without due process of law.

According to the *Random House Dictionary of the English Language*, due process of law is "a limitation in the U.S. and state constitutions that restrains the actions of the instrumentalities of government within limits of fairness."

Black's Law Dictionary offers the following definition: "Due process of law implies the right of the person affected thereby to be present before the tribunal, which pronounces judgment upon the question of life, liberty, or property, in its most comprehensive sense; to be heard, by testimony or otherwise, and to have the right of controverting, by proof, every material fact which bears on the question of right in the matter involved. If any question of fact or liability be conclusively presumed against him, this is not due process of law."

Perhaps the case of *Vaughan v. State* best captures the spirit and intent of due process: "Aside from all else, 'due process' means fundamental fairness and substantial justice."

"Property" and "liberty" are the elements of due process that affect EMS employers and regulators with regard to disciplinary action.

Property

Because an individual's employment or certification is considered his "property" in many cases, state or local governments (or individuals or entities operating under the authority of a state or local government) may not deprive an individual of that "property" without due process.

Who is entitled to due process protection? The courts have held that due process protection applies if contract or administrative regulation standards for retention are specified under state or local law. This means that if any statutory, administrative, or contractual standards for retaining employment (or certification) exist, the individual has a "property" interest in his employment or certification, and these cannot be taken away from the individual without due process.

Doesn't this apply only to public agencies? Prior to about 1980, private employers and their employees were deemed to be outside of the requirements and protections of due process with regard to employment. Employees of private companies were considered to be employed "at will" (at the will of the employer) and had no constitutionally protected employment rights.

Since 1980, the courts have held in several California cases that an implied contract exists between a private employer and his employees. Even though these cases apply only in California, the state tends to be a trendsetter in terms of legal developments.

If the Fourteenth Amendment specifically applies to state and local governments, how can it apply to private ambulance companies? Again, prior to 1980, most private ambulance services in the United States operated in an unregulated environment. Their relations with their employees were on an at-will basis. Now, however, private ambulance companies in many locations are functioning as legal and operational ad-

> "Aside from all else, 'due process' means fundamental fairness and substantial justice."

juncts of local governments, either through regulated monopoly franchises, protected zone arrangements, subsidy agreements, or shared services. These companies are strongly regulated by EMS agencies, including quasi-governmental management entities, and many companies have entered into contractual agreements with employees ranging from labor/management agreements to individual employment contracts.

Consider the following material from the current policy and operations manual of one private ambulance service: "The employee, by virtue of accepting employment, assumes the responsibility to conform to all applicable governmental laws, regulations, ordinances, policies, procedures, and protocols governing emergency medical services personnel, EMTs, and paramedics, including all state, local, and company continuing education and in-service requirements."

In essence, this provision creates a contract between the employer and the employee. Does that meet the standard of the *Board of Regents of State Colleges v. Roth* case, which requires that standards of retention be specified under state or local law, contract, or administrative regulation? Probably so. This company's policy and operations manual creates a contract with the employee and then adopts all applicable governmental laws, regulations, ordinances, etc., as the standards to be met if the employee is to retain his job.

Furthermore, this particular private company has an exclusive franchise in the community it serves, and the city also subsidizes the company. Although there have been no reported cases dealing with the question of a private ambulance employee's "property" or "liberty" interest in his employment, it could be argued persuasively that many private ambulance companies have become quasi-governmental in nature.

This same company has entered into an agreement with its employees' union that includes a provision for "progressive discipline." The progressive discipline system requires that employees receive advance notice, whenever possible, of problems regarding their conduct or performance in order to provide them with guidance and an opportunity to correct any problems. The labor agreement also details the progressive discipline procedure, which includes most of the elements of due process.

Yet even without such contractual links between employer and employee, the structure and intent of current EMS law and regulation in many states seems to treat the private ambulance provider as a quasi-public agency. By being afforded such status, there is a concomitant relationship between employer and employee.

How does the "property" interest apply to medical-control hospitals and EMS medical directors? Although the authority delegated to medical-control hospitals and EMS medical directors may vary from state to state, it generally includes the suspension or revocation of medical command or direction to an individual certificate holder, such as an intermediate EMT or paramedic. In many cases, this is tantamount to suspending or revoking the certificate itself.

To the extent that suspension or revocation of an individual's certification adversely affects his "property" interest in being employed, this infringement may be subject to due process protection. In other words, if the medical director has the power to take away an individual's certificate (or the necessary medical command or direction), thus depriving him of the opportunity to continue working at the same status or level of compensation, that individual's "property" interest in his employment is adversely affected.

To date, there are no reported appellate court decisions involving due process violations by a medical director or medical-control hospital. On the other hand, a recent Minnesota case, *The County of Hennepin v. Assn. of Paramedics* (which did *not* involve due process violations), held, in essence, that an EMS medical director cannot be forced to permit a person to work under his license when he believes that the person is not competent to function as a paramedic.

The Hennepin case illustrates the extensive powers conferred upon medical directors. It also assumes that paramedics are working under the license of their medical director—a legal and factual question that has never been fully explored, and the answer to which could vary from state to state. Even in Minnesota (the state in which the Hennepin case was decided), it would be a mistake for a medical director to assume that this ruling relieved him of the responsibility to afford due process in future cases of discipline.

In time, the courts will be asked to rule on whether disciplinary action by a medical-control hospital or EMS medical director has met the minimum standards for due process. Given the potential for harm to the "property" interests of certificate holders, it is highly probable that the courts will formally impose certain requirements upon medical directors. Most likely, these requirements will include pre-action procedural due process similar to that spelled out in *Skelly v. State Personnel Board* and post-action evidentiary review hearings as defined in *Arnett v. Kennedy.*

Are due process requirements necessary when placing an employee or certificate holder on probation? Probably not. The Skelly pre-action procedure is generally required only in cases of significant punitive action, such as discharges, demotions, or lengthy suspensions. Disciplinary actions, such as warnings, reprimands, performance evaluations, or suspensions of fewer than five days, are not considered significant enough to warrant the pre-action procedure.

Even in situations in which a pre-action procedural due process hearing or a post-action evidentiary review hearing is described in state law or regulations and is made available in cases of certificate suspension or revocation or when renewal of a certificate is denied, such hearings may not be required in cases of lesser discipline, such as probation or written or verbal reprimand. Careful study of applicable state laws and regulations may be necessary to clarify this issue.

On the other hand, it could be argued that imposing probation on an individual's employment or certification may have adverse economic consequences (e.g., loss of opportunities to work overtime, suspension of transfer and time-off privileges, denial of promotional opportunities, and ineligibility for step-pay increases). If an otherwise benign imposition of punishment carries with it secondary economic consequences for the individual, it may be prudent for the employer to conduct pre-action or post-action hearings, even though they may not be formally required.

What if the public needs immediate protection from the actions of certificate holders? On occasion, it may become apparent that a certificate holder represents an immediate threat to the public. If, based on a review of credible evidence, the medical director or the certifying agency finds that such an individual represents an "imminent threat to the public health and safety," he may suspend the individual's certificate immediately.

The key to such action lies in the word "imminent." The immediacy implied by that word justifies taking action without the customary pre-action due process procedure. However, it is imperative that the medical director act only on credible evidence (which generally means detailed written information) rather than on gossip or undocumented verbal reports.

Even when the medical director deems that immediate suspension is necessary to protect the public health and safety, the individual's employer should place him on paid leave until the facts can be presented in a post-action evidentiary hearing. By keeping the individual on paid leave during the process, his "property" interests are less likely to be injured.

If the evidentiary review is conducted properly and if it confirms that the suspension (and possibly a subsequent revocation) was warranted by the facts, due process requirements are considered to have been met, and the individual can be removed from the payroll. If the evidentiary review determines that the suspension was not warranted, no injury will have been suffered by the certificate holder, since he remained on the payroll during the process.

The U.S. Supreme Court addressed this issue in a Connecticut case as follows: "Before a person is deprived of a protected interest, he must be afforded opportunity for some kind of hearing, except for extraordinary situations where some valid governmental interest is at stake that justifies postponing the hearing until after the event."

Why should an employer pay an employee whose certification is suspended and who can't work? Technically, the employer might get away with not paying an employee whose certification has been suspended. Indeed, some labor/management agreements in the EMS field specify that the employee must have a current certificate in order to receive compensation. This is a short-sighted view, however, that is likely to cost the employer more in legal fees, administrative time, and general disruption in the workforce.

Experience from the law enforcement field can be instructional. If a police officer is charged with misconduct, he is almost always placed on paid leave until the allegations can be examined. The officer (usually represented by legal counsel) is then given an opportunity to make a written or verbal statement, witnesses may be examined and cross-examined, evidence can be evaluated, and a decision is reached by an unbiased administrative panel.

If the administrative panel conducts a proper hearing and concludes that the officer was not at fault, his "property" (employment) rights will not have been breached. If the panel concludes that the allegations are correct, due process will have been afforded, and disciplinary measures can be implemented.

Liberty

What exactly is the "liberty" interest? The Fourteenth Amendment prohibits any state or local government from depriving any person of life, liberty, or property without due process of law. In California, the courts have consistently held that, in cases in which the discipline involves charges that stigmatize the employee's reputation, the substantive right to liberty may be implicated to provide the employee with due process rights, even if the employee is found to have no property right in his job, as in the case of a temporary or probationary employee.

The liberty interest cases only involve terminations. Also, in these cases, the liberty interest is not an issue if the employee is charged only with incompetence or inadequate performance. If, however, the employee is charged with immoral or dishonest conduct, he has the right to a hearing that affords him an opportunity to clear his name.

In order for the information that stigmatizes the employee's reputation to be considered damaging—and thus raise the liberty interest—it must be dispersed to others. If that information is discussed in a closed meeting and is not broadcast, reported, or shared with the public or the community, it does not impinge on the constitutionally protected liberty interest.

In the fairly recent case of *Murden v. County of Sacramento*, a temporary deputy sheriff's liberty interests were implicated because his discharge was based on charges of misconduct as well as incompetence. The court, however, ruled that the employee had been afforded an adequate opportunity to clear his name without a full evidentiary hearing, since the employee was notified of the charges, allowed to explain his conduct to the officers making the termination decision and file a written response, and allowed to appeal to a higher-ranking officer before the termination was effective.

Can the liberty interest be implicated in the discharge of employees of a private company or members of a volunteer organization? Thus far, the courts have limited its application to employees of public agencies.

The Mechanics of Due Process

What are the mechanics of due process? In California, the landmark Skelly case spells out certain minimal due process procedures required of public agencies (and possibly private companies operating in a quasi-governmental capacity) *before* serious disciplinary action against "tenured" employees is taken. Again, although this is a California case and the courts of other states are not obliged to follow it, it has withstood many challenges, and the requirements it imposes on employers are fair and reasonable. If the Skelly procedures are followed in any other state, it is hard to imagine a court finding those procedures to be inadequate protection of the right to due process. The court ruled in the Skelly case that, as a minimum, pre-removal safeguards must include the following:

- The employee (or certificate holder) must receive a preliminary written notice of the proposed action stating the date that the action will become effective and the specific grounds and particular facts upon which the action will be taken.
- The employee (or certificate holder) must be provided with any known written materials, reports, or documents upon which the action is based.
- The employee (or certificate holder) must be accorded the right to respond orally or in writing (or both) to the proposed charges.

What is meant by "tenured" employees? The Skelly case involved a physician who was employed by the state board of education. Among other allegations, Dr. Skelly's supervisor claimed that he had taken more time than allowed for his daily lunch breaks. He was considered a permanent employee and, according to the agency's own rules, such employees could not be dismissed or disciplined except for good cause. For purposes of the Skelly safeguards, "permanent" and "tenured" status is considered the same.

Typically, in cases of discharge, due process requirements apply only to permanent employees. Probationary and "exempt" (at will) employees, who may, under the employing agency's rules, be terminated for any or no cause, are not legally entitled to such pre-action due process procedures (nor to a subsequent post-action evidentiary hearing).

Some important exceptions involve cases in which a probationary or exempt employee's reputation may be stigmatized by the disciplinary action. Some of these cases involve arbitrary, long-term, at-will private-sector employees, while other cases involve peace officers. These cases and the exceptions are beyond the scope of this article.

How does such status apply to EMS training institutions and certifying agencies? Although there have not yet been any reported cases specifically on this point, reasonable analogies may be drawn. For example, an EMS trainee, or applicant for an EMS certificate, probably has no due process rights to a diploma or certification. If a trainee is dismissed from the course, or if the applicant is denied a certificate, he probably has no right to a pre-action process or a post-action evidentiary hearing.

On the other hand, once an individual is certified, his property interest in his certified status most likely solidifies, particularly if the certificate is essential to gaining and maintaining EMS employment. In such cases, the property interest in the certificate would seem to be as tangible as the property interest in employment itself. Therefore, it can be reasoned that certificate holders are as much entitled to due process protections as are permanent employees.

Do due process requirements apply to all disciplinary actions? No. According to one informed industry source, in order for due process requirements to apply, the disciplinary action must be deemed "significant punitive action." Warnings, reprimands, improvement-needed performance evaluations, and suspensions of five days or fewer may be administered without affording the Skelly-type pre-action process. Of course, the employing agency is free to establish its own procedures for such minor disciplinary action, and it may provide for either pre-action processes and/or post-action reviews. Typically, these procedures occur through a grievance process.

Conclusion

There can be no dispute about the responsibility of every member of the EMS team to ensure and protect the high quality of emergency medical care. In pursuit of that quality, positive, non-punitive efforts to improve attitudes and behaviors should be an integral part of QA programs. When all else fails, however, or when a certified EMS worker represents an imminent threat to the public health and safety, it may be necessary to impose formal discipline.

Central to our way of life in the United States are the freedoms and rights guaranteed by the U.S. and state constitutions. Among the most vital are those constitutional provisions that restrict or limit the ability of government (or its agents) to interfere in the lives, property, or liberty of its citizens. To the extent that we have a property right in our employment (or the certification that is a prerequisite to employment), we are entitled to due process.

As a limitation on power, the requirement for due process imposes certain responsibilities on those who are in a position to discipline EMS workers. Such responsibilities are not unreasonable, although they may require some study, careful planning, and unemotional administration.

While Fourteenth Amendment due process rights were previously available only to employees of public agencies, there has been a trend toward expanding the protection to those situations in which an actual or implied contract exists between the private employer and his employees.

To the extent that an EMS medical director can impose discipline on an EMS worker, and where that discipline could adversely affect the worker's "property" interest in his employment, the medical director is obligated to respect the worker's due process rights. While specific procedures may be contained in the statutes or case law of various states,

Source

Reprinted with permission from JEMS, *July 1992. James O. Page is an attorney and the publisher and editor-in-chief of* JEMS. *He served as the executive director of the ACT (Advanced Coronary Treatment) Foundation, and in 1973 was appointed by the governor of North Carolina to create and lead that state's EMS agency.*

one widely accepted standard for due process is the Skelly pre-action procedure, as defined by the California Supreme Court.

Fortunately, incidents that require formal discipline do not often occur in EMS systems. Unfortunately, when discipline is imposed, those who impose it usually have little experience with the process. In many cases, the due process rights of the employee (or certificate holder) are overlooked or ignored.

Generally, people don't appreciate the importance of due process until their rights to property, their employment, or their professional reputations are at risk.

Discipline with due process is possible and desirable, although putting it into practice requires time, thought, and extra effort. It is a complex and sometimes frustrating process. But due process serves as a necessary balance of power in a free society. If there is ever a question as to whether it is worth the effort, we should remind ourselves that due process has always been the first target of despots, dictators, and totalitarian regimes.

Important Note

This article was prepared to serve as an example to assist EMS personnel, their employers, regulators, and representatives in understanding the constitutional principles, statutory provisions, and regulatory requirements with regard to formal disciplinary action. This article should not be considered a substitute for legal advice. Disciplinary action, and the response to or defense of such action, must be individually tailored to meet the needs of each individual situation.

Employers, volunteer membership organizations, medical-control hospitals, medical directors, and certifying agencies should obtain the advice of competent counsel before imposing discipline that might adversely affect the constitutionally protected liberty or property rights of an individual. Employees, members, or certificate holders who may be subject to disciplinary action should obtain the advice of competent counsel before responding to such disciplinary action or attempting to defend themselves.

It is not the purpose of this article to create a legal advantage for either side in cases of discipline. Rather, it is intended to "level the playing field" and help create an environment in which the interests of all parties (including future patients) will be dealt with fairly. In cases in which discipline truly is necessary, and the discipline process truly is fair, the facts will prevail, and the truth will lead reasonable people to an appropriate resolution.

Despite the fact that most states have adopted official processes, procedures, and structures for employers administering formal discipline, this article attempts to treat the subject generically. Information contained in this article should be used in connection with local statutes and regulations and, where local statutes and regulations differ or conflict with any statements made in this article, local statutes and regulations must prevail.

References

Arnett v. Kennedy, 416 U.S. 134 (1974).

Bishop v. Wood, 426 U.S. 341 (1976).

Board of Regents of State Colleges v. Roth, 408 U.S. 564 (1972).

Boddie v. Connecticut, 401 U.S. 371, 379 (1971).

Burris v. Willis Ind. School District, 537 F. Supp. 801 (1982); affirmed in relevant part, 713 F.2d 1087 (1983).

Cleary v. American Airlines, 111 Cal.App.3d 443, 168 Cal. Rptr. 722 (1980).

County of Hennepin v. Assn. of Paramedics, 464 N.W.2d 578, Minn, App. (1990).

Jablon v. Trustees of the Cal. State Colleges, 482 F.2d 997, 9th Cir. (1973); 414 U.S. 1163 (1974).

Lubey v. City and County of San Francisco, 98 Cal.App.3d 340, 159 Cal. Rptr. 440 (1979).

Murden v. County of Sacramento, 206 Cal. Rptr. 699, (1984) (petition for hearing before California Supreme Court pending).

Perry v. Sindermann, 408 U.S. 593, 609 (1972).

Pugh v. Sees Candies, 116 Cal.App.3d 311, 171 Cal. Rptr. 917 (1981).

Shimoyama v. Board of Education, 120 Cal.App.3d 517, 174 Cal. Rptr. 748 (1981).

Skelly v. State Personnel Board, 15 Cal.3d 194, 124 Cal. Rptr. 14, 28 (1975).

Vaughan v. State, 456 S.W.2d 879, 883 (1970).

Walker v. Northern San Diego County Hospital District, 135 Cal.App.3d 896, 185 Cal. Rptr. 617 (1982).

Wilkerson v. City of Placentia, 118 Cal.App.3d 435, 173 Cal. Rptr. 440 (1981).

Williams v. Department of Water and Power, 130 Cal.App.3d 677, 181 Cal. Rptr. 868 (1982).

An Overview of Federal Labor Laws Impacting EMS

Mark Flaherty

Labor attorney Mark Flaherty provides information on key federal laws that every EMS leader should be familiar with before accepting a supervisory position. The article provides a framework for asking questions about what state laws apply to your particular EMS situation.

THE MOST WELL-KNOWN and often-used category of federal employment law consists of those laws designed to protect applicants and employees from discrimination in employment. Most states have laws patterned after the federal statutes described in this article. Thus, it is important for EMS leaders to be familiar with these laws, and the new laws that will inevitably be passed.

Title VII (of the Civil Rights Act of 1964)

Conduct prohibited. Title VII, as it is commonly known, prohibits discrimination on the basis of race, national origin, color, sex, or religion. Title VII further prohibits an employer (or labor organization) from retaliating against an employee (or member) because that person has made a charge of discrimination, complained about a practice that he believes is discriminatory, or assisted in the investigation, proceeding, or hearing related to a charge of discrimination. Sexual harassment is included under Title VII as prohibited discrimination based on sex.

Enforcement. Title VII is enforced by the Equal Employment Opportunity Commission (EEOC). Employees may make charges of discrimination to the commission, which then investigates the charges and determines whether there is probable cause to believe that the employee has been a victim of prohibited discrimination. Charges must be brought within 180 days of the most recent act of discrimination, or, in deferral states (those states that have an agency similar to the EEOC established by the state or a local subdivision), within 300 days after the most recent act of discrimination.

Once the EEOC has completed its investigation, it will issue a determination, finding that there is either "probable cause" to believe that discrimination occurred or "no probable cause." The charging party (complaining employee) must file suit within 90 days of his receipt of the determination, which includes a "notice of right to sue." When the EEOC finds that there is probable cause to believe discrimination has occurred, the EEOC may file suit against the employer on the employee's behalf.

Remedies. In general, for conduct that occurred before November 1991, an employee was awarded only equitable remedies if a court found the employer discriminated against the employee as alleged. Equitable remedies include lost wages, costs of suit and attorneys fees, and reinstatement. Since the 1991 Civil Rights Act went into effect, employees may now also receive compensatory and punitive damages, subject to certain limitations.

Section 1981

Conduct prohibited. Section 1981 is a part of the Civil War Reconstruction Era laws, and it provides that all persons of every race shall have the right to make and enforce contracts, to sue, and to receive equal benefit of all laws. Making and enforcing contracts is defined to include the making and enforcing of employment contracts. All forms of discrimination based on race are prohibited through the right to make and enforce contracts. Only race-based discrimination claims may be brought under Section 1981.

Enforcement. Section 1981 provides for a private cause of action, that is, a lawsuit almost always brought by the person alleging discrimination through private counsel. It is not enforced by the EEOC but may be enforced by the U.S. Department of Justice—although it rarely is.

Remedies. Remedies for violations of Section 1981 include actual, compensatory, and punitive damages. With the amendments that resulted from the Civil Rights Act of 1991, Title VII now provides all of the additional remedies that Section 1981 once solely provided, and it is likely that Title VII claims will include most claims that were previously brought under this law.

The Age Discrimination in Employment Act

Conduct prohibited. The Age Discrimination in Employment Act (ADEA) prohibits discrimination in employment for people over 40 years of age. The ADEA also contains prohibitions against retaliation. Thus, it protects not only persons over 40 but also persons who have protested or opposed any practice that they believe constitutes age discrimination, or who have made a charge, testified, or assisted or participated in the investigation, processing, hearing, etc., of a claim of discrimination based on age.

Enforcement. Claims of age discrimination are made to the EEOC, which conducts the investigation and makes the same type of findings described in connection with Title VII. The time limits for bringing charges and filing suit were amended by the Civil Rights Act of 1991 to be identical to those provided in Title VII.

Remedies. Remedies that may be available to an employee include back pay, liquidated damages (for willful violations of the ADEA), attorneys fees, and reinstatement or front pay (in lieu of reinstatement). Compensatory and punitive damages are not available under the ADEA.

Additional requirements. In 1990, Congress passed the Older Workers Benefit Protection Act (OWBPA), which amended the ADEA. In particular, the OWBPA invalidates written releases of age discrimination claims unless certain specified and detailed procedures are followed in obtaining those releases and a certain amount of time is given to the employee to consider the release, discuss it with counsel, and have a change of mind after execution of the release.

The Americans With Disabilities Act of 1990

Conduct prohibited. The Americans With Disabilities Act (ADA) has five sections or "titles," one of which, Title I, prohibits an employer from discriminating against a qualified individual with a disability. Under this law, an employer is required to make reasonable accommodation for the disability of an employee or qualified applicant unless the employee would be a danger to himself or others in the workplace, as long as these accommodations would not impose an undue hardship upon the employer. Undue hardship is determined on a case-by-case basis, and involves an evaluation of the cost of the proposed accommodation, the financial resources of the employer, and the type of accommodation requested or required.

The ADA prohibits employers from requiring pre-employment physicals of disabled persons, unless such physicals are required of all new hires. A physical may not be required until after a conditional offer of employment has been made. That offer may be withdrawn on the basis of a disability *only* if the employee would present a current risk of serious danger to himself or co-workers. Employees with communicable diseases are not considered to present such a risk.

All medical examination and related information must be kept in files separate from employee personnel files and must be kept strictly confidential.

Current users of illegal drugs and current alcoholics are not considered disabled. However, persons who have successfully completed rehabilitation programs or have otherwise successfully rehabilitated themselves from illegal drug use or alcoholism are protected.

An employer is still free to prohibit the use of alcohol and illegal drugs in the workplace, and to prohibit employees from working under the influence of alcohol and/or illegal drugs.

Enforcement. The EEOC will investigate charges of discrimination in employment on the basis of disability.

Remedies. The remedies are those provided under Title VII, that is, back pay, front pay (where appropriate), compensatory and punitive damages, and attorneys fees.

Civil Rights Act of 1991

Scope. In 1991, Congress amended several anti-discrimination laws by passing the Civil Rights Act of 1991. Basically, this act provides that employees claiming discrimination may try their cases before a jury. In addition, it increased the amount and types of damage awards that may be granted to employees under Title VII to include compensatory and punitive damages. It further clarified the burden of proof in some discrimination lawsuits. Expert witness fees may also be assessed as attorneys fees in these cases. The act permits employees to challenge a seniority system when they are affected by it, as well as when it is adopted. It clarifies that all types of racial bias in employment are prohibited by Section 1981. Finally, it extends coverage of Title VII to U.S. citizens employed by U.S. companies abroad.

Enforcement. Since the Civil Rights Act of 1991 amends several statutes and does not make any new prohibitions, there is no agency assigned to enforce it. In general, it affects mostly laws that are enforced by the EEOC.

Remedies. The Civil Rights Act of 1991, among other things, greatly expanded the remedies that an employee or former employee may recover against an employer upon a finding of discrimination. Compensatory and punitive damages may be awarded on a sliding scale, depending on the size of the employer. For employers of 100 or fewer employees, the compensatory and punitive damages are generally limited to $50,000. For employers with more than 100 but fewer than 201 employees, the limit is $100,000. For employers with more than 200 but fewer than 501 employees, compensatory and punitive damages are generally limited to $200,000. For employers of more than 500 employees, the cap is $300,000. Back pay, interest on back pay, and front pay are not included as compensatory damages, and the caps on compensatory damages do not apply to past "pecuniary" losses such as medical bills.

Employee Protective Laws

Other federal labor laws affecting employers in the EMS industry are employee protective laws. These include the following.

The Fair Labor Standards Act. The Fair Labor Standards Act, administered by the U.S. Department of Labor, requires that employees be paid a minimum wage. It also requires that overtime be paid to non-exempt employees who work over 40 hours a week. It "exempts" certain salaried employees from overtime payment, namely executives, administrators, and professionals. Case law holds that EMS employees other than true supervisors and managers do not need any of these exemptions and therefore are paid hourly and entitled to overtime. The Fair Labor Standards Act also prohibits an employer from making deductions from an employee's pay that would reduce the employee's hourly rate below the minimum wage in any workweek. The FLSA prohibits retaliation against an employee who brings claims for wages or overtime, or alleges a violation of the FLSA by his employer.

The Occupational Safety and Health Act. The Occupational Safety and Health Act requires all employers to provide a safe workplace for their employees. The act is administered by the Occupational Safety and Health Administration (OSHA), which can impose penalties on an employer of up to $70,000 per violation.

In addition to the general duty to maintain a safe workplace, OSHA requires that employers adopt and administer certain programs:

• A hazardous materials program to teach employees about

Source

Original article. Mark Flaberty is a partner in the law firm of Husch & Eppenberger, which has eight offices in the Midwest. He represents ambulance services and fire departments nationwide in labor relations matters.

the hazardous materials in the workplace and what to do in case of a spill, leak, etc.

- A lockout/tagout procedure to be utilized when servicing or repairing certain types of electrical equipment
- A program to limit employee exposure to bloodborne pathogens that includes training employees about the hazards of bloodborne (and airborne) pathogens that may be encountered in their work, providing hepatitis B vaccines for all employees who desire them, and adopting and enforcing safe work practices to prevent the spread of bloodborne diseases. Covered employers (and the EMS industry is always covered under at least the first and third regulations) must have written programs available for OSHA's inspection, must retain training records and records of vaccinations, etc., and must keep a log of all exposures, among other things.

The Occupational Safety and Health Act also prohibits retaliation against an employee who has brought claims of unsafe working conditions or work practices to the attention of OSHA.

The National Labor Relations Act. The National Labor Relations Act permits employees to engage in "concerted, protected activity," which includes selecting representation by a collective bargaining representative (a union). The National Labor Relations Act prohibits any form of retaliation against an employee for engaging in protective, concerted activity, as well as for refusing to engage in protected, concerted activity. The National Labor Relations Act is administered by the National Labor Relations Board (NLRB).

These labor laws have been enacted to protect employees from discrimination and to ensure the health and safety of all employees. It is the responsibility of all managers to understand the intent of these laws, how they are enforced, and the impact they have on any EMS system.

AT A TIME WHEN ORGANIZED LABOR in most industries is on the decline, the trend toward unionization in the EMS field is fairly strong and getting stronger. "Prehospital providers understand the life-and-death importance of their professions," said Jeffrey Keeton, president of NEON, a national EMS employee organization made up of nearly 25 unions. "They want to improve services, earn respect, and make a living, and they're turning to organized labor as a means of upgrading the profession. EMS workers understand that if they want to get the respect other emergency services professionals have, they'll have to fight for it. The best way to do that is collectively."

Although many management/labor relationships are strained at best—and bitterly adversarial at worst—representatives of both sides are working hard to build solid foundations of trust, cooperation, and progress. Both are realizing that communication, mutual understanding, and respect are critical. Efforts are under way in many emergency services organizations to heal old wounds and hammer out solutions that will satisfy everyone.

Like the EMS industry itself, unionization within the field is fairly new; nearly all major developments have occurred within the past two decades. While more prehospital workers seem to be unionizing, it's not a coherent, centralized movement. A majority of paramedics nationally are also firefighters, and they are represented by the International Association of Firefighters (IAFF).

In August of 1991, nearly 65 percent of full-time firefighters were union members, according to Garry Briese, executive director of the International Association of Fire Chiefs (IAFC). A wide variety of smaller unions also exist, some EMS-specific and some attached to larger labor organizations. (For instance, when Pittsburgh's EMS union was formed in 1976, it was affiliated with the national steelworkers' union. It became independent several years later.)

This fragmentation has resulted in the lack of a strong, unified voice, and that, said Keeton, is why NEON was formed. "There were a number of professional organizations but no umbrella labor group," he said. "NEON acts as an information clearinghouse for EMS labor unions, supports local groups, and takes positions on national EMS issues."

Although there are many exceptions, EMS unions are especially prevalent in the Northeast and other parts of the country with strong industrial union traditions. Big cities are perhaps more likely to be organized than small towns and rural areas, and municipalities are far more unionized than private ambulance services. But the EMS organizations most likely of

Getting Behind Unions

Nancy Bell

Are unions getting stronger or weaker in EMS? Freelance EMS writer Nancy Bell answers that question and outlines the issues employees cite when they organize.

Wages are big on most bargaining tables around the country.

all to unionize, according to Briese, are those in which management has been unresponsive to the concerns of paramedics and EMTs.

"Union formation reflects management's failure to work with employees toward change," he said. "Unions don't just appear. They're there for a reason—to protect workers because management hasn't been responsive."

Tom Montoya, chief of the Albuquerque, N.M., Fire Department, said management/labor relations there are best characterized as adversarial and confrontational and that they've "never been otherwise." The problem, he said, stems from differing perspectives on money and service. "EMS workers are highly dedicated to providing service to the street and management is, too, but we have to look at delivering services in a cost-effective manner, while EMS people seem to think services should be delivered without concern for cost."

Dave Marra, president of the 160-member Fraternal Order of Professional Paramedics in Pittsburgh, noted that it has taken a long time for the wounds to heal after a nasty strike five years ago. "There were bad vibes for a long time, but now we're trying to change labor's attitude of mistrust. I think we're on the road to open lines of communication. We just want to negotiate a fair contract, and the best way to do that is to be up front and open."

Boston's situation is similar. "In the past, both sides were unclear about their goals and direction, and the situation was antagonistic, but we've let down the barriers and allowed the communication process to begin. EMS is such a new field. We're still evolving and coming into our own," said Neal Braverman, a lieutenant with Boston Emergency Medical Services.

Boston's EMS union structure may be fairly typical of most municipalities. The superintendent, deputy superintendent, and middle management are on the management side, while captains, lieutenants, paramedics (both field and communication), and EMTs are EMS union members. Local 636, founded in 1987, has 189 members who pay dues of $10 a week. Braverman, a former union vice president, noted that it's difficult to get union members to participate in running the organization.

"A lot of people feel they're entitled to protection for $10 a week without being involved. We did 102,000 calls last year, and people who have stressful, difficult jobs like ours want to go home to their families when they get off work."

Main Issues

Wages

What are the main issues that arise in EMS management/labor negotiations? Wages are big on most bargaining tables around the country. "Pay is nearly always an issue, especially when management looks at EMS workers as less than professional," said Keeton of NEON. "Wages in the field started low years ago, and though EMS workers are now well-educated, licensed, and credentialed, pay hasn't kept pace. In Detroit, for example, the most highly trained EMS professional makes $3,000 less a year than the lowest paid firefighter: A fully licensed paramedic earns $34,000, while an entry-level firefighter makes $37,000. A lot of managers attempt to justify the situation by trying to position EMS work as a steppingstone to fire or police service or nursing, but EMS is an end-all profession in its own right."

Pittsburgh's situation is similar. "We're part of the Public Safety Department, along with police and fire," Dave Marra said. "We make less money (between $8 and $14 an hour) because we're seen as less important, and we're newer and smaller."

As confounding as the situation is to union members, management is frustrated, too. Dr. Paul Paris is medical director for Pittsburgh's Public Safety Department and president of the National Association of EMS Physicians (NAEMSP). "It's frustrating to be medical director because I'm caught between union and management. I want to be a strong advocate for paramedics and their needs. They're underappreciated and underpaid. I'm sympathetic to that inequity, yet I'm in a position to be realistic about the city's cost constraints as well."

Braverman of Boston EMS believes unions make a mistake when they focus too much on the issue of wage parity with fire and police. "Don't compare yourself with others," he advised. At negotiations time, "tell them why you're good at what you do and why you need what you need."

Staffing

Staffing is another big bone of contention. Albuquerque, for instance, recently experienced some major changes in EMS philosophy and staffing levels that left both union members and Fire Chief Montoya frustrated. "We went from three people on a rescue unit to two," he explained. "Personnel are 95 percent of a unit's expense. We figured out that if we saved 18 people a year over the life of a rescue vehicle, we'd save $35,000 to $40,000 annually in salary per person, or $5 million over five years. The unions felt they were losing positions, but on the management side, we've got to work within cost containment parameters."

Safety

Safety is the third of the big three management/labor issues. "We deal every day with sick, injured, and distraught people, individuals on alcohol and drugs, the mentally unstable, and those with life-threatening diseases," Keeton pointed out. "EMS professionals are sometimes shot at or assaulted, too. We need as much protection as we can get."

Braverman noted that Boston's EMS union fought for years for bulletproof vests and finally got management to supply them, but they're not ideal. "I was one of the top fighters for the vests," he said, "but most people won't wear them because they're so uncomfortable. I almost passed

> "EMS professionals are sometimes shot at or assaulted. We need as much protection as we can get."

Employee assistance programs (EAPs), peer support efforts, critical incident stress debriefing (CISD) teams, and other programs to help EMS personnel cope with the extreme stress of their jobs are being promoted by many unions.

out doing CPR recently with mine on. Yet they're essential. I've been shot at but not hit, so it's not a matter of *if* a bullet will hit me but *when*."

In addition to vests, EMS professionals are now being supplied with gloves, masks, goggles, and other devices to protect them from diseases such as HIV infection and hepatitis. Educational programs are also proliferating. "Whoever would have thought that the most hazardous material out on the streets would be blood?" Braverman reflected.

A recent incident in Tampa, Fla., illustrates the severity of the problem. In December 1988, Tom Reale, a Tampa Fire Department paramedic, revived a three-month-old child with mouth-to-mouth resuscitation. He later learned the baby was infected with HIV. The child subsequently died, and Reale claimed he developed post-traumatic stress disorder and a blood phobia as a result of the trauma and lack of information and protection. (Tests showed he had not contracted AIDS.) In December 1991, his bid for retirement with a full disability pension was turned down. Although Reale is a union member, the organization, according to policy, did not become involved in the pension dispute but will step in if Reale needs help getting his job back, said IAFF local 754 President Bob Weiss.

Hepatitis B vaccines are another hot issue. The shots can cause physical reactions, and the EMS union in Albuquerque is pushing for an educational program to help employees decide if they want to take the shot with its risk of side effects or accept the chance of contracting the illness itself on the job. The issue of whether management makes the vaccines mandatory is tricky, according to Briese. "Only half of EMS workers take advantage of the shots," he said. "Management wants to do everything possible to protect employees, but if they make the shots mandatory, unions will probably file grievances. It's a dilemma. Unions push for safety, then when management does what they think is right to comply, labor doesn't always like it."

Health

Another thorny issue, said Briese, is mandating fitness and weight standards. "Sixty percent of all deaths in the fire service are due to heart attacks, yet it's difficult to mandate policies to cut down that risk." Unions, he said, protest when standards get tight. Keeton of NEON noted that disability insurance is critical, too, as back injuries in EMS work are extremely common.

Emotional disability in the form of burnout, critical incident stress, and cumulative stress is another area of current dissension between management and EMS unions. Employee assistance programs (EAPs), peer support efforts, critical incident stress debriefing (CISD) teams, and other programs to help EMS personnel cope with the extreme stress of their jobs are being promoted by many unions, according to Braverman in Boston, who has been at the forefront nationally in creating and promoting EMS peer support programs.

"There is still a lot of resistance in management to recognizing that

EMS is a very difficult and stressful occupation," Keeton noted. "I call it 'planned ignorance.' If management admits how tough it really is on the street, they'll have to deal with it."

Grievances

Finally, personal grievance issues often cause disagreement between labor and management. Most are handled on a case-by-case basis rather than as a matter of formal policy, as unions support members in their formal complaints. This presents a problem for management, according to Dr. Paris of Pittsburgh. "Unions are obligated to represent their membership, and as a result, they often defend medics blindly—without logic or all the facts. This setup prevents management from dealing with disciplinary grievances in the best possible way."

Past Influence

What difference does it make, pro or con, when EMS managers are former union members or paramedics who have come up through the ranks? Responses are mixed. Ken Kramer, chief of the Pinellas Park Fire Department near St. Petersburg, Fla., thinks his past makes a difference. "My staff knows I was a paramedic, and I grew up in the Midwest with a union father. I've been active both in a printer's union and the firefighter's union, so I have an understanding of where paramedics are coming from and what unions are trying to accomplish."

Tom Montoya, Albuquerque fire chief, on the other hand, sees it differently. "I was not a paramedic, but when people say I don't understand their needs, my rebuttal is that my role here is to run the system as a whole the best way I can."

Braverman sees the issue from both sides. "When union members are promoted to management, their goals are the same, but they come up against roadblocks from their superiors. They're still the same people and they care just as much, but they get beaten down by the higher-ups and crushed from both sides." Politics, he added, form a critical component in how Boston EMS is run. "Most union members don't know how much management has really advocated for them behind the scenes because of confidentiality. I've often seen where management could have stood in the way of something, but didn't."

The Bright Side

There are some encouraging signs of EMS unions and management working together. "We have a good working relationship with our firefighters' union," said Kramer of Pinellas Park. "I have a participative style of management, and I sit down with the union president and discuss plans. We don't always agree, but we've gotten to the point where we can agree to disagree. The relationship hasn't always been good, and that's why they unionized in the first place. Things are much better now."

Source

Reprinted with permission from Emergency, *April 1992. Nancy Bell is a freelance author in Tampa, Fla. She writes frequently about healthcare, mental health, and emergency medicine.*

Albuquerque's union has been instrumental in helping management implement a medical priority dispatching system, which determines call level and the type of emergency assistance required. The Phoenix Fire Department, according to Briese, has established labor/management teams that attack problems together, and their union president attends staff meetings.

What will it take for EMS unions and management to make substantial progress together and forge solid, positive relationships? It will take teamwork, communication, and a genuine willingness to listen to the opposing side's point of view, say those involved on both sides. "It's got to be a win-win situation for everyone," Briese stressed. "Management must be retrained in a participative style. Too much of current EMS management is still predicated on the military hierarchy type of management that's based on power and control. Today's paramedics are extremely intelligent and committed to the profession, and they want to participate in decision making. The first order of business is to reverse the pyramid where, traditionally, the workers form the support at the bottom and the chief is at the top. We need to turn that upside down so the chief is there to support everyone else."

Briese offered a further observation. "Union leaders are often outspoken, aggressive people, and that's why they're attracted to leadership positions. The old saying holds true: You really can catch more flies with honey than with vinegar. Union leaders need to be less dogmatic than some are now, and both unions and management will gain."

Keeton predicted growth in unionization and added that management must begin by regarding the prehospital care worker as a professional with a serious career, not as a person in an entry-level position who is looking for a steppingstone to a better job. "I think EMS unions will become more numerous and stronger. It will just take time, professionalism, cohesiveness, and communication."

Dr. Paris in Pittsburgh ventured this advice. "It's essential for key individuals—medical directors, public safety [officers], and union heads—to step back and look at the whole situation and be more flexible. It's a mistake to adopt too strict and tough an attitude.

"There's no doubt that, nationally, prehospital care providers need to improve their professional status," Paris said. "They're underpaid, overworked, and under a lot of stress. We need more education and safety measures. Management must consider the needs of these dedicated individuals, and unions are one way of achieving that goal."

A Manager's Guide to National Labor Relations Board Election Procedures

Mark Flaherty and Diane Shoemaker

Aside from hearing that 60 Minutes is in the outer office demanding an interview, the call that many EMS managers fear most is that their service is being organized. In the ensuing panic, mistakes are often made that confuse the issues. This article provides information on avoiding the legal "pits" when organizing efforts are made.

FOR VIRTUALLY ALL PRIVATE SECTOR employees, union organizing efforts are conducted under the jurisdiction and rules of the National Labor Relations Board (NLRB). For state employees, or employees of political subdivisions of a state (such as a city or county), a state agency usually serves the same function with procedures that are generally similar to those outlined in this article. Federal employees are under the jurisdiction of the Federal Labor Relations Authority (FLRA).

Although many employees don't want to believe this, most union organizing campaigns are sparked by employees approaching a union, rather than paid union organizers seeking out employees. In the EMS industry, employees often approach the International Association of Firefighters (IAFF), the Service Employee International Union (SEIU), and sometimes the Teamster's union. However, there is no rule requiring that employees in a certain industry be represented by a particular union. Thus, the International Ladies' Garment Workers union, or any other union, is free to attempt to organize in the EMS industry.

Authorization Cards

Once the contact has been made, employees will be given authorization cards and encouraged to get other employees to sign them. The NLRB requires that a union petition for an election to represent employees must be accompanied by authorization cards from at least 30 percent of the employer's regular employees in the requested bargaining unit. However, unions rarely, if ever, file for an election with support from only 30 percent of the prospective bargaining unit members. Most will not file unless they have cards signed by 60 to 70 percent, because a union must win the election by getting a majority of votes from the people who actually vote. It is inevitable that the union will lose some support after it files the petition. Employees who signed cards under pressure from co-workers or friends and employees who change their minds after the campaign is out in the open may not vote for the union.

Once the union obtains a sufficient number of signed authorization cards, it has two options. If it has cards signed by more than 50 percent of the employees in the appropriate bargaining unit, it can request that the employer recognize it as the employees' bargaining representative. This is a fairly rare occurrence, since most employers are unwilling to recognize a union without an election. The union may offer to have the employer review the cards to satisfy itself that more than 50 percent of the employees have signed them, but an employer retains the right to decline to do so and require the union to file a petition and go to an election. In this second option, the union files a petition with the National Labor Relations Board requesting an election in an appropriate bargaining unit. Generally in the EMS industry, the appropriate bargaining unit includes all non-supervisory EMTs, paramedics, and often dispatchers.

Determining the Appropriate Bargaining Unit

The National Labor Relations Board will notify the employer that a petition has been filed, and send the employer a copy of the petition that identifies the petitioned-for bargaining unit. The NLRB then requests that the employer furnish a list of all employees in the job classifications shown in the petition, excluding supervisors. The NLRB checks that the union has made the required 30-percent show of interest, that is, submitted signed authorization cards from at least 30 percent of the employees on the list. The NLRB will also ask the employer if it agrees that the bargaining unit sought by the union is appropriate.

If the employer does not agree that the requested bargaining unit is appropriate, an NLRB examiner will conduct a hearing. Both parties can present evidence at the hearing to support their positions regarding the appropriateness of the requested bargaining unit. For example, if the union requested a bargaining unit only of paramedics (which would mean that only paramedics would be permitted to vote in an election), the employer could argue that the only appropriate unit should consist of both paramedics and EMTs, based on their "community of interest." The employer would then have to show that the paramedics and EMTs work under basically the same conditions, with similar hours of work, wage scales, benefits, policies, supervisors, etc. Because EMTs and paramedics so often work as a team, share the same shifts, follow the same rules, are supervised by the same people, and share other similarities in their terms and conditions of employment, they are usually placed together in a bargaining unit. The NLRB ultimately decides which employees are included in the "appropriate" unit and which are not, but this is often agreed upon by the EMS organization and the union.

From an employer's standpoint, the appropriate unit should be the broadest one possible, permitting the most people to vote in the election and avoiding a situation where the employer might have to negotiate two or more contracts with its employees. In general, the length of time between filing a petition and holding a hearing to determine the appropriate bargaining unit, when necessary, is two to three weeks. The parties then have one week to submit written briefs in support of their positions. A decision is normally forthcoming in two to three weeks. The election is scheduled three to five weeks from the time the decision on who gets to vote is rendered. When there is no dispute about the appropriate bargaining unit, the time between the filing of the petition and the election is generally negotiated between the parties, but is rarely less than three weeks or more than eight.

Avoiding the "PITS"

Once the petition has been filed, the appropriate bargaining unit has been determined, and a date for the election has been set, the parties engage in a campaign for support from the employees that is very similar to a political election campaign (assuming, of course, that the employer wishes to remain non-union). During this time, the employer is prohibited from taking certain actions that might give it an unfair advantage in the election. These actions include granting wage increases, discharging known union supporters, interrogating employees about their union sympathies, threatening to close the company if the union wins, and similar tactics. The forbidden conduct can be summed up as the "PITS."

The "P" in PITS stands for promises. An employer cannot promise employees direct benefits for working against or defeating the union, such as wage increases, improved or less expensive benefits, "clean slates" with regard to discipline, or similar concrete enticements. An employer can, however, promise to address employees' concerns and investigate those concerns. If the "promise" is couched in terms of investigating and resolving problems, it will not be found to be an unfair labor practice.

The "I" in PITS is interrogate. An employer cannot interrogate employees regarding their union sympathies or the union sympathies of other employees. The employer may not ask employees if they signed union cards, or if other employees signed union cards. Generally, interrogations will not be needed. Employees who are supporting the union sport a variety of union paraphernalia, including baseball caps, T-shirts, buttons, etc.

The "T" stands for threaten. The employer cannot threaten to close or sell the business if the union is successful in organizing employees, nor can it threaten employees on an individual basis with job-related punishments or harsh treatment for supporting the union. The employer can, however, predict things like a loss of competitiveness if the operation were to become union, since that is considered a prediction or opinion, not a threat.

Finally, the "S" stands for spy. The employer may not send a management employee, for example, to a union meeting, nor drive by the location where a union meeting is held and take down the license plate numbers of the cars outside. Again, there is no real reason for these actions, since within a short time after a petition is filed, a clear picture will develop of who is supporting the union and who is not, and the level of strength of that support.

The National Labor Relations Board does not prohibit lying in these union organizing campaigns, and unions frequently do. Employers are generally advised not to lie, however, since they have to live with the

Avoid the "PITS":

P = Promises

I = Interrogate

T = Threaten

S = Spy

Unions are not prohibited from making promises to employees— employers are.

employees later. Living with employees after lying to them is often more troublesome and unpleasant than living with a union. Also, unions are not prohibited from making promises to employees—employers are. The NLRB has taken the position that employees are smart enough to realize that the union does not have the power to fulfill its promises. (If the union wins an election, it wins only the right to bargain, not the right to demand or insist upon any particular proposal.) The NLRB has decided that employees should be able to discount the union's promises and view them as mere campaign rhetoric.

The Election

Approximately one week before the election, the employer will receive notices of the election from the NLRB. These should be posted around the premises. The employer is responsible for ensuring that the notices are not defaced with graffiti and must replace notices that become defaced or have markings on them These notices advise the employees of the time, date, and place of the election.

The election is almost always held at the employer's facility. Voting takes place over a period of time long enough to ensure that all employees have an opportunity to vote before, during, or after their shifts. The National Labor Relations Board sends one or more of its employees to conduct the election. Both the company and the union may have at least one observer present to confirm that the voting employees are who they say they are.

At least 10 days before the election, the employer must furnish the NLRB with an alphabetical list of employees who are entitled to vote, along with their home addresses. The NLRB retains that list and provides a copy to the union so the union may contact employees at their homes. That list is checked at the beginning of the election to make sure it remains accurate, and is then used as the official eligibility list.

If an employee whose name is not on the list attempts to vote, the NLRB agent will permit the employee to vote but will place that ballot in a sealed and marked envelope and set it aside until after the count. Both the union and the employer observers may challenge voters as well. Generally, the union will challenge working foremen, such as dispatchers or team leaders, and clerical employees that may be more supportive of management. Employers challenge voters who have been terminated during the election campaign but return to vote even though they are no longer employees. All challenged ballots are put in separate envelopes, marked, and set aside.

When the voting ends, the non-challenged ballots are counted. If the challenged ballots do not affect the outcome (for example, if there are 50 votes for the company, 30 for the union, and five challenged), then nothing is done to resolve the status of those voters, since the ballot tallies will not affect the outcome. If the challenged ballots are sufficient to make a difference, the challenging party will be asked if it is willing to withdraw the objection. If not, the NLRB will investigate the challenges and often conduct a hearing to determine whether or not to count the challenged ballots.

Once the outcome of the election is decided—either at the time the votes are counted immediately after the election or after the resolution of challenges—the NLRB will certify the results. If the majority of voting employees opted for the union, the NLRB will certify the union as the exclusive bargaining representative of the employees. That certification entitles the union to bargain with the employer on behalf of the employees for at least one year. It does not require that the employer enter into a contract with the union. If at the end of the year of negotiations the parties have bargained in good faith but have been unable to reach an agreement, the union may take the employees out on strike. Or if the union has lost the support of employees and they refuse to strike or accept a contract proposal from the company, it may lose its certification as the exclusive bargaining representative.

If the union does not get a majority of the votes at the election (ties go to the employer), then for a one-year period no union can petition for an election in that (or any portion of that) bargaining unit of employees.

When managers understand the NLRB process and avoid the PITS, conflicts can be reduced and management/labor relations might even improve.

Source

Original article. Mark Flaherty is a partner in the law firm of Husch & Eppenberger. Diane Shoemaker, MBA, is a labor relations specialist at the Kansas City, Mo., office of Husch & Eppenberger.

Accommodating Cultural Differences

Strength Through Diversity

Jay Fitch, PhD

It's common knowledge that minorities are underrepresented in EMS. By some national estimates, minorities represent less than 10 percent of the EMS labor force. The percentage of minorities in leadership positions is far less. This article describes barriers, insights gained from one successful EMS program, and five specific ideas to enhance diversity.

THE EMS WORKPLACE IS CHANGING. Today, no EMS/medical transportation organization can avoid the issue of diversity. As white males become a smaller percentage of the labor force, more non-traditional employees are becoming a larger part of the EMS team. Learning to recruit and retain women and persons of color can provide ambulance organizations with unique advantages in the shrinking entry-level labor market.

Diversity means more than affirmative action. Affirmative action implies quotas, which can stir both anger and resistance. Diversity, on the other hand, is a more positive approach. It implies inclusion of all in the EMS workforce of tomorrow.

The percentage of persons of color in ambulance firms is surprisingly low nationwide. Although no firm figures are available, it is estimated that less than 10 percent of the total EMS workforce is non-white. Particularly underrepresented are Hispanics and Asians. The percentage of women in private sector EMS has grown in recent years, however. Even so, paramedic and supervisory positions still reflect the reluctance of predominately white male leaders to share control with persons who are different from them.

Several ambulance services around the nation are developing programs to increase diversity in their workforces. Mercy Services Inc. in Richmond, Va., is one organization implementing such a program. The Mercy program is less than one year old and is led by Pat Booker. Booker easily wins converts with her desire to see people grow. "There are no magic numbers! It's a matter of helping people make a perceptual shift," Booker said. Mercy has developed the Affirmative Action Advisory Board to advise management on issues related to the program.

Several key factors are important to such a program, according to Booker:

• Don't lower standards

- Encourage recruitment by existing staff
- Link into existing municipal affirmative action programs
- Develop a team interview approach that includes minorities
- Be both creative and patient

In its initial diversity efforts, Mercy found that getting the word out to employees that entrance standards were not being reduced was necessary to avoid resistance. It was discovered, for example, that there were a number of licensed EMTs working as orderlies in area hospitals. These individuals simply needed an opportunity to enhance their field skills and experience.

Existing staff were encouraged to recruit persons of color from volunteer rescue squads and other organizations. In addition to the recruiting efforts of Mercy's coordinator, members of its advisory board, and other employees, the city of Richmond's resources were also used to identify potential candidates for an in-house EMT training program.

It is important to rapidly reach a minimum level of diversity so that individuals considering employment with the service see other non-white employees and perceive the service as one that supports diversity. Mercy includes minorities on the interview team. This action speaks louder than lofty corporate platitudes to demonstrate the firm's commitment.

Booker admits that it's not been an easy process. "Some employees don't understand our diversity goals and resent what they perceive to be preferential treatment," she said. "We know that there are some with deep-seated feelings and it's not our goal to change their minds. I believe that they will choose to change as they have a different set of experiences. Our intent is to help all people feel comfortable here."

Barriers to Opportunity

There are numerous barriers to opportunity that non-traditional employees must overcome.

Prejudice is the most obvious barrier in EMS. It subtly permeates organizational policies and practices through unfounded assumptions that non-traditional employees are less motivated or qualified for positions.

EMS can be a lonely, unfriendly place if one is left out of the social interactions that are a support system for most ambulance workers. Many services are downright cliquish. And if you are different, it's hard to penetrate the inner circle of peers.

Lack of organizational savvy can be a limiting factor for some non-traditional employees. Not knowing how to live within an organization can hinder one's ability to jump on the fast track.

The need to balance career and family presents special difficulties. Customary personnel policies geared toward married men with wives at home, penalize female employees. Yet women often won't raise a career/family conflict for fear of being perceived as non-professional.

Backlash is often a result when white men feel threatened by diversity efforts. Instead of competing only with other white males for advancement, they're forced to compete with everyone.

Developing a Diversity Action Plan

An executive committed to enhancing diversity within the organization should consider the following ideas suggested by Ann M. Morrison in her book, *The New Leaders*.

Table 1.1

Differences in Programs and Approaches

Three different approaches can be used to increase diversity in EMS organizations. Affirmative action, valuing differences, and managing diversity programs each have differing goals, motives, focuses, benefits, and challenges.

Variables	Affirmative Action	Valuing Differences	Managing Diversity
Goal	Creation of diverse workforce; upward mobility for minorities and women	Creation of diverse workforce; establishment of quality interpersonal relationships	Management of diverse workforce; full utilization of human resources
Motive (Primary)	Legal, moral, and social responsibility	Exploitation of "richness" that can flow from diversity	Attainment of competitive advantage
Primary Focus	Acting affirmatively; "special" efforts	Understanding, respecting, and valuing differences among various groups in the context of the business enterprise	Creating an environment appropriate for full utilization of a diverse workforce—emphasis on culture and systems (includes white males)
Benefits (Primary)	Creation of diverse workforce; upward mobility for minorities and women	Mutual respect among groups; creation of diverse workforce; upward mobility for minorities and women; greater receptivity of affirmative action	Enhanced overall management capability; natural creation of diverse workforce; natural upward mobility for minorities and women; competitive advantage for companies moving forward on the vanguard; escape from frustrating cycle
Challenges	Artificial; creates own backlash; requires continuous, intense commitment; cyclical benefits	Emphasis on interpersonal relations; low emphasis on systems and culture; low emphasis on "management"; cyclical benefits	Requires long-term commitment; requires mindset shift; requires modified definitions of leadership and management; requires mutual adaptation by company and individual; requires systems changes

Investigate your diversity problems. Don't assume that your organization doesn't have problems just because complaints haven't crossed your desk. Examine statistics in recruitment, promotion, and compensation. Review policies and practices that could contribute to differential treatment. Consider aspects of corporate culture that help or hinder diversity.

Strengthen the commitment. Top management must not only support diversity, but promote it. Using both praise and confrontation, executives must help managers understand their responsibilities in the diversity effort.

Strive for balance. Use a broad-based team approach to recommend diversity solutions for your organization. Seek long-term solutions. To avoid us-against-them feelings, develop programs that visibly benefit the whole organization.

Set goals and demand results. If it doesn't get measured, it won't get done. Be careful not to let numerical goals be perceived as quotas. Use organizational measures to link diversity to core business objectives and long-term organizational survival.

Maintain the momentum. Increasing diversity is a slow, awkward, long-term process. Diversity practices build upon one another. Recruitment alone and one-shot development programs waste energy and resources if not backed by follow-up and support.

Conclusion

There are many advantages to developing a more diverse workforce, including a larger labor pool from which the service can recruit, consideration when bidding on local government contracts, and improved community relationships with diverse patient populations.

Successful medical transportation organizations of the future will have the courage, ability, and willingness to develop well-rounded workforces. And, these efforts will not go unnoticed by local communities. Diversity programs require top management commitment and careful planning, but they will pay off as good business decisions in the years ahead.

Source

Reprinted with Permission from the Ambulance Industry Journal, *January/ February 1993.*

Reference

Morrison, A. M. *The New Leaders.* San Francisco: Jossey Bass, Inc., 1992.

Affirmative Action, Yes... and Hands Off the Standards!

Thom Dick

One of America's most respected paramedics outlines specific ideas that services can use to develop a plan for improved diversity. Now retired from street service, author Thom Dick believes in affirmative action—and quickly adds that it can be accomplished without reducing standards.

IN A TIME WHEN MANY of the earth's people still purchase their simplest freedoms with blood, we have things pretty easy. We're lucky, although not very many of us ever think about how lucky we are. But the credit for our exceeding good fortune doesn't go to our American ancestors—at least not all of it.

The fact is, much of the natural plenty that once brought us power was harvested by slaves from faraway lands—people whose lives we simply took away, without so much as a by-your-leave. From Asia they came, like it or not, to burrow through mountains in search of our precious metals or to pave the way for our rails and automobiles. From Africa we brought shiploads of them to clear the land we had taken from its natives, to tend our crops and livestock, to do our dirtiest work, and to erect our finest buildings.

We thought we were better than they were, better than anybody. If we wanted something, we worked thousands of them to death for it. It was our "manifest destiny" to profit from their labor and their suffering, and in our churches and public meeting places we forgave ourselves— we still do—with glowing oratory and fine rhetoric. Rhetoric is almost always brought into play when the plain truth gets embarrassing. And the plain truth is this: We did some good things, but along the way, we cheated. We lied. We stole things that didn't belong to us.

We owe a great debt, and if we are to become a great nation, we need to try to make it right. But how?

We've made good efforts abroad. During the past 100 years or so, the United States has been far and away the most generous nation in the world. But during that same time span, we've been stingy at home. Despite additional rhetoric that we coined during the '60s and '70s, we still keep the descendants of those same slaves, and members of ethnic minorities in general, safely in their own neighborhoods and social strata. We do that with an elaborate social infrastructure that makes it difficult for people to rise from one social level to another.

Many of us are trying to eradicate these barriers with things like education and equal employment opportunity (EEO) programs, especially when the government tells us to. (Watch out for that word "program," as it usually means that something is temporary.)

As public services, EMS agencies are accountable for something called affirmative action. What does that mean?

It means you need to know your history. You need to understand something about human cultural differences. And, you need to create customized opportunities for people of ethnic, sexual, and social minorities to qualify for positions in every level of your organization. How many people? Usually, you try to achieve a mix that roughly matches the cultural mix in your community (that's the law). Your efforts to make that possible are called affirmative action.

What really happens is a little more rhetorical. In most agencies, affirmative action means that you do nothing at all—until somebody walks through your front door with a minority background, a few certificates, a blood pressure, and an IQ of at least 60. Then, you bend all kinds of rules and hire the person. If you're lucky enough to find enough folks like that one, you call yourself an equal opportunity employer (EOE). Hire a few more, and you can even brag at city council meetings.

That's called tokenism. It's not affirmative at all, and what it actually boils down to is inaction on the part of somebody whose job it is to recruit and manage human resources.

Tokenism is a lie. It's a technique that lazy managers use to cover up their actual lack of commitment to equal opportunity employment. It attracts employees who are essentially worthless, since they're content to accept good money for a simple accident of birth—money that their co-workers have to earn. It's an insult to prospective minority employees, because it tells them they're being hired *despite* their qualifications. Similarly, it's a slap in the face to the remaining workforce, because it tells them that their work doesn't matter.

You can't hide tokenism. It has an odor like acetone—sickly sweet—that no workforce is likely to miss.

No minority employee who stays after learning that he is employed as a "token" is likely to be worth a damn. Not only that, but such employees are nearly impossible to get rid of. Why? Because in breaking its own rules to hire such a person, an agency has already established a fatal precedent. There can be no turning back.

A municipality or contracting agency encourages tokenism in a public service provider by stipulating that its employees must represent its community's minorities on a percentage basis. Percentages, like response times, are only numbers, which means that they're easy to comprehend for people who don't understand anything else about EMS. Gauging an EMS system solely by its numbers is like assessing a patient by taking a blood pressure. It's easy. It doesn't require any imagination, curiosity, or intelligence. And it doesn't tell you a thing about what's going on.

Developing an EEO Plan

The biggest mistake that most EMS agencies make in their approach to EEO—and to EMS in general—is not involving their own workforce in their initial planning, ongoing development, and eventual successes. At best, this produces widespread misunderstanding. More often, it leads to employee resentment, lack of cooperation, and overt resistance—which, in turn, causes systems to fail.

> Tokenism is a lie. It's a technique that lazy managers use to cover up their actual lack of commitment to equal opportunity employment.

EEO needs to be explained to the general workforce in a historical context. People need to know that it doesn't have to result in lowered standards unless an agency allows this to happen. Employees need to understand the importance of their own personal commitment to its success.

Research

A good first step in developing an EEO plan for your organization is to research the ethnic makeup of your community. Ideally, this would be conducted by one or more interested employees, regardless of their normal duties, who might thus be assigned to a task force. They should be responsible for developing a report that

- Traces the area's history and describes where the ethnic components of its population originated and what their roles were in making the community what it has become
- Analyzes the area's current ethnic makeup, including its geographical distribution and social profile
- Summarizes what the law says you must do
- Uses all available information about known factors and likely changes in the community to project trends in the area's ethnic makeup, preferably for the next 10 to 20 years

This task force should be given specific goals and tight deadlines (30 to 45 days should suffice for the total project) to prevent loss of interest by the workforce and to convey that the matter is important.

Next, target the specific minority groups that you think your agency needs. A practical but flexible way to do this is to try and make the agency's ethnic profile resemble that of the community it serves. But, in any event, let the workforce set its own goals.

What Does the Law Say?

What does the law say about affirmative action? Does an agency really have to meet "quotas" of women, the disabled, and other minority representatives in its workforce?

The Equal Opportunity Act of 1972 was clear that federal, state, and local governments, their contractors and subcontractors, and state universities had to increase the proportions of female and minority employees to levels equal to those in the "available labor market." How that is to be achieved has been a subject of continuous controversy.

The quota approach was declared unconstitutional by the Supreme Court in 1978 in *University of California v. Bakke*. But it was upheld the following year in *United Steelworkers of America v. Weber*. That decision referred specifically to private businesses and unions.

In 1984 and 1986, the Supreme Court ruled to protect seniority systems from the scope of affirmative action plans. In 1987, the justices sanctioned the concept of quotas in cases involving companies with a history of *flagrant* discrimination. That same year, the Court upheld the case of a woman who had been promoted instead of a slightly better qualified man. And in 1989, the Court ruled more than once that the burden of proof in a discrimination case should rest on the plaintiff.

A comprehensive analysis of the law is beyond the scope of this article and its author. It would seem, however, that there is no safer approach to affirmative action than one that is based on an honest commitment to the concept, with liberal involvement of the workforce in its development, implementation, and ultimate results.

References

University of California v. Bakke (1978).
United Steelworkers of America v. Weber (1979).

Also, make it known that there will be a system of progressive rewards for employees who become successful "recruiters." These rewards should be available to all recruiters, minority or not, and the system itself should be developed and agreed upon by the workforce. In addition to any rewards, recruiters should be eligible to wear appropriate earned insignia or pins on their uniforms.

At this point, you've developed a team, and your team has devised a set of goals. You now need a mechanism, and the best mechanism you could ask for is already in place. It's your community's school system. The education system's job, after all, is to develop human resources.

Using the School System

Get involved in your school system in the following manner. These steps are not sequential; rather, they need to be conducted concurrently.

Develop contacts at grade schools. Get to know the grade school superintendents, principals, and school board members in your area's minority neighborhoods. Through these contacts, make it standard practice for third grade students to attend organized presentations by EMTs or paramedics, preferably with an ambulance.

Why the third grade? Third graders are good communicators, both in speech and in listening abilities. They've also begun to figure out who they are. And they're old enough to understand you when you tell them what 9-1-1 is all about. But they're also young enough to receive an impression of EMS that they'll never forget.

If possible, the presenters should be minority employees who want to help recruit minorities and who receive special awards for their contributions. Presentations should be no longer than 15 minutes to accommodate the listeners' brief attention spans. The presentations should be geared toward introducing the EMS system and should feature the distribution of some kind of souvenir (e.g., Lifesaver® candy or 9-1-1 stickers) that kids will want to take home with them. Following each presentation, allow time for kids to touch the equipment and ask questions.

Develop contacts at junior high schools. Make similar contacts with school officials at the junior high school level. Arrange to conduct visits with eighth graders. They're beginning to think about high school and are also starting to consider careers.

Try for slightly longer presentations with this group, perhaps as long as 30 minutes. Gear the presentations toward public safety awareness and, if possible, provide visual aids; slides are always good. Teach rescue breathing, talk about safety, and describe the evolution of a typical emergency response. Try to arrange for about 15 minutes of questions and answers.

As before, the presenters should be uniformed personnel, preferably with ethnic minority backgrounds. Why? Because it's important for minority students to see *themselves* in those uniforms—not somebody else.

Five years after you begin contacting third graders, you should see

Mentorship isn't a new concept in education. People have had tutors for centuries, and that's what a mentor is.

evidence of a continuum of understanding in the 14-year-old kids whose first impressions you yourself once planted. Their questions should be fascinating.

Teach first aid at high schools. Basic first aid is a mandatory subject in most high schools. Who teaches it? Probably not EMTs, but why not? Arrange for your agency's people to teach it at your agency's cost.

Basic first aid instructors should be uniformed. They should be good communicators, and they should be committed to recruiting minorities in EMS. That usually means they need to be from a minority group themselves, and they need to be rewarded for their efforts.

Develop contacts at junior colleges. Develop similar contacts at the junior college level. Standard college curricula include advanced first aid and CPR as health education topics, which could and *should* be taught at no charge by EMS people.

Once again, instructors should be uniformed. They should be watching for people who appear to be especially interested in the subject matter. These students should be personally invited to visit the EMS system for guided tours and to possibly enroll in EMT education programs.

Develop an EMT education program. Who teaches your area's EMTs? Are they nurses? "Professional" instructors? Or is it you? Physicians teach physicians, nurses teach nurses, and EMS providers should be able to teach EMS better than anybody.

Develop a comprehensive EMT education program. If your agency is small, share this responsibility with another agency. It may even be necessary in your state for you to team up with an educational institution so that your students can receive the proper credit. Do whatever you need to, but somehow get control of your system's EMT education.

With input from your workforce, provide incentives that stimulate employees to support your "EMS academy" as instructors, lecturers, assistants, and/or recruiters. Maintain close ties with them so that you are constantly aware of bright, enthusiastic EMT students, even if they are having scholastic trouble. The most important attribute of a good caregiver is that he *likes and cares about people.* You can teach almost everything else.

Co-Pilots

EEO plans fail when they foster recruitment via "soft" standards. What they need to do instead is enable an agency to reach down and elevate an individual's competency levels so that he can meet or exceed the same standards as everybody else.

It's probably impossible to make a caregiver out of somebody who doesn't have the heart for it. But if somebody has the *heart,* even in the presence of significant learning obstacles, you can very often fill in the mental elements. That's what "co-pilots," or mentors, do.

Mentorship isn't a new concept in education. People have had tutors for centuries, and that's what a mentor is.

Once a disadvantaged EMT or paramedic candidate is identified, you assign him to work one-on-one with a volunteer, model-caliber professional who is already practicing. Through on- and off-duty coaching, tutoring, and ride-along contact, the two establish a bond and get to know one another. The idea, of course, is that by spending extra time with the mentor, the candidate receives an in-depth understanding of what it means to be a caregiver.

The co-pilot works with the agency's education coordinator to develop

- An overall needs assessment
- An academic history
- A list of goals
- A system for tracking progress
- Agency commitments for the necessary resources

In short, if you follow these suggestions, you will proactively and vigorously create your own human resource market, matched as closely as possible to the ethnic makeup of your particular community. You will do this with the support of your workforce, because these employees own the system (and thus respect it). Further, you will protect the public from risk at the hands of personnel who may not be qualified to practice. And, finally, you will establish a system that is likely to last.

In other words, it's not only better. It's cheaper.

Source

Reprinted with permission from JEMS, *October 1991. Thom Dick retired in 1993 after 23 years as a street paramedic in La Mesa, Calif. He is the author of* Street Talk: Notes from a Rescuer.

Avoiding Sexual Harassment in EMS

Jay Fitch, PhD

Sexual comments and behavior have no place in an EMS environment. But they are present, and many in EMS have not yet realized the seriousness of participating in or condoning such conduct. This article describes common types of harassment that occur in EMS organizations and how EMS leaders can reduce and prevent offending behavior.

NEVER BEFORE IN MODERN HISTORY has the issue of sexual harassment been as highly visible as it is today. The evidence of this is overwhelming: Although Clarence Thomas was confirmed as a Supreme Court justice, the allegedly harassed Anita Hill was martyred in the media; the Tailhook scandal has scuttled many a Navy career; and most people do not regard U.S. Senator Bob Packwood's claim of being "just one of the boys" as an appropriate defense for his persistent sexual transgressions.

The problem is that being "just one of the boys" is no longer adequate defense—if it ever was—for clearly inappropriate behavior. Proof is in the number of lawsuits and criminal complaints that have been filed in recent years. And it is no longer strictly a "women's problem." A superior court jury in California recently awarded $1 million to a male employee who claimed he was sexually harassed daily for six years by his company's director of personnel.

Of particular interest to EMS managers is a 1991 case involving a Minnesota mining company. According to the *Wall Street Journal*, this case was the first sexual harassment class action suit. The claim was that *all* women in that workplace were subjected to a hostile work environment. The presence in the workplace of sexually graphic photos, cartoons, and graffiti was cited as demonstrating a pattern of sexual harassment.

Given the traditionally male dominance of EMS and fire services, it is important for these organizations to be proactive on this issue. EMS managers who do not plan accordingly can expect to suffer low morale, high employee turnover, increased sick leave, reduced productivity, and even costly litigation expenses.

Title VII

Title VII is the anti-discrimination portion of the Civil Rights Act of 1964. Initially, "sexual harassment" was coined to describe sexual advances made by co-workers or supervisors where the victim was demoted, reassigned, given a negative job evaluation, or fired. The term has come a long way from that first definition.

In 1972, the Equal Employment Opportunity Commission (EEOC) was given the power to sue on behalf of workers filing sexual harassment claims. Managers should make no attempt to discourage the victim from filing a complaint with the EEOC, Human Rights Commission local union, or other appropriate federal, state, or local agency. An employee has 180 days from the date of the incident in which to file a claim with the EEOC.

In 1976, a district court in Washington, D.C., ruled that sexual harassment was a form of sexual discrimination prohibited by Title VII. That same year, a *Redbook* magazine survey reported that nine out of 10 respondents claimed to have been harassed in the workplace. Most surveys since then have maintained that between 40 and 90 percent of working women suffer some form of sexual harassment in the workplace—90 percent of which is done by men to women. It is important to point out, however, that most men do not harass; a few men harass most women.

The first EEOC guidelines on sexual harassment were issued in 1980. The Supreme Court unanimously confirmed the employee's right to a work environment free of sexual harassment in 1986. The Gender Equity in Education Act of 1993 is a bill attempting to legislate protection for women. Sponsored by 70 members of the House of Representatives, the bill is designed to be "a response to social forces working against girls, ranging from teacher indifference and discouragement to debilitating sexual harassment."

Supreme Court Justice Ruth Bader Ginsburg, however, in her confirmation hearings before members of Congress, condemned legislation designed to "protect" women in the workplace. She contended that this "protectionist" legislation, particularly in the last 20 years, was ultimately used as a tool to discriminate against women, and cited laws on pregnancy and exposure to hazardous substances as just two areas where this had occurred.

Still, sexual harassment continues to be the most misunderstood and underreported form of discrimination. Both male and female victims respond to sexual harassment in many ways, from denial and self-blame to confrontation or even quitting or requesting a transfer. This can complicate the reporting process.

Harassment Defined

So what constitutes sexual harassment? Remember that harassment is not gender-specific, but most definitions refer to the woman as the victim. A generally accepted definition of sexual harassment includes "situations where women are addressed in a lewd or obscene manner, sexually explicit material or offensive pictures of women are displayed, or when women are touched, pinched, or made to feel uncomfortable.

"Requests for sexual favors, unwelcome sexual advances, and other verbal or physical conduct of a sexual nature constitute sexual harassment when submission to such conduct is made either explicitly or implicitly as a term or condition of an individual's employment; submission to or rejection of such conduct by an individual is used as the basis for employment decisions affecting such individual; or such conduct has the purpose or effect of unreasonably interfering with an individual's work performance or creating an intimidating, hostile, or offensive working environment."

The court should be the last line of defense for any EMS organization.

According to a pamphlet entitled *Women in the Fire Service*, sexual harassment is illegal under federal law, state fair employment laws, local or municipal fair employment laws, state tort laws, and many state unemployment and workers' compensation laws.

Put this into an EMS perspective, as was done in a *JEMS* survey in February 1992, and you get a host of harassment complaints. Incident descriptions included inappropriate comments, sexist attitudes, being touched inappropriately, and being the target of sexual advances. Others who responded to the survey mentioned sexual jokes and pornographic materials prominently displayed as harassment in the workplace.

The survey also pointed out that most respondents (91 percent) felt X-rated movies were inappropriate for the workplace, as were pornographic reading materials (81 percent). But just to complicate matters, most respondents "saw nothing wrong with dating between employees (87 percent), conversations regarding sex (76 percent), touching between employees (74 percent), and coed sleeping quarters (67 percent)." Unfortunately, it is management's legal responsibility to draw a line somewhere.

Management's Responsibility

Police services, fire services, and EMS, three traditionally male-dominated organizations, have seen an increase in the harassment suits brought against them. The court should be the last line of defense for any EMS organization. There are a number of proactive efforts an organization can make in this regard.

Consider the employee who becomes the object of sexually derogatory remarks, jokes, gestures, or written comments. If this situation is brought to the attention of the employer and no action is taken, management can be considered to be condoning the offense.

This is part of Title VII's requirements that working conditions must be free of sexual intimidation and harassment. But management can be held accountable for employee or supervisory misconduct if that conduct can be anticipated. For example, introducing a female co-worker into an all-male department may require extra supervisory support.

Organizations will often take the stance that the incident was an isolated one, that management does not condone these actions, and that the incident was not known or brought to the attention of management. A supervisor's actions, however, are often viewed by the courts as company policy or at the very least as condoned by management. Without a written policy to the contrary and a clear pattern of conduct that upholds the rights of employees, the company is in for a long day in court. Even a written policy may not be enough.

The courts have found that even when the employer establishes an anti-discrimination policy and grievance procedure, and the employee fails to use it, the employer may not necessarily be protected from liability. If the harassment is pervasive, the employer may be assumed to have "constructive" knowledge, according to the *Women in the Fire Service* pamphlet.

The EEOC guidelines emphasize the obligation that employers have in preventing sexual harassment:

> Prevention is the best tool for the elimination of sexual harassment. An employer should take all steps necessary to prevent sexual harassment from occurring, such as affirmatively raising the subject, expressing strong disapproval, developing appropriate sanctions, informing employees of their right to raise and how to raise the issue of harassment under Title VII, and developing methods to sensitize all concerned.

There are also other, more complicated areas in the harassment picture where an EMS organization needs to be vigilant. For example, when a unit is housed in a facility operated by another agency and a complaint is alleged against an employee of the host agency, what is the EMS employer's obligation? Does simply passing the complaint along to the host agency relieve the employer's responsibility? In most cases, it would not. If the complaining employee is transferred, it could be construed as a demotion, punishment, or further harassment. If the host agency is unable or unwilling to change its employees' behavior, the EMS service's choices may be limited to relocating the entire unit to prevent the harassment from occurring or assisting the employee in filing an EEOC complaint and/or suit against the host agency.

From a management perspective, one area of concern is how to determine whether the conduct was truly unwelcome. "The plaintiff-employee who fails to say 'no' or who sends mixed signals may give judges leeway to indulge their personal prejudices about tight jeans, perfume, short skirts, the complainant's crude language, etc., 'causing' or inviting sexual harassment, reminiscent of rape cases," according to *Women in the Fire Service.*

What is amusing to one person may be offensive to another. The courts are still struggling with what type of reaction to offensive behavior is "reasonable." Some courts have acknowledged the difference between women's and men's views of sexual conduct and adopted a "reasonable woman's" standard. But beware: A woman who engages in pranks and sexual stories will have a hard time convincing the court that similar conduct offended her.

A Manager's Defense

The first line of defense is the station officer, line supervisor, or shift supervisor. The crew should be educated on what is and what is not harassment, ideally in conjunction with departmental training and policy. Once harassment has been identified, it is the person in one of these positions that will usually deal with the incident first. And the incident must be dealt with fairly, effectively, and quietly. The complaint must be received with support, not downplayed. Excuses should not be made for

"Prevention is the best tool for the elimination of sexual harassment. An employer should take all steps necessary to prevent sexual harassment from occurring, such as affirmatively raising the subject, expressing strong disapproval, developing appropriate sanctions, informing employees of their right to raise and how to raise the issue of harassment under Title VII, and developing methods to sensitize all concerned."

the perpetrator. Confidentiality is extremely important. Victims will not file complaints if they think everyone in the station will know about it. Even those who are called as witnesses should be cautioned not to discuss this matter with anyone.

Prevent any kind of retaliation. Harassment victims often believe that filing a complaint is futile and only makes matters worse. If the shift supervisor allows these fears to be realized, harassment episodes will only escalate.

If harassment has occurred, follow your department guidelines for disciplinary action. The discipline should reflect the severity of the behavior and the pattern of offense. Efforts to create a harassment-free work environment also pertain to the behavior of visitors to the station, including family members, equipment salespeople, friends, or repair workers.

And don't engage in questionable or harassing behavior yourself. If you do not walk what you talk, you will be ineffective in preventing harassment.

Manager's Advice

These eight items of advice, adapted from *Women in the Fire Service,* should help the EMS manager or supervisor minimize sexual harassment problems.

- Adopt written rules prohibiting sexual discrimination and sexual harassment, and a workable, confidential procedure for filing complaints. This written policy should be well publicized and distributed to all employees and managers.
- Train your personnel—all personnel—on harassment issues. When people ask where to draw the line between friendly behavior, joking, and harassment, ask them to consider the answers to these questions: Is there an equal exchange? Would you be comfortable doing this with your mother or father or to another person of your gender? Would you want to see this on the six o'clock news?
- Use exit interviews as reality checks. A good manager will want to know the real reasons behind an employee's request for a change in status. Just because you do not hear about sexual harassment going on does not mean that it is not there.
- Ensure personal privacy in accommodations, including toilets, showers, and sleeping quarters. Lack of privacy increases the tensions and resentment that lead to harassment.
- Be a role model. Avoid patronizing any group, and correct any stereotyping that occurs. Be aware of and correct behavior that reflects your own prejudices.
- Encourage people to ask questions and to respect the differences among people.

- What you permit, you promote. Do not ignore harassment. To do so sends the message that you are in agreement with the harassing behavior or discriminatory attitudes. Do not place all of the burden for reporting and correcting the problem on the harassed individual or group. Each stage of prejudiced behavior encourages the next; extreme behavior develops when more subtle behavior is permitted to continue.
- Support—do not discourage—people who bring complaints of harassment to your attention. An open-door policy goes a long way toward resolving problems at the earliest time and lowest level, before the employer is faced with an expensive and embarrassing lawsuit.

Taking Action

The EMS manager whose investigation reveals that sexual harassment has occurred should respond with appropriate discipline, which can range from a written reprimand to discharge, depending on the seriousness of the conduct.

While these steps cannot eliminate the possibility that harassment may occur, they will demonstrate to employees that the employer objects to harassment, provides victims with an avenue of informal and internal resolution, and will help to minimize liability in the event of a claim.

New cultural standards are being defined; the workforce is changing from predominantly white men to predominantly women and men of color. New laws and new forms of acceptable behavior are being determined. The policies, practices, and procedures for handling sexual harassment in your organization should be periodically reviewed by qualified legal counsel.

Source
Original article.

Women in EMS: Breaking Through the Glass Ceiling

Cassandra L. Mathew

Author Cass Mathew has experienced EMS from the inside out and from the bottom up. In this original article, she shares the stories of four colleagues, each with her own EMS success story. Both women and men can learn from the common denominators of these successful women.

WHILE EMS IS OFTEN STEREOTYPED as a male industry, more women are attaining positions of leadership and power. Several women I know have broken through the glass ceiling to EMS success. Four of these hard-working colleagues willingly shared the strategies and attitudes that helped them make it in a "male profession."

Dianne Wright

Dianne Wright is the assistant director for administration at Metro Dade Fire Rescue in Miami. If Dianne was in uniform she would be an assistant chief. Her responsibilities include personnel, budget, finance, management information systems, and anything else she can get her hands on.

Her educational background includes bachelor of science degrees in interior design, art history, and environmental studies. Early in her career, she changed jobs every two years just for the fun of it. Dianne worked for engineers, universities, a hospital, and a bank holding company. Throughout these varied experiences, the constant thread was organization and administration.

In 1980, she completed a master's degree in public administration and became the first woman promoted to division chief of public works in Metro Dade. Four years later she was promoted to her current position, which reports to a deputy director. The department has 1,200 employees and an annual budget of $110 million dollars.

One asset to her position is the work she has done with so many people in county government. She also stays in touch with those who have influenced her. Just one result of networking with EMS colleagues is a new reimbursement process she implemented that promises a projected increase of $650,000 in revenue.

Dianne is a generalist who gets involved in everything. Her advice to others: "Learn to absorb lots of information, simplify it, and then use it. Keep your ears open for new things, stay interested, and volunteer for tasks that expand your horizons." This is an excellent networking technique, she claims, which provides learning experiences and the opportunity to spotlight your abilities.

When asked to describe her mentoring style, she said, "I just grab them! If people are willing to learn, I give them books and tapes. When they come into the office, I put everything down and really pay attention to them. I look at them and listen." She constantly emphasizes the value and power of networking.

Dianne strongly encourages everyone to develop effective writing skills. She feels that many people are unable to clearly express their thoughts on the written page. She encourages those who want to advance their careers to volunteer to edit or reread others' work. "It is a great way to learn about the organization and to become an indispensable part of it."

Conversations with Dianne are a whirlwind of facts, ideas, and observations about what is going on around her. She enjoys what she is doing and feels like she has found her niche. As she charts her future, she knows that it will be EMS and healthcare related. She has found an area where she can successfully combine her interests in applied sciences, organization, and administration.

She recently became certified as an EMT, and remarked that the biology necessary for her environmental studies degree came in handy. She plans to work as an EMT and has great respect for those already in the field. "I've got to be a little nuts to do this stuff," she said. There are many who would agree with her.

Dianne has experienced some of the classic gender problems, including lower pay and more stringent entry-level education requirements than those of her male counterparts. The more subtle gender-related issues she describes as "fun." When one of her two young children is ill, she and her husband divide the responsibility of staying home. On occasion, her husband's employer has objected to this arrangement. Once in a while, Dianne is reminded by some of her peers that their wives gave up careers to raise children. In spite of these comments, Dianne does not feel the need to defend her career choices.

She describes herself as a non-radical feminist who rarely allows a demeaning remark to pass without comment. She has found humor to be the most effective method for managing these situations and educating male counterparts about appropriate behavior.

Dianne stresses the need to be professional: "Learn to deal with all work-related challenges, not just offensive language and behavior, with tact. Cooperation and teamwork are essential to success," she said, "so it is important that co-workers are not alienated or insulted."

When asked what she would do differently with her life, she thought for a long time and then replied, "I've had so much fun doing all these things. I still want to be a writer, but I would not do anything differently in my life."

This woman who stumbled into EMS had a parting comment, "Never stop learning."

> "Never stop learning."

Sue Olson

Sue Olson is another woman who stumbled into EMS. Sue is the president and CEO of Metro Ambulance in Parma, Ohio.

Sue worked in the telephone industry for 17 years. She was the

"I listen and build on peoples' strengths and downplay their weaknesses. I am a coach here."

commercial manager of a branch office when she realized that she had crashed into the glass ceiling. With three and a half years of formal business education, she resigned and entered the healthcare environment by way of a temporary staffing company. After six years of working for someone else, she began her own temporary staffing agency.

She met the former owner of Metro Ambulance when her staffing company was hired to do the ambulance service's billing. Metro's owner was frustrated with the increased regulations and requirements necessary to remain competitive in the ambulance industry. At the same time, Sue's company was not meeting her expectations. They worked out an arrangement in which Sue bought Metro.

Sue had no EMS background when she took over the company, but proudly claims that she is now a nationally registered EMT. "This is a business, and I have the people working for me that understand the technical and medical parts of it. We have an excellent medical director. The rest of it is business—business management," she replied when asked if the lack of an EMS background had been problematic.

The words *we* and *us* pepper Sue's conversation and illustrate her team-centered management style. Rarely does she say *I* or *me*. The organization operates with the understanding that there is no room for personal egos. Egos and attitudes are checked at the door on the way into work. The company culture credits teamwork as the cause of its success. Sue consciously creates a work environment in which employees can perform to their maximum level and where turf wars are not permitted. As a result, in less than two years, Sue developed a management team that has assumed all of the operational tasks. She is now able to concentrate her talents on planning, impacting the community, and serving as a coach and mentor to the staff.

When asked how she mentors, she said, "That's just me. I've always been a pep rally kind of person. I listen and build on peoples' strengths and downplay their weaknesses. I am a coach here." Sue is an excellent example of a manager turned leader.

Sue admits that she is not a detail person but an overseer. She attributes the organization's success to her ability to find the best people to do the job and then providing the environment in which they can grow. When the inevitable mistakes are made, Sue turns the situation into a learning experience. New ideas are encouraged—even expected. If they prove to be unsuccessful, it is never considered failure—something else is simply done instead. This atmosphere contributes to the staff's ability to excel, and Sue delights in watching people develop. She has proven over and over again that when individuals are given the opportunity to use their minds and encouraged to take risks, they will attain new goals. "None of us can do it alone, and that makes my job easier," she said.

Sue has been fortunate in her career to have had several excellent mentors, all of which are male. She is grateful for the knowledge they gave her and uses them as role models. Because of them, Sue bristles when asked if she has had gender-related problems in her career.

Always upbeat and positive, Sue has a strong sense of self and what she has accomplished. She does not need to "blow her own horn" because her abilities and talent are easily recognized when she asserts herself. Within one year of joining the Ohio Ambulance Association, for example, she was elected to the board of directors. In that position, the interactions with other owner-operators have been positive. She quickly adds that people in the industry whom she admires and respects have been helpful in providing her with a strong networking base.

One downside to these relationships, Sue explains, is that some members of her peer group were unprepared to deal with how quickly she took a very basic ambulance service and transformed it into a competitive, state-of-the-art, all-ALS service. "We have blown past some of the other owners who have been in the business for years," she said.

Would she do anything differently in her career? No! Her telephone company management training was "by the book" and the next employer taught her the "by the seat of the pants" style. This combination prepared her to go out on her own. "It's all a learning experience and I wouldn't change a thing. My greatest thrill is watching people develop. That is my reward."

Sue's advice to other women in EMS, "Just do it. Find a way to do it and believe in yourself."

Elaine Gorman

Elaine Gorman wears two impressive hats. She is the emergency management director for trauma for the Upper Keys Taxing District and the administrator of the Key Largo Volunteer Ambulance Corps in Key Largo, Fla.

Education is an important presence in Elaine's life. She attended colleges and universities around the world and describes her community college-based paramedic training as "the most unique educational experience I've ever had." She holds a master's degree in clinical psychology and is ABD (all but dissertation) for a doctorate degree in anthropology and archaeology.

She is committed to providing close-to-home, state-of-the-art education opportunities for the members of the rural Volunteer Ambulance Corps. Elaine designed a training curriculum, obtained grant money for equipment, and developed a paramedic scholarship fund to enhance the career development of volunteers who work for the corps.

The importance of education to Elaine is apparent when she describes her approach to mentoring. She advises people to get a broad-based education that includes management and business administration. "Because few individuals remain in the field until the end of their careers, it is important to plan for that later stage of life," she said. For those who

"If a woman is bright and works hard, she can do what she wants to do."

feel intimidated by the thought of management, she adds that the role becomes more comfortable with increased life experience.

Recognizing that not all individuals are interested in management, she recommends education as an alternative. Regardless of where an individual's interest lies, she stresses the need for continuing education. She is delighted that former employees have become nurses and physicians.

Elaine's method for people development includes a "not terribly directive " management style. It is important that the team work together and cooperate. "I try to have people work with me and not for me."

"Get involved" is Elaine's middle name. She is responsible for organizing a grass roots movement that enabled a county with no critical trauma facilities to make definitive care agreements with trauma centers in Dade County, Fla.

Elaine volunteered to manage the program while she maintained a full-time county paramedic position. With no nursing background, she taught herself to read and understand the patients' medical records in order to complete the required utilization reviews. She also learned how to explore funding sources to maintain adequate reimbursement.

She is no longer a volunteer in this position, but a paid county manager working with an administrative assistant. She is passionate about the county trauma program that she worked so hard to establish with her friends and neighbors. She works unselfishly to protect the agency that she considers to be one of her major professional accomplishments.

Elaine says that she doesn't have a lot of male/female hangups. Aware of problems other women have, she said, "I'm comfortable with my intellect and I don't feel threatened, so maybe that comes across. I have had some outrageous things said to me, but respond to them in a way that cannot be pursued. Ironically, the higher up I've gotten, the more gender junk I've seen." Elaine is confident that her five daughters will not encounter the same gender-specific problems found today. From Elaine's point of view, things have come a long way. She said, "If a woman is bright and works hard, she can do what she wants to do."

Her advice to women is to build personal credibility and be professional at all times. In order to build and maintain credibility, she cautions that you must speak from a base of knowledge and not from a desire to make yourself heard.

When asked if she would do anything differently, Elaine says no. She likes who she is and what she does.

Ellen Corey, MD

I first met Ellen Corey, MD, when she was a paramedic student. I lost touch with her for many moons and was elated to discover that I had been hired at the same hospital where she worked.

She is an emergency department physician at Lake Hospital Systems just east of Cleveland, Ohio. She is also the chairperson of the Basic EMT

Continuous Quality Improvement Committee, an active educator, and a provider of expertise for protocol development and continuing education. She publishes articles on a regular basis, rides squad with local EMS organizations, and maintains high visibility throughout the community.

Ellen was a full-time paramedic for Cleveland EMS for over two years before she decided to pursue medical school. To support her undergraduate studies, she worked as an emergency department technician in a busy urban hospital. She decided to become a physician because of her desire for more in-depth medical knowledge. She wanted to know what happened to the patients after the paramedics left them in the ED. Ellen loved what she saw the physicians doing, and figuring out diagnoses remains a fascinating process for her.

One of Ellen's most vivid memories is seeing a female physician aggressively managing a multiple trauma patient, "doing all sorts of things that I was interested in. I remember at the time thinking this would be a good role for women in medicine—on the front lines. That was a big motivator for me."

When she made the decision to go to medical school, her friends thought she was crazy. Even in the toughest of times she never doubted that she would make it. "It was just going to take a little out of me," she recalled. "When someone wants something bad enough, there will always be tradeoffs and sacrifices."

To attain personal goals we all must take risks. One risk Ellen took was dropping her paramedic certification when she began medical school. She did not want to use it as "something to fall back on if the going got too tough." This is only one example of her ability to set goals and remain focused on attaining them.

Who are Ellen's mentors? She described one with affection, "I have a kooky Aunt Dorothy who lives in Connecticut—a psychiatrist. She has been a physician for 30 years, well before the usual medical school class diversity was in place. It never occurred to me that being a woman and physician didn't go together because she had done it very successfully." The lessons learned from Aunt Dorothy were how to balance home and work without sacrificing either.

Ellen admits that she used to spend a great deal of energy on gender issues. At one point in her life she focused on them and lashed out. But then during her residency program, a formal discussion group explored the difference between sexist and sexual. After that eye-opening session, she began to analyze the comments of others and addressed only those issues that she considered sexist. "It helped me balance my sensibilities as a woman in the day-to-day work environment. You can't be hypersensitive or you won't get anything done," she said.

Ellen's major accomplishment thus far in life came at the end of her residency. She was selected by the faculty to receive the Clinical Excellence in Emergency Medicine Award. She is understandably proud of this formal recognition for all her hard work and dedication.

"When someone wants something bad enough, there will always be tradeoffs and sacrifices."

Source

Original article. Cassandra L. Mathew, BSN, EMT-P, is the administrative coordinator at Lake Hospital Systems in Painesville, Ohio. She is also a consultant for Fitch & Associates, Inc.

If she could do it all over again, she would find a way to eliminate the hostilities she felt in her early years. She would address the issues in a more productive way and feels that she would have come to a sense of balance in her life sooner, which would have made things easier. "But balance did happen and everything has worked out," she said.

Ellen's philosophy of life and success is the belief that if you never take a chance, you will never achieve your dreams or accomplish your goals. Her advice: "The hardest part is taking the first step, quitting that job to go back to school or taking that extra part-time job so you can achieve whatever the goal is. You have to take the first step and then you are on your way." Ellen Corey is well on her way.

Common Denominators

After talking with these four remarkable women, I was struck by their many similarities. It is clear that each of them is self-confident and well educated. They value formal education as well as on-the-job training and experience. They are involved in the world around them and continually seek new activities to expand their base of experiences. They have learned how valuable observing others can be and readily share their skills and knowledge in order that others might learn by their examples.

Each has experienced success and disappointment. The not so good parts have been viewed as learning experiences. Each has tactfully handled the "gender junk" in her own way. All have struggled with balancing professional and personal lives. They have established and actively maintain strong support systems in both of these areas. These women recognize that success is not a singular accomplishment.

The conclusions we can draw from these life experiences are that we must stay alert, aware, and get involved. We must learn to set goals, take risks, and pay attention to the things that matter. And most important of all, we must never stop learning.

There are many successful female EMS managers and the numbers are growing rapidly. It is important that those who have "made it" serve as role models to help others along the way. A special thanks to Dianne, Sue, Elaine, and Ellen for sharing a small part of themselves in order do that.

EMS, the Family, and Stress

WHILE WAITING IN AN IDLING ambulance on a night shift last fall, a young paramedic told me the story of how he and his wife had fallen out of love and were planning to divorce. He told of a flaming romance he thought would last forever and how, in just a short time, the relationship had fizzled. The night shift paramedic wanted to know if his work in EMS had contributed to the failure of his marriage. Would the relationship have fared better had he been an insurance salesman or an auto mechanic? I slid down into a more comfortable position in the driver's seat and tried to come up with an answer.

Does an EMS career affect our relationships and marriages? Little attention has been given to this topic industrywide and for good reason; there are no clear answers. Yet many EMS professionals have experienced trouble in their relationships.

This is a message of hope for facing problems honestly, as well as encouragement for staying together in a world that sometimes appears to be falling apart.

Risk Factors

In CPR, identifying the risks, recognizing the signs and symptoms, and focusing on prevention are probably more useful survival methods than pushing on "Annie." So, too, is the case with relationships. We can often gain more from focusing on prevention and recognizing the danger signals than we can from last-ditch efforts.

One hardship we face is living in a society in which people have a tough time with relationships. There are many ways to interpret the numerous statistics on failed marriages, but there can be no denying that a lot of people, who at one point in their lives think they will be life partners, later go their separate ways.

Divorce is a fact that touches us all. Statistically, our marriages are far

Marriage and the EMS Experience

John M. Becknell

Marriage is often stressful when EMS work issues spill over into the relationship. Author John Becknell uses the analogy of teaching CPR to explain risk factors, warning signs, and actions necessary to resuscitate the relationship.

There is a tremendous sense of satisfaction in helping frightened, hurting people, but occasionally the call to help exceeds our ability to integrate the experience.

more likely to end in divorce than were those of our grandparents. And while the experts don't disagree on the fact that many marriages do not make it today, they do have different opinions about why this is so. One 24-year-old woman said of her broken relationship, "I can't believe this is happening. We had a special love, something different from the rest of our friends who got tired of their marriages. Now we're splitting up." Such reports are so commonplace that, without even considering our careers, we have to admit our relationships are under a lot of societal pressures today.

But does our profession further add to these pressures? Specific and definitive research on the correlation between EMS and relationship success or failure is sparse. But from talking with numerous people in EMS careers and from the research on how stressful occupations affect personal lives, I believe there are indeed some significant relationship hazards for those who provide medical care on the streets.

Consider the working day (or night) of the paramedic. The shift is made up of two unique and important components: waiting and going on calls. Now, waiting may sound great to people who don't do it, but most street medics know that waiting can be sheer torture. Sure, you can rest, read, exercise, or watch television, but if you have to do it for very long, waiting is much more fatiguing and frustrating than being busy. In addition, waiting creates risks in several ways.

If the medic has spent the majority of his shift waiting, he is prone to go home in need of a sense of accomplishment, armed with an abundance of energy, and ready to tear into something productive. But it is difficult, after spending a period of time in inactivity, to go home and shift immediately into high gear. It's as if one foot is on the accelerator and the other is on the brake. The paramedic often experiences explosive energy that evaporates quickly into a lazy feeling, making the out-of-uniform medic a real bear to live with. To compound the problem, medics often put unrealistic expectations on themselves after coming off a slow shift, thinking they should be less tired than they are after a busy shift. Many spouses have described this manic behavior as common.

The other part of the paramedic shift is going on calls. Have you ever noticed how rare it is to have a shift with just the right number of calls? Comments such as "feast or famine," "must be a full moon," "we haven't turned a wheel all night," and "I almost shot my partner for a call" seem to pervade this business. Often when you are busy, you are very busy. And when the paramedic is busy going on calls, he is seeing people in crisis situations.

Our society actively pursues a pain-free existence—it is one of our modern values. Yet the medic is constantly encountering the pain that most of our society would rather not see. Fortunately, there is a tremendous sense of satisfaction in helping frightened, hurting people, but occasionally the call to help exceeds our ability to integrate the experience. This happens when the call load is heavy and the time to absorb the aspects of the work is brief, leading us to bring home the frustrations.

Spouses who are not in EMS may be sympathetic, but they simply cannot fully understand the tragedy and sense of helplessness that sometimes follow us home.

When the street medic does come home with a bag of tough experiences, a barrier often arises because of an "experience gap." For the spouse that has not worked in EMS, it is difficult to relate to some of the tragic experiences. I have felt this experience gap in talking with a paramedic friend who was a "grunt" in Vietnam. When he tells of being shot at by an unseen sniper and of fear and death in the steaming, mosquito-infested jungles, I can only sympathize. Because I wasn't there, our conversations often end in an uncomfortable silence.

Talking about frustrations and concerns with EMS partners is the way many find balance in dealing with the tough stuff. It is one way to avoid bringing home our bad runs and management hassles. But one spouse recently said that she occasionally feels left out. She said her medic husband seems closer to some of the people at work than to her. She may be right. Sometimes we do become closer to our partners than to our spouses. Given the amount of time we spend with them and the experiences we share, we're often talked out when we get home and share very little with our spouses.

In addition to these risks, studies show that around-the-clock shifts result in less sleep, a higher susceptibility to illness, and a lower level of job satisfaction. Furthermore, managing a family schedule in conjunction with a varying EMS schedule that requires work on holidays and weekends can be very difficult. My work schedule has had a significant impact on the plans and traditions of my family's holidays. With my children in school and my wife working days, we frequently run on different time systems, which leads to a great potential for misunderstanding.

You've probably heard many times that the number-one conflict issue in marriage is money. And if you like working the streets, chances are you aren't getting rich. In a society in which success is frequently measured by what we have, it is often difficult to stick with something that does not provide the benefits of a rapidly rising pay scale. Many married paramedics I know are working two jobs to help compensate. Plus, the lack of an obvious career ladder in many departments may eventually add the pressure of planning a career change or squeezing more schooling into an already busy schedule.

Managing Risks

Looking at risks is always a paradox of challenge and terror. What can be done about the risks an EMS career poses to our relationships? Being aware of the risks is certainly the first step; conquering any obstacle begins with honestly admitting that the obstacle exists. Simply being aware that relationship risks are present with an EMS career will better prepare us to deal with the individual problems that may arise. Clearly

> In a society in which success is frequently measured by what we have, it is often difficult to stick with something that does not provide the benefits of a rapidly rising pay scale.

Addressing risks and real problems helps us stop blaming ourselves and others. In recognizing risks, the ability to forgive ourselves and each other emerges.

identify the risks you can control and those in an EMS career that you cannot control.

Risk management is easy to talk about, but in reality, it takes a strong plan of action. Here's a real example of how one couple set up some guidelines to minimize their risks. Bruce, a paramedic, and Carol, a bank employee, experienced repeated disagreements and conflicts after Bruce would come home from a long shift. After recognizing the pattern, Bruce and Carol decided that they would schedule a several-hour buffer period after Bruce came home. During this period, Bruce was free to be, feel, and do whatever he wanted. They made an agreement that they would not discuss major matters during this period or put pressure on each other to accomplish anything specific. Carol also agreed to regard Bruce's work as equal to hers even if he had spent a shift without any calls. Bruce began to expend his after-work energy by engaging in some relaxing physical exercise instead of slamming things around the house. Both felt their relationship improved because they faced the risks and made plans for controlling what they could.

In the company I work for, we get together socially to allow the spouses to get a glimpse of our frustrations, fears, wacky humor, and love for each other. I believe this has been a very significant factor in helping them realize just how much more than a job EMS can be. The get-togethers have enabled us to realize that we all share similar frustrations and are not alone in our struggles to stay together.

Addressing risks and real problems helps us stop blaming ourselves and others. In recognizing risks, the ability to forgive ourselves and each other emerges. If we understand the way we are and why our relationships stumble over small things, we can become more tolerant of the daily stresses and begin to see a bigger picture, which will ultimately strengthen our relationships.

When a heart is starving for oxygen, it usually signals its need with some specific signs. People, too, who have serious relationship trouble often describe common symptoms that can precede a breakup and signal the need for action.

Silence. "Something was wrong. The thing we enjoyed most when we first dated was talking. We still talk about who will go to the store and when the house payment is due, but except for the necessary, we don't talk anymore."

Apathy toward making the relationship work. "I've stopped trying to make it work. I don't even know if I want help for the relationship. When I think about talking about it, I don't have the energy."

Non-specific anger toward your spouse that seems to surface frequently. "Inside I feel this raging anger. I don't even know what I'm mad about, but it seems like everything she does makes me furious. I can't even talk without blowing up."

Seeking affection outside the relationship. "Little by little, I found myself wanting to be with someone else."

A continuing feeling of hopelessness about the relationship. "I made a big mistake with this marriage. I know I would have been much happier with someone else. I just don't see how anything can change to make me believe we can make it."

The persistence of any of these danger signs is a signal for some serious action. But it is often easier not to act. Paralyzed with guilt because our love is not perfect, we often deny the problems and hope they will go away. At a minimum, the couple experiencing these signs needs to set aside all other distractions and give serious attention to the relationship.

If progress seems impossible, obtain some professional help; don't make the decision to break up without discussing it with an objective outsider. Many people report that they ignorantly made the decision to quit too soon. Look for a counselor who comes with credible recommendations, and consider more than one. Don't make the mistake of believing you can't afford professional help; divorce is much more expensive. And don't assume that just getting out of the relationship will bring you instant relief. The pain from a failed relationship can last for years.

Finding a good counselor is tough, but start by asking others you trust to recommend someone. Look for a counselor with whom you both feel comfortable, and try to be sensitive to each other's reservations. Your minister, physician, and even phone crisis lines can provide points of entry. Finding a good counselor is a lot like finding a good car mechanic. You have to assert yourself, do some looking around, and ask for recommendations. If you are embarrassed about your marital problems, realize that the acknowledgment of divorce is worse.

Counselors are not cure-alls. In fact, they tell us what we already know. But during counseling, we learn to listen. We discover our own narrowness and learn some rules for handling relationship conflicts. We gain insight into our own personal expectations as well.

This type of article can be like new spine immobilization equipment—great at addressing the need but too cumbersome for practical use in a real smash-up. In a relationship, we need an easy measuring stick to assess needs and recognize when the marriage can use some special attention. From observing couples who are happy and from marriage experts, we can learn three simple aspects of a healthy marriage: commitment, communication, and quantity time.

Aspects of a Healthy Marriage

Commitment to the Relationship

Early last summer, my oldest son was upset at his inability to smack a baseball high into left field during his Little League baseball games. He wanted to hear the cheers of the other boys instead of the silence his strikeouts often produced. After talking with him about his batting, he shamefully admitted that he wanted the glory of hitting a home run but

> From observing couples who are happy and from marriage experts, we can learn three simple aspects of a healthy marriage: commitment, communication, and quantity time.

was not committed to putting in the extra batting practice. He wanted to hear the cheers from the crowds but not do the extra work.

Recently, I visited with a couple who, nearing their fiftieth wedding anniversary, were still happy together. They told of numerous tough times when finances, hard work, and childlessness threatened to tear their relationship apart. They told me that when the fun stopped, they had to retrace their path and confirm their commitment to each other. At times, this was the only thread that held them together.

We talk a great deal about changes, passages, and transitions when we talk about relationships, but we really should be asking ourselves: "How committed am I to making this work?" Commitment is the price tag on every relationship. If you want to pay a small price, you will get little from the investment. Commitment is the belief that the relationship is valuable enough to work at. One marriage counselor I visited stated that his clients always said they were committed to their relationships but were willing to call it quits when faced with even the lowest level of difficulty. Enduring the tough times is the true mark of commitment.

Communication With Each Other

Not long ago, I was on a call where everything that could go wrong did. It was a multiple vehicle/victim accident. My partner and I got separated, and when I reached for my portable, it was gone. An initially stable patient was in trouble, and I needed the suction. As I tried to yell for help, a gasoline engine on a Hurst tool roared to life, and I was left fumbling with the patient's airway.

In those desperate moments, I found myself thinking about the importance of communication. Just as communication is vital in this business, it is also vital for a satisfying relationship. But communication in a relationship is easy to overlook because we are often fooled into believing that simply talking about daily activities will meet our needs. To be fulfilling, marriage must be more than surviving together. We think we know everything there is to know about a person after a while, but we can always learn more about each other.

Family psychologist Dr. James Dobson said he thought he communicated well with his wife until his communication skills were challenged at a Marriage Encounter weekend. (The purpose of the Marriage Encounter program is to promote communication.) Dr. Dobson related how he experienced one of the most meaningful periods of communication with his wife during that weekend. He learned things about her that had completely escaped him in all their years of marriage.

Just as learning to give a report on the radio is tough at first, so is learning to communicate with your spouse. It's an art that is individual and demands an ear as well as a mouth. To begin, it may be helpful to plan a specific time to talk to each other about more than the everyday events of your lives. This can be frightening at first, but if you have a tough time talking, start by writing. The payoff for all of the work you put into a relationship is often realized in the satisfaction and joy of communication.

Quantity Time

Most things in life take more time than we expect them to. We live in a world of timesavers, grateful that travel, cooking, and emergency care are much faster than they used to be. But we have to be careful not to make the mistake of applying advances in technology to non-technological things. It still takes nine months to make a baby; winter is still as long in Minnesota as it has always been; and there is no shortcut to a happy relationship.

Each year, it seems as though I get busier and busier, but I have discovered that my relationship with my wife still takes a quantity of time to stay satisfying. We have discovered that our marriage can take busy schedules for a period of time, but it demands a proportional amount of time back. Much has been said about quality versus quantity time, but the two cannot be separated. Time together cannot be left to chance. Rarely will you be committed or have clear communication if you do not invest time in your relationship.

Commitment, communication, and time together build a platform of respect, and respect is the basis of a satisfying relationship. You may admire, feel sorry for, be turned on by, or be a caretaker of someone else, but you will not be satisfied if respect is not present. Respect grows from the commitment to someone and the appreciation of him or her as a unique person. Ask yourself if you respect the person with whom you live. If you do not, you must start a deliberate journey toward discovering respect for the person you are committed to. Respect is a powerful builder of self-esteem; nothing destroys self-esteem faster than losing the respect of the one closest to us.

Anyone who participates in street resuscitation has thought about the difference between a beating heart and a meaningful life. Just getting the heart going doesn't guarantee a meaningful life. Likewise, in marriage, there is a big difference between survival and fulfillment. Many people today are choosing mere survival, yet deep inside, life's greatest fulfillment comes when we share our life with others.

EMS may pose some unique problems that require special attention, but it is attention to our relationships that will help us discover why we work so hard to preserve this thing called life.

Source

Reprinted with permission from JEMS, *June 1988.*

References

Dobson, J. *Love Must Be Tough.* Word Books, 1983.
"Occupational Jet Lag," *Mayo Clinic Health Letter* (April 1987).

Tackling Stress Management from All Sides

Steven R. Hawks and Ronald L. Hammond

Stress assails EMS workers from many directions. Authors Steve Hawks and Ron Hammond share organizational and individual strategies for combating stress.

IT IS GENERALLY ACCEPTED that EMS-related occupations are extremely stressful. Several studies conducted over the past few years have significantly increased our understanding of the problem.

The high rate of burnout among EMTs and paramedics is often thought to be a direct result of these high stress levels. Burnout is a process, due to job-related factors, whereby an individual loses motivation to perform at maximum capacity, resulting in an inability to concentrate, increased frustration, loss of enjoyment from work activities, and sometimes exhaustion.

In EMS, high burnout rates are also associated with high rates of attrition. The loss of trained EMTs has been reported to be as high as 40 percent after two to five years of employment. Is there anything that can be done about the situation? The answer is yes, if individuals in all levels of EMS are willing to take the necessary steps.

The recent emphasis in EMS stress management has been on shifting the individual's center, or locus, of stress control from an external orientation to an internal one. Positively altering negative internal perceptions will result in improved coping skills followed by a reduction in distress symptoms, regardless of the types of external stressors present.

It has been argued, therefore, that effective stress management in EMS should focus on accepting personal responsibility for altering one's incorrect and self-defeating perceptions, rather than on eliminating external stressors. In other words, since the level of external stressors will always be high in EMS, the only alternative is to control internal attitudes and perceptions.

While individual responsibility is crucial, recent research indicates that equal attention must also be given to stress management at the organizational level, over which the individual EMT or paramedic has little or no control. Of course, lifestyle changes, such as exercising and giving up smoking, can also help.

Good and Bad Stress

For most EMS providers, the thrill of successfully responding to a challenging run is a source of *eustress*, a term coined by Hans Selye, who many consider to be the father of stress theory. Eustress is defined as "a healthy response by the mind and body to a stressor." A certain amount of good stress, or eustress, in our lives is beneficial, in that it provides us with an increased level of positive challenge, motivation, awareness, and creativity. Selye further noted, however, that stress also has a negative side, which he termed *distress*.

Distress overwhelms us and taxes our ability to cope successfully, leaving us with feelings of exhaustion, confusion, hopelessness, apathy, and helplessness. Combining frequent all-night runs with inadequate work conditions, organizational dissatisfaction, relationship problems, poor diet, sedentary living, smoking, and other poor lifestyle habits may produce these types of negative stress reactions.

Interestingly, the presence of identical external stressors can produce different stress responses in individuals based on their unique mental perception of the stressor as being either negative and threatening (distress) or positive and challenging (eustress). Therefore, the external presence of a stressor alone is not sufficient for distress to occur. An inexperienced EMT may experience higher levels of negative stress symptoms when responding on a critical call than might a more seasoned provider. Although both EMTs are exposed to the same external stressor—the critical call—only the less experienced EMT develops negative stress symptoms due to his perception of the event as threatening.

EMS Stressors

A high number of significant stressors have been identified in EMS in an attempt to account for the occupation's high stress levels. The following job-related stressors have been reported as being especially critical: long hours; low pay; little recognition; dealing with dying patients and their grieving loved ones; personal risk to the responder's life; demanding physical labor; guilt resulting from doubts about personal performance; guilt after making a serious error; responsibility for another person's life; limited training; limited career and advancement options; being on call and being expected to go instantly from a state of rest to a state of peak performance; little medical authority in critical situations; interference with one's family plans; poor scheduling; and disillusionment about one's ability to make a meaningful difference in patient outcomes.

EMTs and paramedics are expected to function in an inhospitable work environment. Shifts are long and tiring, the work is demanding, and the emotional toll runs high. EMTs are also at the bottom of the medical ladder; the most experienced, professional EMT or paramedic is subordinate to the newest RN in the emergency department. In the field, an EMT may need to request permission to perform the simplest of procedures from someone with far less experience in prehospital medicine. Additionally, EMTs and paramedics are rarely recognized for their exceptional performances and are often sharply criticized by supervisors, nurses, and physicians if their performances are below par.

In terms of a career ladder, the pay is low and advancement possibilities are extremely limited. Administrative advancement is highly unlikely. According to one estimate, only one out of seven EMTs or paramedics can advance to a field supervisor position, only one out of 21 to the position of operations manager, only one out of 35 to the position

> A high number of significant stressors have been identified in EMS in an attempt to account for the occupation's high stress levels.

Decreased turnover and burnout rates can save EMS organizations significant amounts of money in the areas of training, personnel management, sick leave, employee replacement costs, substitutes to cover shifts, absenteeism, and employee medical costs.

of assistant manager, and only one out of 70 to manager. The other method of advancing within the medical profession—becoming a nurse, physician's assistant, or physician—requires significant additional schooling.

Given these conditions, it is not difficult to understand why there is a high burnout and turnover rate among EMTs and paramedics. No matter how much they love the work, the battle to make a long-term career in EMS is an uphill one. Nevertheless, it should not be made an impossible one.

Combating Stress and Burnout

Some EMS administrators have apparently accepted as fact that, because of the above-mentioned stressors, there will always be a high rate of burnout and turnover among their field personnel. Accordingly, they have geared their operations to accommodate high levels of attrition. Agencies pay minimum wage and work their EMTs and paramedics as hard as possible, knowing that they will only last a year or two anyway. They unwittingly contribute to the problem of EMS burnout, and actually work against their own best interests.

Fortunately, there is another way to approach the situation. Many job-related stressors can be approached by administration, management, and individual field providers in positive, cost-effective ways that can significantly relieve much of the pressure facing EMTs and paramedics. At the same time, these approaches can help the organization achieve its financial aims.

Decreased turnover and burnout rates can save EMS organizations significant amounts of money in the areas of training, personnel management, sick leave, employee replacement costs, substitutes to cover shifts, absenteeism, and employee medical costs. In addition, the result will be a more productive, professional, and well-trained staff, working in a more positive, enjoyable environment.

Accepting the Responsibilities

A review of recent literature on stress and EMS personnel shows that most authors are concentrating on the premise that, in order to cope with stress effectively, the locus of control must be internal, which places all of the responsibility for stress management on the individual care provider.

In the article "Burnout Revisited," R. G. Nixon commented, "We will no longer expect a magic cure for burnout from our supervisors or employers. Since we are responsible for, and in control of, our own lives, it would be unrealistic to expect our employers to provide the cure for our ills. The cure, or better yet, the ounce of prevention, is in our own hands."

It seems clear, however, that successful stress management needs to occur at all levels within the EMS service, not just at the individual level. The most successful stress management programs are those that include both individual and organizational approaches. An excellent study of burnout in the emergency department setting, which appeared in *General Hospital Psychiatry*, presented the following thesis:

> Research to date has emphasized stress and burnout as a problem with an individual locus. Such issues as commitment and hardiness implicitly place the locus of stress within the individual. Although it is obvious that the behavioral results of stress are certainly manifest in the individual, it is also quite possible that these problems exist, in part, at the organizational level. Therefore, interventions designed to reduce or prevent high levels of stress should be designed at both the individual and organizational levels.

Other studies have confirmed that stress within EMS has two distinct components: administrative (organizational) and clinical (individual) stress. Administrative stressors include poor organizational support and recognition, poor attitudes on the part of hospital personnel, low pay, too much paperwork, long hours, inadequate equipment, limited career ladders, and inadequate continuing education.

Clinical stressors involve such things as patient deaths (especially those of children); gory sights; abuse of service; mass casualties; threat of injury, illness, or death to self; feeling responsible for patient outcomes; and dealing with patients with chemical abuse problems.

EMTs and paramedics need to accept responsibility for learning proper stress management techniques to cope with clinical stressors, but management also needs to accept responsibility for addressing and mitigating organizational stressors. Only through such a comprehensive approach can significant improvements be realized in overall stress reduction for EMS providers.

Organizational Strategy

EMS managers and administrators need to evaluate their organizations in terms of the amount of administrative stress they generate for their employees. Then, they must take action to remove as many causes of that stress as possible. While all of the suggestions that follow may not be implemented overnight, they should become part of a long-range stress management plan at the organizational level.

Pay

Low pay is almost always mentioned in conversations about the drawbacks of an EMS career. The pay is undeniably low for several reasons. In most areas, there is an adequate supply of EMTs to replace those who do not like the work or the pay scale. (Although many areas are presently experiencing a paramedic shortage, the pay scale for paramedics also continues to be low.) Initial EMT training is relatively short, inexpensive, and easy to obtain, which creates a large pool of eager applicants.

In addition, the lure of EMS is strong. It is emotionally rewarding to complete EMT training and then work productively in such a demanding

> EMTs and paramedics need to accept responsibility for learning proper stress management techniques to cope with clinical stressors, but management also needs to accept responsibility for addressing and mitigating organizational stressors.

field. EMS is also often seen as a glamorous field. Given these conditions, it is easy to see why the pay is low. In the private sector, compensation for basic and intermediate EMTs actually decreased between 1987 and 1988.

Nevertheless, EMS managers who hope to have their services remain competitive in the future need to recognize that stable, high-quality, experienced employees are essential to their success. In addition, agencies are discovering that increasing pay actually results in long-term savings. High-quality, stable EMTs who make decent wages actually cost the company less in the long run than do underpaid, poorly trained, inexperienced EMTs who only stay for a year or two and then have to be replaced.

Career Advancement

Another sore spot for EMS personnel is the limited advancement potential within the industry. The organizational solution to the lack of an EMS career ladder is far from clear. Perhaps the most direct approach would be enhancement of the on-line EMT and paramedic positions to make them an acceptable career end in themselves.

Workload

One study of stress among paramedics noted that the level of stress significantly increased among those paramedics who averaged more than 600 runs per year. If a paramedic works 10 shifts a month, that averages out to only five calls per shift. This may not seem like many calls, but for those involved in EMS, it is not hard to understand the implications.

Managers and administrators need to recognize that EMTs and paramedics cannot be expected to last long if they are regularly expected to handle 10 to 15 or more calls per shift. An individual can only deal with a certain amount of stress and physical exertion during each 24-hour shift on a long-term basis.

Accordingly, managers need to make sure that call volumes per unit are reasonable and that they are distributed among shifts and units as equitably as possible. Another alternative may be to use eight- or 12-hour shifts (instead of 24) to meet the call demand without overloading crew members.

Recognition

EMS providers are rarely complimented for work well done, yet are quickly reprimanded if they make mistakes. Managers can do a great deal to reverse this. Alternatives include an employee-of-the-month award to recognize outstanding performance, personal letters of recognition to employees who do exceptional work, regular bonuses for steady performers, announcements to the press about incidents handled with unusual competence, regular announcements to hospital personnel (especially in the ED) regarding outstanding EMT and paramedic performances, nominations for state and national EMS awards, and agency banquets of honor. None of these programs is difficult to initiate, exceptionally time-consuming, or expensive, and the payoff in terms of improved agency morale, positive atmosphere, employee satisfaction, and stress reduction will be significant.

Fitness

In addition to reducing stress, company-sponsored fitness programs have been shown to result in cost benefits in terms of reduced healthcare claims, less absenteeism, and lower replacement costs. Employee fitness programs can take many forms, from granting spa membership privileges to providing on-site facilities. One agency uses the local university's fitness equipment and facilities. In any case, exercise programs are a well-documented method of reducing stress, anxiety, and depression, and managers of innovative provider agencies should have little trouble identifying cost-effective ways to make fitness facilities available to their employees.

Continuing Education

A national survey conducted by *JEMS* in 1983 profiled individuals who were planning to leave EMS. One reason cited for leaving the field was the lack of adequate training and education. Some provider agencies have attempted to rectify this by reimbursing tuition spent on continuing education related to the job. Other agencies have sophisticated in-service programs, which bring in qualified experts to explore different emergency medical topics in depth. In any case, individuals in a knowledge-intensive field such as prehospital medicine should be provided with ample opportunities to expand their knowledge and sharpen their skills.

Stress Management

Finally, EMS agencies have the responsibility to train their EMTs and paramedics about stress and how to manage it effectively. Qualified educators and counselors should be called upon regularly to explain the causes, signs and symptoms, and effective management of stress. Individuals experiencing unusually high stress levels or having difficulty coping with their stress should be provided with further instruction and counseling. Provider agencies should also monitor employee stress levels on a regular basis, using a valid, reliable instrument, such as the medical personnel stress scale (MPSS), to determine the specific elements of employee stress and the results of stress-reduction efforts.

In addition, EMS agencies should provide some type of mechanism for relieving the stress that results from responding to emotionally disturbing calls. Time can be set aside for group therapy sessions, which give crew members an opportunity to vent their frustrations, express their concerns, and discuss their anxieties. Critical incident stress debriefing (CISD) should also be used when appropriate and when available. Programs such as these can significantly help employees cope positively with their stress.

Individual Strategy

Once the EMS organization has done all it can to reduce stress levels, the rest is up to the individual. Developing a healthy internal locus of control is still crucial for managing stress effectively.

Lifestyle

Adopting healthy lifestyle habits is perhaps the most effective path to overall wellness. When an individual is healthy, his ability to cope with high stress levels is also significantly enhanced. Specifically, steps to good health include limiting or avoiding the use of alcohol, giving up smoking, getting seven to nine hours of sleep each night (a difficult task when working a 24-hour shift), eating a healthy breakfast, maintaining proper weight, eliminating junk-food snacks, and exercising regularly. The person adhering to these disciplines will be much better able to deal with high stress levels.

Group Support

Discussing negative feelings and expressing fears and concerns to friends and loved ones is very therapeutic in reducing stress. And yet, people in EMS have a tendency to keep their negative feelings to themselves. If opportunities to discuss feelings are not provided by the agency, EMS personnel should seek out a spouse, co-workers, or friends with whom to share the burdens of their EMS work. EMTs and paramedics also need to lead balanced lives and spend adequate time in play and recreational activities unrelated to EMS, as well as quality time with their families.

Cognitive Therapy

The basic premise of cognitive therapy is that mental perceptions result in bodily reactions. According to this theory, understanding the impact our mind has on our body is crucial. It works like this: The mind experiences an event, interprets it, and secretes hormones (based on the feelings and emotions associated with that interpretation or perception) that then create a physiological reaction. As might be expected, viewing events through negative perceptions or through distortions in thinking will lead to an overload of stressful physical reactions. On the other hand, learning to perceive events as positive challenges, rather than negative threats, is a skill that can, and should, be learned and developed to reduce stress levels.

Progressive Relaxation/Mental Imagery

In conjunction with cognitive therapy, progressive relaxation and mental imagery are proven methods of reducing personal stress. Again, these skills can be learned and developed by an individual wishing to reduce his stress level. Visualizing or picturing in the mind a special, favorite place, while using learned techniques to relax the muscles, can significantly reduce stress easily and with little time invested. There is an abundance of literature available that adequately explains these and other self-help methods for stress management, which should be used as a resource for EMS personnel.

Conclusion

High levels of stress occur in all aspects of EMS, resulting in unusually high levels of dissatisfaction and attrition among EMS professionals. While individuals in EMS must take responsibility for developing their own successful techniques for coping with clinical stressors, EMS managers and administrators also need to address and resolve organizational stressors, over which the individual EMT or paramedic has no control.

An EMS agency's future success will revolve around that provider's ability to attract and maintain highly qualified professional EMTs and paramedics. To accomplish this, EMS agencies will need to offer comprehensive stress management programs that address both the clinical and organizational aspects of EMS stress. By doing so, they can maintain the highest quality of patient care and retain professionals in the most cost-effective manner.

Source

Reprinted with permission from JEMS, *September 1990. Steven R. Hawks, EMT-I, EdD, is an assistant professor at Utah State University. Ronald L. Hammond has earned his doctorate.*

References

Allison, E. J., et al. "Specific Occupational Satisfaction and Stresses that Differentiate Paid and Volunteer EMTs." *Annals of Emergency Medicine* 16, no. 6 (1987).

Brownstone, J. E., et al. "Reducing Stress Factors in EMS: Report of a National Survey." *Emergency Health Services Review* 2, no. 1 (1983).

Durham, T. W., et al. "The Psychological Impact of Disaster on Rescue Personnel." *Annals of Emergency Medicine* 14, no. 7 (1985).

France, D. K. "Less Stress." *Emergency* 20, no. 4 (1988).

Hammer, J. S., et al. "Measurement of Occupational Stress in Hospital Settings: Two Validity Studies of a Measure of Self-Reported Stress in Medical Emergency Rooms." *General Hospital Psychiatry* 7 (1985).

Hammer, J. S., et al. "Occupational Stress Within the Paramedic Profession: An Initial Report of Stress Levels Compared to Hospital Employees." *Annals of Emergency Medicine* 15, no. 5 (1986).

Hawks, S. R., et al. "How Does Your Health Rate?" *JEMS* 14, no. 3 (1989).

Hempel, L. S. "Wellness Programs for EMS Personnel." *Emergency Medical Services* 16, no. 2 (1987).

Herbison, R. J., et al. "National EMS Burnout Survey." *JEMS* 9, no. 1 (1984).

Hinds, C. "The Heat of Burnout: How to Reduce Stress." *Emergency Medical Services* 17, no. 10 (1988).

Keller, K. L., and W. J. Koenig. "Management of Stress and Prevention of Burnout in Emergency Physicians." *Annals of Emergency Medicine* 18, no. 1 (1989).

Keller, R. "1989 EMS Salary Survey." *JEMS* 14, no. 3 (1989).

McSwain, N. E., and M. B. Skelton. "Burnout—Real or Imagined?" *Emergency Care Quarterly* 1, no. 4 (1980).

Mitchell, J. T. "Stress: The History, Status and Future of Critical Incident Stress Debriefing." *JEMS* 13, no. 11 (1988).

Mitchell, J. T. "The 600-Run Limit." *JEMS* 9, no. 1 (1984).

Nixon, R. G. "Burnout Revisited." *Emergency Medical Services* 16, no. 1 (1987).

Selye, H. *Stress Without Distress.* Philadelphia: J. B. Lippincott, 1974.

Shaffer, M. *Life After Stress.* Chicago: Contemporary Books Inc., 1983.

Steinmetz, J., et al. *Managing Stress Before It Manages You.* Palo Alto, Calif.: Bull Publishing Co., 1980.

Zun, L., et al. "Emergency Physicians Stress and Morbidity." *American Journal of Emergency Medicine* 6, no. 4 (1988).

Critical Incident Stress Debriefing Part I: The History, Status, and Future of CISD

Jeffrey T. Mitchell, PhD

Critical incident stress debriefing teams are saving careers and the very lives of EMS workers throughout the nation. Jeff Mitchell reviews the key concepts of CISD in this important two-part article, a must-read for every EMS leader.

IN JANUARY 1983, *JEMS* published the first article on critical incident stress debriefing (CISD). It started a nationwide and worldwide trend among emergency service organizations of developing programs that would assist emergency personnel before and after they encountered distressing events on the job. The goals of CISD are twofold: to lessen the impact of distressing critical incidents on the personnel exposed to them, and to accelerate recovery from those events before harmful stress reactions have a chance to damage the performance, careers, health, and families of emergency services personnel.

The CISD program did not simply fall out of a journal article, however; it had some roots in history. Before that landmark article was written, there was a long CISD development process, which started in 1974 when I was a regional EMS coordinator in Maryland. Nine years of development went into the CISD program before the concept was presented publicly in the 1983 article.

Human ideas are rarely formulated by themselves; many human experiences and subtle influences interact with one another until a new idea evolves. Thus, the new idea actually has a foundation in many other ideas that have been shared between people over decades—perhaps even centuries.

The CISD process is one of those concepts. It evolved out of the experiences and influences of many individuals and organizations. Four major influences can be pinpointed as the foundations of the CISD process:

- Military experiences
- Police psychology
- Emergency medical services
- Disasters

Military Experience

Combat stress reactions have been recognized since 603 B.C. For example, historians report that the American Civil War produced thousands of combat stress victims. But by World War I, new methods were being used to assist soldiers suffering from severe stress. It was found that quick treatment of these soldiers in field hospitals near the front lines was far more effective than delayed treatment at distant hospitals. While approximately 65 percent of those who received immediate psychological treatment for stress were able to return to combat duties, less than 40 percent of those who were given delayed treatment in distant areas were able to return to combat.

Rudimentary debriefings, provided by Dr. W. Glenn Srodes on Utah Beach during the D-Day invasion in World War II, were found to be quite helpful to stressed combat troops. Many were able to return to their duties after brief discussions with psychological support personnel. World War II units without psychological "first aid," on the other hand, sustained significant personnel losses, as distressed personnel had to be evacuated to distant treatment centers. Delays in treatment resulted in very few men returning to effective military duty.

The Israeli Defense Forces can be credited with the first effective research on psychological first aid and group psychological debriefings. It was noted in the Israeli studies that rapid intervention near the front lines, involving group as well as individual support, reduced the incidence of serious psychological disturbances, especially post-traumatic stress disorder, by as much as 60 percent.

Police Psychology

Police psychology units form the second major influence on the development of the CISD concept. Police psychologists came into the emergency services in the mid-1960s. Although the majority of police psychologists worked with individual officers and not groups, they contributed a great deal to the understanding of stress effects on the police services and their families. Police psychologists have added tremendously to knowledge about the personality profiles of emergency workers, specifically police, and have recommended the best types of psychological support services.

Police psychologists use a number of support strategies that have influenced the development of the CISD process. These include family support services, educational programs, post-shooting trauma teams, peer support officers, and group debriefings.

Emergency Medical Services

EMS organizations began developing psychological support services for staff members in 1972, with the first programs based in large hospitals and trauma centers. The services for staff members were an offshoot of the services provided for traumatized victims and their families. Those early efforts by hospital-based social workers and psychologists on behalf of overburdened and overstressed staffs pointed to the need for support services for field personnel as well as hospital-based personnel.

Nancy Graham, MS, of Los Angeles, was among the first hospital-based mental health professionals to see the need to reach out beyond the hospital to those who worked in the field. Her lectures and articles supported the development of the CISD concept.

Disasters

The last major influence on the CISD process was the occurrence of disasters. During the past 10 years, the National Institute of Mental Health has sponsored numerous studies on American disasters and has supported the development of several important documents that clearly point to the need for psychological support services, in particular, debriefings for police, fire, and emergency medical personnel. But even before these documents were published, disasters were showing themselves to be so extraordinarily powerful that few emergency workers escaped without significant stress reactions. Since large groups of emergency personnel experienced the same type of stress, it was believed that group debriefings would do much to eliminate the common belief among disaster workers that they are either unique or abnormal if they experience distress after working at a disaster.

One person who felt strongly that group debriefings were important to alleviate stress in emergency personnel was Captain Chip Theodore of the Arlington County, Va., Fire Department. In 1982, he worked at the scene of the Air Florida Airlines crash in Washington, D.C. He and his personnel were extremely stressed by that incident, and Captain Theodore pushed for the development of the first CISD team in the United States. The Arlington/Alexandria CISD team came into existence one year later, and the team continues to function today.

CISD Teams

Since 1983, hundreds of CISD teams have been established throughout the United States. A number of states have statewide teams. In addition, teams now exist in four other countries—Canada, Australia, Norway, and Germany. In all, the teams have provided more than 4,500 debriefings to thousands of emergency personnel in events ranging from single-victim auto accidents and shootings to full-scale disasters, such as the Ramstein, Germany, air show catastrophe.

Three Phases of CISD Development

The CISD concept has passed through two development phases during the past 14 years. In the first phase, CISD was conceptualized in 1974, implemented in various forms, and publicized in the 1983 CISD article in *JEMS*. In the second phase, CISD strategies and tactics were refined, and teaching strategies and course content were further developed. In fact, a consistent training course was developed, so the basic protocols for CISD teams across the nation are very similar, if not identical.

The third phase of CISD development is the evaluation of the process and further refinement, which are yet to come. This does not mean that debriefing evaluations have not yet been conducted; it simply means that CISD evaluation is new and that much more must be done.

The first evaluation studies are being undertaken by Dr. Robyn Robinson of Melbourne, Australia, who in 1986 conducted the largest stress-related study of emergency services ever. Preliminary data in her current study indicate that the majority of emergency personnel (fire, police, and ambulance) who attended debriefings in Melbourne throughout one year thought the sessions were helpful. In fact, the more serious the incidents, the more helpful the debriefings were perceived to be. In addition, Dr. Robinson found that most debriefing attendees thought their group (unit or squad) benefited from the debriefing process even if they, as individuals, only experienced a minimal amount of personal help. Seventy-five percent of those who participated in Dr. Robinson's preliminary study cited three main values of CISD:

- Expressing oneself and being reassured that one's reactions are normal
- Learning from others and mobilizing one's own coping behaviors
- Gaining a greater understanding of critical incident stress

Many emergency personnel also reported that they experienced a lessening of stress-related symptoms after a debriefing. Even the few negative comments did not indicate that the debriefings were not helpful; instead, these respondents made suggestions for improving the debriefing process and the communication between the CISD team and those being debriefed.

Dr. Robinson's research is exciting and promises to shed greater light on the CISD process. Her final report is likely to be filled with data and conclusions that will guide CISD teams into the next decade.

Further Support for CISD

Recent studies at Harvard University have lent further support to the provision of immediate intervention after traumatic events. Dr. George Everly suggests defusings and debriefings within 24 to 72 hours of a critical incident (see Part 2 of this article, "Development and Functions of a CISD Team").

While rapid initiation of defusings and debriefings help block a serious cognitive misinterpretation of the event, misinterpretation of the *personal* meaning of a critical incident may produce the very serious psychological disorder called post-traumatic stress disorder. Dr. Everly points out that in cases in which help for extremely traumatic events was provided within three weeks, the costs for treatment of a severely traumatized person were about $5,000. If help was delayed beyond three or four weeks, however, a severely traumatized person (or his organization) might face bills of approximately $200,000 to achieve recovery.

It is obvious that the third phase of CISD development has just begun. Much more research will be needed in the future to ensure a stable place for CISD teams as support for emergency services personnel. The challenge for CISD teams lies in developing research projects that do not violate the important services of CISD teams or the confidentiality of debriefing participants.

> Many emergency personnel reported that they experienced a lessening of stress-related symptoms after a debriefing.

The first and most important issue is a continued emphasis on pre-incident stress education. The more information people have on stress and its effects, the better they can recognize stress and seek help when they become overwhelmed.

The Future

Research is not the only challenge to CISD teams in the upcoming years. Other issues must be given careful consideration, or the CISD process will be doomed to failure.

The first and most important issue is a continued emphasis on pre-incident stress education. This has always been a mainstay of the CISD process. The more information people have on stress and its effects, the better they can recognize stress and seek help when they become overwhelmed. Administrators and instructors have to recognize the essential nature of stress training and commit themselves to continued support of it. Otherwise, they will spend more time and resources on rehabilitating people who might have avoided or lessened their stress with appropriate training before the events.

The next important issue is administrative support for emergency personnel. Even the best CISD teams will be frustrated and ineffective if they are forced to work in an environment in which administrators do not support their most valued resource—their personnel.

Another challenge for CISD teams is to stick closely to the CISD model, which has been carefully designed to assist emergency personnel and has been tried on many incidents with notable success. Significant changes in the tried-and-true methods may cause additional damage to emergency personnel. For instance, if a CISD team tries to make a debriefing into a psychotherapy session, which it was never designed to be, emergency personnel may be left more distressed than if help was not provided at all. On the other hand, CISD teams must make considerable efforts to keep up with new developments in the field of stress. These teams need to adapt to new information while holding tightly to proven CISD strategies.

Conclusion

When first mentioned in 1983, CISD was a new, relatively unresearched psychological and educational process designed to mitigate the effects of stress and accelerate the normal recovery process of emergency personnel. Many scoffed at the idea of emergency personnel discussing in a group how a critical incident had affected them. Few thought the concept would last.

Today, however, CISD teams are being woven into the fabric of emergency service organizations in several countries. Not everyone has become a believer; some actively resist CISD. There will probably always be doubters and resisters, and not everyone in every instance will benefit from CISD. Sometimes, personnel may need more help than a debriefing alone can provide.

But the evidence is beginning to mount that CISD teams have been successful in assisting many emergency personnel. The teams have advanced from a clumsy, unsophisticated developmental stage into a more organized, structured, and efficient stage. Hopefully, they will become integral and permanent parts of emergency service units as they repeatedly prove their value in assisting emergency personnel who are just too valuable to lose.

References

Appel, J. W. "Preventive Psychiatry." In *Neuropsychiatry in World War II.* Eds. A. J. Glass and R. J. Bernucci. Washington, D.C.: U.S. Government Printing Office, 1966.

Appel, J. W., G. W. Beebe, and D. W. Hilger. "Comparative Incidence of Neuropsychiatric Casualties in World War I and World War II." *American Journal of Psychiatry* 102 (1946): 196-199.

Bailey, P. "War Neuroses, Shell Shock and Nervousness in Soldiers." *JAMA* 71 (1918): 2148-2153.

Breznitz, S. "Stress in Israel." In *Selye's Guide to Stress Research.* Ed. H. Selye. New York: Van Nostrand Reinhold Co., 1980.

Brown, M. W., and Williams. *Neuropsychiatry and the War: A Bibliography with Abstracts.* New York: National Committee for Mental Hygiene, 1918.

Cohen, R., and F. Ohearn. *Handbook for Mental Health Care of Disaster Victims.* Baltimore: Johns Hopkins University Press, 1980.

Epperson, M. M. "Families in Sudden Crises." *Social Work Health Care* 2, no. 3 (1977).

Epperson-Seboier, M. "Response." In *Role Stressors and Supports for Emergency Workers.* Ed. B. Green. Washington, D.C.: Center for Mental Health Studies of Emergencies, U.S. Department of Health and Human Services, 1985.

"Glenn Srodes, 79, Dies, Chief of Staff of Hospital." *Pittsburgh Post Gazette,* 14 July 1984.

Graham, N. K. "Done In, Fed Up, Burned Out: Too Much Attrition in EMS." *JEMS* 6, no. 2 (1981): 25-31.

Graham, N. K. "Part 2: How to Avoid a Short Career." *JEMS* 6, no. 2 (1981): 25-31.

Green, B., ed. *Role Stressors and Supports for Emergency Workers.* Washington, D.C.: Center for Mental Health Services, 1985.

Hartsough, D. M., and D. Garaventa Myers, eds. *Disaster Work and Mental Health: Prevention and Control of Stress Among Workers.* Washington, D.C.: Center for Mental Health Studies of Emergencies, U.S. Department of Health and Human Services, 1985.

Mitchell, J. T. "Critical Incident Stress." In *Proceedings from a Conference on Dealing with Stress and Trauma in Emergency Services, August 7-9, 1986.* Ed. R. Robinson. Melbourne, Australia: Social Biology Resources Center, 1986.

Mitchell, J. T. "Rescue Crisis Intervention." *EMS News* 4, no. 3 (1976): 4.

Mitchell, J. T. "The Psychological Impact of the Air Florida 90 Disaster on Fire-Rescue, Paramedic and Police Officer Personnel." In *Proceedings of the First International Assembly on Emergency Medical Services, Baltimore, Md., June 13-17, 1982.* Ed. R. A. Cowley. Washington, D.C.: U.S. Department of Transportation, 1982.

Mitchell, J. T. "When Disaster Strikes . . . The Critical Incident Stress Debriefing Process." *JEMS* 8, no. 1 (1983): 36-39.

Mitchell, J. T., and H. L. P. Resnik. *Emergency Response to Crisis.* Bowie, Md.: R. J. Brady Co., 1981.

Nakanomiya, J. "History of War Medicine in Japan." *National Defense Medical Journal* 22 (1975): 67-73.

Nordlicht, S. "Effects of Stress on the Police Officer and Family." *New York State Journal of Medicine* 79, no. 3 (1979): 400-401.

Pugliese, D. "Psychological Pressures, Media: Israeli Defense Forces Confront Soldiers' Frustrations." *Armed Forces Journal International,* 28 May 1988.

Raphael, B. *When Disaster Strikes: How Individuals and Communities Cope with Catastrophe.* New York: Basic Books Inc., 1986.

Reese, J. T., and H. A. Goldstein, eds. *Psychological Services for Law Enforcement.* Washington, D.C.: U.S. Government Printing Office, 1986.

Salmon, T. W. "War Neuroses and Their Lesson." *New York Medical Journal* 109 (1919) 993-994.

Solomon, Z. "Front-Line Treatment of Israeli Combat Stress Reaction Casualties: An Evaluation of its Effectiveness in the 1982 Lebanon War." *Israeli Defense Forces Journal* 3, no. 4 (1986): 53-59.

Taylor, A. J. W., and A. G. Frayer. "The Stress of Post-Disaster Body Handling and Victim Identification Work." *Journal of Human Stress* 8, no. 12 (1982): 4-12.

Critical Incident Stress Debriefing Part 2: Development and Functions of a CISD Team

Jeffrey T. Mitchell, PhD

DURING THE PAST TWO DECADES, mental health professionals have gradually become aware of the stresses that negatively affect emergency personnel. As a result of this increased awareness, several classifications of mental health professionals have developed an interest in emergency workers. Consider the following:

Entrepreneurs. The "entrepreneurs" see emergency personnel as just another business deal. They generally have little understanding of the population they serve and make no special provisions for the emergency worker. Their main concern is to cultivate positive relationships with administrators so they have the best potential for developing a lucrative contract.

Glory seekers. The "glory seekers" are nowhere to be found unless an event that attracts the media occurs. Then, they suddenly appear as "experts" and lap up as much exposure as possible during the incident, quickly fading away when the excitement dies down.

Number crunchers. The "number crunchers" do not see genuine research as a tool to help emergency service workers but instead as a way to complete a degree, get published, or draw attention to themselves. They usually appear suddenly, demand a lot of survey data from emergency workers, and disappear without a trace of feedback to those who have spent time completing the surveys.

Well-meaning but unknowing. The "well-meaning but unknowing" mental health professionals have not taken the time to learn that emergency personnel are normal people reacting to abnormal events. They use non-directive or "psychiatric" interventions on emergency people, which will not work. They are generally clumsy in their approach to emergency response personnel and unable to establish a connection because they have failed to learn about the special personalities and needs of emergency workers.

Dedicated and trained. The "dedicated and trained" professionals understand the unique personalities of emergency personnel and the special jobs they perform. They take the time to go through special training, read about emergency personnel, and ride along with them on calls. They keep a low profile, are not primarily motivated by money, and perform careful research that aims at bettering emergency workers.

Most emergency personnel have encountered all these types of mental health professionals in the course of their careers. They will agree that the dedicated and trained type is the best to have on a critical incident stress debriefing (CISD) team and that the wrong type of mental health professional is usually worse than no help at all.

CISD Teams

CISD teams are made up of dedicated and trained mental health professionals who combine their expert knowledge and talents with specially trained peer support personnel drawn from the emergency service's ranks. The CISD team is essentially a partnership between the two groups with a common goal—the reduction of critical incident stress in emergency personnel.

CISD teams serve emergency personnel in any organization. They provide services to hospital-based emergency personnel and critical care personnel, as well as firefighters, police officers, and EMS providers. Individuals are not charged for these debriefing services.

The makeup of a team is roughly one-third mental health professionals and two-thirds peer support personnel. Most teams have 20 to 30 specially trained people, chosen for service after they have applied and been interviewed by the team leadership.

The average team serves a community of about 100,000 people and is activated for major stressful events six to eight times a year. There may also be a number of smaller events that require the services of one or two peers and, occasionally, a mental health professional. Caution should be exerted not to establish too large or too small a team since team members won't want to be over- or underused.

Another point to keep in mind when establishing a team is the size of the area served. Since mental health resources are limited, it is recommended that a team serve a region encompassing several jurisdictions. The majority of current CISD teams encompass several jurisdictions and all emergency agencies within them.

Serving more than one jurisdiction is important for several reasons. First, it is not a good idea to formally debrief your friends and fellow workers because it is too emotionally draining. Second, supervisory staff members may join the team and are always more helpful to people outside their own organizations because of management issues that may arise. Third, the debriefing attendees feel more comfortable when receiving services from people they do not see or work with regularly.

General Functions of a CISD Team

CISD teams function in three areas: pre-incident, incident, and post-incident.

Pre-Incident CISD Functions

The pre-incident functions have always been an essential part of CISD team activity and include the following.

Educating line personnel about stress, stress recognition, and stress reduction. Education should include material on critical incident stress and how it differs from non-emergency stress, as well as a description of the CISD team and how to use it if the need arises.

> CISD teams are made up of dedicated and trained mental health professionals who combine their expert knowledge and talents with specially trained peer support personnel drawn from the emergency service's ranks.

Educating command staff members about stress and its effects on them and their personnel. This segment should include specific information on field strategies for stress control during a crisis. Commanders should also know the capabilities and limitations of the CISD team and how to initiate services during and after a critical incident.

Developing stress management protocols for field use. If guidelines are written down and practiced, they are more likely to be followed. The protocols should list guidelines for commanders on items such as the optimal length of work time, frequency of rest periods, maximum time at the scene, food, shelter, replacement of gloves, and the use of the CISD team members during major events.

Providing spouse and family education programs. Spouse and family education programs enhance the quality of life for emergency personnel and the people important to them.

Developing supplementary programs. Individual counseling programs, employee assistance programs, chaplain services, and disaster intervention plans should be organized, as well as any other programs helpful to emergency responders.

CISD Functions During an Incident

On-scene support services. During the incident, a debriefing team is involved in providing on-scene support services that assist obviously distressed personnel. The team advises and counsels command staff and gives direct and indirect support to the victims until other appropriate agencies can be mobilized to provide services.

Defusings. These are shorter, unstructured debriefings that encourage a brief discussion of the events and significantly reduce acute stress. Defusings are done anywhere from one to three hours following the incident, often at the station, and generally last from 30 minutes to an hour. Only those crews most affected are involved; not all workers from the scene attend, as would be the case in debriefings.

If the defusings are not accomplished within 12 hours, a full formal debriefing is the next alternative and takes place approximately three days after the incident. A well-run defusing often eliminates the need for a full formal debriefing. Even if both are necessary, a debriefing held three days to a week after a defusing usually is more beneficial than one held without a defusing, as people are more willing to talk during a debriefing when first presented with a supportive defusing shortly after the incident.

Demobilizations. These are reserved for large-scale incidents only and take the place of a defusing. Immediately after emergency units cease and disengage from operations at a major incident, units are sent to a large meeting facility, where they are met by mental health professionals. Unlike the defusing or debriefing, personnel are not requested to discuss the incident. Instead, the mental health professional assigned to their unit provides a 10-minute presentation on the typical effects of critical incident stress and the signs and symptoms that may appear. The personnel are given as many practical suggestions for stress management as possible, along with an opportunity to ask questions or make comments. The mental health person assigned to the group remains available to privately discuss the situation or people's reactions. Talking to other mental health professionals at the debriefing center is also an option. Chaplains may be present at the debriefing center and are available if an emergency person would prefer to discuss something with them. No one is required to talk unless they choose to.

All of the personnel being demobilized are given an opportunity to get something to eat and relax before returning to duty or home. They are encouraged to rest during the transition from a major event back to routine duties. The entire demobilization process should be completed within 30 minutes, and two-thirds of that time should be allotted to rest and eating.

Post-Incident CISD Functions

Once an incident is over and defusings or demobilizations are complete, emergency personnel enter a phase lasting about 24 hours in which they generally prefer not to discuss the situation with outsiders. Many private thoughts emerge as crew members attempt to sift through the details of the incident. Often they are concerned with whether protocols and procedures were followed exactly, and they may be required to write reports or go through preliminary investigations. They are usually not ready to deal with whatever feelings may have arisen during the incident.

Emergency responders usually do not benefit from CISD during this 24-hour period because their reactions are too intense to absorb the important messages presented in a debriefing. What is usually more important is to provide individual support to those people showing the greatest need and to provide advice to the command staff trying to plan for the support services required.

Following a crisis, emergency workers are likely to close ranks, preferring to talk with individuals in the unit or participate in small group conversations related to the event. These conversations are called "initial discussions," and CISD teams usually have little involvement in them. However, peer support personnel, including those involved in the incident, are trained to watch for telltale signs of distress in their fellow workers: irritability, excessive humor, increased derogatory remarks about one another, significant changes in behavior, and withdrawal from others. If these signs of distress become apparent, peer support personnel contact the CISD team coordinator, who may initiate the setup of a formal CISD.

Formal CISD

The formal CISD is a psychological and educational support group discussion that uses a specially trained team of mental health professionals combined with peer support personnel. The main objectives of CISD are to mitigate the impact of a critical incident and accelerate the return of personnel to routine functions after the incident.

> The main objectives of CISD are to mitigate the impact of a critical incident and accelerate the return of personnel to routine functions after the incident.

Events that require a CISD include the following:
- Any event that has significant emotional power to overwhelm usual coping mechanisms
- Line-of-duty deaths
- Serious line-of-duty injuries
- Emergency worker suicides
- Disasters
- Unusually tragic deaths of children
- Significant events in which the victims are relatives or friends of emergency personnel
- Events that attract excessive media attention
- Events that seriously threaten the responders' lives

Because overuse of CISDs dilutes their effectiveness, they are reserved for only those events that overwhelm the usual coping methods of emergency personnel.

Before a debriefing is held, all of the coordination associated with the debriefing is finished, including the announcement to those involved and the setup of the room. Also, the CISD team reviews the incident by reading the reports and newspaper clippings and viewing photographs or videotapes of the incident. Many CISD teams visit the scene before conducting a debriefing.

Once the debriefing begins, it follows a carefully designed structure that progresses through seven phases and provides important stress reduction information. While participants are not required to speak, they are encouraged to discuss various aspects of the incident that distressed them. The whole process usually takes two to three hours to complete.

During the debriefing, personnel should not be required to respond to calls; others in the system need to fill in for them. Also, only those involved in the incident should attend, including command officers. If the critical incident affected various types of emergency personnel at the scene, a joint multi-agency debriefing is often held. It is important, then, to pick peer support personnel for the CISD team from each of the services. If an incident involves only EMS personnel, however, it is important to choose EMS peers, since EMS people are more likely to trust fellow workers. The same concept holds true for police and fire personnel.

Introduction. The CISD begins with an introduction from the CISD team members, at which point they state that the material to be discussed is strictly confidential. It should also be emphasized that the CISD is not an operations critique. Attendees are then told what to expect during the debriefing and are ensured that the CISD team's major concern is to restore people to their regular routine as soon as possible, with minimal personal damage. The basic rules of the debriefing are explained before the team members move into the next phase.

Fact phase. The second phase of the CISD is the fact phase, in which people are asked to describe what happened at the scene. This is a relatively easy phase for emergency personnel because they are used to talking about the operational aspects of an incident.

Thought phase. Once the incident is described, the debriefing team leader leads the discussion into the thought phase of the process. The usual question asked in this phase is "Can you recall your first thoughts once you stopped functioning in an automatic mode at the scene?" This helps people personalize their experiences; the events are no longer a collection of facts, but individual, meaningful recollections of how each worker personally experienced the incident.

Reaction phase. The fourth phase of a debriefing is the reaction phase, the point at which people can describe the worst part of the event for them and why it bothered them. If a critical incident has any significant emotional content attached to it, it will usually be discussed during this phase. It can occasionally become a heavy emotional phase of the debriefing but is not necessarily intense.

It is not the CISD team's objective to promote emotional behavior but to foster discussion so recovery occurs as rapidly as possible. This phase allows people to discuss the worst parts of an incident in a controlled environment that encourages the venting of thoughts and feelings associated with the event and prepares personnel for useful stress reduction information.

Symptom phase. The fifth phase of the CISD process is the symptom phase. The group is asked to describe stress symptoms felt at three different times. The first are those symptoms experienced during the incident; the second are those that appeared three to five days after the incident; and the last are symptoms that might still remain at the time of the debriefing. Changes in symptoms, as well as increases and decreases in symptoms, are good indicators to the mental health person of the need for additional help for some attendees.

Teaching phase. The next phase of the CISD process is the teaching phase. The CISD team members furnish a great deal of useful stress reduction information to the group. They also incorporate other information, such as a description of the grief process, how to promote communication with spouses, and how to help one another through the stress.

Re-entry phase. The seventh phase of the debriefing process is called the re-entry phase. Personnel may ask questions at this time. The team gives a summary, and the CISD is concluded.

After debriefing, the CISD team remains at the debriefing center to talk with those needing individual assistance. Referrals are made for counseling if necessary.

Finally, the CISD team holds a post-debriefing meeting to quickly review the debriefing and discuss ways to improve their functions for future debriefings. However, the main reason for meeting is to make sure that everyone on the team is all right before going home—hearing about the pain that others have experienced may bring about some pain for the debriefers themselves.

Teams need to be carefully developed, protocols need to be expanded and improved, and team members must be given the very best training.

Follow-Up Service

All defusings, demobilizations, and debriefings must receive follow-up services. Follow-ups usually begin 24 hours after the debriefing. The many ways follow-up can be achieved include

- Telephone calls to individuals
- Discussions with commanders
- Visits to the stations
- Sending peers to see that personnel are doing all right
- Educational programs
- Individual counseling sessions
- Spousal support services
- Other activities as the needs arise

Other CISD Team Considerations

Simply reading this article in no way gives anyone the ability to perform a CISD. *Minimum* training time for a CISD team is two days, with continuing education on a regular basis. A CISD is ineffective without trained peer support personnel.

Likewise, a CISD team without mental health professionals is not only ineffective but dangerous. Mental health professionals are necessary to provide leadership and supervision. They also possess diagnostic skills and recognize problems that are more serious than stress alone. Missed symptoms may cause an emergency worker to commit suicide.

It takes a special task force at least six months to one year to properly organize a CISD team in most communities. All CISD teams should have the same training and operating protocols, and these should be developed in writing so they are interchangeable.

People should be accepted on CISD teams because of their competency—not because of politics.

CISD teams survive and are successful if they meet regularly, cross-train (mental health personnel should ride on emergency units for field exposure), and provide continuing stress education to field personnel.

Much has already been written about CISD teams and their development. Review the protocols and the accomplishments of other teams before developing a team in your region.

Conclusion

CISD teams have experienced phenomenal growth in the last several years, overcoming many problems and achieving many successes. They have assumed an important position within emergency services organizations and are likely to continue their support services into the future.

Teams need to be carefully developed, protocols need to be expanded and improved, and team members must be given the very best training. There are many challenges associated with the development and operation of a CISD team. Dedicated people are needed to ensure the stability and success of the teams as they provide the valuable service of healing the helpers.

Additional information on CISD teams can be obtained from the International Critical Incident Stress Foundation, 5018 Dorsey Hall Drive, Suite 104, Ellicott City, Md. 21042; (410) 730-4311.

References

Duckworth, D. H. "Professional Helpers in Disaster Situations." *Stress Medicine* 2: 315-323.

Harris, V. "Working with Families of Emergency Services Staff." Paper presented at the conference Dealing with Stress and Trauma in Emergency Services. Melbourne, Australia, August 1989.

Hartsough, D. M., and D. Garaventa-Myers, eds. *Disaster Work and Mental Health: Prevention and Control of Stress Among Workers.* Washington, D.C.: Center for Mental Health Studies of Emergencies, U.S. Department of Health and Human Services, 1985.

Kennedy-Ewing, L. *Delaware County Critical Incident Stress Management Program, Operational Guidelines.* Media, Pa.: Delaware County Department of Human Resources, 1988.

Mitchell, J. T. "Critical Incident Stress." In *Proceedings from a Conference on Dealing with Stress and Trauma in Emergency Services, August 7-9, 1988.* Ed. R. Robinson. Melbourne, Australia: Social Biology Resources Center, 1986.

Mitchell, J. T. "Critical Incident Stress Management." *Response, The Magazine of Emergency Management* (fall 1986): 24-25.

Mitchell, J. T. "Effective Stress Control at Major Incidents." *Maryland Fire Rescue Bulletin* (June 1987).

Mitchell, J. T. "Recovery from Rescue." *Response, The Magazine of Emergency Management* (fall 1982): 7-10.

Mitchell, J. T. "Teaming Up Against Critical Incident Stress." *Chief Fire Executive* 1, no. 1 (1986): 24, 36, 84.

Mitchell, J. T. "The Psychological Impact of the Air Florida 90 Disaster on Fire-Rescue, Paramedic and Police Officer Personnel." In *Accidents, Civil Disorders, Natural Disasters, Terrorism.* Eds. R. A. Cowley, S. Edelstein, and M. Silverstein. Washington, D.C.: Department of Transportation (DOT HS806302), 1982.

Mitchell, J. T. "When Disaster Strikes . . . the Critical Incident Stress Debriefing Process." *JEMS* 8, no. 1 (1983): 36-39.

Stauffer, E. "Role of Chaplains in Support of Emergency Personnel." Paper presented at the conference Stress, Helping the Helper. University of Maryland, May 1987.

Source

Reprinted with permission from JEMS, *November and December 1988. Jeffrey T. Mitchell, PhD, is the developer of critical incident stress debriefing (CISD) intervention and is the president and co-founder of the International Critical Incident Stress Foundation. He is a clinical associate professor of emergency health services at the University of Maryland and has authored more than 75 articles on stress, CISD, disaster psychology, and crisis intervention. He is also the primary author of four books on related topics.*

EAPs: Easy Answers to Paramedical Stress

Carolyn S. Garcia

Employee assistance programs can and do mitigate the stress that affects EMS workers. The following articles by Carolyn Garcia and Kevin Armstrong describe EAPs and discuss how to implement these programs in EMS organizations.

IN EMS, STRESS IS PART of the daily routine. This constant emotional and physical drain results in increased incidences of failed or troubled marriages, alcohol and drug abuse, and chronic stress for responders.

For an answer to its own cry for help, EMS has taken a cue from the business community that, for years, has provided its employees with employee assistance programs (EAPs) to help them deal with their problems.

Members of today's EMS community suffer from the same problems the business community does: finances, career-advancement stress, depression, lack of personal physical fitness, drug testing, governmental regulations, and life's everyday problems.

In 1988, counselors and fire and EMS personnel from all over the United States gathered for a national conference in Fort Worth, Tex., to exchange ideas and discuss the strong and weak points of existing EAPs.

The conference, sponsored by the International Association of Fire Chiefs Foundation (IAFCF), provided a forum for fire and emergency services personnel to question qualified officials about everything from AIDS and other infectious diseases to drug testing.

These officials presented some startling statistics. Approximately 20 percent of the U.S. workforce is dealing with problems that affect their job performance. For fire and EMS personnel, the percentage may be higher, according to Marla Zipin, former EAP coordinator for Fairfax County, Va. It is estimated that 40 to 80 percent of all illnesses that cause employees to miss work are stress-related.

"EAPs are a way to salvage people who would otherwise lose their jobs or drain the company of productivity," Zipin said. "EAPs should be considered a necessity rather than a company or department benefit."

According to Zipin, some key components for any EAP are confidentiality, employee education, evaluation, stress reduction, and overall prevention of more serious problems.

But while an EAP addresses a number of issues and problems, its primary focuses are stress and substance abuse, since most job-related employee problems stem from these. However, one of the valuable things about EAPs is that they can be designed to fit a service's specific needs.

Setting Up an EAP

The first step in setting up an EAP is to write a policy statement. Administrators must set clear goals for their program. For example, the Fairfax County Fire and Rescue Department's general policy statement reads, "The purpose of the employee assistance program is to assist employees to cope effectively with personal or job stress. In addition, the EAP aims to retain valued employees, increase job effectiveness, and encourage a positive work climate."

In addition to a general statement, individual policy statements should be set for chemical dependency, confidentiality, disability claims, and fitness for duty.

Next, decide which EAP services will be provided. These may include clinical services, education and training, and program evaluation.

Clinical services provided through an EAP can be consultations, referral services, and short-term counseling.

Educational services help familiarize employees with the services provided, thus encouraging early identification of problems and self-referral. Training for supervisors enables them to understand how the system works and helps them to recognize employee problems early.

Program evaluation is an important part of any EAP. This evaluation should explore the program's efficiency, both operationally and financially.

Employees may either refer themselves to the program or be referred to it by a supervisor. The families of EMS personnel may also initiate contact. All EAP communication, however, must remain confidential as outlined in the service's confidentiality statement.

There are three types of supervisory referrals: employee-initiated, job performance, and disciplinary diversion.

An employee may initiate discussion about a personal problem with a supervisor, and the supervisor, in turn, may recommend that the employee use the EAP.

Job-performance referrals should be based solely on job-performance problems—EAPs are not designed to make diagnosticians or detectives out of supervisors.

Disciplinary-diversion referrals provide an alternative to serious disciplinary action. Before choosing this avenue for correcting an employee's performance, however, check with the EAP to ensure such a referral is appropriate.

"It's not the supervisor's job to act as counselor," Zipin said, "but it is his job to evaluate job performance."

A Look at Stress

Research shows that stress affects memory; the ability to reason, decide, and communicate; motor-skill coordination; and interpersonal relationships. Someone once said that all humans want "to love and be loved, and to work and be productive." We now know that stress can steal one's ability to fulfill these needs.

A critical incident stress debriefing (CISD), especially in EMS, is one area where an EAP can curb stress, according to Bill Bratvett of the Psychiatric Institute of Fort Worth.

> "The EAP aims to retain valued employees, increase job effectiveness, and encourage a positive work climate."

"A CISD can mean the difference between saving a person's emotional stability or not," said Bratvett.

In addition to CISDs, research shows there are other methods for battling stress: relaxation, physical exercise, confronting problems, and employee effectiveness profiles.

Overall good health, too, is becoming more and more important. In addition to smoking bans and physical fitness requirements, many services require pre-employment drug testing.

Drug or substance-abuse testing, however, opens a Pandora's box

EAPs: Designed for Success

Kevin T. Armstrong, MA

Establishing an EAP within an EMS agency is an all-encompassing project; the "healthy" skepticism held by most emergency responders toward new ideas can put the skids on the most worthwhile endeavor. On the other hand, when supportive of an idea, their dedication and hard work can almost ensure its success. Involvement must come from the ranks. If the golden rule is followed (i.e., the one with the gold sets the rules), administration may not win the support of the workers. The finest EAP on the books, handed down to emergency workers from up high, is worthless if it isn't used.

Initially, an EAP must be designed to meet agency needs. EAP providers have a tendency to rubber-stamp programs that work for the general public. However, to be effective, mental health counselors and educators have to be knowledgeable about the general personality types of emergency responders. EAP providers have to spend time in the rigs, on the streets, and in the classrooms to know the group they're serving. Inappropriate mental health services can actually be worse than no service at all.

There are vast numbers of counseling theories and styles. Some work well for certain individuals and groups, while others would turn people off from ever seeking counseling again. The qualifications of employees of EAP provider agencies may also vary greatly; there can be obvious differences between providers at the

bachelor's, master's, and doctorate levels. Are they licensed or certified in your state? Potential EAP providers and emergency response personnel have a lot of preliminary research and work to do before program planning can begin.

Referrals

When establishing the EAP referral process, self-referral and referrals by concerned friends should be emphasized rather than supervisor referrals. However, supervisors should refer employees when problems aren't recognized or referred by others. Furthermore, any special training provided for supervisors should be open to all personnel so people who care about an individual can best refer him for help when needed. Issues affecting job performance are everyone's concern.

Credibility

What chance would a psychologist have if he stepped into your station—first time in the shark tank—to explain what services he could provide for you? Probably little, if any. This reminds me of a story about city council candidates who were seeking support from firefighters. When one candidate was asked about his platform for public safety agencies, he stated that his priorities were to fix bumps and cracks in the sidewalks and broken playground equipment at the parks. Obviously, the candidate had little of legal issues. These include possible violation of personal privacy rights, violation of the Fourth Amendment, which provides protection against unreasonable search and seizure, and violation of the Fourteenth Amendment, which guarantees due process of law.

Before starting a drug-testing program as part of an EAP, talk to administrators of other services to learn how they set up their programs, what kinds of tests they use, and what, if any, problems they've encountered.

"Alcoholism and substance abuse are diseases and potential terminal illnesses," said Terry Cowan, executive director of the Workers Assis-

knowledge of the issues deemed important by his firefighter constituents.

All of the academic degrees in the world won't ensure credibility if people can't relate to one another. Police psychologists and some mental health folks specializing in fire and EMS have committed themselves to experiencing life in the field so they can effectively counsel EMS personnel. These EAP providers have spent time in the rigs, on the streets, in the classrooms, and at the stations. In doing so, they've opened many doors and established trust while truly assisting employees with their mental health needs.

Confidentiality

Once a trusting relationship is established between mental health providers and EMS employees, work is required to maintain it. Any breach of trust can easily end emergency workers' use of the program. Although no professional would willingly breach confidentiality, each has to have and share a thorough knowledge and understanding of the potential loopholes. It's nice to think that all mental health services are confidential, yet some important gaps remain that affect confidentiality.

Counselors keep written records of sessions with almost all clients. Some keep extremely detailed notes, while others record basic information to understand the flow of sessions. Records can be subpoenaed in a court of law or by deposition, and insurance companies will often require a diagnosis or label for treatment. They also may require records of sessions.

Do these records now become the property of the insurance company? How many hands do they pass through during the confirmation, filing, and review process? What is the extent of the insurance company's contractual relationship with your employing agency? If seen through a hospital-based service, are these records part of your medical records? Most of us have seen charts routed all over a hospital. Fiscal and program accountability dictate the need to keep training records and use statistics. However, these stats can easily be kept without using individual names or other identification.

Answers to questions like these should strengthen your program—all of the cards will be on the table. Alternative ways of accomplishing goals can then be found if necessary, and no surprises will await you.

It is obvious that many EAPs currently serving emergency response agencies are helpful and have beneficial aspects. Yet programs custom-designed by qualified, credible mental health specialists and emergency service personnel from all ranks will be far more effective. It is possible to have entire agencies benefit from an EAP rather than just a few individuals. When they do, you will find EMTs and firefighters knocking on your door to tell their EAP stories.

Source

Reprinted with permission from JEMS, *January 1990. At the time of original publication, Kevin T. Armstrong, MA, was a paramedic/firefighter with the Olympia Fire Department in Olympia, Wash. He holds a master's degree in psychological counseling* tance Program of Texas. "Forty percent of industrial accidents involve substance abuse, and 90 percent of inmates in the Texas Department of Corrections have a history of substance abuse."

Job performance statistics on substance abusers are sobering, says Cowan. Substance abusers are 16 times more likely to be late to work, three times more likely to apply for sick benefits, three times more likely to have accidents, five times more likely to file for workers' compensation, and two and a half times more likely to miss work than non-abusers.

How to Pay for an EAP

Once the service has decided it needs an EAP, the next step is to convince the city or county government to fund it.

Diane Breedlove, a CPA with Breedlove and Co. in Houston, says the first step in this process is to put specific goals in writing. Breedlove, who is also a training officer with the Klein Volunteer Fire Department, says departments should develop objectives that can be measured in time, money, and productivity.

An important goal is increased productivity through improved health. "To measure success, you need measurable objectives such as reducing absenteeism by 15 percent or decreasing the number of off-the-job accidents by 10 next year," Breedlove said.

The department must then design a program to meet the stated goals. This, Breedlove adds, requires research, investigation, planning, teamwork, and asking for help from those knowledgeable in EAPs. The person in charge of the project will want to write specifications much like a service does for procuring equipment.

"You already believe you ought to provide assistance to your employees for human reasons," Breedlove said. "That fact, however, is hardly a convincing argument for those who make decisions about spending money."

There are several financial reasons for implementing EAPs. According to Breedlove, the average employee misses five days of work per year. Employees abusing drugs or alcohol miss 22 days. Other troubled employees miss 12.5 days per year.

Ten percent of Americans suffer from alcoholism, another three to seven percent from drug abuse, and still more from other mental health problems, she says. That means that for every 100 employees, administrators can expect 10 to be alcoholic and at least seven to be troubled.

If these 17 employees earn an average of $23,000 a year, that's a loss of $20,470 to absenteeism in one year, not including fill-in costs or losses in efficiency. Turnover is another costly problem. An eight- to 10-percent rate is not uncommon, according to Breedlove. And this rate may be higher for EMS personnel.

The expense of replacing employees is high. Some predict that a new employee works at 50 percent efficiency the first six months of employment and at 75 percent efficiency the next six months. There are also recruiting and interviewing costs; hiring costs like physicals, testing, and background checks; and training costs.

The service's records can provide the statistics necessary to promote the need for an EAP. How many employees missed zero to five days? How many missed more than five days? What compensation were they paid? What was paid for fill-in time? How many employees had accidents? How many people terminated employment? How much money was paid in medical benefits? How much has the insurance coverage increased?

The cost of an employee assistance program depends on its design. An internal program will require a director's salary plus support staff and overhead costs. It may be more economical to contract with a provider.

Many mental health providers offer six to 10 visits per year per person for $20 to $50 per employee, Breedlove says. A small organization can expect a larger per capita cost than a large one.

Take a look at the service's insurance policy. Will the insurance provide for employee participation in the EAP? Part of the program's success, Breedlove says, depends on the ability of employees to afford recommended treatment.

Private industry EAPs have a long enough history to provide a basis for prediction. According to Breedlove, United Airlines estimates that over the work life of an employee (23 years), it saves $16.95 for each dollar invested in its EAP.

Some providers provide services on a co-risk basis, requiring some of the costs up front and the remainder based on the increased pool at the end of the year. There may be grant money to begin a program. Several years ago, the city of Houston got a $40,000 grant from the Texas Commission on Alcohol and Drug Abuse to fund its program.

To find out about grants, EMS administrators should contact their local council of government or planning commission and check the Federal Grants Register at their city library. The Foundation Directory lists private foundations and the grants they offer. Local university research faculties are usually skilled at writing grant applications and may be willing to help.

Rank the programs in order of priority. Decide what is most important. Compare the costs of an EAP with the costs of *not* having one. Describe everything in numbers.

"If you believe in EAPs, invest in a good program," Breedlove said. "To continue to justify a program, one must know the results—the impact."

Source
Reprinted with permission from JEMS, *November 1988. At the time of original publication, Carolyn S. Garcia was the editor of* Texas Firemen Magazine *and the public information officer for the State Firemen's and Fire Marshals' Association of Texas.*

Reference
Facts and supporting data for this article were taken from oral and written presentations at the 1988 EAP conference in Fort Worth, Tex., which was sponsored by the International Association of Fire Chiefs Foundation.

Pay Now or Pay Later: A Look at Substance Abuse in EMS

Scott Bourn, RN, and Michael G. Smith, EMT-P

Substance abuse is an increasingly common mechanism among medical workers for coping with stress. EMS staffs are particularly susceptible. How does substance abuse happen? Whose problem is it? How can it be prevented? These are some of the questions answered in this article.

MAYBE THE PROBLEM DOESN'T EXIST. Perhaps the periodic stories we hear about impaired paramedics are just that—stories. Or maybe there are a few deranged individuals out there who will die or be fired before they hurt anyone. Maybe the problem of substance abuse is limited to other health professionals, such as physicians, physician's assistants, or nurses. After all, articles about substance abuse in these groups are appearing in various journals more frequently.

On the other hand, is it just possible that we have chosen to ignore this problem by looking the other way? If we do have a substance abuse problem, who will find it? The media? For an industry that has worked as hard as EMS has to be recognized as a profession, the impact of such a revelation would be the loss of *years* of trust-building. Therefore, possibly a better alternative is for us to determine whether we have a problem and, if we do, to get on with paying the price to remedy it. If we sit back and ignore substance abuse in our profession, when it finally does rear its ugly head, we'll still have to pay the price. Only then it will be a bigger price—in dollars, credibility, and professionalism. The choice is ours: Pay now or pay later.

The Scope of the Problem

You would have to have spent the past several years on another planet not to have been exposed to the growing concern regarding substance abuse. The "Just Say No" campaign initiated a nationwide effort to educate the children of America to the hazards of illicit drug use. Mandatory drug testing is one of the hottest topics around and has impacted everything from the federal government to the National Football League. It has also become a topic of discussion among various health professions and the transportation industry. But what about in EMS?

The use of drugs in EMS may be better understood if it is examined in the context of a larger problem that affects all of the healthcare professions. Substance abuse is a major occupational hazard for healthcare professionals, with members having a *two to three times greater risk for drug addiction than the general population*. While the exact numbers of impaired professionals are not known, estimates of alcoholism in medicine vary from three percent to 15 percent of the workforce. An estimated five percent of all nurses are addicted to alcohol or drugs, a percentage that translates to a staggering 40,000 to 75,000 in the workforce. Higher rates of abuse are also documented in the veterinary and dental professions.

As in the population at large, alcohol tops the list of abused substances in the medical profession; 66.4 percent of impaired physicians are alcoholics. Demerol, Valium, and amphetamines are the next most abused drugs. The cost of substance abuse in these groups is phenomenal; an impaired employee who earns approximately $18,000 per year will cost his employer $50,000 to $75,000 annually in decreased efficiency, sick leave, overtime (to cover shifts), workers' compensation, and replacement personnel. And this figure does not take into account the potential for treatment error or decreased patient safety, loss of public image, or possible litigation due to negligence while impaired.

What happens to impaired professionals? Physicians and nurses have both developed fairly sophisticated methods for identifying and helping impaired practitioners. Medical practices are carefully monitored by state pharmacy boards and the Drug Enforcement Administration (DEA) due to the physician's role in dispensing medications. According to C. J. Shanaberger, a paramedic, attorney, and investigator of physician and nursing malpractice for the state of Colorado, most cases of physician drug abuse are identified by those two watchdog agencies. Drug problems in the nursing profession are usually identified by the hospital that employs the nurse based on medication count irregularities or reports from colleagues. According to Shanaberger, abuse is rarely noted by patients.

What happens after a problem is identified? Generally, the first action is to notify the board of medical examiners or the nursing board. The licensing board responds by notifying the individual involved. An investigation of the facts surrounding the allegation follows; if reasonable grounds exist to suggest substance abuse, the board files a complaint against the individual. A hearing board is then asked to analyze both sides of the issue, and the hearing judge makes a recommendation to the licensing board.

The first recommendation usually includes having the individual enter a voluntary treatment program, a number of which are available in most states for impaired nurses and physicians. These programs are specifically oriented to the substance abuse problem in the medical profession and provide feedback to the licensing board. Often the board suggests a period of supervised practice, which entails having another professional monitor the individual's medical care, with periodic written reports to the board. Regular updates on rehabilitation and blood/urine screening may also be required as prerequisites for continuing to practice. In all cases, the focus is on maintaining a safe practice and returning the individual to his profession.

What about EMS? No research is available to document the prevalence of substance abuse in our profession. But why should we be any different? We share with our colleagues in medicine a number of risk factors for substance abuse, as well as access to controlled substances. As the incidents presented in this article demonstrate, there *is* substance abuse in EMS. The only question is why it happens and what we're going to do about it.

> An impaired employee who earns approximately $18,000 per year will cost his employer $50,000 to $75,000 annually in decreased efficiency, sick leave, overtime (to cover shifts), workers' compensation, and replacement personnel.

How Can It Happen?

During a recent conversation with a young female paramedic, she confided that her sister had left a small amount of cocaine in her freezer after a party one night. It stayed there for a number of days, but one morning after a late night out, the paramedic decided to have "just a line" to get her up for her shift. "What could it hurt?" she thought. "Just one line—that won't affect my judgment."

Well, the cocaine didn't last long, and soon she had purchased more. Before too long it wasn't just before her shift, but it was first thing after her shift as well. "After a while," she said, "I was making up excuses for my partner to swing by my house during mid-shift . . . 'I think I left my upstairs window open, and it looks like rain.'"

Fortunately for this woman, she realized what was happening to her and quit. But for so many of the people we read about in the newspaper and in magazines, things don't work out as well, and their lives and jobs are destroyed.

Why does anyone abuse drugs? And what substances are included in the description of substance abuse? All sources agree that the most abused drug is alcohol. Ranked as the number-four health problem in America, alcoholism affects 4.9 percent of the population, according to the World Health Organization.

Regardless of the substance abused, most theorists propose that there are three principal reasons why people become addicted. The first is *psychological need.* This need makes an individual susceptible to the belief that drugs or alcohol will minimize or eliminate the needs or pain of life. The stress of EMS, frustration about the job, pain from the tragic nature of our work—these are prime examples of the tensions we all experience. Many individuals who are susceptible to abusing drugs believe that using certain substances will either remove the pain or decrease its impact on their lives.

The second factor leading to substance abuse is *social or peer pressure.* The social climate of many EMS organizations, including hospital, fire, and ambulance groups, is one of working hard and partying hard. This attitude not only makes drinking and drugs acceptable—it makes non-use unacceptable. Individuals who don't or won't participate are often labeled as outsiders and are excluded from the group, frequently resulting in their leaving for an organization with a different social climate.

Some departments may have bars in the firehouse or regular group drinking or drug sessions after work. One group was famous for its "parking lot parties," which occurred in a parking lot across the street from the facility. These parties would be attended by nurses and paramedics coming off duty—and often lasted several days as one shift ended and another began.

The final risk factor linked to substance abuse is *access to substances of abuse.* In EMS, this access may take many forms. A bar in the firehouse makes drinking very easy. Having close and continued access to physicians makes it simple to get a prescription for back pain. A second prescription may be obtained by seeing a different physician in a different ED. Because we have collegial relationships with most of our emergency doctors, they very rarely question our symptoms or investigate whether we have seen another physician.

The presence of controlled substances in our units and in the hospital makes access to narcotics also fairly easy and the temptation formidable. Prescription pads are everywhere. Because we are part of the system, our presence in the medication room of the ED is rarely questioned. And it is often easy to conceal drugs missing from an ambulance or stockroom for a long period of time—making it difficult to determine what crew lost the medications. The result: EMS personnel have extremely easy access to medications.

Who's Got a Problem?

A bright young EMT on the way to paramedic school confided to his medical adviser that he was worried—he thought he may have a drinking problem. While he never drank on duty, he spent much of his off-duty time drinking heavily. Then, when scheduled to return to work, he was hung over and often overslept, resulting in a late arrival. However, he was most frightened by another factor: When he got drunk, he sometimes used cocaine with friends—an activity he would never do otherwise. He was concerned that he was becoming an alcoholic and wondered what he should do.

Substance abusers aren't demons. They're often nice, intelligent professionals we know. For this reason, one of the difficulties in discussing substance abuse is defining who has a problem and who doesn't. How much of a substance is too much? Is abuse acceptable as long as it doesn't occur on duty? Or is a hungover individual a problem at work?

There are no absolute answers to these questions. What is universally accepted is that substance abuse can occur with any intoxicating substance, be it licit or illicit, drugs or alcohol. The crux of having a drinking or drug problem is a *loss of control over the substance* and losing control of yourself in the process. Unfortunately, the lack of clear signs and symptoms for substance abuse makes it easy for an affected individual to rationalize the problem by reasoning that he doesn't have all the "signs and symptoms" or can "quit anytime." But there are some common warning signs that point toward a substance abuse problem (Box 1.3).

Clearly, warning signs are just guidelines; everyone with one or more of these signs is not an addict. Nevertheless, assessment of substance abuse, just like every other kind of assessment, is based on an index of suspicion. These signs should increase your suspicion that you or someone around you has a substance problem. But what should you do if you see these signs in others? At what point, legally, morally, or ethically, do we

> Substance abusers aren't demons. They're often nice, intelligent professionals we know.

Box 1.3

Warning Signs of a Substance Abuser

Substance Abuse in an Employee or Partner

- Chronic tardiness (from being hungover or still impaired)
- Financial problems that are not apparent and don't seem proportional to visible obligations, such as rent or car payments (from buying drugs or alcohol)
- Volatile mood swings, including anger, tears, defensiveness, or depression
- Inability or unwillingness to confide in others; this is especially noticeable if the individual was once close to a partner or friend and now pulls away
- Frequent sick calls to work
- When possible, sick calls are made by spouses, roommates, or others (so the individual does not have to confront or discuss problems with employer)
- Use of dark glasses or long-sleeved clothing in inappropriate settings (to cover bloodshot eyes, dilated pupils, or needle marks)
- Always tired; sleeps a lot during the day
- Disappears for periods of time into the

take the responsibility to intervene in our partner's or an employee's life if we suspect a drug or alcohol problem?

Intervention Strategies

As far as emergency medicine goes, intervention is a daily process. We intervene during crisis situations involving a variety of situations ranging from traumatic injuries to medical emergencies, usually for patients who seek our help willingly. However, when we're talking about a person who is chemically dependent, we're talking about a different matter. These people usually are not seeking help willingly, primarily because they do not think they have problems. Denial and delusion are the hallmarks of this illness, and many patients believe they can fix it on their own—but rarely, if ever, does this occur.

Sandy Maher, RN, BSN, is the unit nursing director of the Mercy Alcohol and Drug Rehabilitation Program at Mercy Hospital in Des Moines, Iowa. "These folks get good at giving excuses for their behavior," she reported. "As the disease process continues, there are more and more occurrences, and finally they can't even keep the stories straight." She continued, "Even when confronted with the problem, they believe it's no big deal and that they can take care of it themselves."

But that rarely happens. Once a problem with alcohol or substance abuse has been identified, our focus should be on directing the individual toward professional help in the form of a substance abuse program. We may be helpful, concerned, or supportive, but *one thing we are not is substance abuse counselors*. A deep dependency relationship with an alcoholic or drug abuser more often than not leads to increasing difficulties for both parties and often doesn't help the abuser. The key is to get the individual to *professional* treatment.

What kind of treatment is appropriate or available? Alcoholics Anonymous and Alanon are good programs that are available in most communities. In addition, a wide variety of employee assistance programs are in place in many hospitals, municipal fire/ambulance organizations, and large private ambulance companies. These programs offer a variety of alternatives, from in-patient treatment facilities for substance abuse to individual therapy. Our role is to help the substance abuser into treatment and then be his friend.

And what if you see these signs in yourself? First, your honesty is to be admired. Recognition of a problem is the first, most difficult step. Discuss your problem with someone you trust who can help you. A supervisor or medical adviser is usually a good place to start; both should know how to help you get in contact with an appropriate program or expert. This conversation will be scary for both of you but hopefully not as scary as having to cope with such an overwhelming problem alone. The EMT who went to his medical adviser recognized his own problem—the hardest part. And, while it is not fair to say that his problem is over (he is and will always be an alcoholic), he has taken steps to combat the "scariest thing that has ever happened to him." By joining Alcoholics Anonymous, he has accepted responsibility for his addiction—and its treatment.

Mandatory Drug Testing

The topic of mandatory drug testing has certainly been an item of much discussion. From professional athletes to pilots to truck drivers, few people—especially those entrusted with the safety of the general public—have managed to avoid this controversy. More often than not, the rationale for testing has been to avoid the resulting litigation if an accident is caused by an individual under the influence of an illicit drug. And, while reducing a company's exposure to a huge financial insult is indeed an item of concern, it is just the tip of the iceberg. Consider the potential impact to an EMS provider found guilty of causing an accident or of mistreating a patient while under the influence.

We spoke with John Murray, past president of the National Association of EMTs (NAEMT) and currently the director of Travis County EMS in Texas, about his views regarding mandatory drug testing. "If an ambulance is involved in an accident and obvious fault on the part of the ambulance driver is identified," said Murray, "mandatory drug testing could be considered. However, I'm not supportive of arbitrary testing at someone's whim."

Obviously, if drug testing is used for harassment or to simply pry into someone's personal life, the testing takes on an entirely different meaning. How can the public's trust and safety be ensured without violating the rights of the individuals caring for them?

In a recent issue of *Success* magazine, Brian Zevnik, editor-in-chief of the Alexander Hamilton Institute, a New York publishing company, stated, "There is no other area on the corporate front today where lawsuits are filed more frequently and more expensively than in employee privacy." While the legal causes of action run the gamut from discrimination and defamation to wrongful termination, the underlying theme of the litigation remains the same—the employee's right to privacy. The Alexander Hamilton Institute recently published a book titled *Privacy in the Workplace*, which suggests taking the following steps before administering any drug testing.

- Limit testing at hiring to very special situations, such as those in which workers' jobs involve a significant risk to other employees or the public at large.
- Test only when there is strong evidence of abuse, such as impaired job performance.

Box 1.3 (cont.)

bathroom or garage—somewhere alone
- Sudden change in grooming; weight loss
- Excessive use of perfume, aftershave, or breath fresheners to hide odor of alcohol or smoke
- Secretive phone calls

Substance Abuse in Yourself

- Social activities revolve around drinking, smoking, or taking drugs
- You feel better while taking drugs than when sober
- You do things while taking drugs that you would never do when sober (such as taking other drugs, dancing on tables, having extramarital affairs)
- You feel physically bad when you don't get high (withdrawal symptoms), and call in sick more frequently than in the past
- You feel isolated from everyone
- You feel like you have little in common with co-workers, that they are too "square"
- You feel like you can't stop and that you have no control over your drug habits—or your life

Adapted from Gleason, S. C. *Diagnosing Substance Abuse.* 3rd ed. Des Moines, Iowa: Mercy Press, 1986.

- Be certain that the employee is aware that he is being tested specifically for drugs.
- Keep all tests confidential.
- Confirm all positive results by giving the employee an alternate test. Because some of the less expensive drug tests have a high error rate, a more accurate test should be conducted on those who test positively.
- Offer rehabilitation through an employee assistance program to those who test positive. If they refuse, you can take further action.

Using these criteria, what role (if any) is there for drug testing in EMS? We certainly fit into the category of employees who have significant public trust and risk for harm if personnel are impaired. The International Association of Fire Chiefs (IAFC) is a 115-year-old organization that represents fire chiefs throughout the nation. In an interview with Garry Briese, the executive director of the IAFC, he related his organization's policy on drug abuse and testing in the fire service. In addition to discouraging drug use by chiefs and line personnel, the policy makes the following statement regarding drug testing: ". . . the IAFC supports and encourages its member chiefs and fire and related emergency service organizations to establish drug testing programs for entry level and on a regular, periodic, or as-needed basis."

The NAEMT is a much younger organization, which is also acutely concerned with substance abuse among emergency services personnel. While much of the organization's energy has been spent on the type of issues necessary to initiate a credible, respected national organization, NAEMT President Janet Head, RN, MS, REMTA, reports that the NAEMT will be looking at the substance abuse issue "in the near future."

Paying the Price

It's true. There is substance abuse in EMS. And it is probably not going to go away. Like an individual confronting an addiction, recognizing the problem is the first step. To carry the analogy one step further: There are no quick-fix, easy solutions. So we'd better get started.

We have a long way to go. Our colleagues in medicine have excellent mechanisms for detecting abuse, a system for treating it, and access to a number of specialized treatment programs. Currently, we in EMS have few—if any—of these tools in place. But they are available, and we must use them to conquer this problem. In conclusion, Janet Head, the president of NAEMT, said it best: "There should be a two-part approach to substance and alcohol abuse. To begin with, we should take care of the folks who have a problem. We must also develop strategies for preventing the problem from occurring in others."

Acknowledgment

We would like to thank the many people who shared their personal problems, fears, and perspectives on addiction with us. They are among the best in our profession; we commend them for their courage.

References

Dimoff, T. *Substance Free*. Akron, Ohio, 1987.

"Drug Testing Without Abuse." *Success* 28 (October 1987).

Gleason, S. C. *Diagnosing Substance Abuse*. 3rd ed. Des Moines, Iowa: Mercy Press, 1986.

Haugland, S. M. *Alcoholism/Chemical Dependency*. Lecture outline. Des Moines, Iowa: Iowa Methodist Medical Center, 1988.

Haugland, S. M. "Intervention Strategies." *Iowa Medicine* (1986): 113-114.

Naegle, M. A. "Creative Management of Impaired Nursing Practice." *Nursing Administration Quarterly* 9, no. 3 (1985): 15-16.

O'Connor, P., and R. S. Robinson. "Managing Impaired Nurses." *Nursing Administration Quarterly* 9, no. 2 (1985): 1-9.

Talbott, G. D., K. V. Gallegos, and P. O. Wilson, et al. "The Medical Association of Georgia's Impaired Physicians Program: Review of the First 1,000 Physicians." *Journal of the American Medical Association* 257, no. 21 (1982): 2927-2930.

Source

Reprinted with permission from JEMS, May 1988. Scott Bourn, RN, MSN, REMT-P, is president of Scott Bourn Associates, Inc., of Broomfield, Colo. A frequent contributor to JEMS, he is a writer, lecturer, consultant, and educator. He also practices as an emergency nurse at Denver's University Hospital. Michael G. Smith, REMT-P, is director of the paramedic program at Tacoma Community College in Washington. He lectures frequently at national conferences and is the author/editor of "Tricks of the Trade," a regular column in JEMS. He has been a paramedic for more than 17 years.

Case 1

What's a Supervisor to Do?

This "real-life" example is from my own supervisory experience. It illustrates many of the judgment calls supervisors and managers must make in dealing with people and with the human resource policies of an organization.

As you read the case, think about what steps should have, or could have, been taken by an effective supervisor. Reflect on the information presented throughout this section of the book as you answer the questions at the end of the case. Keep in mind that the case questions have no clear-cut right or wrong answers. They are designed to stimulate your thinking process.

—Jay Fitch

Bob HAD BEEN A GOOD EMPLOYEE during his three years with the service. His clinical assessment and judgment skills were excellent. The medical director had recently commended his thoroughness in response to my note about Bob's upcoming performance appraisal. Bob seemed to have good customer service skills and to get along well with his peers. However, in the past three months, a subtle change had taken place.

The shift on duty before Bob's complained, "He is *always* late." When I approached him to informally discuss his tardiness, he was apologetic. He told me he had car problems and was taking his wife to work at the grocery store each morning. He seemed to be genuinely concerned that I mentioned it and promised to do better.

I should have been more specific about my expectations for his future performance, I thought, after the exchange. It was easy to rationalize that I let the issue slide because Bob was such a good employee.

While visiting another station the following day, I inadvertently overheard several crew members discussing Bob. He and another married paramedic apparently had been having an affair, and the other medic had decided to end it. That explains it, I thought. Dragging that emotional baggage to work each day was enough to impact performance. I was sure that my little talk with Bob had set him straight and that he would be on time from now on.

A member of the crew that had complained about Bob's tardiness caught up with me in the hospital parking lot a few weeks later. "I thought you were going to talk to Bob," Jim said. I could tell he was upset and asked, "What's going on?" Jim stonewalled but then said testily, "I told you Bob wasn't showing up on time and you didn't do anything about it."

His partner Alexis walked over and said, "Look, it's not just attendance. Bob's carelessness and personal problems are going to get somebody hurt." Instinct told me something was up, so I probed gently and listened carefully.

Jim and Alexis went on to explain that after they had talked to me several weeks ago, other crew members began to notice things out of place in the trauma kit and airway bag. The oncoming crew told them that several narcotic items were missing when they did their inventory one recent morning. The crew called Bob at home. He was upset but told them not to worry. He had simply forgotten to restock the kit after a late call. Bob told them that he would swing by the trauma center pharmacy and pick up replacements for them. That seemed unusual, but they were extremely busy so they didn't question it.

Bob was at the station when the crew returned. He quickly restocked the kit and, before they could talk with him, the crew received another assignment. The incident made the crew curious. Later, when things were slow, they reviewed the run reports. They were surprised to find that Bob hadn't used any pharmaceuticals on any of his patients the previous three shifts.

This incident was troubling. My mind jumped to three or four negative scenarios, but then I also thought there could be an equal number of rational explanations. I decided to review the investigation algorithm established by the director to guide us in these situations. I headed for the trauma center for a cup of coffee and a few minutes of quiet concentration.

Seeing me walk through the door, the head nurse nodded and said, "We need to talk privately." She told me that one of the staff had reported seeing Bob come out of the trauma room several days earlier with pharmaceuticals. The nurse did not think much about it at the time, but later remembered the incident when a broken seal on the med cart was discovered. Several amps of morphine sulfate were missing. They were sure Bob was responsible. I explained that Bob had some things going on in his personal life, and that we would initiate a formal investigation.

My head started throbbing. It was going to be a difficult day. The head nurse agreed to

provide copies of their internal report, which had already been sent to security and administration. The crew that noticed the missing items were called at home and asked to document the incident and drop the paperwork by the office.

About an hour later, things started to come unglued. Bob showed up at my office door between assignments. He was angry and irrational. He began shouting, "You had no business investigating me and telling the head nurse at the trauma center about my affair." After regaining my composure, I explained that I did not tell the head nurse he was having an affair. I redirected the discussion to the potential theft charges the hospital was considering, and then asked Bob to write an incident report.

Apparently one of the crew members who had been called to write an incident report was a close friend of both Bob and one of the nurses. He called them both to help get everyone's story straight.

Based on the "evidence" and on his irrational behavior, Bob was relieved from duty. When told that there were reasonable grounds to require him to submit to a drug test, he turned white. Then he began to cry uncontrollably.

Bob poured out his story while I listened as non-judgmentally as possible. He had been involved with another medic, and his life came apart when it ended. He began a downward spiral of substance abuse that started with alcohol and sleeping pills and quickly digressed to cocaine and whatever else he could buy or steal. As the conversation went on, he pleaded for his job. "For my family's sake! My wife and kids can't live on her salary from the grocery store," Bob begged.

Frankly, I did not know what to do. There seemed to be grounds to terminate him, but that might only compound the issues. I knew he could not continue to function as a medic. The in-service about the employee assistance program had occurred during my vacation. How did you make a referral to the EAP, anyway?

Other questions came quickly. How would Bob and his family get through this? What was my obligation to Bob as an employee? What was my obligation to the service? If I referred him to the EAP, how would the other medics feel about working with him in the future? Would the medical director continue to extend medical control privileges to Bob, knowing that he had stolen drugs? What was our liability in letting him come back to work? How would we deal with hospital administration and staff? What if this came out in the press? These and hundreds of other questions flashed through my mind as I wrestled with the decision about whether to refer Bob to EAP or simply move toward termination.

After several weeks of in-patient care, Bob was released and entered after-care. It was not an easy road. His family participated in the support group offered by the EAP, and, although it was difficult, they stuck by him. Things at work were rockier. He returned to work after four months. Some of the medics never forgave him for breaking their trust. Others remained angry about the fact that he potentially exposed the service to embarrassment, or worse, to his criminal prosecution.

Within six months, things at work settled down. Bob's life seemed to be back on track. He remained a productive, loyal employee long after I left the organization. Several years ago, Bob attended a management conference where I was speaking. He wasn't sure how to approach me or what to say. After a few minutes of casual conversation, he pulled me aside to tell me how much he appreciated being referred to the EAP. In a low, emotion-filled voice, he told me he had planned his suicide the evening before our conversation that resulted in his referral. I was thankful for Bob and his ongoing contribution to EMS. I was also thankful for the EAP, and the decisions made many years earlier.

Case Questions

1. What policies are in place, or missing, within your organization that might have changed the outcome of this situation?
2. Why didn't management know that Bob was chronically tardy instead of relying on crews to report an infraction? What systems or approaches could be employed to ensure supervisor awareness?
3. What actions, if any, should have been taken against the crew who suspected narcotics were missing but failed to report their suspicions?
4. Was the supervisor's comment to the head nurse about Bob's personal life "out of bounds"? If not, why not? If so, how could the situation have been handled differently?
5. Could the supervisor have limited discussion of the incident by asking the crew members to write the incident report while on duty instead of calling them at home?
6. What course of action would you have taken to explain your actions to your director? The hospital administrator? The press?
7. What was one ethical dilemma the supervisor faced in deciding a course of action?
8. Had Bob not "volunteered" his story, were there enough grounds to terminate him? What are the due process issues involved in this case?

Part Two

Evolving EMS Operations

You cannot step twice into the same place in a river, for waters are continually flowing in.
—Heraclitus

The Greek philosopher Heraclitus might have been speaking about EMS in the 1990s instead of about the world as he saw it 500 years before the common era. Things are "flowing in" at an ever-accelerating pace for the EMS profession. And nowhere is that more evident than in how the EMS system operates.

Modern 9-1-1 emergency service and the increasing use of emergency departments for primary care are multiplying medical transports and creating demands on EMS systems in an era of fiscal constraint. There is no school that teaches how to manage the operational aspects of an EMS system. EMS management requires a combination of hands-on experience and a willingness to learn new ways to accomplish the tasks of the future.

Peter Drucker, a more contemporary leadership philosopher, once stated, "The first test of management competence is productivity." The articles in this section address issues that impact EMS operational productivity. If Heraclitus's statement is a universal truth—and managers and leaders cannot step in the river in the same place—then the authors in this section teach us how to cross the river toward the future while avoiding the deep holes.

—Jay Fitch

Part Two Contents

Understanding Response Times and Planning Resources

EMS Lives or Dies by Response Times

Richard A. Keller

Response times have long been a source of confusion and debate in EMS. Many systems are judged on response time criteria over all other considerations, sometimes unjustly so. In this article, consultant Richard Keller defines response times and explains how to raise the standards of performance.

RIGHT OR WRONG, THE MOST critical measure of an emergency medical service's performance is its response times. Response times are relatively easily quantified and readily understood by the public and the providers. Often this one criteria becomes the sole measure of an organization's performance. However, no single method of measuring response times is accepted and used consistently throughout the country.

EMS response times mean many things to many people. Different starting points are used by various systems, and even the event that stops the clock may differ. Some services start measuring response times from the time the 9-1-1 call is initially answered. Another beginning point for response times is when the 9-1-1 caller or information is transferred to the dispatching center responsible for EMS. Other systems start the response time clock when enough information is gathered to dispatch the appropriate response resources. Still others start the clock when the ambulance crew is initially notified, and some don't begin measuring response times until the unit is actually en route to the scene.

There are almost as many ending points for response time measurements as there are starting points. Some systems stop the clock when the responding unit is in the general vicinity of the incident. Some stop the clock when any responding agency arrives at the scene. Others will not terminate response time measurement until the arrival of ALS resources. Still others require the arrival of a transport-capable ALS unit.

The wide variety of methods used to measure response times distorts any system comparisons. Before comparing one system with another, managers must fully understand what time increments are being measured.

The only relevant response time measurement is from the patient's or victim's perspective. The response time the victim cares about is the time from the onset of the illness or occurrence of the injury until appropriate assistance arrives. EMS systems cannot control the first two increments of this response time: the discovery time and the access time. Discovery time is the time from the occurrence of the event until it is recognized as a medical emergency. The access time is the time from the discovery until the emergency response system is accessed or 9-1-1 is called.

The Increments of Response Time

For EMS systems, the only definition of response time should be from the time the 9-1-1 telephone is answered until appropriate resources arrive at the scene of the emergency. This response time consists of at lease five increments. The first increment starts when the 9-1-1 call is answered and ends when it is identified as an emergency medical incident. This increment is known as the call evaluation. The second increment can be termed caller interrogation. At this point, definitive details regarding the incident, such as location, severity, etc., are elicited from the caller. This period begins when an event is identified as needing emergency medical resources and ends when the decision to dispatch units has been made. The next increment is the unit dispatch time, which is when the resources to be dispatched are identified and notified. These first three increments—call evaluation, caller interrogation, and unit dispatch time—compose the system dispatch time.

The fourth increment is called the "launch time," or is sometimes referred to as the "out-of-chute time." It begins when dispatch notifies the unit to respond and ends when the unit begins progressing toward the scene. The launch time combined with the system dispatch time composes the unit activation time. The fifth time increment is the en route time and begins when the ambulance or EMS unit begins to respond and ends when it arrives at the scene. Some systems go so far as to add a patient access time, which is the length of time from the unit's arrival at the scene until the patient is actually accessed. The sum of all these increments will provide the true EMS response time.

Measuring Response Time

Defining the components to be measured in EMS response times is the first step in documenting performance. But just as important as defining the time increments is deciding how to report response time information. The predominant response time reporting method is the average measurement method. In this method, all the response times for all the incidents or a particular category of incidents are accumulated, and the average is calculated. This average response time is reported for the EMS system.

An alternative method of reporting response times is the fractile measurement method, also known as the percentage compliance method. In this performance indicator, a defined goal or standard is used for the response time. For example, the goal or standard of a system could be 10 minutes for emergency requests. Once the goal or standard has been decided on, a percentage is identified as the compliance level for the service.

> Defining the components to be measured in EMS response times is the first step in documenting performance.

The most commonly used compliance percentages are 90 and 95 percent. Thus, 90 (or 95) percent of the emergency calls should be responded to within 10 minutes. A system would report its percentage compliance level toward the standard. On a month-to-month basis, the percentage of compliance will vary. For example, in one month, 91.6 percent of the emergencies may be responded to within 10 minutes, while in the next month, 92.3 percent of the emergencies may be responded to in that time frame.

Adapting the Percentage Compliance Method

It is much more difficult to achieve 90-percent compliance with a 10-minute emergency response standard than it is to achieve a response time average of 10 minutes.

This makes it difficult for many systems to transition from one response time measurement methodology to another. For example, if a system with an average response time of 8.62 minutes decides to change to the percentage compliance method with a standard of 90 percent within 10 minutes, its performance is going to be viewed as worse in the public's mind. In reality, the average of 8.62 minutes translates to only a 71.9-percent compliance with the 10-minute standard.

The best way to change an 8.62-minute average response time to the percentage compliance method is in phases. In other words, a system can work toward complying first with a standard of 12 minutes and then with a standard of 10 minutes. The goal of the phased-in upgrade is to ultimately achieve 90-percent compliance within 10 minutes. The two phases identify the estimated impact that meeting increasingly stringent compliance standards has on the average response time. In the phase one upgrade, when the service achieves a 90 percent compliance within 12 minutes, the average response time decreases to 7.71 minutes. In the phase two upgrade, when the service achieves a 90 percent response time within 10 minutes, the average response time decreases further to approximately 6.88 minutes.

Figure 2.1 identifies the actual measure of response times on an average basis. The figure demonstrates the percentage of calls that are responded to within a given number of minutes. The black graph line is the projected percentage of calls for a given response time that would occur if the system were to adopt and achieve a standard of 90 percent compliance within eight minutes.

EMS management needs all the information that can be collected to aid in the identi-

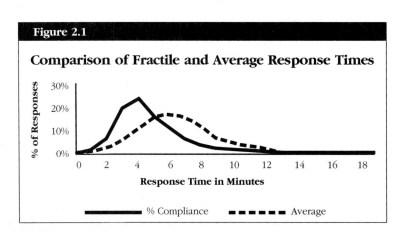

Figure 2.1

Comparison of Fractile and Average Response Times

% of Responses

Response Time in Minutes

———— % Compliance   ▪ ▪ ▪ ▪ ▪ Average

Table 2.1

Response Times in Selected Communities

City	Population	Provider Type	Response Time Average	Fractal Measures Used	Response Times Mandated	How Measured
Houston	1,630,553	FD-cross-trained	5.2 minutes	No	No	Disp-arrive
Phoenix	983,403	FD-cross-trained	4.6 minutes	Yes	No	Disp-arrive
Los Angeles	3,485,398	FD-cross-trained	6.3 minutes	Yes	No	Call receipt-arrive
Philadelphia	1,585,577	FD-cross-trained	8.0 minutes	Yes	No	Call receipt-arrive
Detroit	1,027,974	FD-separate service	6.3 minutes	No	No	Call receipt-arrive
San Antonio	935,933	FD-cross-trained	5.6 minutes	Yes	No	Disp-arrive
San Diego	1,110,549	Private Service	6.0 minutes	Yes	Yes	Transfer by PSAP-arrive

Table 2.2

Public Utility Models

All times are mandated and are measured from receipt of call to arrival at scene.

City	Population	Life-Threatening Emergency Response Time Standard 90% Within	Non-Life-Threatening Emergency Response Time Standard 90% Within	Compliant
Ft. Wayne, Ind.	304,000	8:30	10:30	Yes
Richmond, Va.	210,000	8:59	12:59	Yes
Reno, Nev.	260,000	8:30	12:30	Yes
Pinellas County, Fla.	900,000	10:00	10:00	Yes
Ft. Worth, Tex.	535,204	8:59	10:00	Yes
Kansas City, Mo.	435,146	8:59	12:59	Yes
Tulsa/Oklahoma City, Okla.	1,000,000	8:00	12:00	Yes

fication of strategies to achieve performance improvement. Statistically, the two most valid pieces of information used in response time measurements are the medium response time (in other words the midpoint of all response times) and the percentage compliance measurement. The average response time alone does not provide enough information to make adequate deployment and staffing decisions.

Tables 2.1 and 2.2 include the results of a telephone survey conducted in 1993 to determine how various cities measured and publicly reported response times. The first figure includes systems that measure on an average response time basis, and the second figure includes public utility models, which contractually mandate a percentage compliance within a given standard. The particular standards are identified for the seven communities.

It is important that EMS systems clearly define the entire EMS response time for measurement and reporting. The system should establish realistic response time standards as measured on a percentage compliance basis. Regular reporting of these key performance indicators should occur in order to define realistic expectations in the community and to monitor the provider's performance.

Source

Original article. Richard A. Keller is a partner at Fitch & Associates, Inc. He is nationally known for his work in EMS system operations, reimbursement, and design. He is a principal author of the book EMS Management: Beyond the Street, *2nd ed.*

System Status Management: The Strategy of Ambulance Placement

Jack Stout

System status management can be a formal or informal system of determining where your EMS resources should be. Former EMS consultant Jack Stout coined the phrase to describe a process that every system has but doesn't always know how to use. This landmark article established the criteria for understanding the basics of system status management.

SOME OF THE MOST EARTH-SHAKING concepts seem merely interesting when they first emerge into view. Some go nearly unnoticed. The force and impact of the idea may change our lives without us ever knowing that the particular idea was what did it.

The well-known Eisenberg studies certainly caught our attention, but did you know that those studies are subtly but powerfully impacting the very structure of the ambulance industry? Legally imposed response time standards are no longer arbitrary or entirely subjective. The courts are upholding ordinances with stringent response time requirements based, in part, on the Eisenberg studies. The right of private ambulance companies, or public agencies for that matter, to deliver life-threatening response times has been seriously weakened. The life expectancies of low-performance ambulance organizations, and even entire classes of ambulance systems, have been dramatically shortened by the new knowledge. Almost unnoticed, these forces have been set in motion.

In the February 1983 issue of *Medical Care*, Dr. C. Gene Cayten and others upped the ante even further with the publication of a research project summary entitled, "Clinical Algorithms for Prehospital Cardiac Care." This article, perhaps with less fanfare than the Eisenberg studies, is another blockbuster. Whether an EMS system should go to the trouble of developing and documenting detailed step-by-step procedures for patient care instead of relying more heavily on paramedics and medical control physicians to "invent" algorithms on the spot used to be a matter of "professional preference." While the debate is bound to go on, Cayten's evidence is on the side of planned and documented clinical procedure.

As our infant industry matures, we are learning that some ways are better than others, and that everything isn't a matter of opinion. Eisenberg showed us that, for certain patient conditions, both fast BLS and slow ALS are deadly. Dr. Cayten and his colleagues have shown us that well-documented clinical algorithms not only help paramedics retain their technical skills, but actually can be traced with statistical significance to changes in patient outcome.

Gradually, we are learning what some have suspected all along. Life-saving system performance is hard to come by. Smart people with good intentions and expensive equipment are not enough. Our business is more like pro football, guerrilla warfare, or heavy weather sailing; all depend upon recognizing that a variety of events are going to happen very quickly, that your responses to those events must be perfectly selected and executed, and that you can't possibly predict what's really going to happen. Then, you try to predict everything that could happen anyway, figure out what you would do if it did happen, write it down, think it through, prepare yourself, and practice, practice, practice. When things do start happening, you hope most of what you do goes according to plan, leaving you and your crew free to concentrate your intelligence and creativity on a limited and more manageable set of unforeseen circumstances.

The concept common to all of these activities is the goal of reducing, as much as possible, the need to invent protocols and procedures on the spot. Think it through before it happens. Plan the response while the pressure is off, while the advice of others is available, and while mistakes can be made and corrected in the hypothetical—not in a ditch under a car in a foot of water covered with a shiny film of gasoline.

And practice. Cayten noticed that the number of paramedics treating the patient influenced patient outcome, and he had to adjust the analysis to account for this and other variables. But having lots of paramedics at the scene doesn't automatically help the patient. You can't outnumber an attack of ventricular fibrillation. Paramedics make a better team when they all know what's going on, what's next, and how to help. But how many two-tiered systems have even written down, much less practiced, team task descriptions and protocols so that BLS crews know how to really join the team when assisting an ALS crew?

High Performance in Dispatch

The term "dispatcher" is used in the commercial trucking industry and the taxicab industry, and it defines the job of the 18-year-old clerk who sends out the Xerox repair man, the plumber, or the exterminator crew. Back when "as soon as we can, ma'am" was soon enough—the same era when "in the best of hands" and "all that could be done was done" were the measures of good medical care—dispatchers dispatched ambulances, too.

But just as we are learning that highly ordered and practiced action in the field makes for better management of patient care, we are also beginning to learn that the management of the entire system can be dramatically improved by similar refinements in the control center.

I remember a conversation I once had with an experienced dispatcher in a large urban system. I was watching the operation of the dispatch center late one night when I heard the dispatcher say to a telephone caller, "What is your telephone number?" Later, I asked the dispatcher if the caller was phoning from the caller's own home. The answer was "no." The dispatcher had asked, literally, for the caller's own phone number. What the dispatcher wanted to know was the callback number. I suggested that if he wanted to know what number the caller was calling from, he should say, "What number are you calling from?" No other words are as good.

There still exist throughout the country major ambulance service systems, some even ALS, where the conversation between the dispatcher and the caller is more like a chat than anything else. Each dispatcher has

> Paramedics make a better team when they all know what's going on, what's next, and how to help.

System status management refers to the formal or informal systems, protocols, and procedures that determine where the remaining ambulances will be when the next call comes in.

his own approach to the conversation—a far cry from the orderly and reliable telephone protocols (i.e., information-gathering algorithms) of Dr. Jeff Clawson's Salt Lake City Fire Department operation.

Sloppy and extemporaneous telephone protocols generate misunderstanding, faulty information, and missing information, yet the system's entire initial response is based on that information.

In some better managed EMS systems, medically trained dispatchers employ clinically sound and thoroughly thought-out telephone protocols to gather information and to provide the caller with pre-arrival instructions. In multi-tiered response systems, these same protocols guide the selection of ambulances and first responder units. But what about the management of the system itself—the system whose configuration when the phone rings can often make the critical difference? What about the management of system status?

System status management refers to the formal or informal systems, protocols, and procedures that determine where the remaining ambulances will be when the next call comes in. Whether formal or informal, elaborate or simple, written or remembered, every system has a "system status management plan." But does your system status management plan make sense and does it work?

Effective Unit Hour Utilization

Every ambulance system can afford to place only a limited number of ambulances on the street. Because ambulance demand patterns usually follow a weekly cycle, I like to think in terms of "unit hours per week." A "unit hour" is simply a fully equipped and manned ambulance on the street for one hour. A dispatcher trying to match supply with demand must utilize the available "unit hours" in the best way he can to squeeze the highest response time performance possible out of the unit hours available.

At the most basic level, there are two extreme forms of unit hour deployment. At one extreme, the system could run the average number of unit hours available per week all the time, i.e., the same number of ambulances on the streets 24 hours a day, seven days a week. At the other extreme, but not much more foolish, the system could put all the unit hours on the street at the same time for one hour, if it owned that many ambulances.

Since all of the calls don't come in during one hour a week, it would obviously be stupid to use up all of the precious unit hours during one 60-minute period each week. However, demand for ambulance service fluctuates wildly by time of day and day of week, so it wouldn't be much more intelligent to run the same number of units all the time. Somewhere in between is a solution that makes sense. The Demand Analysis Report for Kansas City, Mo., (from the American Ambulance Abstract Service—AAAS) illustrates the normal and unusual patterns of fluctuation, by time of day and day of week, for life-threatening emergency calls, non-life-threatening emergency calls, and non-emergency calls for all the Thursdays for four months ending December 1982.

Taking surplus unit hours off the street when they aren't needed and adding these unit hours during times of overload or wild fluctuation makes sense. But the question of where to put these ambulances remains. If you assume that the geographic pattern of demand is fairly constant, or completely random, chances are you will be wrong, and from some patients' perspectives, dead wrong.

Every ambulance system has a strategy for placing its ambulances, ranging from the Pollyanna approach of giving every ambulance a permanent "home base" and leaving it there except when dispatched, to automated deployment systems, which use different deployment plans for each hour of the day and each day of the week, complete with mini-deployment plans within each hour depending on the number of ambulances then left available in the system.

Maps A and B in Figure 2.2 show the locations of all emergency requests in Tulsa, Okla., over a period of several weeks. The difference is that Map A shows the geographic emergency demand pattern between 9 a.m. and 10 a.m. Thursdays while Map B shows the geographic demand patterns just one hour later on the same day of the week. (This is not a computer model, but rather an actual plot of real emergencies experienced by real patients.)

A "G" on the maps represents a life-threatening emergency where the system responded in eight minutes or less. A "B" (i.e., bad) on the map represents a life-threatening emergency with a response time over eight minutes. An "O" means a non-life-threatening emergency with a response time under 10 minutes, while a "P" (i.e., poor) refers to a non-life-threatening emergency with a response time over 10 minutes.

Notice that during Hour 10 on Thursdays, activity concentrates heavily along the west end of Skelly Drive, with scattered activity in the south-central part of the city, while almost nothing happens up north.

Now compare that with what goes on during Hour 11. There is not much happening on Skelly Drive, but you'd better be ready to head north. You can't cover the north, however, at the expense of the near south.

Maps A and B show how different things look in the same city, on the same day, just an hour apart. Now let's look at the same hour (i.e., Hour 10, 9 a.m. to 10 a.m.) on Fridays. Map C in Figure 2.2 shows the plan that

Figure 2.2

Emergency Demand Patterns

Response Time Limits
(call received to arrival):

Priority 1: G=0–8 min.   B=9 and over min.
Priority 2: O=0–10 min.   P=11 and over min.

Map A: For Day 4—Thursday; for Hour 10

Map B: For Day 4—Thursday; for Hour 11

Map C: For Day 5—Friday; for Hour 10

worked for Hour 10 on Thursdays will be absolutely wrong for Hour 10 on Fridays. Hour 10 on Friday is not only tougher geographically, but Tulsa's Demand Analysis Report (not shown) also tells us that this geographically scattered demand will fluctuate in volume as well. Hour 10 on Fridays is expensive to cover, revenues are mediocre, and the crews must be moved around more than usual to keep things covered.

A more sophisticated system status plan is simply a plan for dealing with different demand patterns by basing the around-the-clock deployment of unit hours and the geographic deployment of remaining units available upon the historical, geographical, and time-of-day fluctuations in demand patterns. Of course, for some hours in some areas, there is almost no pattern to be found. The "O's," "B's," "P's," and "G's" are scattered, and demand volumes hit everywhere except on the average. But this, too, is a type of pattern—the toughest of all to deal with. We are forced to get out the checkbook, spread out our units, and when the last unit is all we've got, park it near a freeway exchange where it can't get to any location very fast but can cover the whole city with some reliability.

When I go through this process, I get my latest AAAS maps and demand analyses, along with several other useful reports, and sit down with the most experienced dispatchers and street people I can find. I show them the maps and the demand analyses for one hour of the day, one day of the week, and ask them the following question: "Knowing the frequency and fluctuation of demand for this hour, and seeing the maps of historical demand and response time performance, if you only had one ambulance left in the system, where would you like it to be located?"

This, as it turns out, is an amazing question. The "system status committee" may often argue and struggle for some time to come up with an answer. They pick a spot and then someone notices that, at that time of day, the ambulance would be upstream of the hotspot, and in rush-hour traffic. Someone else notices that another location would be downstream from traffic relative to a potential hotspot, but would have a difficult time reaching the occasional call on the other side of the city. But notice carefully: If it takes this much analysis and discussion to make the decision when the pressure is off, when all the data is available, and when the most experienced people in town are making the decision, how on earth does anyone think a single dispatcher, under pressure, with no time, limited information, and six calls in progress, is going to do any better?

When we are finished figuring out where one ambulance should be if it's the only one left and it's 4:30 p.m. on a Friday, I ask what should be done if there are two ambulances left, then three, then four, and so on.

Then we figure out, at each level of remaining capability, which ambulance posts have the lowest priority, and should therefore be used for dispatching non-emergency calls. This effort helps to preserve the best possible remaining coverage while minimizing post-to-post moves.

We also recheck the demand fluctuation for that hour, and ask ourselves what level of vehicle coverage is so low that non-emergency dispatches should be suspended until another unit comes back into service. Finally, we "make a wish" as to how many ambulances we think would be necessary for safe and effective coverage during that hour of the day on that day of the week—i.e., how many "unit hours" shall we "spend" on this one of 168 hours of the week?

When this is done, we move on to the next hour. Another 167 "plans" later, we have a pretty good idea of what the best and most experienced dispatchers and street people in the system think should be done. We find some hours in which the volume of demand fluctuates wildly and the geographic distribution takes on no pattern at all. During these hours, we know coverage will be expensive and difficult; we will have to make up for the losses somewhere else.

We also find hours where demand volume is highly predictable and where geographic patterning is relatively concentrated. During these hours, coverage is easier to achieve. And, if the system depends heavily on fee-for-service revenues, the "profits" made during that hour will help cover the "losses" incurred in other hours.

If the whole thing sounds difficult, boring, frustrating, and not worth the effort, you are beginning to understand. High performance is hard to come by unless money and "unit hours" are no object. Even with a blank check on unit hours, real high performance may still elude a system. In any case, when we are finished with the process, everything is written down and displayed in a flip chart or entered into a computer programmed as a system status management aid (i.e., Micad or Minicad). The result is the beginning of a "system status plan."

When complete, this plan serves dispatchers as a sort of algorithm for on-line management of system deployment, just like a clinical algorithm guides a field paramedic. It minimizes seat-of-the-pants redeployment, and benefits from the experiences of many instead of a few. Perhaps best of all, its effectiveness can be measured and evaluated, and the plan can be continually improved and fine-tuned. As long as every dispatcher does his own thing, there is no "plan" to evaluate—only dispatchers.

Every System Has a Plan, However Silly It May Be

Before we first began our work in Kansas City, the plan then in use, though not written down anywhere, went something like this. . . .

There will be 14 ambulances on the street, 24 hours a day, seven days a week, for a total of 2,352 unit hours of coverage a week. Every ambulance crew shall be on a 24/48-hour shift, shall show up for work at a permanently assigned ambulance post, and shall relieve the crew on duty either on time or whenever that crew returns to its post. There shall be no rules governing suspension of non-emergency transfer work or out-of-town dispatches. If there are 13 calls in progress and only one ambulance left in the system, it's acceptable to send the last ambulance out of town or to a non-emergency transfer call, even though the emergency load may be about to peak. Furthermore, if the only ambulances left in the system are stationed at the most remote and least active posts, while all the other ambulance crews in the system are working their tails off, it won't be necessary to relocate any of the remaining ambulances, especially if it is late at night and the outlying crews are asleep. Finally, whenever any ambulance completes a run, its crew shall return to its permanently assigned post, regardless of whatever else may be going on in the system at the time. If a dispatcher would like to experiment from time to time by relocating ambulances during a shift, no rules will prevent and no policies will guide such experimentation. If the crews get mad because of the inconvenience or if the fuel bill rises noticeably, who knows what will happen.

The multi-million dollar ambulance company that used this plan is now out of business. But this "plan" is not all that uncommon. It is easy to see why systems using system status plans like Kansas City's now-discarded plan usually don't write them down. This plan and variations on its theme, had been used in Kansas City for years, even in the presence of a million-dollar-plus federal grant to centralize dispatching of the old multiple provider system.

Most systems use formal or informal plans that lie somewhere in between the old Kansas City model and the most sophisticated models. Unfortunately, most are far closer to the old Kansas City model than to the higher performance end of the spectrum.

Deployment Isn't Everything

Our first experience with really sophisticated system status management was the result of being squeezed between a stringent city-imposed response time requirement and an increase in union wages of several hundred thousand dollars. Revenues were fixed, costs were going up, and response time performance *had* to be maintained. We had no choice except to squeeze more performance out of fewer unit hours per week.

Our second experience with system status management occurred when we were asked to help a system equalize an otherwise good response time record throughout various neighborhoods of the city. An effective and primarily black consumer group demanded an investigation of that system's response time performance in the poorer neighborhoods of the community. We were initially called in to perform that investigation, and the data showed that while the black community was receiving comparatively good response time performance, it could have been better. But surprisingly, there was a remote and wealthy neighborhood experiencing chronic response time performance problems. It seemed to us that response time performance could be better equalized throughout all areas of the city using some of the deployment and management techniques we had recently developed elsewhere.

We went through the whole process with dispatchers and field people, and after some reshuffling of crews, posts, and shifts, a new system status plan was installed. The result was an improvement in overall response times, and an even greater improvement in equality of performance throughout the city. (That system had focused its attention, partly by the ordinance, on average response time performance—a practice we now know results in more life-threatening response times for patients at the dangerous end of the distribution curve, and also promotes geographic inequity in response time performance.)

Everyone was generally pleased with the initial results, and after a few months of operating with the new system, fine-tuning began. Using more AAAS maps and reports, we began to identify problem times of day and neighborhoods that needed extra attention. We started by locating areas and times of day where we apparently had surplus production capacity. (AAAS "solution maps" highlight areas and times/days where response times are unusually fast and where the eight-minute maximum is virtually never exceeded. The purpose is to locate surplus unit hours that can be reassigned either geographically or by time of day to cover peaks and overload conditions.)

As we proceeded with this fine-tuning process, we ran into some really stubborn performance problems that didn't seem to be solved by any amount of ambulance coverage. Looking more closely at the records of these specific runs, we began to learn that the problem wasn't always a lack of ambulances, or even a lack of *nearby* ambulances.

With the help of our Micad computer aid, we were able to recreate a record of the status of the system at the time any given call came in. That is, we could produce a report that told us, for example, that when the problem call came in at 12:35 a.m., there were seven ambulances in the system, one with mechanical problems, two on emergency calls, one on a non-emergency call, and the remaining three ambulances available for dispatch—one at Post 12, one at Post 13, and one en route from County Hospital to Post 3. With that kind of information available to us, we could then take a look at the dispatcher's vehicle selection and the conformance of the system with the original plan. When we were short of ambulances when a call came in, we could begin to find out why.

Sometimes the problem was simply a lack of sufficient ambulances to achieve coverage or the placement of remaining ambulances in the wrong locations, but not always. We began to identify a whole list of factors that impacted response time performance, some of which cost money to deal with, but most of which did not.

If money is no object and you have a response time performance problem in some neighborhood or during some time of day or day of the week, you can simply buy another ambulance, hire another crew, and add another "unit hour" at the right time and place. Sometimes that will solve your problem, and sometimes it won't.

Ambulance system response time performance is not good or bad, in general. If you are having response time problems, they are almost

Ambulance system response time performance is not good or bad, in general. If you are having response time problems, they are almost always occurring at some times of the day or days of the week but not at others, and problems often repeat themselves in fairly predictable geographic patterns.

always occurring at some times of the day or days of the week but not at others, and problems often repeat themselves in fairly predictable geographic patterns. These patterns are obscured by the fact that *where* the response time problem is occurring will change depending on *when* it is happening. Since only a handful of systems have a way of combining and displaying this information for analysis, and since most systems rely heavily on averages, few of us have learned to see response time problems in a diagnostically useful way.

If I have no prospect of increasing system costs to solve the problem, then I must exhaust every possibility for solving the problem before I resort to adding equipment and crews, or even to going through the hassle of revising schedules and shift assignments. I must first pinpoint the time and location of the problem, and then proceed to diagnose the causes. Only then can I devise a solution. The process I use relies extensively upon statistical information from the AAAS reporting service, and I follow a step-by-step path that is too lengthy to be detailed here. However, several of the most productive steps can be described as follows:

Define the problem specifically. I must know exactly when and where the response time problem is occurring before I can begin to diagnose it. Is there a pattern?

Bonafide system overload? Was the dispatcher out of ambulances when the call came in? Were the available ambulances too far away? If so, why? Where were all the other ambulances at the time, and what were they doing?

Plan followed or violated? Did the problem occur because the system status plan is faulty or because the plan wasn't being followed?

Dispatcher error? Was the nearest ambulance dispatched? Were the routing instructions accurate? Is the crew or dispatcher unfamiliar with that neighborhood? One AAAS report analyzes response time performance by *dispatcher* by district or neighborhood to detect performance problems that may be the result of a given dispatcher's lack of familiarity with a specific neighborhood. For example, white dispatchers may spend less time in black neighborhoods than in other parts of the city, and therefore be less familiar with primarily black neighborhoods. If that is the problem, no amount of extra ambulances will solve it.

Are unit hours being wasted? Even though plenty of ambulances are on duty at that hour given the number of calls received, is availability still lacking for some reason? A report from the AAAS was designed to detect hospitals whose methods of receiving patients excessively delay ambulance crews. As a result of this particular report, a "uniform hospital drop policy" may be developed and adopted by all hospitals, reducing unnecessary out-of-service time to the tune of thousands of dollars in lost unit hours per year.

Another report analyzes hospital drop time by senior paramedic. There is no "right" time at the scene, and there is no "right" hospital drop time either. Every call is different. But when you are looking at 40 or 50 runs per medic, and one medic averages twice as long at the hospital as everyone else in the company, it's worth a conversation. Most medics in our systems are used to these reports, and posting alone seems to do the trick. But the first time we ran these reports, the numbers were all over the place.

If you think all hospitals are about the same in hospital drop times, think again. In one city, we found a hospital that averaged triple delays in drop times, no matter who the medics were. This added up to over $150,000 per year in lost unit hours due to that hospital's methods of accepting patients. Other AAAS reports detect bad habits that hurt system performance. I call one report the "paramedic honey locator" report, since it can detect a paramedic who is normally fast in hospital turnaround time, but who routinely takes longer at a particular hospital that is normally fast for everyone else. I presume the presence of a "honey."

Equipment failure? Are the units plagued by equipment failures? How long does it take to get a unit back in service? How often does one ambulance assist another because the latter's cardiac monitor won't work, etc.?

Demand pattern change? Has the demand pattern begun to change for this location and time of day or day of week? Is there a seasonal fluctuation that we can prepare for? Was there a special event that we failed to account for?

Traffic flow problem? Were the units upstream when they should have been downstream?

Out-of-chute time? One standard AAAS report routinely displays average times from unit alert to en route status, organized by senior paramedic name and number. For life-threatening calls, this time should be under 30 seconds on the average, and never over one minute. Lost time leaving the chute can never be made up, no matter what you do. In one case, we found what should have been obvious to everyone—an ambulance post location where the crew quarters were on the second floor and at the other end of the hall from where the ambulance was parked. We moved the crew quarters and solved the problem. Sometimes our work isn't very sophisticated.

Dangerous non-emergency cutoff level? Is the problem repeatedly happening when several non-emergency transfer runs are in progress? Could the problem be fixed by simply raising the non-emergency cutoff point to a safer level?

Change post locations? Could we solve the problem simply by moving an existing ambulance from a less frequently utilized post location into the problem area? This is the simplest move, since it requires no reshuffling of shift schedules. However, care must be taken since you may simply relocate the response time problem to the other side of town. The AAAS solution maps help make this decision by locating neighborhoods where problems rarely occur and where response times are extra rapid. We will deliberately adjust the system to eliminate emergency re-

When a system begins to implement system status management, the past plan of deployment is normally so poorly documented, poorly conceived, poorly followed, or all three, that it makes no sense to use the past system as a basis for refinement.

sponse times over eight minutes, even if doing so results in a slight increase in either overall *average* response times or slightly decreased coverage in an apparently over-served neighborhood.

When a system begins to implement system status management, the past plan of deployment is normally so poorly documented, poorly conceived, poorly followed, or all three, that it makes no sense to use the past system as a basis for refinement. Most of the time, you can do better by simply abandoning the past structure in favor of an initial system status plan developed by your most experienced dispatch and field personnel, utilizing the process discussed earlier in this article, together with the essential displays of demand pattern history.

Every time we have tossed out an old deployment plan and replaced it with a new system status plan, the improvement has been instantaneous and dramatic. For example, Kansas City (a 100-percent paramedic system providing both emergency and non-emergency work) has managed consistent improvements in response time performance, both citywide and by the city's mandated councilmatic districts, while shrinking unit hours per week to 1,600 hours.

The system had to drastically cut either unit hours or wages, due to a declining city subsidy and a badly needed, commercially financed $2.5 million total equipment replacement. In that city, late runs cost the operator $10 per minute in payment deductions, and chronic late runs would cost the entire contract. Under such circumstances, performance is almost inevitable, or at least mandatory.

Implementation of the first sophisticated system status plan (SSP) usually requires a major reshuffling of ambulance post locations, shift schedules, compensation plans, crew change methods, inventory control, and just about everything else that is sacred in an established ambulance service. This reshuffling can be traumatic.

Furthermore, during the earlier stages of the plan, there will be quite a few seemingly unnecessary post-to-post vehicle movements, mostly occurring in the middle of the night when a 24-hour crew is trying to sleep. Dispatchers will tend to delay a post-to-post move if another crew is nearly ready to clear from a hospital. If these delays are too frequent, the SSP isn't being tested at all. The result might be that you finish a difficult two or three months of initial experience only to find out that you have not actually implemented the SSP. You can't be sure whether the problems you are still having are the result of the SSP or the result of not following the SSP. If you don't follow the SSP, you can't fine-tune it.

Fine-tuning your system status plan is, I think, fun. In the first round of planning, everything was based on the expert judgment and prediction of the most experienced people available, with benefit of detailed demand maps and demand analyses. The second time around, adjustments to the plan can be based on the initial plan's actual results.

During fine-tuning, you can shift some posts around, shift some unit hours around, and take numerous steps to simultaneously reduce unnecessary post-to-post movement while squeezing out any remaining performance problems.

In most systems, you will need about three months of data per fine-tuning cycle, which means that you must stick with the current plan as closely as possible. Of course, the initial plan should be watched very closely during the first few weeks to detect any obvious flaws that may need mid-course correction. In this case, it is good to "stay the course," but not at all costs. If a mid-course change is necessary, the important thing is for it to take the form of a change in the plan—not an authorized departure from the plan. That way, subsequent data can be used to assess the effectiveness of the revised plan—not the old plan that was abandoned.

With enough time and experience, and enough quarterly fine-tuning efforts, the plan will begin to take on seasonal variations, and will account for special events such as the Fourth of July, Christmas, New Year's, and Rolling Stones concerts. After a year or so of development and fine-tuning, you will have squeezed, poked, and prodded all of the performance you can out of your system, at least in terms of response time performance per unit hour. From then on, small semi-annual adjustments should do the trick, and probably without fanfare or too much gnashing of teeth.

The reality of instituting sophisticated system status management is considerably harder than you might think. Dispatcher duties and responsibilities are more than doubled. Dispatchers of moderate ability will not survive. (The new job is so different that we hate to call these people "dispatchers"; we prefer "system status managers.") The dispatcher training program must involve extensive off-line simulations. Our system status manager certification test covers Salt Lake City-type telephone protocols, medical vocabulary, and a compressed 200-run system simulation covering every conceivable complication. Certification requires zero-defect performance.

We have had to completely overhaul labor contracts and shift schedules, compensation programs, and bonus plans. We adapted a shift bid process from the way TWA bids flights for flight attendants.

We use eight-hour shifts, 10-hours shifts, 12-hours shifts, 24/48 shifts, and hybrids. In one city, a strike nearly occurred due to the loss of some 24/48 shifts, while in another, labor got mad because some eight-hour shifts were being lost to 24/48. In another case, crews had actually purchased homes near their permanently assigned posts. We eliminated permanent post assignments.

But the ultimate purpose of sophisticated system status management is very simple: We want our ambulance crews and equipment to be located where and when they are needed as often as humanly possible.

> The ultimate purpose of sophisticated system status management is very simple: We want our ambulance crews and equipment to be located where and when they are needed as often as humanly possible.

Failure Guaranteed Four Ways

If system status management is such hot stuff, where has it been all

System status
management, done
properly, takes a
whole lot of work,
requires constant
attention, may strain
labor relations, and
is really easy to
screw up.

this time? The uncomfortable but grownup answer is that organizations learn to do what makes money or what it takes to survive. You can count on one hand all the cities that fine their ambulance providers for poor response time performance. Government operations almost never compete for survival, and there's always the average response time to hide behind.

System status management, done properly, takes a whole lot of work, requires constant attention, may strain labor relations, and is really easy to screw up. No wonder no one developed it until they had to.

There are probably hundreds of ways to prove that system status management won't work in any city. But there are four ways that are guaranteed to make it fail.

Try buying part of it. An organization will make system status management work when its financial stability and very existence depend upon it. Under any other conditions, system status management is just too much trouble. If you really want good system status management, turn over your dispatching and field operations to a qualified operator, hold that operator financially accountable for every late run, forget average response times and focus on maximums, and be ready to bury the operator for chronic performance failure. Then forget about system status management, and you will get it.

As I always say when asked by private ambulance operators how the city wants the dispatching done, no one cares how many ambulances you put on the street, how you dispatch them, or what you do with the money the city pays to you. When the phone rings, the city wants a qualified paramedic talking to the caller, a full-blown paramedic ambulance on the scene within eight minutes 90 percent of the time, and superb equipment and performance, and it doesn't care how you do it. If you can put a guru on a hill who can get two ambulances to handle thirty thousand calls a year, go for it. But screw up a little, and it's 10 bucks a minute. Screw up a lot, and you're out of business.

Separate dispatching from operations. The absolute key to system status management is the operation of the dispatch center and the quality of dispatch personnel. The company that does the dispatching and the company that runs the ambulance have got to be the same company, and it's that company that must be responsible for developing, revising, and implementing the system status plan. It's just too complicated to work any other way. If you think it isn't that complicated, then you clearly don't understand, and you will probably never know what went wrong.

Try it with employees who care little about their patients and less about their company. People get used to the old ways. Low performance is less work than high performance. I know for a fact there are ambulance personnel who have deliberately delayed an emergency response for the sole purpose of "proving" that the new plan won't work and that more unit hours are needed. These people are, perhaps without realizing it, dedicated to their company's failure. And they will jeopardize their patients to make a point.

These are the same people who, rather than helping to work out the bugs, wag their fingers at dispatcher error, make anonymous calls to reporters in hopes of making their company and its effort to improve performance look foolish, and were recently caught driving 35 mph, with red lights and siren on, in light traffic on an open road on the way to an emergency. If you have such people in your company, you have a choice: Get rid of them or cater to them. As long as they are on your payroll, they have the power to prove you wrong. I have seen them do it.

Try computer simulation. I do not recommend or support the use of computer simulation models to determine ambulance coverage patterns and post locations. Such models rely too heavily on theoretical travel times to optimize distribution. Our experience has convinced us that a committee of experienced dispatchers and street people can out-perform a computer simulation every time if they are provided with the demand pattern statistics, demand maps, and other informational tools. These tools combined with human judgment and experience can take into consideration traffic flow patterns, complex street names or number-ing systems, familiarity with areas, and a hundred other factors that go far beyond the scope of practical computer simulation.

Conclusion

When thinking about system status management, keep in mind that regardless of how you staff and deploy your ambulances, you are using a system status plan. System status management isn't good or bad—it is inevitable. Your plan may be simple and stupid, complex and stupid, simple yet effective, or possibly even complex and even more effective.

There are many good reasons for sticking with a more simplified approach to system status management. Only the best managed organi-zations with the most dedicated personnel should even attempt to use the most complex and sophisticated models. But almost every system can benefit from thinking things through with the maps, demand analyses, and other reports, even if the result is an elegantly simple but more ef-fective approach to deployment.

Source

Reprinted with permission from JEMS, *May 1983. Jack Stout is an advisor to the Business Council at Med Trans. For 25 years, he was president of The Fourth Party, an EMS consulting firm that designs and implements EMS systems.*

Deployment as an Employee Stress Factor

Jay Fitch, PhD

How much is enough and how much is too much are questions that many EMS managers ask when it comes to deployment. The author details potential liability for EMS organizations and describes the eight job loading factors that can increase or decrease the impact of deployment stress in your system.

A NUMBER OF SERVICE MANAGERS have asked if stress should be a factor when considering unit hour utilization ratios and developing deployment plans. Stress and fatigue can be factors, as they relate to both psychological and physiological pressures experienced at work.

Well-planned, reasonable staff utilization is necessary if accidents are to be avoided. This is an important issue, as demonstrated by a case that occurred in Portland, Ore. A jury held the McDonald's Corporation liable for a traffic accident caused by a teenager who fell asleep at the wheel on his way home after working at one of their restaurants most of the night. Here are the facts, as reported by the Associated Press:

> Eighteen-year-old Matthew Theurer was a senior in high school and had been regularly working long hours at McDonald's. On the day in question, he went to school and then to work. At both school and work, he complained of fatigue. His McDonald's schedule was a peak productivity/split shift. . . . He worked from 3:30 p.m. until 8 p.m., took off four hours, and then returned from midnight until 8 a.m. Shortly after leaving work that morning, his car crossed the center line and collided head-on with a car driven by the plaintiff, who suffered severe leg injuries in the crash. The McDonald's employee was killed. The jury awarded $400,000 to the plaintiff—$170,000 in actual damages for medical expenses and lost wages and $230,000 in punitive damages. The jury verdict indicated that McDonald's was negligent in allowing the youth to work too many hours without rest before the accident.

Undoubtedly this decision will be appealed by McDonald's, but imagine trying to defend your ambulance service in similar circumstances—when an accident occurs in the 46th hour of a "mandatory overtime" shift.

Fatigue and stress related to deployment are intertwined but are not the same. Medics have told me that system status management causes stress. I don't buy it! That statement is the equivalent of a physician, who uses multiple exam rooms in which to see patients, saying that effective use of his time causes stress. However, there are multiple stressors in EMS. Despite all the talk about stress, most people don't understand it very well. And many employers don't want to deal with it. Yet a recently published national study conducted by Northwestern National Life Insurance Company indicated that workplace stress caused 34 percent of workers to seriously consider quitting their jobs last year. And 69 percent said stress makes them less productive. The study went on to say that organizations with supportive policies have less than half the burnout rate of those without such policies.

EMS work can be stressful, and poor deployment practices can add to that existing stress. Psychological stressors vary from person to person. Your body and mine react essentially the same when invaded by bacteria. Yet we may react very differently to a confrontation with a snake, having a co-worker yell at us, or being in an ambulance on post for 18 out of 24 hours.

There are four types of classical anxiety typically related to employment. In most EMS situations, all four are present. In systems that use very aggressive deployment plans, these four types of anxiety may be aggravated.

Time stress. Time stress is that anxiety associated with the fact that we must do something before a deadline. The pressure to "make" response times is an example of time stress that individuals in EMS systems often feel.

Anticipatory stress. Commonly known as worry, anticipatory stress is a feeling about an impending event. Many experience this in the months prior to recertification exams. Being on-post for long periods of time anticipating an assignment could also be stressful for some workers.

Situational stress. Situational stress is the result of finding yourself in a situation beyond your control. Related to deployment, this type of stress occurs when there are simply not enough resources, and the employees find themselves in a confrontation with nursing staff due to being chronically late.

Encounter stress. Anxiety about dealing with one or more people whom you find unpleasant is called encounter stress. Sometimes, too much interaction can cause encounter stress. If an employee works a high-demand, emergency-only unit day after day, without adequate days off, signs of encounter stress may be apparent.

Job Loading Factors

There are eight job loading factors that have been consistently identified by organizational psychologists in recent years. These job loading factors have been shown to be applicable to a variety of industries. We've combined these widely accepted theories with our practical experience in EMS deployment to provide the following tips for reducing the impact of stress in a high-productivity system.

Workload. Make sure the workload is reasonable. Specific efforts to monitor and adjust the workload are important in high-productivity systems. Sophisticated computer-aided dispatch systems provide a constant prompt for communications personnel concerning the number of assignments each crew has completed.

Physical variables. In a high-productivity system, the individual's physical comfort during a long shift can be a major consideration. EMS leaders should design vehicles for increased comfort. For example, cloth seats, tinted windows, noise reduction packages, oversized air conditioner units, and AM/FM cassette players should be considered standard features. MedTrans' San Diego County units are outfitted with hot and cold drink dispensers and built-in color televisions for the crew.

Job status. A perceived lack of job status can be a major stress factor. Avoid derogatory terms like "driver" or phrases like "he's just an EMT." The poor physical conditions of crew quarters and furnishings are often a negative statement about the individual's job status.

Accountability. Most of our work involves such a high risk element in performance and such a limited degree of control that we tend to operate in an accountability overload mode most of the time. One of the most helpful techniques for combating accountability overload is to provide high levels of involvement and control over non-clinical tasks. Equipment committees, which have decision-making authority within a certain dollar volume for capital equipment, and an employee scheduling group are both good examples.

Task variety. Only doing transfers or only doing blood and guts trauma can negatively impact job satisfaction levels. We've learned that variety helps. This is one of the reasons full-service systems have become increasingly popular. In these all-ALS, full-service systems, crew members handle both critical and routine calls. Another approach in larger service areas is to pair urban and rural units on the schedule so that there is a regular mix of urban and rural assignments.

Human contact. This means nothing more than occasional satisfying transactions. We've found that rural or low call volume units may need to be stationed in areas that provide higher contact. For example, one EMS service we have worked with leases space from a county library. Another has a crew station in a rural health clinic.

Physical challenge. Unfortunately, very few people in EMS are actually in good enough shape to safely do their jobs. To avoid back and other injuries, opportunities for physically challenging the staff are needed. Many clients have added workout equipment at low-priority posts. There are a number of isometric exercises that can be done in the cab of a unit while on post that also fill this need.

Mental challenge. Brain activities are needed to keep people psychologically involved with the job. When there is no productive mental activity required, staff members can focus negative mental energies on the company. One of the most effective ways to address the need for positive mental activity when on post assignments is to utilize a series of 15- to 30-minute continuing education assignments designed to be completed while on duty.

There is one additional deployment stress factor that should be considered by ambulance services. It involves partners. Who an individual works with may also be a stressor in a high deployment system. The working relationship between partners can impact both attitudes and productivity. When partners are well matched, they can usually tolerate more than those partners who do not enjoy being together. While an organization should strive for equity in its shift bidding and unit assignment policies, it should also provide flexibility within those policies to accommodate partner matches and mismatches.

Conclusion

Increasing demands for ambulance service and limited resources require increased productivity. Employers can reduce stress factors related to deployment by using creative alternatives to reduce job loading factors.

Source

Copyright © 1991, Fitch & Associates, Inc. Reprinted with permission. This article appeared in the Ambulance Industry Journal.

Burning the EMS Candle: EMS Shifts and Worker Fatigue

Russ McCallion,
EMT-P, and
Jim Fazackerley,
EMT-P, MPP

EMS workers experience a variety of shift schedules. Some schedules and off-duty lifestyles are incompatible with management's goal of putting alert medics on the job. The effects of sleep deprivation and the liability associated with poor scheduling practices make this article a must-read if your staff is burning the EMS candle at both ends.

- A SAN FRANCISCO BAY AREA police officer notices an ambulance stopped in the middle of an intersection with its red lights and siren on. Thinking that the crew may have been called to the scene of an accident, the officer approaches the ambulance and finds both crew members asleep in the front seat.

- The paramedic driver of an ambulance that is transporting a critical patient reaches the hospital. When he opens the back door of the ambulance, he discovers not only that the patient is still unconscious, but that his partner is asleep on the jump-seat.

These are just a few of the horror stories that have recently emerged from a single region in California. Are they isolated incidents of EMS worker fatigue, or is there a more pervasive—yet officially unrecognized—problem of employee fatigue caused by overwork and poorly conceived EMS staffing schedules? Alarming incidents of sleep-deprived inattention to duty have generated major workplace changes in other areas of healthcare, as well as in industry at large. Although EMS agencies may only occasionally be concerned with chronic fatigue afflicting prehospital personnel, the growing body of sleep research, healthcare precedents, and liability promises to wake them from their slumber.

A Sleep-Deprived Society

Sleep researchers agree that, although the typical adult requires approximately eight hours of sleep per night to function most effectively, most people in this country are skimping, sleeping six to seven hours. The result is chronic sleep deprivation.

William Dement, PhD, director of Stanford University's sleep research center, believes that most Americans no longer know what it feels like to be fully alert. In an increasingly busy 24-hour-a-day society, the problem continues to escalate. Up to 20 percent of the American workforce is now scheduled to work evenings or nights or have rotating shifts that confound natural sleep-wake cycles.

Catastrophic industrial accidents offer grim testimony to the growing threat posed by sleep-deprived workers. Sleep experts contend that it is not surprising that large disasters, such as those at Bhopal, India; Three Mile Island; Chernobyl; and on the Exxon Valdez happened after midnight, when workers were most likely to be drowsy.

Sleep deprivation is a pervasive problem in everyday settings as well. The U.S. Department of Transportation estimates that as many as 200,000 annual traffic accidents may be sleep-related. For truck drivers, the accident risk is at least 10 times higher between 4 a.m. and 6 a.m. David Dinges, PhD, a sleep expert from the University of Pennsylvania, noted, "Human error causes between 60 percent and 90 percent of all workplace accidents, depending on the type of job, and inadequate sleep is a major factor in human error, at least as important as drugs, alcohol, and equipment failure."

The Effects of Sleep Deprivation

Although sleep deprivation surveys of EMS workers have not yet been published, other public safety organizations have attempted to quantify the problem. In one survey of police officers, 80 percent reported that they had fallen asleep at least once a week while working night shifts.

An even closer comparison to the EMS workplace may be reflected in studies examining the effects of extreme fatigue on medical residents and interns, who are often scheduled to work as many as 120 hours per week. Not surprisingly, sleep-deprived residents were found to make more treatment errors than those who were well-rested. In addition to the effects of fatigue on a person's intellectual abilities, changes in personality, particularly loss of humor and increased ill temper, were also noted. Sound familiar?

One study showed that, for medical residents, the loss of only one night's sleep resulted in a drop in test scores on medical knowledge from approximately a third-year-resident level to a first-year level. Another study, applicable to EMS personnel, found that, when sleep-deprived residents examined EKGs for abnormalities, they made significantly slower assessments with significantly more errors than when they were rested. But contrasting results from other studies suggest that doctors can contend with sleep deprivation as long as their tasks are of short duration. One unanswered question is whether the relatively brief duration of prehospital tasks also insulates fatigued EMS personnel from making serious mistakes or omissions in care.

New York State recently passed legislation regulating the work hours of residents and interns, possibly paving the way for similar regulation throughout the healthcare industry. The legislation limits residents to an 80-hour workweek (averaged over four weeks) and limits them to 24 consecutive hours on duty. In large part, the New York legislation passed because of an uproar following the death of Libby Zion, an 18-year-old woman who died of an undiagnosed but treatable infection that was missed because of inadequate medical supervision and resident fatigue.

Similar legislation has been defeated in California due to opposition from the California Medical Association and hospital associations. The groups opposed the legislation because it would result in increased costs in hospital staffing; they felt that "self-regulation" by the hospitals was sufficient.

EMS Staffing Patterns

What harm might EMS providers be bringing to themselves and to their patients because of their staffing patterns? While EMS systems operate under a wide variety of shifts and schedules, including eight- and 10-hour shifts, they also incorporate the more grueling 12-, 24-, and 48-hour shifts, even in high call volume regions (Table 2.3). Also of concern are those systems that still rotate prehospital personnel between shifts, thereby forcing sudden adjustments from day to swing to night shifts.

Many EMS systems continue to impose no limit on the number of hours that personnel can work in a given time period; recently, in the San Francisco Bay Area, one paramedic worked 307 hours out of the 336 possible hours in a two-week pay period. And, in areas where there are "limits," they seem to be set unrealistically high. For example, with the approval of a supervisor, Los Angeles City paramedics can voluntarily work as many as 120 hours without relief.

Officials from the U.S. Department of Transportation, the California State EMS Authority, and the National Association of EMS Directors acknowledge that there may be problems with EMS staffing patterns but either deny having the ability to regulate the issue or state that it is a management problem best handled by EMS providers themselves.

Some employers appear reluctant to set standards for staffing or to allow standards to be imposed on them from outside agencies. If mandatory limits are imposed on employee hours, there may be a resultant increase in pay per hour, thereby increasing personnel costs and hence their cost per unit hour. Also, if the number of hours at work is regulated, there may be a loss in scheduling flexibility. Certainly, if there is a sched-

Table 2.3

Examples of Variable Staffing Patterns

Agency	Mandatory Length of Shifts	Hold Over	Maximum
Los Angeles City F.D.	24 hours	48 hours additional	120 hours straight
NYC*EMS	Eight hours, fixed	Yes, eight hours	16 hours straight
San Jose, Calif.	24 hours	Yes, 25 hours	49.5 hours straight
Vancouver, B.C., Canada	Rotating, 10-hour day, 14-hour night	No, mandatory eight-hour rest period	10 to 14 hours maximum
San Francisco	10 or 12 hours, fixed	Yes, up to 10 hours	20 hours straight
Johnson County (Overland Park, Kans.) Med Act	24 hours straight	Yes, up to 12 hours	36 hours
San Mateo County (Calif.) Baystar	10, 12, or 24 hours	Yes, up to 50 percent of shift	48 hours straight
Kansas City, Mo. (M.A.S.T.)	Varies	No	14 hours straight

uling gap on an ambulance that uses 24-hour shifts, it is easier to simply force the employee to hold over into what could become a 72-hour shift than to find a replacement and move personnel around.

Implementing Change

Brenda Steffan of the American Ambulance Association points out that many private "high-performance systems" have addressed the fatigue factor when awarding contracts by limiting workloads through the number of consecutive hours worked (typically 24 to 36 hours) and the amount of rest required between shifts (at least eight hours or two-thirds of the prior shift's number of hours). Voluntary changes in personnel practices, such as unit rotation based on call volume and responding less-busy units when feasible, have also helped alleviate shift fatigue.

Rick Keller of Fitch & Associates, a Platte City, Mo., organization experienced in establishing EMS systems, believes that it is "the employer's responsibility to look out for the workforce's shift schedules. The employers can't abrogate their responsibilities." According to Keller, the length of shifts is a quality-of-care issue that should be a medical decision, designed to maintain optimal quality of care.

In at least one community, a serious incident effected change. A manager of one midwestern EMS service admitted that "people became pretty focused on the problem" of fatigue because of a serious injury accident involving an EMT who had fallen asleep at the wheel of his ambulance, which was responding with lights and siren. As a result of the accident, the local physician advisory board now mandates maximum shift lengths for crews.

EMS innovator Jack Stout, founder of an EMS consulting firm called The Fourth Party, predicts that, within two to three years, labor unions and management within some U.S. EMS systems will come to an agreement on workload standards, which could spread throughout the industry. According to Stout, these standards will take the form of maximum percentages of on-duty time during which crews can respond to calls or other assignments.

Ironically, some of the greatest opposition to changing or regulating staffing patterns often comes from the very employees whom the regulations are supposed to protect. Twenty-four-hour shifts are probably not the best staffing system for most urban EMS services, but, as Keller points out, many EMS responders do not want to lose those "great" schedules.

Many employees like working shift schedules that allow them to "trade" themselves into 72-hour shifts so that they can then take a week off. Still, Keller believes that employees must ask themselves, "Are these shifts reasonable?" A potential problem with this staffing pattern is when some employees become "overtime hounds," snatching up every available extra shift. Some EMS personnel moonlight by taking on other jobs or split their work among different jurisdictions and cumulatively end up working excessive hours.

The length of shifts is a quality-of-care issue that should be a medical decision, designed to maintain optimal quality of care.

Fatigue Takes its Toll

The question remains: What quality of medical care is being delivered by these chronically fatigued workers? Sleep research suggests that, with clear-cut critical patients, responders can probably mobilize themselves to overcome fatigue. But on the more subtle "gray area" calls—the man found down outside of a bar or the young patient with abdominal pain—responders may not be able to deliver the same safe, compassionate care at 3 a.m. as they would at 3 p.m. The tendency to become uncaring and irritable with patients, not to mention other public safety personnel, can also result in complaints and, ultimately, lawsuits, even if the care delivered was technically competent.

In addition to possible compromises in patient care, the toll on EMS employees from chronic fatigue should be addressed. Health problems, insomnia, weight gain, depressed immune systems, and depression can all result from work-related fatigue, as can safety problems, particularly while driving. One study showed that evening- and night-shift workers had twice the auto accident rate off duty as people who work during the day. Additionally, those who work evening and night shifts are particularly prone to chronic fatigue and sleep disorders, which can begin to affect one's home life as well. Over an extended time period, fatigue and sleep deprivation can result in the burnout, substance abuse, or loss of an otherwise competent employee.

Taking Steps Toward a Solution

Within the complex challenge of efficiently providing 24-hour EMS, is there an optimal shift schedule that can help alleviate the problems of fatigue and sleep deprivation? According to Marty Klein, PhD, president of Synchro-Tech, a Lincoln, Nebr., company that specializes in setting up shift and staffing schedules for clients such as Boeing, utility companies, and hospitals, there is no best shift schedule. Rather, shift lengths should depend on employee age, marital status, commuting distances, and personal preferences. Once established, employees need to adjust their lifestyles to match their work shifts.

According to Klein, poor schedule design can lead to burnout, chronic stress, and increased workers' compensation claims, resulting in high employee turnover and higher operational costs. And most sleep experts, such as Klein, do not support 24-hour shifts for EMS workers unless they work in very slow systems. To work a 72-hour shift, according to sleep disorder expert Phillip Westbrook, MD, is "crazy; it's denying our evolutionary biology."

As part of a more humane schedule, Klein advocates 12-hour shifts, either from 6 a.m. to 6 p.m. or vice versa. These shift times allow most employees to avoid commuter hassles, and they can also avoid circadian-rhythm problems that often develop with later night shifts (e.g., 9 p.m. to 9 a.m.), as the last part of the shift launches them into bright daylight—

causing confusion in the body and insomnia for the worker. Another reason that Klein supports 6-to-6 shifts is that employees of both shifts should be able to eat dinner at home, thereby facilitating social and family interactions.

Sleep experts agree that some of the worst schedules are those that rotate between days, evenings, and nights, as these schedules plunge the body into a constant state of confusion. Such schedules are particularly

How to Survive Working Nights

Obviously, someone has to work on the rigs during evenings and nights. For EMS workers who are assigned to these shifts, several things can be done to fend off the negative effects of shift work.

- Allow time after your shift—whether it's an evening, night, or 24-hour shift—to unwind and relax before trying to sleep. Rather than force yourself to sleep, get up and do something until you become drowsy.
- Exercise to reduce stress, release endorphins, and tire muscles, all of which lead to a deeper sleep. Exercise—like a hot bath—raises the body's temperature, however, so it should be done a few hours before attempting to sleep.
- Avoid stimulants, such as nicotine and caffeine, during the last several hours of a shift. Remember that caffeine can be found not only in coffee, teas, and colas, but also in chocolate and many over-the-counter prescription drugs, including aspirin. While a depressant, alcohol can also cause sleep loss.
- Eating simple carbohydrates, such as cookies or a small candy bar, can stimulate the body into producing tryptophan, an amino acid from which serontin is made. Serontin helps ease the body into sleep.
- Create a better sleeping environment. Keep the room cool and dark, to make your body think that it's night. Try to pick a quiet room in which to sleep, and make sure it's well-insulated with carpets and drapes. Run an air conditioner or a "white-noise" machine to drown out extraneous sounds. Unplug the phone and doorbell, and put up a "Do Not Disturb" sign on the front door.
- Educate your family and friends about your need for sleep so that they'll minimize interruptions. You also need to make lifestyle decisions regarding which social or family functions, such as your child's baseball games, you can attend and which you have to miss.
- When working a straight night-shift schedule, create an "anchor period" of sleep around which you schedule the remainder of your sleep hours. For example, if you get off at 7 a.m., always set aside four hours, from 8 a.m. until noon, for dedicated sleep time, regardless of whether it is a workday. If you're coming off a night shift, sleep from 8 a.m. until 3 or 4 p.m.; if you're off duty, don't go to sleep until 2 or 3 a.m., and sleep until noon.
- If you work nights on a straight, non-rotating basis, don't try to revert to a regular day-shift lifestyle on your days off.
- Sleep difficulties, no matter what their duration, should be taken seriously. If you experience such problems, consult a physician who specializes in sleep disorders. For physician referral, contact the National Sleep Foundation, 122 South Robertson Boulevard, Suite 201, Los Angeles, Calif. 90048.
- Remember, shift work is a lifestyle and not just a work schedule, so don't fight it. Learn to live with it.

References

Hauri, P., and S. Linde. *No More Sleepless Nights*. Chicago, W. B. Saunders, 1990.
Klein, M. *Chrono Care Handbook: A Personal Lifestyle Guide for Health Professionals Who Work Shifts*. Lincoln, Nebr.: Synchro-Tech, 1988.

Source

Reprinted with permission from JEMS, *October 1991. At the time of original publication, Russ McCallion, EMT-P, was a supervisor with the San Francisco Department of Health's Paramedic Division and vice president of the San Francisco Paramedic Association. Jim Fazackerley, EMT-P, MPP, was a field paramedic with the San Francisco Department of Health's Paramedic Division.*

difficult when the shifts rotate every week. According to Klein, if rotating shifts are an absolute necessity, there should be at least three weeks between each rotation.

Once schedules are designated, employers have a responsibility to educate their employees and their families in how to live with their particular schedule. Similarly, employees have a responsibility to not "overbook" themselves with family activities, extra work, or school, which may cause them to come to work already fatigued. The practice of trading shifts should also be limited if it causes personnel to work lengthy shifts.

Additionally, employers must monitor employees carefully for signs of fatigue. EMS managers can also attempt to spread the workload more equitably by rotating crews or redistricting zones. And, due to liability reasons, if someone complains of being overfatigued, management should consider sending the worker home.

Allowing shift-fatigue problems to lie dormant can lead not only to reactionary legislative cures and incident-related policymaking but also to exposure to litigation. For example, an Oregon court has already established that employers are responsible for monitoring employee fatigue; a large award was upheld against the McDonald's Corporation for a fatigue-related auto accident involving an employee who had just gotten off work late at night after a split-shift. Other cases have recently been decided in the same fashion.

More than anything else, the issue of liability may force EMS employers to re-examine the way in which they schedule workers. Employers and employees alike must be aware of the consequences of the shift patterns being worked. It appears inevitable that increased scrutiny will be visited on this area of EMS, thereby forcing additional regulations. The only question remaining is whether such regulation will come from inside or outside of the EMS industry.

References

Angier, N. "Cheating on Sleep." *New York Times,* 15 May 1990.
Brody, J. "Personal Health." *New York Times,* 5 July 1990.
Friedman, P. "The Intern and Sleep Loss." *New England Journal of Medicine* 285 (1977): 201.
Garza, M. "Courts Are Finding Employers Liable for Accidents Due to Fatigue." *EMS Insider* 18, no. 5 (1991).
Hauri, P., and S. Linde. *No More Sleepless Nights.* Chicago: W. B. Saunders, 1990.
Jacques, C. M., et al. "Effects of Sleep Loss on Cognitive Performance of Resident Physicians." *Journal of Family Practice* 30: 223-229.
Keller, R., Fitch & Associates. Interview by author, 30 July 1991.
Klein, M. *Chrono Care Handbook: A Personal Lifestyle Guide for Health Professionals Who Work Shifts.* Lincoln, Nebr.: Synchro-Tech, 1988.
"Limits on Intern's Schedules Killed." *San Francisco Chronicle,* 7 August 1990.
Stout, J. Interview by author, 12 August 1991.
Toufixis, A. "Drowsy America." *Time* (December 17, 1990): 78-85.

A POORLY DESIGNED PARAMEDIC schedule can significantly affect morale and enhance burnout. Even a good schedule can have a psychological effect due to the frequently needless calls that are still transported because the patient does not have a vehicle or cannot be left alone. These types of calls tend to make medics feel unappreciated for two reasons: The patient thinks the medic owes him a ride; and the boss expects the medic to reduce the company's liability (abandonment).

The volume of calls answered and miles traveled by paramedics can be physically exhausting. Scheduling that requires a person to work the hours designated to supply the service must be changed to a more cooperative effort between management and the person the schedule affects the most—the medic. Medics should be supplied with a schedule that does not consume their family life or cause fatigue, yet will meet the service's demands. This can be done by making the medic's schedule flexible enough that hours can be switched with another medic when something comes up and time off is needed. Also, care should be taken to reduce the number of consecutive days a medic works.

The first step to effective schedule development is defining objectives. That might sound silly because we obviously need to staff our equipment in order to answer calls. However, medics—and the community—have additional needs that should be considered.

In most systems, the peak demand is usually a quantity of hours during the day. With that in mind, your resources should increase (e.g., more ambulances on the road) during those hours. Even though resources are increased, the demand on these medics will be greater than on those medics working nights. So consider making the shifts shorter for medics working the system's high call volume hours.

Because many systems give paramedics or EMTs the responsibility of scheduling, address the scheduling process in the same manner that you would assess a patient.

Primary Assessment

Gather enough information to exclude serious and immediate problems that can affect the patient and your staff. These problems include the following:
- Crews are not eating.
- Crews are not getting off duty on time.
- Exceptions increase at shift changes.
- One ambulance has significantly more calls than another working the same shift.

Different Scheduling Strokes for Different Folks

Jim Brodie

EMS manager Jim Brodie outlines the steps he follows to develop a workable schedule. His step-by-step approach, using the analogy of a patient assessment scenario, makes the process of scheduling understandable.

- Ambulances are not being restocked.
- Ambulances are not being inventoried.
- Late arrivals are occurring on scheduled calls/transports.

The steps for gathering information to detect these problems are assessment, compiling information, and communication.

Assessment

The needs of the patient include

- Rapid response times on emergency calls
- Scheduled transfers
- Patients waiting to be returned
- ALS vehicle availability

The needs of the medics include

- Crisscrossing units to facilitate post moves
- Meal times
- Getting off duty on time
- Completing paperwork
- Time to restock equipment
- Long-distance transports

Considerations and concerns of the system include

- Excessive response times
- Units not available
- No flexibility for scheduling transfers
- The needs of the patient, medics, system, department, and company.

Compiling Information

After the assessment, key information must be collected.

First, the call volume should be collected and reviewed. The necessary information pertaining to the volume includes the date, time, and location of each call.

Next, review the calls that do not meet the response time standards established by the organization. These should also be analyzed by date, time, and location.

Finally, review the number of hours medics work per week, the lengths of their shifts, and their days off in the current schedule. Include in your analysis the preferred schedule the medics are requesting.

After you examine this information, put it together to form a baseline utilization ratio. This will give you an idea of the system's production. You need to know the production of the system to determine what the workload currently is. Also try to determine at this point if the information you have compiled is going to meet budget expectations.

Communication

The last step of the primary assessment is communication.

The objectives of the schedule should be discussed with all personnel. The discussion should be two-way—the medics' input is extremely important in this stage of the process.

It is also important to share the information you are researching. When you do this, the staff will recognize that you are putting the schedule together to meet the call demand. In addition, you will be educating them on how you make that match-up and providing proof that it is not solely a budgeting decision.

Secondary Assessment

In this part of the assessment process, detailed historical (call volume statistics) and physical (staff input) findings are compiled to determine the needs of the system as a whole.

There are four steps in this stage: inspection, palpate, auscultation, and percussion.

Inspection

Analyze all data gathered pertaining to the call demand and the hours medics work per week. At a minimum, three months of this data is necessary to make informed decisions. If possible, use the past 12 months.

Palpate

Get a feel from the community and staff on how they think the system's schedule should work. The community will be concerned with response times, unit availability, and cost of the operating system. The staff will be interested in the units on duty, the response utilization ratio, the length of shifts, and the number of shifts per week.

Auscultation

Listen to the customer and staff. If you ask, customers will tell you what they think of the staff. The supervisor or manager should determine if some of the customer complaints are the result of staff fatigue.

Percussion

Bounce your ideas off the staff. Make every effort to resolve difficult or poorly conceived ideas before you put them in place. The best way to do this is with small task teams, an agenda, and clearly defined objectives.

Plan of Action (Treatment)

After deciding what the results should be, how do you determine the number of vehicles and people you need?

Vehicles

Based on the number of responses you anticipate, determine if you have enough vehicles to respond to the calls. This sounds pretty simple; however, consider some additional points that you may have overlooked before you decide.

- How many responses can one vehicle make in one hour?
- How many vehicles are needed to provide coverage that will meet your response time requirements?
- How do you know how productive your units are? Why do you need to know?

These questions can be answered through the following methods.

To answer the first question, determine the location of the calls for that time of day and where they were transported. Then measure the total time on task (call received to in-service). This is done by adding the lines for all calls together and dividing by the total number of responses. This figure will change based on the number and types of calls.

For the second question, try this formula: Add the average number of responses (rounded off to the next highest whole number) to the number of vehicles it takes to cover the response area. This number will equal the number of vehicles you need for that hour.

To solve the third question, use this formula to determine the how and why of unit production. You need to find the following:

- Total time on shift (each unit)
- Total time on calls (transports and dry runs)
- Total time on post moves

Divide total time on calls and on post moves by total time on shift. This will give the percentage of the shift that is producing call volume or covering the system (other than stationed at a post).

Example: Medic 2

Worked 500 hours	30,000 minutes
Total time on calls	10,000 minutes
Total time on post moves	5,000 minutes

30,000 divided by 10,000 = 33.0%
30,000 divided by 5,000 = 16.6%

33.0% + 16.6% = 49.6%

The Medic 2 unit is actively participating in the system 49.6 percent of the time. In other words, for about one-half of its time on duty, the unit is on assigned tasks.

The production formula not only tells you how often the units in your system are active, but also gives you an idea of how many more calls or movements your system can effectively handle without fatigue becoming a factor. An acceptable percentage for a system is decided by you and your staff and should be periodically evaluated.

Personnel

This is the easiest of all the tasks. Staffing is largely, but not solely, based on budget. The number of hours personnel work a week is usually decided by the accountant. The number and length of shifts should be decided by you and your staff. Don't get wrapped up in the old myth that if there are fewer emergencies, it's all right to let personnel work longer shifts. Your staff will be just as tired behind the wheel on a non-emergency run as they are in the back of the ambulance on an emergency.

Don't learn the hard way—let your people have input in creating the schedule. Give them guidelines and they will do most of the work for you, and probably be a lot happier.

The success or failure of your schedule is based on everyone. The challenge to all managers and directors of operations is to take concepts on the effectiveness of 12- and 24-hour shifts, as well as highly productive ambulances, and successfully use them in their own systems.

As the term EMS says, this is a service business, but while you're working on the schedule, think of the business as manufacturing. In manufacturing, you are producing a product, or "widget." You need to determine how to put out a quality product, and make sure that you are sufficiently staffed so that quality is not compromised by overworked, tired personnel. Secondly, you need to make sure that you don't have too many people, so the company isn't wasting resources or sacrificing financial stability.

This is how the EMS/manufacturing analogy works:

- SSM controllers take the orders.
- They send the invoice to the plant manager.
- The plant manager sets up the number of machines needed to fill the orders (schedule).
- The schedule lets everyone know how many machines (ambulances) need to be working (each machine needs two technicians).
- The machines are given the orders (calls).
- Quality improvement inspects the final product (patient transport and care).
- Administration judges performance by input from QI and by the total number of widgets produced compared to how well the factory is running.

I am not suggesting that patients are widgets or our field and dispatching jobs are that simple. However, you have to understand that you are serving a lot of people. Don't forget about the two primary people the scheduler serves: the patient and the caregiver. You owe it to both to do what is best for all. Taking the time to establish or change the schedule to make it as effective as possible is not only important but should be required of everyone who is charged with this responsibility.

Source

Original article. Jim Brodie is the director of operations for Mercy Ambulance in Ft. Wayne, Ind. He has over 19 years of experience in EMS.

Emergency Medical Dispatch, Communications Centers, and Computers

Dispatch Life Support: Establishing Standards that Work

Jeff J. Clawson, MD, and Scott A. Hauert, AEMT

Dr. Jeff Clawson is considered the inspiration behind modern EMS dispatch techniques. In this article, he outlines the standards medically accepted as "dispatch life support." His methods, now universally accepted as EMD, have saved thousands of lives in the past 15 years.

IN THE EMERGENCY MEDICAL services world where seconds count, acronyms help keep things simple and direct. Acceptance of these shortened versions of names or products is assured when the acronyms can stand by themselves without explanation. EMT is one such example. EMD (emergency medical dispatcher) is still relatively new, in existence less than a decade. It won the battle against EMS-D (emergency medical services–dispatcher), which rolled easily off no one's tongue and is now obsolete.

A new acronym was recently coined to establish an identity for, and enhance understanding of, a new key component of EMD. DLS, which stands for dispatch life support, represents the knowledge, procedures, and skills used by trained EMDs to provide care via pre-arrival instructions to callers. It consists of those BLS and ALS principles that are appropriate for use by emergency medical dispatchers.

But isn't this really just basic life support in disguise? The answer is a resounding "no." Each item serves as an example of how these standards relate to the role of the medical dispatcher.

The core of BLS, CPR, and ACLS revolves around the standards and guidelines developed by the American Heart Association (AHA), which are tailored for EMS providers. Unfortunately, difficulties arise when these guidelines are applied directly to medical dispatching.

The consistency of care and acceptance brought about by these much-needed standards created order from the chaos that previously existed in these areas of EMS. However, to some extent, blind acceptance of the standards, coupled with their limitations in certain situations, has caused significant difficulties when the standards are applied directly to pre-arrival instructions given by EMDs.

These problems often surface when medical control physicians adopt and review pre-arrival instruction protocols, and find that they appear to deviate from current guidelines, such as those of the AHA. Actually, the medical director's real dilemma is in attempting to understand the special limitations that are inherent in the dispatch situation, not in the pre-arrival instruction protocol itself.

Since the AHA changed its recommended airway control maneuvers to the chin-lift and jaw-thrust methods in 1987, some people believe that continuing to include the head-tilt method in dispatch protocols is unsound. However, from a dispatch perspective, it is not, which further reveals the limited application of these standards to dispatch.

The National Association of EMS Physicians (NAEMSP) stated in its *1988 Consensus Document on Emergency Medical Dispatching,* "Training and recertification [of EMDs] in basic life support, as is appropriate to application by medical dispatchers, is necessary to maintain and improve this unique, and at times, lifesaving, non-visual skill." NAEMSP's more recent position paper on EMD makes this distinction more specific by defining this area as dispatch life support.

Challenges for Dispatchers

The AHA's BLS standards are designed for the teaching of physical procedures in person to a willing student, often over many hours. Although the creators of these standards could not have foreseen the limitations placed on dispatching, the guidelines do recognize the need for some flexibility.

Still, certain obstacles present themselves to dispatchers when applying these standards. Thrust in the role of "instructor," the dispatcher must teach the caller (an unwilling student) a physical procedure in a matter of seconds, without visual aids of any kind or even any opportunity to practice.

Obviously, this means there is no in-person verification that the procedure is properly performed or that it is performed at all. If the limitations of a given process are understood up front, the procedure can be molded to effectively meet the needs of the user while still creating the desired results. This, unfortunately, has not yet been done; no currently published BLS standards were designed with the dispatcher's situation in mind.

Although the chin-lift method of airway control is not difficult to perform, dispatchers must recommend that callers use the simplest method of securing a patient airway, as long as it is safe and effective. Since most cardiac arrest situations require that airway management (as instructed by the dispatcher) only briefly precede mouth-to-mouth resuscitation as a precursor to CPR, the more complicated chin-lift instruction is not as feasible in a dispatch setting. The jaw-thrust method is also not practical when conveying instructions to callers who have no assistance.

The head-tilt method of airway control, however, can be easily taught to an untrained caller in the following manner: "Put one hand on his forehead, your other hand under his neck. Lift up on the hand under his neck and push down with the hand on his forehead. This will open his

During the evolution of citizen CPR, it was discovered that, if training instructions were too complicated and confusing as to the sequence of CPR, people might hesitate and delay the procedure.

airway." There is nothing basically wrong with the head-tilt method. In fact, any street practitioner has probably personally experienced its effectiveness. Of course, EMDs are taught to be aware of the hazards of neck manipulation if the patient has sustained a significant mechanism of injury. Fortunately, this scenario is less likely to occur, as most callers reporting traumatic incidents have not remained on scene.

Callers need simple, easy-to-understand "verbal pictures" to follow. During the evolution of citizen CPR, it was discovered that, if training instructions were too complicated and confusing as to the sequence of CPR, people might hesitate and delay the procedure. This concern first surfaced many years ago when the initial process for doing CPR differed in witnessed versus unwitnessed arrest situations. One might think that people would, if confused, decide immediately that either method was better than doing nothing at all. But this is not always the case, as people sometimes hesitate or, even worse, give up.

Although this cannot be observed firsthand at the scene of an actual citizen CPR case, the fact that it occurs in practice on mannequins supports the contention that it occurs in the confusion of a real crisis. This delaying mental trap has been appropriately termed "paralysis by analysis."

DLS Guidelines

There are several other examples that illustrate the problems of applying BLS training taught in a controlled environment directly to medical dispatching. The following are important concepts that are not present in BLS guidelines, but are essential to DLS:

- A seizure or convulsion may be a symptom of the onset of cardiac arrest. Any patient 35 years or older who presents with a seizure as the chief complaint should be assumed to be in cardiac arrest until proven otherwise. This is a statistical probability that occurs with some regularity.
- Cardiac arrest in a previously healthy child should be considered to be caused by a foreign body obstructing the airway until proven otherwise.
- Dispatchers should be trained to identify obvious death situations (as defined by medical control), mobilize the response accordingly, and give limited pre-arrival instructions.
- If the victim is unconscious and breathing cannot be verified by a second-party caller, the victim should be assumed to be in cardiac arrest until proven otherwise.
- EMDs should assume that bystanders have inappropriately placed a pillow under the head of an unconscious victim, until proven otherwise, and ensure that it is removed.
- BLS protocol for choking victims should be modified to reflect that EMDs recommend a specific number of thrusts, rather than stating a range of six to 10 thrusts. The present guidelines contain no basis for deciding during the crisis how

Seeing the AHA Standards from a Medical Dispatch Perspective

The following are excerpts from the American Heart Association's "Standards and Guidelines for Cardiopulmonary Resuscitation and Emergency Cardiac Care," published in the *Journal of the American Medical Association*, June 6, 1986.

Emergency cardiac care. Basic life support is that particular phase of ECC that either 1) prevents circulatory or respiratory arrest or insufficiency through prompt recognition and intervention, early entry into the EMS system, or both, or 2) externally supports the circulation and respiration of a victim of cardiac or respiratory arrest.

Standards and guidelines. The 1980 standards and guidelines were intended to 1) identify a body of knowledge and certain performance skills that are commonly necessary for the successful treatment of victims of cardiorespiratory arrest or of serious or life-threatening cardiac or pulmonary disturbance, and 2) indicate that the knowledge and skills recommended or defined do not represent the only medically or legally acceptable approach to a designated problem, but rather an approach that is generally regarded as having the best likelihood of success in view of present knowledge.

Standards and guidelines. The standards and guidelines were not intended to imply 1) that justifiable deviations from suggested standards and guidelines by physicians qualified and experienced in CPR and ECC under appropriate circumstances represent a breach of a medical standard of care, or 2) that new knowledge, new techniques, or clinical circumstances may not provide sound reasons for alternative approaches to CPR and ECC before the next definition of national standards and guidelines.

Basis for changing recommendations. In some subject areas, sound data had accumulated, and changes were recommended on that basis. In other areas, while the experimental data were not conclusive, changes were recommended on

the basis of clinical evidence or in order to improve educational efficacy.

Standards and guidelines. "Loose constructionists," while realizing the need for uniformity and consistency, have believed that more flexibility is needed for two principal reasons: 1) New knowledge and innovation are ongoing, and failure to permit flexibility can result in delay of potentially lifesaving advances; and 2) The physician prerogative for discretionary action may be threatened by overly rigid standards, particularly because the term has important legal, as well as medical, overtones.

Emergency cardiac care. Emergency cardiac care is dependent for its success on laypersons' appreciation of the critical importance of activating the EMS system as well as their willingness to initiate CPR promptly and their ability to provide it effectively.

Basis for changing recommendations. Final decisions took into account not only which technique or adjunct or therapy was the most correct, but also how the public could best be served, which brought into the decision making such factors as safety, effectiveness, teachability, and ease of sequencing into related maneuvers.

Public education. Other changes for improving retention should include simplification of the sequences of BLS and inclusion of only one method of managing foreign-body obstruction in the adult.

Public education. There are many reasons why lay individuals do not become involved in performing CPR. These include lack of motivation, fear of doing harm, inability to remember exact sequences, and poor retention of psychomotor skills.

Reasons to withhold CPR. Few reliable criteria exist by which death can be defined immediately. Decapitation, rigor mortis, and evidence of tissue decomposition and extreme dependent lividity are usually reliable criteria. When they are present, CPR need not be initiated.

Source

Reprinted with permission from JEMS, July 1990. Jeff J. Clawson, MD, is the originator of the medical priority dispatch system and has been referred to as the "Father of EMD." He is currently the director of research development for Medical Priority Consultants, Inc., and is outgoing president of the National Academy of Emergency Medical Dispatch. He is also the medical director for Gold Cross Ambulance Service. Scott A. Hauert, AEMT, was director of training for the National Academy of Emergency Medical Dispatch and Medical Priority Consultants, Inc., both in Salt Lake City.

many to use. This simplification will eliminate any confusion and subsequent hesitation on the caller's part.

- The Heimlich maneuver should be the primary treatment for infants, children, and adults who are choking.

Many readers will assume that EMDs are aware of these concepts. But most of this information is not directly taught to the majority of EMTs and paramedics and is not covered in the current EMT and paramedic textbooks. Addressing these omissions highlights the need for dispatcher-specific training.

The psychology behind pre-arrival instructions is currently undergoing some unique and very useful expansion. As callers' actions can now be predicted to a reasonable extent, EMD protocols need to reflect these new understandings. There is no question that DLS is different from BLS, just as EMDs are different from EMTs—not better or worse, but different. You don't get "apples" by training people to be "oranges." Likewise, you won't get good guidelines for baking apples by using the recipe for peach cobbler. The next step in solving this problem seems an obvious one: Medical dispatch experts, line dispatchers, and the standard setters must work together in creating sound DLS guidelines.

The AHA has correctly stated, "Basic life support can and should be initiated by any person present when cardiac or respiratory arrest occurs." Furthermore, "the most important link in the CPR-ECC system in the community is the layperson."

In the future, every time the requirement of BLS is mentioned in the AHA Standards and Guidelines, it should be preceded by a reference to DLS. And every discussion of the layperson being an important link in the initial provision of emergency cardiac care should emphasize the dispatcher's role as teacher of that layperson. Until this is accomplished, no standards or guidelines, regardless of how well-intentioned, will best serve people in crisis who need immediate, but realistic, dispatch life support intervention.

References

National Association of EMS Physicians. "Consensus Document on Emergency Medical Dispatching." *JEMS* 13, no. 11 (1988).
National Association of EMS Physicians. "Position Paper: Emergency Medical Dispatching." *Prehospital and Disaster Medicine* 4, no. 2 (1989).
"Standards and Guidelines for Cardiopulmonary Resuscitation and Emergency Cardiac Care." *JAMA* 255, no. 21 (1986).

Modern Priority Dispatch

Jeff J. Clawson, MD, and Robert L. Martin

Modern dispatch standards, protocols, and practices are detailed in this article by two authors who are experts in the field. Included is an important segment on quality assurance practices.

EMS SYSTEMS THROUGHOUT the world are continually faced with an uncomfortable dilemma—that of providing prompt and appropriate EMS response in the face of rising costs and increasing demands. Many urban areas have been experiencing a steady 10-percent increase in emergency calls each year without any concurrent increase in personnel and equipment. Adding to the dilemma is continued abuse of the system by a sizable number of callers demanding emergency service in non-urgent situations.

Over the past 15 years, EMS has continued to evolve and, in general, to improve. This improvement is exemplified by the move from untrained mortuary services and first aid vehicles to emergency medical technician (EMT) ambulances and, finally, to advanced life support (ALS) paramedic systems. The expertise of the emergency responder has been significantly upgraded. With EMTs now receiving hundreds of hours of intensive training and paramedics often more than 1,000 hours, it is obvious that education is considered vitally important in the EMS world—that is, until we consider dispatcher training.

At the center of our modern, well-trained, specialized, and expensive EMS configuration is the emergency dispatcher, who in many cases has not been given even a single hour of relevant emergency medical instruction. The dispatcher occupies an absolutely essential role in EMS, deciding how, who, when, and even whether or not to respond. But for many years, emergency medical dispatchers (EMDs) have remained the weakest link in the EMS chain of response.

If EMS is to continue to meet the challenges of tomorrow, it must effect positive change today. To do this, it must ask two significant questions. First, in this era of tight fiscal restraints, are EMS managers making the most efficient use of their human and material resources in dispatch and response? And second, are EMS dispatch and consequent unit response done with regard to sound medical evaluation and prioritization?

A Dispatch Standard

In some areas of the country, it is common dispatch and response practice to send the closest available ambulance or first responder, as well as ALS paramedics, on all EMS calls. In addition, most response procedures still require red lights and sirens en route to the scene for all incidents. Many even use them on all transports.

Some claim the advantage of this type of response philosophy is that those in dire need will receive not only the most basic help immediately but also the most advanced help as quickly as possible. This,

The medical priority dispatching system (MPDS) has enabled the different agencies to meet the rising public demand for EMS without over-burdening already stretched resources.

however, is the case in most incidents regardless of dispatch philosophy. And for the majority of EMS providers, a "maximal response policy," coupled with fiscal restraints, severely taxes limited resources.

Increased call volume without a concomitant increase in the number of EMS units and personnel ultimately begins to strain agencies with a maximal response policy. Wear and tear on the units and equipment becomes increasingly apparent, mechanical breakdowns become more frequent and dangerous, and the increased stress begins to take its inevitable toll on personnel.

Many cities and EMS centers, however, have implemented another dispatching method to handle and prioritize these calls. This program, known as the medical priority dispatching system (MPDS), has enabled the different agencies to meet the rising public demand for EMS without overburdening already stretched resources.

The development of MPDS and EMD training, initially done in Salt Lake City, combined with the more recent development of standards and certification by the National Academy of Emergency Medical Dispatch and the issuance of position statements by organizations such as the National Association of EMS Physicians, has led to nothing short of a revolution in EMS dispatch. The increased focus has led to further definition of medical dispatch standards, the concept of medical call prioritization, and more formal but intelligent medical control.

Protocol

At the basis of the MPDS system is the manual priority card system. This system consists of the initial entry-level protocol card, 32 pairs of dispatch priority cards, plus eight telephone treatment sequence cards. Each caller complaint category is listed in alphabetical order for quick reference. The card index reflects either a symptom or an incident categorization of problems and therefore avoids the pitfalls of diagnosis-oriented dispatch.

If diagnosis is used as an index, the dispatcher must diagnose or accept the caller's diagnostic opinion before selecting the appropriate card for response. Since diagnosis is considered the most difficult of all medical skills, requiring the traditionally least medically trained individual in an EMS system to diagnose as an initial step for response selection is clearly a medically unsound process.

Once a dispatch priority card has been selected, the EMD continues the interrogation by asking key questions. These questions have been medically determined to be the minimum amount of interrogation necessary to adequately establish the correct level of emergency medical response, including EMT versus paramedic and routine versus red-lights-and-siren responses.

While key questions, pre-arrival instructions, and dispatch priority determinants remain constant from one locality to another, the dispatch priority section of each card must reflect a given agency's varied ability to respond, ranging from single-unit volunteer squads to the multiple-level response of major metropolitan fire departments and EMS agencies. Dispatch priorities become necessarily more complex for more sophisticated systems. Each individual area's situation should be studied carefully before various responses are assigned to each determinant. These response assignments are medical control decisions and should be made in conjunction with medical control and EMS physicians prior to implementation of the dispatch system.

The determinant subsection reflects lines of separation of different preplanned levels of response. For example, in Salt Lake City's paramedic system, chest pain in a 10-year-old would not evoke the same level of response as in a 57-year-old, just as hives with no difficulty breathing would require a less urgent response than when breathing difficulty is present.

In Practice

In an actual MPDS response, each call is immediately evaluated through a programmed, medically approved interrogation sequence that uses questions to determine the chief complaint or incident type. Within the first 30 seconds, the potential critical status of the patient's condition is determined. If consciousness and breathing cannot be confirmed by a second-party caller, a maximal response is sent prior to any further questioning or interaction. If the victim is determined to be conscious and breathing, however, the interrogation is continued for another 20 to 30 seconds while the specific patient problem is more clearly identified and appropriate response selected and initiated. The chief complaint, age, consciousness, and breathing status are thus considered the "Four Commandments" of medical dispatching, much as vital signs are considered the essential informational elements for the field practitioner.

The preprogrammed key question interrogation component of the MPDS is essential even for those systems not prioritizing calls, since the questions are geared to the more objective identification of those conditions requiring pre-arrival telephone assistance. It has been clearly proven, for example, that it is feasible to dispatch less than an ALS paramedic on many EMS incidents and to drive without red lights and sirens not only during transport, but also during initial response. The simple logic behind such a system is based on the medical fact that every EMS call of distress does not require the same response.

An agency may decide initially to provide paramedic response or maximal response to all incidents for purposes of legal protection. At some point, however, this agency may be unable to defend the delayed or unavailable ALS response to an adult victim of chest pain or severe trauma when that unit is tied up responding to a simple fractured arm or other BLS-level call.

In addition, with emergency vehicle-related accidents in North

The preprogrammed key question interrogation component of the MPDS is essential even for those systems not prioritizing calls, since the questions are geared to the more objective identification of those conditions requiring pre-arrival telephone assistance.

America estimated into the tens of thousands, it is medically unsound and managerially unsafe to require a red-lights-and-siren response on all incidents. This exposes crews to the additional hazards of a full emergency response, just to arrive one or two minutes earlier for a non-critical patient. In order to ensure medical appropriateness, managers must include "dispatch literate" physician medical control as an integral part of their medical dispatch protocol system.

Training the EMD

Emergency medical dispatcher training is being initiated throughout the United States and Canada. At the forefront of national EMD certification and training is the National Academy of Emergency Medical Dispatch, formed in 1988 to bring about nationwide improvement in EMD training standards and recognition, and to meet the pressing need for a national standard of training, protocol, certification, and recertification. The academy now offers individual, regional, and international EMD courses, seminars, and conferences on MPDS, thus continuing the growth in EMD that has taken place over the past 10 years as priority dispatching has become more commonplace.

Under MPDS, a typical 24-hour EMD training course consists first of a brief review of course objectives, basic dispatch techniques, equipment, and essential regulations and codes. The role of the EMD is then defined, and the MPDS concepts are discussed in detail. In this discussion, students are taught the system's three core components: key questions, pre-arrival instructions, and dispatch priorities, the last of which includes predetermined response configuration and driving modes.

The Four Commandments of medical dispatch are reinforced as essential interrogational elements in the MPDS and the absolute baseline of information to be obtained and relayed on every call. In this key question component, the importance of obtaining symptoms such as "chest pain" rather than making a judgmental diagnosis such as "heart attack" is emphasized. The answers to the key questions then lead to the appropriate pre-arrival instructions and also establish the correct (standardized) level of emergency medical response known as the dispatch priority. While maximal response is permitted "when in doubt," the number of such situations is greatly reduced, thereby simplifying dispatch decision making while making it safer and more efficient.

At the heart of the EMD certification course is the ALS-level (and MPDS-experienced) instructor review of the medical symptom or incident type priority card. This includes a basic review of the problem involved, discussion of the additional information section of the protocol, the significance of each key question, and a brief explanation of pertinent pre-arrival instructions. The medical (as opposed to political or geographical) priorities of dispatching are stressed for each caller complaint. Approximately half of the course must be taught by an EMD-literate, ALS-level instructor.

Dispatch Life Support (DLS)

An integral part of dispatcher training is that of pre-arrival instructions. The NAEMSP has stated in both its consensus document and its position paper on emergency medical dispatching that "pre-arrival instructions are a mandatory function of each EMD in a medical dispatch center." These instructions are not only an essential element of the MPDS, but they are also a logical improvement in dispatch.

In preparation for the role of giving lifesaving instructions to the caller, EMDs are trained in dispatch life support (DLS), which contains many elements of BLS, including CPR. The instructions range from basic head-tilt airway maintenance and the Heimlich maneuver to phone-instructed CPR. Also included in the training are hemorrhage control by direct pressure, treatment of small burns, eye flushing, removing pillows from behind the heads of unconscious victims, and prehospital obstetrical do's and don'ts, as well as actual childbirth assistance.

An important learning experience for the EMD trainees and a highlight of the certification course is the introduction of the non-red-lights-and-siren response concept for many calls previously believed to be dire emergencies by untrained dispatchers. After explaining that abdominal pain and fever in a 17-year-old male who probably has appendicitis is not a prehospital medical emergency and requires neither a red-lights-and-siren nor an ALS/paramedic response, dispatchers often respond, "Why, after all these years, haven't we been told that before?"

To round out the basic MPDS certification course, students attend a practical session of treatment and interrogation using carefully designed mock cases (including CPR and choking scenarios). This is designed to give the EMD experience and confidence in using the new manual card or computer-assisted priority dispatch system and to see the newly taught concepts in action.

MPDS and EMS

So what are the advantages to the EMS or fire service manager of having certified EMDs in the dispatching system? Quite simply, such certification training eliminates the need to hire—in addition to regular dispatchers—registered nurses or other ancillary medical personnel to perform medical dispatching functions. Also, the call evaluation and prioritization provided by certified EMDs are more standard and consistent and are comparable to the operating procedures followed by police officers, firefighters, and paramedics. In terms of time and money, the 24-hour basic EMD certification course is less expensive to provide than EMT training, which, although longer, is not even vaguely dispatch-related and has been proven to be much less useful to the dispatcher.

The concept of priority dispatching by trained EMDs goes hand in hand with the system of tiered response, which is dispatching only the care that is reasonably needed. The concept is also continuing to grow through-

In preparation for the role of giving lifesaving instructions to the caller, EMDs are trained in dispatch life support (DLS), which contains many elements of BLS, including CPR.

out the United States. In Utah, for example, more than 500 dispatchers have received EMD certification training. Additionally, more than 400 municipalities and thousands of individual agencies in 48 states and five Canadian provinces have adopted the dispatch system for their own use.

Positive Effects

What results can an MPDS program deliver for a municipality? In Salt Lake City, the system has reduced the number of fire department responses by more than 33 percent. Non-urgent BLS incidents are now handled by contracted, EMT-staffed private ambulance teams. The estimated cost savings of the program appear to be substantial, especially considering that one-third of Salt Lake City's medical calls now require no response by the fire department at all. In addition, the city's fleet management reported that its emergency vehicle accident rate was initially reduced by 78 percent.

Salt Lake is only one of many examples in which correctly implemented MPDS has made significant contributions in providing quicker, more efficient EMS response. Paramedics nationally have reported significantly improved response information, as well as more appropriate use of their highly skilled time.

Some areas in EMS in which a properly initiated MPDS could have positive effects include the following:

- Decreased liability exposure (in more than 10 years experience)
- Decreased response time to zero minutes (pre-arrival instructions)
- Decreased emergency medical vehicle accidents
- Decreased burnout of field personnel
- Decreased red-lights-and-siren runs
- Improved medical control at dispatch
- Improved dispatcher professionalism
- Improved relationship of dispatch center to elements of the field
- Addition of a continuing educational environment to dispatching
- Increased dispatcher morale
- Increased dispatcher pay
- Increased quality of the dispatch employee
- Increased defensibility of dispatcher's actions and employee standards
- Increased standardization of care, interrogation, and decision making
- Increased number of lives impacted
- Increased appropriateness of medical care through correct response

- Increased resource availability, especially ALS
- Increased safety of response personnel at scene
- Increased arrival knowledge of response personnel
- Increased cooperation with associated public safety systems, law enforcement, and fire departments

Making the Change

Sound planning is the key to success in starting any MPDS. Once the decision is made to effect a change, a thorough system evaluation should be made, including the collection and review of present and past information about the existing system. This not only clearly defines where the system is at the present time, but also provides the objective justification for change.

The implementation process should include input from all appropriate sources: operations managers, EMS managers, dispatchers, field and private providers, training personnel, and physician medical control. Planning (including timetables for training and startup) should be detailed and should involve a phased implementation scheme to optimize the process. Each step of the implementation process should be clearly defined in terms of objectives, action plans for meeting objectives, associated training process required for each phase, and identification of the people responsible for all activities.

There are three generic prerequisite ingredients for a successful system implementation:

- A progressive EMS provider administration
- Strong, involved physician medical control and direction
- Municipal government understanding and support of planned training and response protocol changes

For many cities and emergency medical systems, localization of the dispatch priority section will also require an unprecedented justification of response modes and unit selection. Now is the time to review and revise older policies calling for full emergency response to all incidents. The use of strong medical control over the past 10 years' experience with MPDS has redefined dispatch and response procedures and has definitively determined that in a sizable number of incidents, the use of red lights and siren is unnecessary and puts EMS personnel at preventable risk.

In establishing routine versus emergency response assignments, the following questions should be considered during any MPDS protocol implementation.

- Will time make a difference in the outcome? In other words, is the problem a true time-priority case requiring a response of less than five minutes? This includes cardiac or respiratory arrest, airway problems, unconsciousness, severe trauma, hypovolemic shock, or a true obstetrical emergency.

- How much time leeway do you have for that type of problem?
- How much time can you save driving with red lights and sirens?
- When the victim gets to the hospital, will the time saved be significant compared with the time spent waiting for care such as X-rays, lab tests, and so on?

Again, it is important to emphasize the need for strict medical control in developing alternate response policies. However, the savings in the amount of fuel used, in stress to personnel, in vehicle wear and tear, in the prevention of hazards to personnel and to the public on the road

Medical Control Gets Tough With EMD

Jeff J. Clawson, MD

The National Association of EMS Physicians (NAEMSP) was founded in 1985. From the beginning, its mission statement made clear the need for adequate medical control in all aspects of EMS: "The growing importance and increasing sophistication of emergency medical service systems have led to a greater need for the physician, as patient advocate, to assume a role that would ensure the patient's right to the best care possible."

EMS physicians in general have recognized medical dispatch as the last major component of EMS systems to be identified and appropriately defined. According to NAEMSP, "The involvement of EMS physicians in the world of dispatch is relatively new but unquestionably essential."

The NAEMSP has taken a leadership role by recently developing consensus documents to be followed by more definitive position papers on key issues in EMS. In recognizing that the activities of medical dispatchers are crucial to the efficient operation of an EMS system, NAEMSP stated, "The 'health' of many EMS systems can be gauged by the appropriateness of training, protocol, and medical control of dispatchers." This statement was made as part of a general rationale for the development of their recently approved *Consensus Document on Emergency Medical Dispatching.*

The NAEMSP has taken an important stand. Medical directors, with their inherent responsibility for ensuring safe activities within EMS in general and for medical dispatchers specifically, should be taking the lead in establishing the first published national-level standard. The medical/legal ramifications of inadequate EMS dispatch services impact everyone from the agency to the medical director, field practitioners, and ultimately the patient. Dispatch is the means by which appropriate medical care is assigned and directed to the victim. Indeed, the EMD can even initially provide that care remotely through the caller.

The NAEMSP has taken a major step in establishing fundamental medical control at dispatch through the creation of this document. It sets not only professional, organizational, and supervisory responsibilities for medical dispatcher programs, but establishes the "moral necessity" of certain dispatch interventions on behalf of the victim. Recommendations for ongoing quality assurance and risk management processes are made and encouraged to be in place after initial training. Finally, the eventual governmental certification of medically supervised EMDs is stressed as a method of ensuring that these goals are met in the future.

Note: The complete formal version of the EMD Consensus Document is available from NAEMSP National Headquarters, Center for Emergency Medicine, 190 Lothrop Street, Suite 113, Pittsburgh, Pa. 15213, (800) 228-3677.

will prove well worth the initial investment of time and effort in adopting more realistic, reasonable, and clearly defined dispatch procedures.

Quality Assurance

Without sound quality assurance, a new dispatch program or an older, poorly functional system will remain an "event" rather than a healthy, sustained "process." Recent EMS literature has described the 11 QA elements of medical dispatch. These include dispatcher selection and evaluation; orientation programs; initial EMD training; continuing dispatcher education; dispatch protocol data generation; medical dispatch case review; medical control and EMS physician involvement; certification; recertification; a risk management program; and refusal, suspension, or revocation of certification.

Conclusion

Hundreds of localities have discovered what was originally proven in Salt Lake City in 1979 when MPDS was in its infancy. That is, many dispatchers were performing in the role of EMD without the benefits of either dispatch-specific medical training or medically sound protocols in dealing with the problems that constituted their daily routines. To correctly use dispatchers as members of the emergency medical team, it is necessary to upgrade their skills through EMD training courses and certification programs.

The benefits of the medical priority dispatching system are far-reaching. Through dispatch-specific education and practical experience, the EMD is able to more accurately interrogate the caller, provide more pertinent information to responders, give direct aid to patients through the callers in a safe and efficient manner, and make sound, sensible decisions about EMS responses. In addition, the system as a whole allows for preplanned, safer responses (fewer units responding in the red-lights-and-siren mode), fuel and energy savings (fewer units used when possible), and the reserving of ALS teams for ALS emergencies.

If EMS is committed in its quest to provide dynamic and responsive care to the citizens it serves, continued reassessment is necessary to plan for the increasing demand that will inevitably be placed on providers in the future. The establishment of a comprehensive MPDS should be one of the primary steps taken to maximize the most efficient use of our human and material resources in the provision of high-quality, safe, and effective patient care.

References

American College of Emergency Physicians. *Principles of EMS Systems: A Comprehensive Text for Physicians.* Ed. W. R. Roush. Dallas: American College of Emergency Physicians, 1989.

Clawson, J. J. "Dispatch Priority Training: Strengthening the Weak Link." *JEMS* 6, no. 2 (1981).

Source

Reprinted with permission from Emergency, *January 1990. Jeff J. Clawson, MD, is the originator of the medical priority dispatch system. Robert Martin was the director of publications for Medical Priority Consultants. He has worked closely with Dr. Clawson during the refinement of the priority dispatch concept and is an expert in medical priority dispatch logic systems.*

Clawson, J. J. "The Maximal Response Disease—Red-Lights-and-Siren Syndrome." *JEMS* 12, no. 1 (1987).

Clawson, J. J. "Medical Dispatch Review: 'Run' Review for the EMD." *JEMS* 11, no. 10 (1986).

Clawson, J. J. "Medical Priority Dispatch—It Works." *JEMS* 8, no. 2 (1983).

Clawson, J. J. "Quality Assurance: A Priority for Medical Dispatch." *Emergency Medical Services* 18, no. 7 (1989).

Clawson, J. J. "The Red Lights and Siren Response." *JEMS* 6, no. 2 (1981).

Clawson, J. J. "Telephone Treatment Protocols: Reach Out and Help Someone." *JEMS* 11, no. 6 (1986).

Clawson, J. J., and K. B. Dernocoeur. *Principles of Emergency Medical Dispatch.* Englewood Cliffs, N.J.: Brady/Prentice Hall, 1988.

Kuehl, A., ed. *EMS Medical Directors' Handbook.* C. V. Mosby Co., 1989.

National Association of EMS Physicians. "Consensus Document on Emergency Medical Dispatching." *JEMS* 13, no. 11 (1988).

"Position Paper: Emergency Medical Dispatching." *Journal of Prehospital and Disaster Medicine* 4, no. 2 (1989).

ANY COMPUTER-AIDED DISPATCHING (CAD) system should reduce call response times and enable dispatchers to support EMS personnel in the field. These goals are achieved by providing a calculated response to service requests and dispatching the appropriate resources.

This article describes different systems available for computer-aided dispatching. As with anything else, the more bells and whistles you buy, the more the system will cost. You can buy a simple records management system or the most ornate system available on the market today.

One of the most important applications for computers in EMS is their use in dispatching operations. Gone are the days of writing information on cards and time stamping an ambulance's every move. Instead, computers track all information, search databases for critical details, and make recommendations for dispatchers on the closest responding units or on pre-arrival instructions for medical emergencies.

When selecting a CAD program, it is important to look for a system that is user friendly. The middle word in "computer-aided dispatching" is "aided." Computers are intended to make the dispatcher's job easier, not more difficult. Key characteristics of user-friendly systems are anticipation of dispatcher errors, painless correction of such errors, helpful screen messages, clear on-screen instructions for all features, and well-written documentation.

Most manufacturers claim their CAD programs are user friendly, but in reality, some packages are friendlier than others. Dispatchers often differ in experience, expectations, and work habits, too. A CAD program that one dispatcher finds extremely complicated, another will enjoy using. The only way to find out if the software is user friendly is to use it. Properly ergonomically designed hardware and user-friendly software can reduce eyestrain, headaches, and backaches, raise productivity, and decrease turnover.

Your system should be geared for reduced keystrokes and instantaneous access to critical information. Good CAD programs use color and reverse video flashing to alert dispatchers to high-priority information.

Emergency personnel should be provided with pertinent information before their arrival at the scene. Many CAD systems recommend the most appropriate emergency vehicle either through suggested apparatus response or a tracking system, such as an automatic vehicle locator (AVL) or a global positioning system (GPS). If the vehicle recommended is not the closest, a manual override feature should allow the dispatcher to enter the correct vehicle into the computer.

A computer system should always provide a current status display of all emergency vehicles in the fleet. If possible, out-of-service vehicles

Understanding Computer-Aided Dispatching and Interfaces

Gary G. Ludwig,
MSM, EMT-P

Gary Ludwig is the author of the workbook, Computers in EMS and the Fire Service. *This article, adapted from the book, outlines key components of EMS computer and automatic vehicle locator systems. It separates the basics from the bells and whistles, and aids the reader in becoming a more informed buyer of these expensive tools.*

Any computer-aided dispatching system should facilitate the training of dispatchers.

should be one color, vehicles in service and in quarters should be another, and vehicles in service and on the street should be a third color. Information—about a vehicle on the scene of a shooting too long, for example—should show in reverse video after a preset period of time.

Many CAD systems can interface with various informational components. For ease of data entry, 9-1-1 data from the ANI (automatic number identification) and ALI (automatic location identification) should be automatically dumped into the system without someone having to rekey it.

Other computer systems have the ability to produce geographic information from a database. The geofile function of a CAD system can do data searches for cross streets or physically draw a map on the dispatcher's screen, pinpointing the site of the emergency. Other communication centers can take this map and project it onto a large screen so other dispatchers can also view the location of the incident.

Mobile computing is another interface feature. It provides for field data entry and an inquiry system that operates on portable computing devices. The software permits incident entry in a real-time environment. An ambulance arriving at a scene, for example, need only hit the arrival key on a portable computer to update the communications center. Constant voice communications between field units and the communications center are reduced. Some private hospital-based ambulance services have a device called a keyboard data terminal (KDT) that accesses the main computer at the hospital to provide a patient's medical record at the scene.

Hardware and Software Considerations

The CAD hardware and software vendor selected should be responsible for the complete design and installation of all equipment.

The design should include past reliability of the entire system in other agencies of comparable size. Another area of concern is the speed of your dispatchers when operating the system. A CAD system that causes the dispatcher to stumble from screen to screen searching for the right keys could slow your dispatching process considerably. In one CAD program, over 180 different five-letter commands had to be typed in to update information in the computer system. Remember, user-friendly systems are a must in high-tension dispatching procedures.

Any computer-aided dispatching system should facilitate the training of dispatchers. Managers need to realize that not all dispatchers are computer literate; some dispatchers may even suffer a fear of computers. Therefore, training dispatchers on the use of the CAD system should be uncomplicated. When a needs analysis is done for a CAD system, it is highly recommended that the dispatcher be involved in the initial discussion and planning. Even if some dispatchers have never had experience with computers and know nothing about computer-aided dispatching, they should be encouraged to express and discuss their ideas. Their thoughts and recommendations may not make any sense, but the goal is to make them feel a part of the system and the decision-making process.

9-1-1

The use of a single three-digit phone number for all emergencies began in England in 1937. The number 9-1-1 was chosen in the United States because no existing area codes or exchange prefixes began with those numbers. Since then, most major cities and populated areas in the country have gone to the 9-1-1 system. Officials estimate that installing 9-1-1 can shave 30 to 60 seconds off any emergency call.

A computer system should be compatible with your 9-1-1 system. It would probably be best to speak with your telephone representative to get a format of the 9-1-1 data stream coming into your PSAP (public service answering point). It is very important that your computer system capture the 9-1-1 data and dump it directly onto the dispatcher's screen.

A computer system should be able to interact with the existing computer systems your agency already possesses. Some EMS agencies may have a billing computer system for their responses and transports to hospitals. The CAD system should be able to transfer data that the billing computer can interpret and use for invoicing purposes. Data entry personnel should not have to rekey pertinent information into the billing system when it is already found in the CAD system.

The CAD system should have room for future growth. The needs and expectations of an EMS agency are constantly changing. For example, a service may want to add four more dispatcher consoles to the system because of an expected increase in call loads. The CAD system should be designed to accommodate this growth. Also, compatibility between the CAD system and the mobile data terminals (MDTs) needs to be considered when the bid is awarded.

CPU

Any CAD system purchased should have enough processing power to handle the volume of incidents, the ancillary file searches, and the number of terminal devices proposed for the communications center. Insufficient processing power will lead to slow data responses and screen updates. Commands entered into the CAD system should be measured by maximum response time (MRT) in seconds, and should be required in 99.5 percent of all transactions. For instance, a search and display of basic information from a geographic file containing cross streets, zip codes, hazard information, and response districts should not take more than two seconds during peak load conditions. The status change and display of any unit should take no more than one second. A CAD system that takes 15 seconds to search these databases can hinder the dispatching process.

A CAD system should be fault tolerant. This is particularly important because a CAD system is operating continuously with an extremely critical function. Even a few seconds of computer downtime can be

Remember that your CAD system will undoubtedly operate 24 hours a day, seven days a week. The goal is to use only equipment that will experience the longest, most useful life, fully supported by the industry.

disastrous. Therefore, the system should maintain an uptime ratio exceeding 99.5 percent.

Many EMS agencies create a fault-tolerant system by having two main computers constantly processing information. One computer will usually do the processing and mirror the information to the other computer, along with writing information to a hard disk. If the first computer fails, the second one will maintain the system until the first one can be repaired.

When requesting a bid from a vendor, specifications should indicate that all hardware should include standard, unmodified models in current, regular production (not Beta test units) by leading manufacturers. Remember that your CAD system will undoubtedly operate 24 hours a day, seven days a week. The goal is to use only equipment that will experience the longest, most useful life, fully supported by the industry.

Printers

No CAD system is complete without printers, which are necessary to produce hard copies of information. They are also necessary to capture data from query applications and current activity within the system.

It is not necessary to have a printer connected to each workstation in the communications center. With networking systems, all dispatchers can share one printer. If more than one printer is in the room, the printer of choice can be selected.

Monitors

The preferred computer-aided dispatching system should use color monitors displaying a minimum of 640 x 480 VGA. The monitor should be able to display various colors, dual intensity, reverse video, blinking, blanking, and underlining, and it should be capable of transmitting protected and unprotected fields. A protected field displays information that cannot be overwritten by the dispatcher. For instance, a dispatcher may time-stamp the arrival of an ambulance at the scene. The field should be write-protected so that no one can go back and change it by typing in a new time.

Flashing modes, such as reverse video flashing, should be reserved for exceptions, such as a high-priority incident, failure of a field incident to respond within preset parameters, or alert/hazard notifications.

The monitor's size is especially important if plans are to mount it in the dispatcher's console. Consoles now have modular designs to adapt to changing technology. Consoles need to be ergonomical, modular, and highly flexible. It is likely that the size of most computer monitors will increase by 30 to 40 percent over the next decade. These larger monitors will place information from three or four monitors onto one screen.

Monitors should be either freestanding or mounted in the dispatcher console. If the monitors are freestanding, they should have tilt and swivel adjustments.

The monitors should have a bonded, non-reflective surface or faceplate to minimize reflection from ambient light sources and to prevent implosion. Many hardware vendors sell or provide anti-glare glass screens that cut down the glare significantly. The dispatcher should be able to adjust the brightness with a variable control. Finally, the monitor should be placed at eye level to reduce dispatcher neck strain.

Keyboards

The dispatcher's terminal keyboard should be divided into four distinct areas. These four areas enable the dispatcher to use a variety of simple, one-keystroke programming functions to accomplish a task. The areas are

- Main typewriter keys ("QWERTY" design)
- Cursor control keys
- Numeric key pad
- Function keys

The keyboard should be equipped with "up," "down," "left," "right," and "return" keys. The dispatcher should be able to move the cursor to any position on the screen except for protected areas.

A minimum of 12 function keys should be programmed with one-button commands for the most frequently required tasks. These may include inputting confirmed 9-1-1 data, time-stamping a call, accessing a help menu, or routing a request through the system to a call-waiting screen.

Keyboards may be placed either on a pull-out tray or a keyboard shelf off the work surface. Since keyboards reduce the amount of available work space, the best design is to put them below the work surface or near the monitors at a 33-degree angle. If you have a policy that allows your dispatchers to eat and drink in your communications center, plastic keyboard protectors are a must.

Operating Software

The software vendor should furnish and install the operating system and all the utility programs required for the CPU and CAD system. The software should also be commercially available, fully supported by the manufacturer, mature, and the most recent version.

The vendor should provide information on file updating and maintenance procedures, including purging. Purging is eliminating certain files or records on command or at a specific period, such as a date or at the two-year mark. File maintenance capabilities should be restricted to designated individuals via password identification to ensure file security and control.

The system must have full file integrity safeguards at the record level. File management/maintenance software should permit full file backup/archive and recover/restore utilities. Some software systems allow file maintenance capabilities to be restricted to a certain terminal position with the proper password entry.

CAD Software

A vendor should provide an EMS organization with the specific types of programs and modules being used. Most vendors have preprogrammed software packages. Vendors should agree to make modifications to the existing "canned" packages, because slight modifications are usually necessary to fulfill the needs of the EMS organization.

Before any computer-aided dispatching system is programmed, the vendor should sit down with representatives from the EMS organization and provide printouts of what the screens will display. This is usually a good time for the EMS agency to make recommendations or changes—before the programming is done. However, the vendor should agree to make moderate or minor software modifications without cost after the system is installed and operational. A minimum time period of six months should be allowed for these modifications.

Key Requirements of a CAD System

It is very important for a CAD system to survive in the face of conditions that would create downtime in most other computer systems. This is why the CPU and the disk file should be redundant. An uninterrupted power supply (UPS) should maintain your entire system, including all workstations, until your building's generator kicks in and powers the computer system.

All CAD systems should operate in real time. If the operating system does not provide real time, the CAD system will need a central time generator, external or internal to the computers. The central time generator is designed to keep accurate time, down to the second, on every workstation within the CAD system.

The dealer should fully describe any plans to make your system fault tolerant. Fault tolerance means that the system is able to sustain itself in the event of electrical, CPU, or hard disk failure. The vendor should describe the system's ability to switch the data from one computer to another or to sustain the system electrically.

Another concern should be the recovery time in the event of failure. A recovery time that involves a repairman coming out Monday morning for a failure that occurred on Friday night is unacceptable. Your maintenance agreement should specify a time period in which the company must respond. This time period should indicate a company response to your phone call during your working hours, not theirs.

Key CAD System Facilities

Every computer-aided dispatching system should provide a full set of dispatcher capabilities, including a comprehensive CAD management reporting system that supports EMS operations and facilitates administrative information retrieval. Before buying any CAD system, make sure the vendor provides you with details on what information you will be able to retrieve.

EMS managers will obviously want to track a call from dispatch to when the equipment is back in service. However, managers often fail to ask for reports that can impact their service. Detailed reports should provide the chief of an EMS agency with Medic 1's average response time to any scene during the last fiscal year, or the average time an ambulance spends at hospitals after delivering patients.

All incident reports should be kept in an hour, minute, and second format. Without the seconds, what may look like two minutes to get to a scene may have only taken 62 seconds. Most computer-aided dispatching systems track time in a 24-hour format (military time).

Dispatchers should be able to work with multiple calls and enter data on separate incidents simultaneously.

Visual and audible alarms are important tools that alert the dispatcher to key occurrences during a dispatch process. These alarms, located at the dispatching console, should reflect time-related conditions on equipment status. If a vehicle has been dispatched but has not provided an acknowledgment or an en route signal within one minute, a visual or audible alarm should alert the dispatcher.

Alarms should also alert the dispatcher when an address matches an instruction file. An instruction file contains special information about a particular address. For example, the instruction file may indicate that a baby at this address is on a SIDS monitor and appropriate equipment needs to be brought in.

Visual or audible alarms should also be displayed at the dispatcher's console when an address matches information contained in a hazard file. This may be any hazard, not just hazardous materials.

The historical file is another tool that can be of value to dispatchers and responding personnel. The historical file also matches addresses, and displays every past response and the nature of the calls. The historical file should be preset to show all responses for the last 30, 60, 90, or 120 days, or even longer.

Additionally, audible and visual alarms should be provided in the communications center to indicate failures of any major components of the CPU, including power transfers and interruptions.

The CAD system should capture and maintain a journal of all transactions. Any information recorded should include originator and destination information, as well as the time down to the second.

The system should periodically record the journal on magnetic tape. Information backups should be done at the end of every business day. Full backup of both recorded information and the actual CAD program should be done once a week, and the magnetic tape should be transported to another site for storage. The tapes can then be used to reconstruct the system database in the event of damage or destruction to the CAD system.

Tell your software vendor how long you wish to store data. If your agency does 70,000 calls a year and you want to store two years worth of data on your computer before writing the information to magnetic tape for permanent storage, make sure the vendor knows.

The system should have the flexibility to allow for easy and quick reassignment of functions and units to other terminals. This would be necessary if a dispatcher needed to take over for another dispatcher suddenly required to support a high-intensity, short-term incident.

The CAD system should be able to accept hardware identification and emergency alerting signals from voice radio units or MDTs (mobile data terminals) in the field. This identification must be displayed to the dispatcher in real time. The requirement for rapid, simultaneous display of voice transmission and digital and voice assignment is very important.

Electronic mail is a beneficial feature in bigger systems where dispatchers operate in large or separate rooms. It also has benefits for dispatchers who work different shifts. An electronic mail software package within the CAD system can deliver messages to and from dispatchers.

CAD Interfaces

Any CAD system should support a number of key interfaces that enhance an integrated command, control, and communications facility. Some interfaces include

- ANI/ALI and call sequencer
- Mobile data terminals
- Master time generators
- Other computer networks
- Hard copy printers in the communications center or in ambulance houses
- Remote terminals
- Pagers or tone-activated radios
- AVL (automatic vehicle locator)
- Digital communications
- Computerized status maps

CAD System Functions

The CAD system should have a sign-on and sign-off procedure that will activate and deactivate all terminals. These procedures should use a personal identifier (helpful when accumulating statistics in the communications center) and a position identifier. The personal identifier, usually a dispatcher number, is provided by the dispatcher. The position identifier is automatically provided by the terminal when the dispatcher enters information. These identifiers will appear in the record of all calls handled through the terminal. The end result is that terminals are limited to authorized transactions. Dispatchers can be similarly limited, and unauthorized attempts to bypass the system can be recorded and reported.

Every system should provide a sign-off procedure. Another dispatcher signing on at an active terminal will automatically log off the existing personal identifier and replace it with the new personal identifier for future transactions.

Incident Number

Incident numbers are important for tracking and identifying a specific call. The CAD system should automatically assign a sequential number to a dispatching incident. The calendar year is usually at the beginning of a case number, creating an incident number like 92-15675.

Help Functions

A computer-aided dispatching system should provide help functions accessible by a simple keystroke, like hitting F1. The help function should provide a brief description of the data requirements for all fields in the system. The help function should also include a general description of system operations, file listings, and file access.

Call Taker Entry Processing

The call taker or dispatcher evaluates the nature of the rescue or medical incident, and usually assigns a coded number to a call. An overdose may be coded 113, or a shooting 345. Coding an incident helps when information is retrieved. If every call were text written, a heart attack could be "heart attack," "MI," "myocardial infarction," etc. Generating a year-end report would be a nightmare. With a three-number code, a manager directs the computer to look for all 113's for the year-end report. Other computer-aided dispatching programs provide a written description of the code, when entered. Most CAD systems have a priority pre-assigned to a specific type of call. If three transfers and a heart attack come in at the same time, the heart attack would have a pre-assigned priority higher than the transfers.

The CAD screen should provide a field for entering a short narrative. Narratives might include the current condition of a patient in a medical situation, hazardous information provided by the caller, etc.

The date of the incident should be automatically assigned in a protected field on the screen. Most systems have an internal clock with a date timer that will provide this information.

All times should be placed in protected fields provided on the screen. Usually a simple keystroke, such as hitting F3, will automatically time-stamp the field. Times usually recorded are

- Time phone call was received
- Time phone call was put into the computer for dispatching
- Time unit was dispatched
- Time unit confirmed the call
- Time unit was en route
- Time unit arrived on the scene
- Time unit left scene for the hospital
- Time unit arrived at the hospital
- Time unit was in service

A computer system may have to record other pertinent information, including what the first unit on the scene reported or what hospital a patient was taken to. Other EMS agencies require that the ambulance provide a code for the nature of the medical incident when a patient is transported to the hospital.

Management reports help allocate resources and personnel, develop budgets, and validate inquiries.

Most CAD systems require the dispatcher to identify the unit or units handling a call. Other CAD systems search a preprogrammed database and produce a recommendation of which units to send.

CAD Support Files

Some files supplement the dispatcher's job but are not related to the CAD function. The dispatchers, from within the system, should have access to a telephone directory for a number of people and agencies. The directory might include numbers of all hospital emergency rooms, numbers of contacts at a business containing hazardous materials, or the home, business, pager, and cellular phone numbers of key public safety personnel.

A manager's security file should contain the names, passwords, and levels of authorization of all those who use the CAD system. Updating, changing, and retrieving records should be restricted to specific persons or keyboard positions. At least two management personnel should have the password to access this file. No computer-aided dispatching system should ever rely on only one person to function effectively and efficiently.

Some EMS agencies choose to track hospitals in their response area that are on diversions. If a hospital is currently on a diversion, the information should display on the dispatcher's screen in order to alert the ambulance transporting to that hospital.

Reports

Management reports summarize the data recorded in the operations process. After a call is completed and moved to storage, the information should be retrieved to generate management reports. Management reports help allocate resources and personnel, develop budgets, and validate inquiries.

Communications Center Performance Report

The CAD system should provide reports on all activities in the communications center, including comprehensive reporting on the process, personnel, and equipment used to provide services. Management needs to call up these reports on a real-time basis.

Call Taker Activity Report

The call taker begins all services in the communications center. Management needs to track

- Call taker identifications
- Terminal position identifications
- Number of 9-1-1 calls received per position
- Number of incidents entered by call taker

Running totals on this data are required, as are averages for the current year and for the same period during the preceding year. Additionally, management should be able to track information by the total number of calls per hour, shift, and day for daily, weekly, biweekly, monthly, or yearly periods. With this information, a manager can make personnel and resources decisions for a more productive communications center.

Dispatcher Management Reports

Management also needs to generate data on the dispatching process, including average time periods for dispatching, unit acknowledgment, arrivals, and when units are available for assignments. This information should also generate reports that vary from hourly to yearly periods.

Daily Incident and Statistical Report

This report is composed of all EMS calls within the previous 24 hours. Some agencies generate this report automatically at a specific time every day, at several designated printers. A portion of this report summarizes events from the previous day. This report also contains "exceptions" that have occurred within the last 24 hours. Exceptions can include incidents where a crew was not dispatched or en route within the preset time.

Time Computations

Unfortunately, EMS organizations are not usually judged on how well employees splint a fracture or start an IV, but on how fast they can get to a scene. So time tracking is an important part of record management. Some necessary time-elapsed computations include

- Total elapsed time from initial receipt to clearance of incident
- Dispatcher elapsed time from the receipt of the call until call is dispatched
- Acknowledged elapsed time from dispatch until the unit's responding transmission
- Responding time elapsed from initial dispatch until the time of arrival on location
- Call arrived on location time elapsed from initial receipt of call by the call taker until the first unit arrives on scene
- On location time elapsed from arrival on scene to the time the unit is available, returning to quarters, or responds to a hospital
- Responding to hospital time elapsed from when the unit departs the scene and is responding to the hospital until it arrives
- Unavailable at hospital time elapsed from when the unit arrives at the hospital to the time when it is available for assignment

The computer system should provide everything from daily to weekly, biweekly, monthly, and yearly averages for these elapsed time categories, including year-to-date and year-to-month totals. These times should also be retrievable in whatever manner requested. For instance, you might want to know the entire department's average response time or just Medic 3's average response time to the scene of any emergency.

Running Cards and Preplans

Computer-aided dispatching can either be a records management system, or it can provide "aid" to the dispatcher and responding crews with vital information. Information retrieval can make the difference between an efficient and effective service or just a functional one that may put personnel at risk by not providing key details. Some departments may be smaller and rely on another agency for dispatching. Running cards and preplans can help supplement any department with critical facts before arriving at the scene. In the anticipation phase of any call, the more information available, the better the planning.

Running cards and preplans are designed to supplement dispatchers and emergency personnel with predetermined staging and role information. Your department should be able to retrieve information at the dispatcher's position and at the equipment housing quarters.

Running cards and preplan information should include the following:

- Business name
- Owner name
- Occupants
- Street address
- Box number
- Hazards phone number
- After-hour company representative name and phone
- Cross streets
- Map coordinates
- Inspection information
- Preplanning instructions
- Constraints for construction or traffic problems
- Directions to the scene
- Mutual aid information

System Status Management

System status management (SSM) uses extensive data analysis to aid dispatchers when positioning ambulances for optimal use of personnel and resources. While all services use some form of SSM, this computerized management technique is almost essential for private ambulance services who contract with government municipalities. Most government contracts require an ambulance to be on the scene within, for example, eight minutes 90 percent of the time. With computers projecting where the next call might be, dispatchers move units appropriately to provide optimal response times.

This strategy for continuously managing resources available in the system at a given time can shave minutes off any response time. By moving ambulances to various locations throughout the day, a system can improve the probability of an ambulance being near an incident.

System status management requires the development of a system status plan (SSP), designed by a team of system status planners. The team is usually made up of line, staff, and management position employees. An SSP is developed by first reviewing grid maps of the city showing all calls, their locations, and response times. Calls are plotted on 168 maps, equating to each hour of a seven-day week. The planners can then look at maps from 16 different weeks over an 18-month period for the same one-hour time of day. Some services make transparent maps so they can be overlaid for ease of use. Based on the highest call volume, recommendations are made on where to base ambulances awaiting a call.

Once the data has been analyzed and recommendations are made for posting ambulances, the information is fed into a computer for a graphic display of recommendations or posts.

Pre-Arrival Instructions

In communication centers where licensed and medically trained personnel are not available to provide pre-arrival instructions to callers, software is available that either interfaces with your current CAD or can be dedicated to a specific personal computer in a "stand-alone" mode. Training in pre-arrival instructions, medical priority dispatch protocols, and good communication skills are a must for this line of work.

It is not uncommon to hear stories of dispatchers teaching people over the phone how to do CPR, deliver babies, or control bleeding.

These pre-arrival software packages follow an algorithm for delivering instructions to the caller. The dispatcher may ask if the patient is breathing or not breathing. The questioning and instructions will follow one set pattern if the patient is breathing, and another route if the patient is not breathing. The dispatcher often provides pre-arrival instructions to the caller, and the computer informs the dispatcher how to prioritize the assignment.

Mobile Data Systems

The use of equipment like status message units and mobile data terminals enables EMS agencies to consolidate their computer and radio communication systems into a single data network. This network provides immediate access to vital information available through CAD systems and their interfaced computer databases.

Some of the primary purposes for using status message units and mobile data terminals are

- Reduced radio channel activity
- Better security
- Improved resource control
- Dispatched information displayed in vehicle

Any computer-aided dispatching system must be easy to use and must provide quick, accurate emergency response data to dispatch personnel.

- Reduced dispatcher workloads
- Improved status monitoring
- Access to incident information, preplan information, or building schematics

Status Message Units

Status message units (SMU) function as if they were hooked up to the main computer in the communications center. The status message unit operates as a terminal or peripheral to a CAD system.

These units usually rely on a mobile radio system to transmit information to and from the SMU. The information is transmitted over the same frequency as voice transmissions.

SMUs usually have a control head the same size as a radio control head. One or two rows of buttons will send a preset message to the communications center when pushed. For example, if a unit arrives on the scene, the paramedic pushes the preset button indicating that the unit has arrived. The status of the mobile unit is automatically updated in the communications center.

Some departments use SMUs in the dispatching process. For example, an alarm is received in the ambulance quarters about a shooting. The paramedics, when heading out the door, hit the preset button indicating they have received the alarm and are en route.

Since voice and data are transmitted over the same radio frequency, a piece of hardware in the communications center called a controller is used to differentiate between voice transmissions and data bursts from the SMU.

Mobile Data Terminals and Computers

A mobile data terminal or computer is the same as a status message unit except that it operates on a separate radio frequency from voice transmissions. A mobile data terminal or computer has a keyboard and screen, and paramedics type a message and determine where to send it. All data transmissions are recorded in a permanent record.

MDTs and MDCs have the ability to access other computer systems to obtain files or retrieve information. EMS personnel use their terminals for finding hazardous material information or patient records, and for sending electronic mail between offices, vehicles, or dispatchers.

Maintenance Agreements

Unless you are a computer programmer, wrote the computer program that your system operates, and can repair computer hardware, you will probably need a maintenance agreement with your hardware and software vendor. How much maintenance support you will need should be negotiable with your vendor. The vendor should provide you with a certain period of warranty or guarantee for the products without any charge.

Maintenance service to hardware and software must be performed and available on a 24-hour, seven-days-a-week basis within a specified period of time. Make sure that the specified time is in your working hours.

Your agreement should also provide for a time period in which the vendor has to have the repair completed. Leaving this time period open-ended could result in a week or more of downtime for your computer system. Even with a redundant system, you want to specify that all repairs are made in eight to 16 hours. If the repairs are hardware-related and cannot be made within the specified period of time or if repairs have to be made off-site, your vendor should supply you with working equipment of greater or equal value, at no cost to you.

If software and hardware vendors jointly enter into a project, obtain in writing which vendor will be the service contact in the event of a failure.

Some vendors do not charge an annual maintenance fee, and many provide an 800 number so your call is free. These features are used as marketing techniques to get you to buy their product.

Conclusion

Any computer-aided dispatching system must be easy to use and must provide quick, accurate emergency response data to dispatch personnel. The CAD system should track all calls for service, the locations of the calls, and pertinent information, including all times associated with the calls. The system should also provide critical supplemental data to the dispatcher.

Source

Original article. Gary G. Ludwig, MSM, EMT-P, is deputy chief of EMS for the city of St. Louis. He is the author of Computers in EMS and the Fire Service.

Are EMS Communications Still All Talk?

Steve Adler

In this article, the manager for Motorola's EMS and fire markets describes different communications technologies available to the EMS manager. Steve Adler makes the communications options understandable, even for non-technophiles.

- COMMUNICATIONS DEVICES with voice, data, and color video
- Communications devices that respond to voice and touch commands
- Communications flexibility between responding agencies
- Patient databases for EMS response
- Automatic vehicle location systems for effective response selection and routing

All of these capabilities, and more, are within the vision of today's emerging communications technologies.

Public and Private Communications

There has been, and continues to be, a plethora of changes in public and private communications. New wireless systems are being developed. Public systems designed for personal use are being implemented for both short- and long-range telephone access. And there is a movement away from wired to wireless (or untethered) radio systems, from mobile to portable systems, and from local to regional systems.

Automatic channel assignment, or trunking, radio systems have already been developed for more efficient use of the radio-frequency spectrum. Automatic assignment is designed to nearly eliminate interference among users of the same frequencies and is especially effective in urban areas, where radio users often must compete for valuable channel space.

The effect of a trunked system is similar to that of a bank queue: All of the patrons form a single line, and the first available teller serves the person at the front of the queue. The advantage of this system is that it optimizes the use of tellers serving customers or of radio channels serving users.

Extending this trunking technology, which has been used in telephone systems for a long time, to two-way radio and adding features for rapid access and priority levels has made an ideal system for shared-system users.

The microprocessing computer's impact on communications is also being seen. New technology has improved radio, telephone, and computer systems and the interconnection and exchange of information between them. Sending data over analog communications circuits has become a highly sophisticated process. Digitizing voice transmission is now commonplace in telephone-switching equipment and in some digital transmission systems. Point-to-point fax transmission has become a worldwide success.

Today's digital radio systems for one-way and two-way data applications, such as display paging and database access, will soon be joined by new digital radio technologies, allowing integrated digitized voice and data capabilities. With these new capabilities, EMS systems of the future will have improved voice communications as well as improved text and graphics communications and color video transmission.

Both telephone and radio systems are moving toward integrated analog and digital communications systems, which are sometimes referred to as ISDNs, or integrated services digital networks. In the United States, public safety radio interests and the federal government are already developing new digital systems.

This blitz of radio technologies will impact each element of the EMS communications system, particularly citizen access, dispatch, medical control, and interagency contact.

Citizen Access

Both the efficiency and methods of citizen access vary widely throughout the United States and the world. In many communities, citizen access has been improved by the implementation of a central access number, such as 9-1-1. The primary advantage of a central access number is that callers have one easy-to-remember number for access to emergency services in a given geographic area.

Standard 9-1-1 systems route all calls from a single city, county, or region into a central location, known as a public safety answering point (PSAP). Newer enhanced 9-1-1 (E-9-1-1) systems not only route all calls into a central location but also provide automatic number identification (ANI) and, in some cases, automatic location identification (ALI). ANI systems display the telephone number from which the call is made, while ALI systems display both the number and the address of the caller. Call takers can also tell whether calls come from cellular telephones, residences, schools, businesses, or a variety of pay-telephone locations.

Thirty-four states now have statutes requiring 9-1-1 access to emergency services. In addition, many states provide radio call boxes along highways and freeways for motorists to call or signal for emergency assistance. Several types of highway call boxes are currently in use, including new cellular voice call-box systems in California, older UHF two-way voice highway radio call-box systems in Connecticut, and highway call boxes that use microwave relays to connect to 9-1-1 answering centers in Alaska. Non-voice highway radio call boxes are used in Florida, and some areas also have highway call boxes wired through the telephone system to PSAPs.

New public communications systems are constantly being developed to improve citizen access. These include personal communications provided by systems like the CT2 expanded cordless telephone, the digi-

The primary advantage of a central access number is that callers have one easy-to-remember number for access to emergency services in a given geographic area.

Medical control will be more easily connected with the field, using more efficient private shared radio systems or via simple interconnection between private radio systems and local public systems.

tal European cordless telephone, and the worldwide low-orbit satellite cellular service.

Dispatch

Dispatch systems continue to improve as capability is increased and sharing among municipal, county, and state agencies grows. Many local systems serving single agencies have grown into regional shared systems, resulting in improved communications for each participating agency.

The advent of public safety trunked systems is the driving force behind this trend. In these systems, multiple agencies can share a common infrastructure, providing improved communications range and new features for each agency. A major feature of these systems is that each agency operates and controls its own usual communications and has its own "talk groups" for handling EMS, police, and fire operations. A talk group is a group of people (a receiving hospital and a paramedic team, for example) who frequently speak to one another and are assigned a radio channel on demand. Another key feature is that the common infrastructure allows for the creation of new multiagency talk groups either on a planned basis or as required by multiagency incidents.

In addition to adequate voice communications for dispatch, expanded information is now available to assist in the dispatch process. Computer-aided dispatch (CAD) and automatic vehicle location (AVL) are two of the newer dispatch tools gaining widespread acceptance.

The new digital radio technologies also provide integrated communications services via a single radio. Voice-, data-, and telephone-interconnect capabilities, with their dynamically different usage characteristics, will be served in one multi-feature digital radio, resulting in the integration of data and voice.

Medical Control

Medical control communications needs are unique to EMS. While many prehospital events can be handled by EMTs or paramedics with standing orders or protocols, some of these events require consultation between field personnel and the physicians at the hospital or patient-receiving location. A majority of these cases require this communication at the time of patient assessment under conditions particularly difficult for wireless communications. Patient locations in buildings and roadside ditches are typical of EMS situations that result in poor communications.

Future EMS systems will have sophisticated mobile-access systems to facilitate medical control communications. Medical control will also be more easily connected with the field, using more efficient private shared radio systems or via simple interconnection between private radio systems and local public systems.

As sensor technology improves for field use with patients, digitized outputs from these sensors will be rapidly communicated to host-computer systems for analysis and display. In addition to color video from a patient location, multilead EKGs, blood pressure, blood gases, respiration, internal temperature, and other vital signs will be communicated to points of medical control.

Interagency Communications

Interagency communications continue to improve, using both the private shared radio systems and new public communications systems. The development of more flexible private shared systems will provide unique access and priority features among public safety agencies and public utilities during events that endanger lives and property. Already, public safety agencies are insisting that new communications technology developments include migration capabilities in communications products, which will allow a system to change gracefully and economically from analog units to digital units. These migration features also provide for interoperability between older neighboring systems and the newer digital systems.

EMS Spectrum Management

The EMS radio spectrum in the United States is regulated by the Federal Communications Commission (FCC). Currently, EMS radio systems are licensed under the Special Emergency Radio Service (SERS), which they share with a variety of non-medical service eligibles.

EMS radio systems, with many restrictions, are eligible in SERS for 20 VHF low-band frequencies, 13 VHF high-band frequencies, 10 paging-only frequencies in the VHF low band and UHF band, 24 UHF frequencies (four UHF frequencies for vehicular repeater access, two UHF dispatch MED channels, and eight UHF medical communications MED channels), and some 800-MHz channels that are shared with other public safety radio services.

The FCC has proposed that a new Emergency Medical Radio Service (EMRS) be established that would only include as eligible those actually involved in the delivery of emergency medical treatment.

VHF EMS Radio Systems

VHF low band and high band were the first frequency ranges used for EMS. Hospitals and ambulances continue to use the Hospital Emergency Administrative Radio (VHF high-band HEAR) systems. EMS communications outside major metropolitan areas rely on VHF-FM systems. The FCC includes special provisions for VHF high-band cardiac-telemetry use outside of the 50 largest U.S. metropolitan areas.

UHF Radio Systems

FCC action in the late 1960s and early 1970s initially allocated five UHF frequencies for EMS and later allocated the UHF complement of frequencies available today. The EMS UHF channel allocations—having separate 5-MHz-spaced transmit and receive frequencies—permit UHF systems to operate as full duplex, which means that they can send and receive messages simultaneously. Many EMS professionals prefer to use duplex UHF EMS systems because they are similar to a telephone and provide simultaneous transmission and reception at the base station and with ambulance crews using a duplex radio or two or more simplex radios. With simplex radios, users transmit while keying the radio on and then unkey the radio to receive transmissions.

In addition to duplex-system operation, UHF systems can penetrate buildings better than VHF, resulting in better radio coverage in urban and suburban areas.

800-MHz Public Safety Trunked Systems

The newest frequency bands used by public safety users, including EMS, are 800-MHz channels. Both the frequency spectrum available and the types of systems implemented in this frequency range encourage shared use.

Public safety planning advisory committees, established by the Associated Public Safety Communications Officers (APCO), exist in each state and territory and in a few large metropolitan regions. These committees are charged with developing regional plans to license users in the 800-MHz public safety frequency bands. If EMS agencies wish their needs to be addressed by these committees, they will have to ensure that they send representatives to the board in a timely fashion. Many regional plans have already been accepted by the FCC, primarily in metropolitan areas, in which the demand for additional channels is greatest.

Provision for radio-frequency trunking is part of all 800-MHz public safety plans, and, in fact, trunking is still only permitted by the FCC in the 800-MHz band. Trunking systems in UHF frequency bands are in use today by government agencies and users in other countries.

Wide-Area EMS Communications

Wide-area communications are provided in VHF (800-MHz) and UHF (450-MHz) systems using point-to-point communications systems as well as a variety of radio-relay techniques. Satellite receiver systems, vehicular repeaters, and microwave links are three methods most commonly used for coverage of wide areas.

Many EMS regions, for instance, use two or more base sites, with repeaters and satellite receivers for countywide coverage. Pinellas County, Fla., uses a combination of microwave links and radio base stations for its countywide system. Mountaintop relay systems are used in many states, including Alaska, California, Idaho, Nevada, New Mexico, and Ohio.

Cellular Radio Telephone

Cellular radio telephone service is now available in most urban areas in North America, and some cellular systems are expanding into rural areas. A vast majority of rural areas, however, still do not have cellular telephone coverage. Implementation of a cellular system is extremely costly, and system expansion depends on the rate of radio telephone demand in the area. In other words, many subscribers are needed to spur the development of cellular service in suburban and rural areas.

Although few EMS agencies use cellular radio telephones exclusively or as their primary EMS communications system, the use of cellular telephones for EMS communications is viewed by many as an alternative to dedicated EMS communications systems. Cellular service is attractive for EMS purposes because, like a regular telephone, it provides duplex voice communications. Autodialing features and hospital telephone features, such as three-way calling, simplify some cellular EMS operations.

Cellular telephone use, however, can be a disadvantage in EMS systems when disciplined access to medical control is bypassed and crews do not follow existing transport protocols. A more critical disadvantage for EMS is that priority access usually is not available with cellular telephones. Major accidents, fires, disasters, and even family-oriented holidays cause cellular systems to become busy and, in many cases, inaccessible. Also, because cellular communications are one-to-one, operations using multiple cellular-equipped field units can be difficult to coordinate. This coordination is particularly difficult during a mass-casualty event because, unlike many radio systems, each call is discrete and cannot be monitored by other members of the response team.

Even though priority access is not yet available, cellular radio telephones are effective in many EMS situations. Cellular radio telephone access to hazardous materials information sources, poison control centers, and at command posts during major disasters is useful. Even in daily EMS responses, a cellular telephone is a useful addition to dedicated EMS radio communications.

Satellite Communications

Land-based radio systems for rural areas are expensive. The infrastructure cost per person in rural areas is extremely high because of the wide areas covered and low population densities. Thus, radio satellite communications systems, which now provide coverage for large parts of North America, may be more economical and useful for some EMS operations. These commercially available systems, which can now incorporate ground stations and transportable stations, provide voice, data, and video communications. There are even plans to provide low-earth orbit (LEO), worldwide land-mobile satellite communications. The first of these LEO systems, called Iridium, will support handheld portable radio telephones.

Air Medical Communications

Helicopter and fixed-wing air medical services responding to emergencies need air-to-ground radio channels for communication to hospitals and ground ambulance services. Unlike commercially available air-to-ground communications that use frequencies allocated for that

Communications
are a vital element
of EMS and can
be significantly
improved with the
proper use of
technology.

purpose, EMS airborne communications frequencies must share the current SERS frequencies allocated for land-based systems.

Also, when airborne radios use an EMS radio channel, the transmitted energy covers a wide area and may interfere with other EMS communications on that channel. To prevent this occurrence, current FCC rules permit aircraft public safety communications only on a secondary (non-interfering) basis, which allows for air-to-ground service communications with restrictions on transmitter power. Establishing a new EMS air-to-ground spectrum, along with coordinated assignments, would do more to eliminate this interference and would reduce the restrictions on air-to-ground communications.

EMS Communications System Plans

Successful EMS systems must have effective communications. A combination of state and local planning is required to create, implement, and support EMS communications systems. All state EMS programs should have comprehensive EMS communications plans that include current and future EMS communications system development.

To implement these plans and to take advantage of new communications technologies, all state and local agencies should inventory their present resources and re-evaluate their needs-assessment programs. They can use their findings to drive the development of specific future plans for EMS systems and their use of UHF MED channels, VHF high-band frequencies, VHF low-band frequencies, and 800-MHz public safety channels.

Conclusion

Communications are a vital element of EMS and can be significantly improved with the proper use of technology. Improved voice, data, and video communications can improve each of the important EMS communications links: citizen access, dispatch, medical control, and interagency coordination. Private radio systems serving EMS providers can be even more closely and seamlessly linked to public systems. And faster, more effective patient service can be provided with new communications technologies applied to EMS systems.

Depending on factors such as geography and demographics, however, some technologies may be more appropriate or cost effective than others in meeting the needs of a particular area. To achieve full success and utilization of new technology in EMS, providers should take part in the ongoing process of evaluating new communications tools and implementing those that can provide improved communications services.

References

Addendum I to Highway Safety Program Manual Volume II, DOT HS 802 976, Communications Manual. Washington, D.C.: U.S. Department of Transportation, National Highway Traffic Safety Administration, June 1978.

Archambault, S., and F. Pethel. *EMS Communications Compatibility Studies*, DOT HS 803 858. Washington, D.C.: Systech Corp. for U.S. Department of Transportation, National Highway Traffic Safety Administration, November 1978.

Barnes, G. "PCN vs. Microwave: The Spectrum Battle." *Telecommunications* (December 1991).

Comparison of State 9-1-1 Legislation and Standards. Dallas: Texas Advisory Commission on State Emergency Communications, 6 March 1992.

Hall, J. A., et al. *Emergency Medical Services Communications System Technical Planning Guide*, NTIA SP 79 3. Washington, D.C.: Systech Corp. for U.S. Department of Commerce, March 1979.

Johnson, M. S., and R. Tredwell. "Rural EMS Communications." *Emergency Medical Services* 20, no. 8 (August 1991).

Public Health Service. *Emergency Medical Services Systems Program Guidelines*, DHEW 79 2002. Washington, D.C.: U.S. Department of Health, Education and Welfare, August 1979.

U.S. General Accounting Office. *Report on State and Local Emergency Medical Services Programs*, GAO/HRD-86-132. Washington, D.C.: U.S. General Accounting Office, September 1986.

Source

Reprinted with permission from JEMS, May 1992. Steve Adler is the director of business strategy for Spectrum and Standards, a part of Motorola's Land Mobile Product Section serving public safety, EMS, and fire markets.

Who Calls the Shots? EMS Operations Control and the Role of the Communications Center

Robert E. Suter, DO, MHA, EMT-P

Communications centers exert an expanding control over a number of operational aspects of emergency services. They have increasingly become a significant management tool as well, challenging the role traditionally held by field supervisors. This article by Dr. Robert Suter examines the traditional role of the communications center and proposes a theory that places the center at the "hub" of management decision making.

ONCE IGNORED BY HEALTHCARE and management theorists, emergency medical service has begun to attract attention to its traditional policies and practices. Long-standing notions about job qualifications, job responsibilities, organizational structure, and operations control are being challenged by alternative approaches such as system status management (SSM), computer-aided dispatch (CAD), and emergency medical dispatch (EMD). One important characteristic of these new models is their emphasis on the role of the communications center in controlling operations. Convincing arguments for these systems have been advanced, and they have been implemented successfully in many areas.

Despite these developments, variations of the traditional model, which minimizes the importance of the communications center and emphasizes control by field supervisors, still characterize many, if not most, EMS systems in the United States. While this probably is due to a natural resistance to change and local political concerns, data supporting the new systems unfortunately are only anecdotal. Except for superficial comparisons, the traditional and alternative approaches have not been examined in light of accepted management theory and principles. Therefore, this article will analyze the communications center and operations control from a theoretical standpoint to determine where in an EMS organization control is exercised most naturally, and how these findings could impact management effectiveness.

Control Theory

Control is necessary for the effective management of any organization. It can be defined as the intervention and action necessary to promote appropriate behavior. The key term is intervention, since it is what distinguishes control from planning. To exert control, managers must have the ability to communicate effectively with employees. When confronted with problems or unique situations, there must be mutual access between supervisors and employees.

Since the focus of this article is operations control, it is important to separate operational from administrative control. Operations control focuses on "line management," the supervision of those producing the organization's primary services. Classically, this occurs through constant observation. Since EMS does not allow continuous observation, EMS operations control is inherently more complicated, and hence does not lend itself easily to comparisons with other fields.

Operations control may be categorized in several ways. One major classification scheme distinguishes between direct and indirect control.

Direct control is accomplished by communications with appropriate individuals, and is more characteristic of EMS operations control. Indirect control is accomplished through the use of conceptual tools like budgeting. The other classification scheme divides feedforward from feedback control. Feedback control is retrospective in nature. It involves proactively establishing standards, and then retrospectively using performance data to design corrections needed to prevent the reoccurrence of deviations. Feedforward control is future oriented and attempts to prevent problems before they occur. It is characterized by analysis of important data and assessment of variations followed by timely action.

EMS control systems should be feedforward in nature and use direct control techniques.

Ideal EMS Control

Cybernetics is the science of control, including the study of how control should be exercised and of the flow of information necessary to achieve it. When applied to EMS operations, it is clear that to prevent irreversible adverse outcomes, EMS control systems should be feedforward in nature and use direct control techniques. The common requirement of both is effective communication with personnel. Furthermore, this communication should be real time, occurring as events are actually happening. Only after real-time communications are established can feedforward operations control be attempted.

Problems With Traditional EMS Supervision

In the small to medium-size services that constitute the majority of EMS systems, the field supervisor is the primary person responsible for controlling EMS operations activities. The supervisor obtains control information by observation, inspection, evaluation, and monitoring of the two-way radio frequency. Control is exercised by on-scene verbal orders, written evaluations, and communication by radio or telephone. While none of these techniques is particularly unusual, control theory identifies several potential problems.

First, the opportunity to observe crews is extremely limited. Second, inspection and evaluation are feedback techniques. Perhaps most important, however, is the reality that a field supervisor cannot always maintain contact with crews.

The inability of EMS field supervisors to maintain constant contact with crews stems from communication barriers inherent in EMS systems. Call information is filtered by the communications center and may be incomplete. This may result in a misleading assessment of ongoing events. Physical and technological barriers also play a part. In a large geographic area, mobile VHF radio units have a limited ability to communicate with each other. Supervisors may not be able to hear communications from subordinates. If supervisor input is desired, messages must be relayed, a cumbersome and time-consuming process that can be complicated or delayed by multiple events. The numerous distractions involved in a supervisor's normal activities also complicate effective monitoring of communications.

Even without distractions or technical limitations, supervisors frequently do not have sufficient control information, because the type of data transmitted is limited due to the public monitoring of radio frequencies. The need to transmit sensitive information may delay supervisor input until telephone contact can be established. This particular problem can complicate communications with those requesting service, ambulance crews, and senior EMS management.

The Role of the Communications Center

The importance of communications to control leads to continued focus on the communications center. Nearly all EMS communications networks are "wheel" systems with the communications center as the "hub." Management theorists describe wheel communications systems as characteristic of centralized management structures in which managers deal with the external environment, and then order subordinates to accomplish specific tasks.

Besides being the anchor of all real-time operational communications, the communications center is the initial point of contact with the external environment. It serves as a message center—the point of transfer of information between telephone and radio or vice versa.

The Message Center Function

Since EMS crews are dispersed over a large area, consistent, real-time communications are achieved only by radio or telephone. The communications center is the focus of this activity, since it is the only organizational asset that can transfer information between radio and telephone to maintain real-time communication.

The importance of real-time communications raises questions about the amount of effort required to maintain it, as well as the amount of time dispatchers perform other communications tasks. To provide information on the time spent performing these various tasks, the communications tapes from one medium-size, midwestern EMS agency were evaluated. The results are shown in Table 2.4.

Table 2.4

Dispatcher Communications Time-Use Analysis

These data were obtained from the communications center tapes of a "traditional" EMS system during a randomly selected 72-hour period. The system was a third-service public agency providing comprehensive EMS including all ALS response. At the time of the study, seven ALS units made approximately 6,000 responses per year in a 600-square-mile area with a population of 180,000.

Type of Communication	Minutes	Percent Total
Routine traffic—radio	41.8	9.9
Routine traffic—telephone	7.6	1.8
Information request—radio	6.0	1.4
Information request—telephone	64.0	15.5
Emergency call traffic—radio	47.9	11.4
Emergency call traffic—telephone	82.1	19.5
Non-emergency call traffic—radio	10.1	2.4
Non-emergency call traffic—telephone	25.1	6.0
Relay to/from supervisor—radio	36.8*	8.8
Relay to/from supervisor—telephone	96.9**	23.3
Totals	**418.3**	**100.0**

Explanation of Terms
- Routine traffic: Acknowledging status notification, etc.
- Information request: Non-call inquiries concerning status of other units, road information, or similar information.
- Emergency call traffic: Anything concerning acceptance, handling, or processing of an emergency call.
- Non-emergency call traffic: Anything concerning acceptance, handling, or processing of a routine transfer.
- Relay to/from supervisor: Any communication in which the dispatcher relays a message involving the on-duty field supervisor and a third party.

* At least four messages were clearly urgent, requiring immediate action to prevent unfavorable events. In two cases the delay in establishing contact with a supervisor was substantial.
** At least two messages were clearly urgent, requiring immediate action to prevent unfavorable events.

Prehospital and Disaster Medicine © 1992 Suter

While it was anticipated that relaying information to and from supervisors would account for a significant amount of time, the actual numbers were startling. Dispatchers spent nearly one-third of their communications time relaying information to field supervisors. Most of this was by telephone, and thus was not related to the distance limitations of VHF radio. An average of two messages per day were very urgent in nature, and, in at least one-third of these critical cases, the delay in relaying messages was substantial. While the results of this tape analysis may not be apply to every EMS system, the study demonstrated that in some systems, the dispatcher may merely be an extra layer in the overall communications process.

Source of Real-Time Control

The message center function potentially has significant negative implications on operations control by field supervisors in most EMS systems. Despite this, EMS managers must realize an even more important fact about the communications center. It is where information is transformed into action. Therefore, it is the natural source of real-time control.

No one has a finger on the pulse of the EMS system to the extent that the individuals staffing the communications center do. It is from this site that deviations from plans are most readily detected and that the greatest impact on real-time operations performance can be exercised. Decisions made by dispatchers consistently have more impact on system response performance than any other factors. By receiving requests for service, triaging, assigning crews to calls, and ordering ambulance movements to reconfigure the system, the EMS dispatcher assumes responsibility for action and decision making that is identical to theoretical descriptions of management functions.

Dispatcher decision-making responsibility does not end with these tasks. In the response phase of EMS, real-time information transmitted from the communications center provides specific task directives, information on policies or procedures, and data on response and transport performance, also in-line with management characterizations.

Authoritarian Control

In most EMS organizations, crew input is not desired in the response phase of operations. Policies indicate a preference for dispatcher judgment in an effort to avoid the time loss associated with questioning assignments. This makes communication from the communications center to crews conform to a downward communication pattern.

Reliance on real-time EMS dispatcher discretion creates an absolute control situation between dispatchers and crews comparable to "authoritarian" leadership or "MacGregor's Theory X." These leadership theories describe situations in which immediate unquestioning obedience to orders is expected. The EMS crews receive orders from the communications center in the form of terse radio messages, which are autocratic in character and authority-based.

This authority also applies to outside requests for assistance. The EMS dispatcher has extensive responsibility for real-time policy interpretation on emergency calls, and must take actions that initially are not subject to approval by a supervisor. While, theoretically, field supervisors can override assignments, this rarely occurs due to the relatively limited information available to them. In traditional systems, unless blatant errors are made, bad decisions are not addressed until the time for effective corrective action has passed. The consequence is a corresponding loss of real-time control by operations managers.

Counter-Arguments

Despite these facts, some may argue that supervisor loss of operational control to the communications center is a misguided notion. Many systems attempt to anticipate potential response scenarios and use computer dispatch programs or develop multiple decision trees for communications center personnel to follow. These algorithms attempt to improve management control by limiting decision making by non-supervisors. Further, the communications pattern between dispatcher and crews might be described as "cross-wise" information sharing instead of downward.

While there is some merit to these counter-arguments, there are real problems. Computer programs or decision trees alone are inadequate to provide in-depth control because of unpredictable chance events that occur routinely in EMS systems. Therefore, the impact of computer programmers or decision trees on dispatchers is limited. This is true particularly in light of the distinction between plans and controls. Controls require efforts to compel events to conform to plans; they don't mean the development of the plans themselves.

The case for cross-wise communications also is problematic. From a control perspective, the concept of cross-wise communications rests on the assumption that subordinates keep supervisors informed of important activities and refrain from making commitments beyond their authority. While EMS dispatchers attempt to observe these limitations, they do not occur consistently on a real-time basis, and only are achieved by feedback. Since operations control in EMS settings requires real-time communication, any approach that utilizes feedback cannot provide the ideal level of control.

An Alternative Approach: System Status Management

The concern over the importance of communications in EMS operations has led to several valuable developments including computer-aided dispatching and emergency medical dispatch training. More relevant to this discussion of control, however, is system status management.

The primary causes of poor performance in direct control settings are a lack of expertise, knowledge, or judgment on the part of those implementing plans, and environmental uncertainty. Since system status management recognizes real-time communications as a critical control asset, it attempts to minimize these factors by developing hourly status plans, using resource utilization theory, and employing paramedic-level "system status coordinators" instead of "dispatchers" in the communications center.

By acknowledging the controlling nature of the communications center, SSM attempts to follow the Principle of Organizational Suitability, which states:

> The more that controls are designed to reflect the place in the organization where responsibility for action lies, the more they will facilitate correction of deviations from plans. Deviations from plans must be the responsibility primarily of managers who are entrusted with the task of executing planning programs. Since it is the function of an organizational structure to define a system of roles, it follows that controls must be designed to affect the role where responsibility for performance of a plan lies.

One area of EMS operations control remains problematic even with SSM. While system status coordinators are responsible for the performance of "the system," they are usually not designated as supervisors, and therefore are not line managers. In these settings, medics are expected to follow orders given to them by persons who are not above them in the organizational structure. Dispatchers or coordinators must give orders without independent authority to enforce compliance. This may create confusion and even resentment among both groups of employees.

To minimize this confusion and improve control, several large systems have added actual operations supervisors to the communications center. This includes at least one large system where supervisors perform the dispatch duties themselves instead of monitoring the actions of EMDs.

Analytical Recommendations

It should be obvious that even in traditional systems, the EMS dispatcher has a great deal of power over the EMS system. Decision making in the form of choosing between alternative actions is inherent in the tasks performed by the communications center. The EMS dispatchers have clear real-time decision-making authority, and everyone who has authority has power.

Although alternative approaches are in place in some large systems, the trend has moved away from the no-training model toward a minimum of EMT or EMD certification. In most EMS agencies, however, the persons staffing the communications center are still the least trained and lowest paid employees in the organization. In light of management theory, this is a curious tradition.

Historically, the dispatchers' lineage can be traced to the messengers of ancient times. Prior to telephone communications, police and fire dispatchers were the precinct desk sergeant or fire captain who greeted those requesting assistance. Electronic means of communication initially did not change much. Equipment operators merely transmitted messages dictated

The EMS dispatcher has a great deal of power over the EMS system. Decision making in the form of choosing between alternative actions is inherent in the tasks performed by the communications center.

to them by supervisors. Over time, the straightforward nature of police and non-EMS fire services allowed semi-independent dispatcher function. When EMS developed, superficially there was no difference in using untrained EMS dispatchers. The fact that most other public services using "untrained" dispatchers located operations supervisors with them was forgotten. Things that made EMS dispatching different—call triage, larger per unit geographic service areas, privacy of key information, pre-arrival instruction, and infrequent or inconsistent on-scene supervision—were unrecognized.

The preceding theoretical analysis has shown that the communications center is where responsibility for real-time performance of EMS operations plans is found and where control is best exercised. It is the only place from which deviations can be corrected on a real-time basis with the flexibility to ensure that the controls will be effective despite unforeseen events.

Of the current formalized approaches to EMS control, the one that comes closest to the cybernetic ideal is SSM. Even it, however, falls short of satisfying the principle of organizational suitability, when the communications center staff does not include line managers. Therefore, in SSM or any other system, adding an operations supervisor to the communications center staff is the simplest way to meet the requirements for improved EMS control.

Unfortunately, many EMS agencies cannot justify staffing the dispatch center with more than one person. To provide ideal levels of control, these small and medium-size systems must challenge their traditional ideas about the job status of the dispatcher. Organizational structures should be modified to elevate the position to a line management position with supervisory authority over ambulance crews. Individuals filling these positions should be experienced paramedics trained in the unique features of medical priority dispatch and in using computer-enhanced system status management.

While the communications-center-based operations manager theoretically is the most important in the organization, reliance on this individual to provide all supervision may be unwise, except in the smallest agencies. Systems benefit from some direct feedback control over routine station activities and by having the capability for on-scene control. Depending on the size of the system, this may be accomplished by having at least one field supervisor, or a crew chief system, or both.

In systems with communications-center-based supervisors, the existence of field supervisor positions generates another possible control improvement. By rotating between field and communications center assignments, operations supervisors can increase their effectiveness by enhancing their control of human factors that influence system performance. In this manner, they can maintain a better appreciation of all aspects of leadership, management, and control within the EMS operations system.

Conclusion

This theoretical analysis of EMS operations control has challenged the importance and status of communications center personnel in traditional agencies. Despite current organizational structures to the contrary, the communications center is the critical means of exerting effective control in any EMS system. Whether in large systems using EMDs with on-site operations managers or in smaller systems with actual supervisor dispatch, implementation of communications-center-based supervision should improve operations control. By eliminating the message relay process and enhancing communications flow, operations supervisors can exercise real-time control over each crew and the system as a whole in a manner that approximates the feedforward ideal. Within this framework, any agency can establish a near ideal approach to EMS operations control.

Acknowledgment

The author wishes to thank his wife, Brenda Suter, RN, for her skillful assistance with the preparation of the manuscript, and John Johnson MD, FACEP, and James Adams, MD, for their thoughtful reviews and suggestions.

References

Baker, J. R., and K. E. Fitzpatrick. "Determination of an Optimal Forecast Model for Ambulance Demand Using Goal Programming." *Journal of Operational Research Society* 37 (1986): 1047–1059.

Barton, G. K. "The Wait for an Ambulance." *JEMS* 11 (1986): 67–70.

Benveniste, R. "Solving the Combined Zoning and Locations Problems for Several Emergency Units." *Journal of Operational Research Society* 36 (1985): 433–450.

Clawson, J. "Telephone Treatment Protocols." *JEMS* 11 (1986): 43–47.

Haimann, T. *Supervisory Management for Health Care Organizations*. 3rd ed. St. Louis: Catholic Health Association of the United States, 1984.

Hirsh, H. "Does Curtailment of Emergency Ambulance Rescue Constitute Abandonment?" *Hospital Physician* 20 (1984): 22.

Hough, T. G. "View from the Street-System Status Management." *JEMS* 11 (1986): 48–50.

Kanenetzy, R. D., L. J. Shuman, and H. Wolfe. "Estimating Need and Demand for Prehospital Care." *Journal of Operational Research Society* 30 (1982): 1148–1167.

Koontz, M., C. O'Donnell, and H. Weihrich. *Management*. 8th ed. New York: McGraw-Hill Co., 1984.

Kresky, B., and M. Henry. "Responsibilities for Quality Assurance in Prehospital Care." *QRB* 12 (1986): 230–235.

Levey, S., and N. P. Lamba. *Health Care Administration*. 2nd ed. Philadelphia: J. B. Lippincott Co., 1984.

Liebner, J. G., R. E. Levine, and H. L. Dervitz. Rockville, Md.: Aspen Publishing Co., 1984.

Page, J. "The Police Dispatch Syndrome." *JEMS* 11 (1986): 4.

Rakich, J. S., B. B. Longest, and K. Darr. *Managing Health Services Organizations*. 2nd ed. Philadelphia: W. B. Saunders Co., 1985.

Saunders, C. E. Interview by author concerning the San Francisco EMS System Communications Center, 15 June 1991.

Stout, J. "Computer-Aided What?" *JEMS* 11 (1986): 89–94.

Stout, J. "System Status Management." *JEMS* 8 (1983): 22–32.

Uber, K. "Emergency Dispatch Training." *JEMS* 11 (1986): 48–50.

Warner, D. M., and D. C. Holloway. *Decision Making and Control for Health Administration*. Ann Arbor, Mich.: Health Administration Press, 1978.

White, S. L. *Managing Health and Human Services Programs*. New York: The Free Press, 1984.

Source

Reprinted with permission from Prehospital and Disaster Medicine, *October-December 1992. Dr. Robert Suter is the chief of the Department of Emergency Medicine/ Acute Care at Eisenhower Army Medical Center, Fort Gordon, Ga.*

Vehicle and Equipment Maintenance

Emergency Vehicle Maintenance Goals

Lee Reeder

In a relatively short period, emergency vehicle maintenance has evolved from an ugly stepsister to a valued member of the EMS family. In this article, Lee Reeder describes the changes in certifications, standards, and environmental issues that are impacting vehicle maintenance programs now and will affect these programs in the coming years.

In January 1985, AUTHOR and former EMS consultant Jack Stout issued a challenge to EMS fleet management professionals: Approach emergency vehicle maintenance as if people's lives depend on it.

Stout's article ("Ambulance Maintenance: Aircraft Standards Should Prevail," *JEMS*, January 1985) used major issues and findings from a first-ever national maintenance symposium, which identified critical needs in emergency vehicle fleet management (now known as the Emergency Vehicle and Fleet Management Conference).

A lot has changed since that article was published, but many of those same issues are being addressed around the country, others are not, and some new issues have surfaced. How far has emergency vehicle maintenance come since that gathering in 1985? The following were the major issues identified at that first maintenance symposium:

- Record-keeping systems
- Inadequate standard service programs
- Fleet standardization
- Fleet size
- "Failsafe driving" program
- The switch to diesel engines
- Custom modifications of new equipment

Since 1985, other pressing issues have moved to the forefront of emergency vehicle fleet management, including environmental and health regulations, liability concerns, tight budgets, and a greater emphasis on preventive maintenance. These issues do not alter the goal of limiting critical failures, but they have changed the shop environment in which that goal is realized.

The Role of Management

Stout wrote in 1985 that what most distinguishes successful firms from less successful firms are a thousand little things done right. This attention to detail is what makes the difference in limiting critical, life-threatening failures. And this type of pursuit begins with management.

During the 1993 Emergency Vehicle and Fleet Management Conference in St. Louis, it became clear that although many ambulance services and agencies were embracing continuous quality improvement, the emphasis was often on reforming EMT field performance quality assurance programs rather than widening the scope to other critical needs, such as overhauling fleet management and maintenance. The irony is that true preventive maintenance is identical to the philosophy of continuous quality improvement: Build quality performance into the beginning of a system instead of inspecting later and "fixing" defects. However, fleet maintenance is often one of the last areas in which process improvement is begun.

Although effective emergency vehicle maintenance programs can save organizations thousands of dollars per year in costs and lost revenue, such programs are far from universal. Kent Klausing, warranty manager for Road Rescue of St. Paul, Minn., emphasizes the importance of giving priority to the "fix it before it breaks" philosophy of preventive maintenance. He is surprised by the number of emergency vehicle maintenance shops nationwide that have not implemented preventive maintenance programs. "Administrators who operate these services are starting to learn that, if you do certain things, it's actually going to save money in the long run and [extend] vehicle life," he said.

The Environment

Undoubtedly, the resurgence of environmental awareness in the 1990s is having a great effect on emergency vehicle fleet management. While some services are taking the initiative to be environmentally aware, all are being affected by environmental laws and regulations.

"There is legislation everywhere," said Frank Allison, of the International Mobile Air Conditioning Association (IMACA). "I'm not saying that it isn't right, but it's been a horse that politicians can ride and wave an environmental white hat. City, county, and state legislation is now being written all around the country."

And some of the laws affecting fleet maintenance come as a result of international agreements. The global push to reduce ozone-depleting chlorofluorocarbons (CFCs) has resulted in an accelerated phaseout of the common refrigerant R12 and the subsequent switch to R134A. This transition has brought changes in hardware, maintenance procedures, training, and certification. All mechanics who work on air conditioning systems must receive certification from instructors licensed by an accredited organization such as IMACA. They must follow stringent new environmental guidelines for air conditioning service and refrigerant recovery and recycling.

Local, state, and federal regulations are affecting fleet management

> Attention to detail is what makes the difference in limiting critical, life-threatening failures.

with concerns that range from waste-oil and other hazardous materials disposal to air quality. Environmental regulations on paint booths and body shops are so strict that having such a capability is now financially not feasible for many shops.

Another environmental issue that will affect emergency vehicle maintenance will be the imposition of tighter controls on engine emissions. According to mechanical engineer John Mueller of the EPA's Emission Control Technology Division, "The urban ozone problem is the most pressing problem we have." Mueller says that solving the problem, which manifests itself as smog, will only be accomplished through tighter tailpipe emissions standards. Changes in hydrocarbon and particulate emissions standards are expected to result in engine modifications designed to provide more efficient air and fuel handling and better oil control.

And environmental regulations will continue to cause radical changes in emergency vehicle fleet management. "In the not-too-distant future, I see ambulances that are all-electric, which means no gasoline engines and no diesel," said Charlie Epps, president of ambulance manufacturer Excellance.

Liability and the Law

Several ambulance manufacturers, who were panel members at a recent EVFM conference, cited crash injury protection, safety, and pathogen contamination as liability concerns affecting both manufacturers and customers. Mel Globerman, chief of the Vehicle Engineering Branch of the Automotive Commodity Center for the U.S. General Services Administration, which produces the KKK-A-1822 specification for ambulances, says that because of new federal Occupational Safety and Health Administration (OSHA) regulations on bloodborne pathogens, the patient compartments of ambulances must be designed to be much more easily cleaned than in the past. Globerman adds that cabinets must be stripped of linings that are not easily cleaned of bloodborne pathogens.

Globerman also warns that OSHA regulations on bloodborne pathogens affect all vehicles regardless of the KKK-1822 specification revision that they meet, and that modifications may be necessary to avoid stiff fines. "Get a copy of those OSHA regulations, read them carefully, and see how they're going to affect you," Globerman said.

Robert Johnson, head of customer relations for Road Rescue, said, "It's very challenging for the manufacturers to respond to the new technologies that are out there and to absorb the new regulations, whether they come from OSHA, KKK, or whatever." Johnson adds that because of this fact, it is even more critical today that fleet managers work closely with manufacturers to develop specifications that will serve the organization well.

Globerman and others on a recent EVFM panel also warn against asking for specifications that affect the health and safety of EMS workers and patients. "Don't force a manufacturer to do something that's not right," Globerman said. "It'll come back to haunt you."

Rob Eisterhold, production supervisor for Osage Ambulance of Linn, Mo., says that manufacturers and customers alike have to keep "common sense in design" in mind, particularly with regard to design elements that might cause injury, such as cabinet placement. "The big thing is the safety and well-being of the people in that vehicle," Eisterhold said.

Keene Schaaf, regional sales manager for Wheeled Coach of Winter Park, Fla., also extends this warning to those who make their own modifications after delivery of the vehicle. He says that services making unauthorized modifications to the ambulance must realize that by doing so, they "have taken that saddle of liability off our horse and put it on [theirs]."

Globerman believes that liability should be in the minds daily of people responsible for equipping and maintaining emergency vehicles. "Maintenance is no longer an issue that you can bury," he said. "You certainly don't want to put your head on a chopping block for an attorney."

Record-Keeping Systems

The 1985 article pointed out that there was not an industrywide standard for record-keeping, and there still is none. Since that time, the explosion in affordable computer technology and computer literacy has made that goal more attainable and has created many new options for fleet managers.

Evaluations from the latest EVFM conference showed that participants of the fleet management track were no longer interested in basic computer information. They wanted in-depth training in software that would enable them to track preventive maintenance and document vehicle maintenance histories in order to improve system performance. One of the greatest benefits of increased computer data collection capability is that fleet managers are better able to approach administrators with hard facts and bottom-line statistics that show the need for capital improvements, personnel, and training in the shop.

Training and Education

During the 1993 EVFM Conference, 70 members of a quality improvement workshop identified downtime as the number one opportunity for improvement in emergency vehicle fleet maintenance. A 20-member focus group in the workshop was asked to identify causes that got in the way of the ultimate goal of decreasing downtime. The following are the highest ranking causes listed by the group:

- No standard operating procedures
- Lack of trained managers
- No early reporting of problems
- Insufficient training
- Crew error

Armed with understanding about the vehicles, dispatchers are much better able to diagnose vehicle problems in the field and take appropriate action.

- Vehicle abuse
- Inefficient preventive maintenance program design
- Staff failure to do checks
- Ford

It is interesting to note that of these nine items, seven are training issues and the other two are linked to training issues, which indicates that training is an excellent place to start in decreasing downtime. It has also become a serious liability issue.

"Nobody ever told me about this." Bill Leonard, executive vice president of Medical Transportation Insurance Professionals in Phoenix, says that this quote is a frequently heard and potentially damaging comment made by drivers in accident investigations. In the EVFM quality workshop, the majority of the fleet managers present reported that they have direct responsibility for training new drivers during orientation and for continual driver training. This means that many fleet managers are potentially liable not only for incidents caused by maintenance procedures, but for driver problems.

Eric Maloy, owner of East Tex Consulting Specialists and a veteran emergency vehicle fleet manager, says that comprehensive driver orientation for EMTs can pay off. "I found that by giving that orientation, I saved thousands of dollars," he said. Maloy says that most of the savings comes from preventing such common incidents as backing into trash dumpsters. Maloy urges that dispatchers also receive an orientation to the vehicles from both operational and mechanical standpoints. "When your dispatchers have more understanding about what's actually going on with the vehicles," he said, "they can help your maintenance department a great deal." Armed with understanding about the vehicles, dispatchers are much better able to diagnose vehicle problems in the field and take appropriate action.

Manufacturers as Educators

In Stout's 1985 article, he commented that ambulance manufacturers were not invited to be part of that first national gathering of fleet managers and mechanics. "During this first symposium, we decided against inviting equipment manufacturers, mainly because we didn't want the meeting to turn into a forum for salesmanship," Stout wrote. Since that time, however, the manufacturers have become a vital part of the EVFM conference.

Ambulance and chassis manufacturers recognize the positive effect that education and awareness have on effective maintenance and resulting customer satisfaction. Consequently, these manufacturers are making themselves more accessible as educators for the consumer, both during and after vehicle delivery. The manufacturers have won widespread praise from fleet managers for their efforts.

Mark Vance, a maintenance supervisor with Sullivan County EMS in Blountville, Tenn., says he has taken advantage of the emphasis on manufacturers as teachers. "One of the problems we were having was a lack of education," he said. After some searching, his service discovered and began sending its mechanics to Ford-sponsored mechanics classes in Cincinnati and in Louisville, Ky.

Rick Harms of Ford's Modified Vehicle Engineering Branch says that supervisors should contact their district Ford representatives for information about these free training programs, which are conducted by Ford district service engineers or heavy-truck engineers. Besides providing training, Harms says that the program "gives you somebody to call when you get into a pinch."

Vance learned about the training program from his local Ford dealer. "It has been very beneficial to us," he said.

Klausing, of Road Rescue, says that some ambulance manufacturers are providing similar training, usually in response to requests rather than as part of a formalized program. "We're becoming more and more professional in this industry," Klausing said. "The manufacturers have learned that we have to respond to you. We can't give you this product and say 'Here you are—have fun with it.'"

Jim Overstreet, who sells ambulances both nationally and internationally for McCoy Miller of Elkhart, Ind., says the company recommends that vehicles be accepted at the plant and that administrators responsible for accepting vehicles send their maintenance people to McCoy Miller to spend a few days learning from McCoy Miller technicians.

Fred Schimmel, a member of the engineering staff at Mobile Medical in Decatur, Ind., says that one problem he has found with the smaller emergency service agencies is that no one seems to take responsibility for maintenance. He stresses that it is critical to delegate responsibility for vehicle maintenance to someone who will take the time to become familiar with the owner's manual and ask questions of the technical representatives. He says that an EMS organization does itself and the ambulance manufacturer a great injustice by conducting a one-hour delivery. According to Schimmel, the purpose of making a more in-depth visit is "not just taking delivery of the vehicle, but understanding what you took delivery of."

Globerman agrees. "This is a mutually advantageous position," he said. "The manufacturers have a vested interest in you having a good vehicle, because they come out smelling like a rose when you're happy. But it's certainly in your interest to ensure that you totally understand the vehicle."

Starting Out on the Wrong Foot

While recognizing that they have a duty to the customer, manufacturers also stress that the relationship should work both ways. When the performance and longevity of costly emergency vehicles are concerned, the bottom line is large amounts of money. Ambulances can begin siphoning funds from a service the first day they come on line. Such losses often are ignored because they are generally considered part of the cost of being in the ambulance business. Sometimes, these expensive behe-

> It is critical to delegate responsibility for vehicle maintenance to someone who will take the time to become familiar with the owner's manual and ask questions of the technical representatives.

Reputable ambulance manufacturers are caught between trying to serve the needs and wishes of customers and providing reliable vehicles with realistic electrical specifications.

moths are quickly destroyed by something as simple as lack of attention to detail. And, more often than not, the fault for these losses lies with the purchaser—the one who has the most to lose—rather than the chassis or ambulance manufacturer.

Excellance President Charlie Epps said, "As much as we'd like to build perfect ambulances, they are built by humans and they are machines, and there are going to be some problems."

Schaaf says the biggest problem routinely plaguing the ambulance industry is electrical overload. "Each year we get the same speech, but we have progressed to the point where we need to take logical, professional, and analytical decision-making approaches to equipping our ambulances," he said. "We continue to get request after request to equip vehicles that simply obliterate the electrical output of those systems."

Engineer Fred Schimmel says it is not easy to inform a customer that the requested specifications will result in an electrically overloaded vehicle. He says that in a majority of such cases, the customer argues: "Our other vehicle used to have it on there. Why doesn't it work now?" Schimmel says that trying to convince the customer that the other vehicle truly did not "work" is even more difficult. "They may be going through a set of batteries in a few months, and they may have starting problems consistently," Schimmel said. "But they've accepted it."

Therein lies the quandary: Reputable ambulance manufacturers are caught between trying to serve the needs and wishes of customers and providing reliable vehicles with realistic electrical specifications. Another factor in this dilemma is every manufacturer's fear that the customer will go elsewhere to find a manufacturer that will put anything on the vehicle just to make the sale without regard to the vehicle's long-term serviceability.

"We all know the severity of that problem because it does one thing: It makes you so disappointed in the vehicle that you don't come back and buy our vehicles again," Schaaf said to the audience at the 1992 EVFM conference. He adds that when requests are received for vehicles that will be electrically overloaded, it is the manufacturer's responsibility to discuss workable alternatives. "Let's work together as professionals and solve the problems," he said.

Schimmel stresses the importance of managing the emergency vehicle electrical system. "I would like to have all of the bells and whistles on my own unit that I use out in the field," Schimmel said, "but it's just not practical." He says that EMS organizations often don't want to invest the time and money into electrical management, such as modifying the electrical system or adding multiple battery packs.

Cooperation in emergency vehicle maintenance also puts a burden of responsibility on the end user, according to Globerman. "The hardest thing you're going to have to do as a customer is to separate the real need from the perceived need," Globerman said. "Is bigger always better? Do you really need that medium-duty chassis for an urban application when you have a squad truck running with you for patient extrication? Generally, if you don't need something, bigger is not better, and you may want to think twice about asking for more."

The education and awareness of professionals involved in vehicle maintenance and fleet management have become crucial for services struggling with limited budgets in hard economic times. This is especially true for smaller and medium-size services, which are particularly vulnerable to the costs of excessive vehicle downtime.

All services want to get the most out of their major purchases, and maintenance is a key determinant of vehicle life. When asked what kind of vehicle life could be expected from a diesel ambulance chassis, Excellance President Charlie Epps replied, "Many people with excellent maintenance programs are able to run [their vehicles] between 100,000 and 200,000 miles and still get good service out of them. So much of the life of the ambulance is determined by how well you maintain it."

But it is often the manufacturers who take the heat for problems caused by the purchaser. And many such problems often start with unreasonable expectations of what a vehicle should be able to do.

Globerman says that through the work of the Ambulance Manufacturers Division (AMD) of the National Truck Equipment Association, the ambulance industry has made great strides in the levels of vehicle quality, service, and integrity, resulting in better vehicles. This improvement in the ambulance industry also opens the way for more cooperation between manufacturers and EMS organizations to ensure that ambulances remain on the road longer.

"The vehicles are not just thrown together anymore," Globerman said. "You just can't take this piece and that piece at random because it looks sharp and tell the manufacturer to put it on the vehicle and have him tell you that it's going to be the greatest and most reliable vehicle, because it's not," he added. Globerman says that everything that is added to the vehicle affects the weight, electrical load, center of gravity, or various other vehicle systems. "For every action you take, there is a reaction, and the reaction is not always in your best interest," Globerman said.

> "So much of the life of the ambulance is determined by how well you maintain it."

The Near Future in the Ambulance Industry

One development in the ambulance industry is the advent of a General Motors (GM) ambulance prep package. "Ford pretty much dominates this industry, so I can tell you that we're taking steps to try and change that." said Michael Bailey of GM Truck and Bus Engineering in Warren, Mich. He says that through attending national conferences and working with members of the ambulance industry, GM is gaining an understanding that will help it serve the needs of the emergency vehicle market. Bailey hopes that GM will not "reinvent the wheel" but will instead "pick up where things are today and bring it forward." He predicts that competition from GM's new package will be healthy for the industry.

Manufacturers will continue to adapt their products to meet the needs expressed by people in the industry rather than "force-feeding" EMS providers an ambulance design.

According to Bailey, an improved electrical charging system will be central to the GM package. "When we offer our ambulance prep package, one of the key elements it certainly will contain is a high-output electrical charging system," he said. "That's been missing, and we haven't really had an ambulance prep package. That's what we're seriously going after right now, and the electrical charging system is probably the heart of that package."

Several manufacturers commented that the future of ambulance design will be dictated by the industry itself and not by the manufacturers. "We're going to go where you're going," said Schaaf of Wheeled Coach. He says that manufacturers will continue to adapt their products to meet the needs expressed by people in the industry rather than "force-feeding" EMS providers an ambulance design.

Industry Change Drives Fleet Change

Ron Burnham, chief of the Red River, N.M., Fire Department, reports that a Taos County survey found that 92.6 percent of their EMS calls were non-life-threatening. That leaves about seven percent in which the ambulance is doing strictly what it was intended to do. Statistics such as these are driving changes in out-of-hospital care around the country.

Evolution in the traditional role of EMS will likely also have a great effect on ambulance design and maintenance. The move toward providing more primary care and performing expanded treatment skills in the field will perhaps mean that some emergency vehicles operate as an emergency department or physician's office on wheels, while some continue to provide traditional EMS, but with expanded capabilities. A great number of vehicles may not even be designed with patient transport as a primary function.

"We've seen ambulances grow bigger and become essentially an extension of the hospital emergency room in a lot of respects," said Herman, who predicts that the trend will continue, resulting in ever larger ambulances. However, he added that he doesn't expect Ford to increase the gross vehicle weight rating in the near future. "So if the ambulances are to get bigger and carry more," Herman said, "we have to make our bodies lighter." He says this will be accomplished by using aluminum and other lightweight materials throughout the box and in the cabinetry. According to Herman, this also may result in the use of honeycomb or sandwich construction on the modular bodies to reduce weight.

"All manufacturers would agree that we're going to be building quite a few medium-duty chassis ambulances," said Epps of Excellance. He added that due to the increased manufacture of such vehicles, "I also think we are going to be facing problems that have been reconciled on some of the current chassis that are in high use." He says services are pleased with the longer life of the chassis and engines and the higher payloads of the medium-duty vehicles. Although such vehicles don't have an application in every service, "there are a lot of places that can put them to good use," Epps said.

Specifications for ambulances are also being overhauled by the Ambulance Manufacturers Division of the National Truck Equipment Association, which is made up of representatives of more than 90 percent of the ambulance manufacturers in the nation. The AMD, which has played an ever-expanding role in developing federal ambulance specifications, is developing a new standard for ambulances. In late 1993, the standard went out for three months of public comment. "Our goal with the new standard is to make it more performance-oriented rather than [based on] design," Epps said. "We want to try to provide the opportunity for more innovation in the industry."

Just as specs have changed, so have the rules. As emergency vehicle fleet managers strive to eliminate critical failures, they will be doubly challenged by strict environmental regulation, tight budgets, training needs, and new technology. The challenge for them will be not only to manage, but to lead.

Source

Original article. Lee Reeder is the special projects coordinator for Jems Communications. He has planned the educational programs for four Emergency Vehicle and Fleet Management conferences and has published fleet management articles in JEMS *and* Ambulance World, *an Australian EMS publication.*

Maintenance of Defibrillators in a State of Readiness

Roger D. White, MD

As more sophisticated technology is employed on ambulances, services must take greater care to ensure that the devices are properly functioning. Litigation arising from field failures have underscored the importance of the information presented in this article by Dr. Roger White, one of the early leaders in prehospital care.

SINCE 1984, THE U.S. FOOD and Drug Administration (FDA) has utilized the Medical Device Reporting (MDR) system as a mechanism for reporting adverse incidents associated with the use of medical devices, including external defibrillators. The frequency and content of these reports prompted an FDA-conducted five-state study of defibrillator user training and maintenance practices for both devices and batteries. The study also included inspection and testing of defibrillators and batteries to assess their state of maintenance.

A detailed review of the reports and of the five-state data confirmed that in the majority of cases, adverse incidents were related to improper defibrillator operation and maintenance, prompting the FDA Center for Devices and Radiological Health to launch an educational effort directed toward those who operate and maintain defibrillators. Proper maintenance of batteries (both nickel-cadmium and sealed lead-acid) was a major component of the educational thrust, because battery failure was identified as a recurrent and preventable problem. In an effort to correct the diverse types of incidents being reported, checklists were developed by the FDA for both manual and automated defibrillators. The checklists are designed to cover the spectrum of reported problems related to both device and user.

The advent of more stringent FDA adverse incident reporting regulations, coupled with increased use of defibrillators in diverse settings with varying usage frequencies, would seem to give a major impetus to the regular use of these checklists wherever defibrillators are employed.

Overview of Issues

Case report 1. Emergency medical technicians attended a 45-year-old man in cardiorespiratory arrest. The semi-automated defibrillator analyzed the rhythm and advised a shock. When the device completed charging and advised shock delivery, the shock control was pressed, but no shock was delivered. The unit continued to display a message to shock the patient. Several attempts were made to discharge the defibrillator with no success. The patient was not resuscitated. A service representative confirmed failure to complete a charge. A failed main board on the device was replaced.

Case report 2. After attaching a semi-automated defibrillator, the operator depressed the "analyze" control. A shock was advised and the device began to charge, but the power shut off before a full charge was attained. Reportedly, the device gave no "low battery" message before shutting off. No spare batteries were available. The patient was not resuscitated. A biomedical engineer subsequently confirmed that the battery in the defibrillator was in a discharged state.

Case report 3. A corporate nurse attended a company employee who collapsed in ventricular fibrillation. Defibrillation was attempted, but the device failed to complete a charge. The patient was not resuscitated. A service representative found the batteries to be in a depleted state. The battery charger was examined and was found to have an open fuse.

Case report 4. A user reported that the defibrillator would not charge to the selected energy level. The service representative identified a defective energy-select switch. He also noted that there was a large crack in the case and that sand had entered the device.

These cases are excerpts from four of 580 reports of presumed external defibrillator malfunction reported to the U.S. Food and Drug Administration in 1991 through its Medical Device Reporting system. They represent a cross-section of the major types of problems encountered and reported by defibrillator users. The increasing application of early defibrillation, and therefore the placement of more defibrillators in a wide variety of settings (often with low usage rates) will only accentuate this problem unless a standardized procedure is adopted to ensure a maximum state of preparedness for operation on the part of both operators and defibrillators.

In December 1984, the MDR regulation became effective, requiring manufacturers or importers of medical devices (such as defibrillators) to report to the FDA all incidents in which such devices may have caused or contributed to a death or serious injury. Manufacturers or importers also were required to report incidents in which devices malfunctioned and, if the malfunction recurred, would be likely to cause or contribute to a death or a serious injury. Under this regulation, manufacturers or importers become aware of such information from users (individuals or institutions), from published experiences in medical or other scientific journals, and from their own research, testing, and servicing of devices. In events in which death or serious injury occurs, the regulation mandates that a report be submitted to the FDA by telephone no later than five calendar days after initial receipt of event information and by written report within 15 days of initial receipt.

Between December 13, 1984, and November 30, 1988, 495 external defibrillator adverse incident reports were received by the FDA through the MDR system at a constant rate. This frequency prompted the FDA's Center for Devices and Radiological Health (CDRH), Office of Training and Assistance, to conduct a five-state study of defibrillators and defibrillator users. Data were collected from emergency medical services systems and from hospitals. The first portion of this study focused on defibrillator users and examined such areas as training and retraining, maintenance practices, and battery care. The second part of the study consisted of inspection of the defibrillator and testing of its performance.

Several areas of concern and recommendations for improvement emerged from this study.

Battery maintenance was identified as a major problem; the final five-state survey report in August 1988 recommended improved dissemination of information on battery care, including development of criteria for proper battery use and maintenance. Other recommendations included research and development (to improve defibrillator design and maintenance) and establishment of a uniform standard for "hands-on" continuing education to enhance user training. The latter recommendation reflected the observation in the five-state study that many problems attributed to defibrillators were related to improper operation or maintenance of the devices and their batteries.

During a similar time period, ECRI (formerly the Emergency Care Research Institute), by means of its Problem Reporting Network, received 156 reports of problems related to external defibrillators. ECRI is an independent, nonprofit organization that has maintained the voluntary Problem Reporting Network for health devices since 1971. Again, improper defibrillator maintenance and operator use were identified as frequent causes for reports of malfunction.

Based on the disturbing frequency of reported device malfunction and the observations in the five-state study of errors in defibrillator and battery maintenance and in operator use, the FDA convened a Defibrillator Working Group in 1989 to address these problems and to develop educational strategies that would encompass both defibrillator and battery maintenance and use of the device. The working group was instituted as an educational program within the Office of Training and Assistance of the CDRH. A detailed report on this background information and the preliminary recommendations of the working group were published in 1990. The working group included physicians, nurses, emergency medical technicians, biomedical engineers, and defibrillator and defibrillator battery manufacturers.

Commentary

Several projects were undertaken to ensure a maximum state of readiness for defibrillators and their users. These included a teleconference in 1990 that addressed a wide spectrum of problems and solutions, with emphasis on preventive maintenance. High priority was given to the creation of checklists for both manual and automated defibrillators. It was believed that regular use of such checklists would help prevent the types of defibrillator problems being reported to the FDA and observed in the five-state study. In addition, use of such checklists would familiarize the user with defibrillator operation, including knowledge of the backup supplies and their location, presence of the medical documentation system, the state of charge of the batteries, and the actual operation of the defibrillator. A rhythm simulator was used with automated external defibrillators to determine the response of the rhythm-detection algorithm to both treatable and non-treatable rhythms.

Initial field pilot testing of the checklists was performed in Dallas, Houston, and Seattle; revisions were made based on this experience. The final versions for both manual and automated defibrillators reflect pilot testing assessment in prehospital EMS systems in Washington, Ohio, Iowa, Texas, Florida, Connecticut, and Virginia. Pilot testing included first responders, emergency medical technicians-basic, and emergency medical technicians-paramedics. Metropolitan and rural EMS systems—private, municipal, and volunteer—contributed to the final phase of pilot testing. Thus, the checklists (developed by the FDA's Defibrillator Working Group) represent the input of a broad base of field EMS personnel and operations (Figures 2.3 and 2.4).

Several recommendations need to be emphasized.

First, it is essential that the users of the defibrillators being assessed actually perform the checks. This is necessary if a major function of the checklists is to be fulfilled—maintaining thorough user familiarity with all aspects of defibrillator function and operation.

Second, it is recommended that the checklists be used with every shift change, however frequently that occurs. This recommendation is intended to ensure that all personnel who assume responsibility for use of the device will have an opportunity to assess its (and their own) state of preparedness for operation. For volunteer services, a maintenance schedule can be developed to provide for a daily defibrillator check. Such a schedule should ensure that all volunteer personnel participate in use of the checklists.

Third, the use of the checklists should be understood to be in addition to, and not in any way a replacement for, regularly scheduled, more detailed maintenance checks as recommended by the manufacturer. Batteries, in particular, need specific maintenance procedures. Nickel-cadmium batteries should undergo reconditioning (usually deep discharge/charge cycling three times) every 90 days, and their capacity should be assessed after the discharge/charge cycle. Lead-acid batteries should be kept in a fully charged state and recharged after use. Lead-acid batteries are best kept connected to a charger when not in use; if left in a discharged state for long periods, they can be damaged. Manufacturers' periodic maintenance recommendations need to be followed to maintain both defibrillator and batteries in optimal condition.

Fourth, under the "supplies" section, some items may be carried separate from the device itself. Such separation is acceptable, provided all supplies listed and applicable for the specific device are immediately available.

Fifth, with manual defibrillators in which the remote defibrillation option using adhesive pads instead of paddles is employed, a capacitor charge/discharge cycle using a rhythm simulator can be used.

A commitment to the regular use of these checklists should reduce

Figure 2.3

Checklist for Use With Automated Defibrillators

Automated Defibrillators: Operator's Shift Checklist

Date: _____ Shift: _____ Location: _____
Mfr/Model No.: _____ Serial No. or Facility ID No.: _____

At the beginning of each shift, inspect the unit. Indicate whether all requirements have been met. Note any corrective action taken. Sign the form.

	OK as Found	Corrective Actions/Remarks
1. Defibrillator Unit		
Clean, no spills, clear of objects on top, casing intact		
2. Cables/Connectors		
a. Inspect for cracks, broken wire, or damage b. Connectors engage securely		
3. Supplies		
a. Two sets of pads in sealed packages, within expiration date b. Hand towel c. Scissors d. Razor e. Alcohol wipes f. Monitoring electrodes g. Spare charged battery h. Adequate ECG paper i. Manual override module, key, or card j. Cassette tape, memory module, and/or event card plus spares		
4. Power Supply		

a. Battery-powered units
  (1) Verify fully charged battery in place
  (2) Spare charged battery available
  (3) Follow appropriate battery rotation schedule per manufacturer's recommendations
b. AC/battery backup units
  (1) Plugged into the outlet to maintain battery charge
  (2) Test on battery power and reconnect to line power		

5. Indicators/ECG Display		
a. Remove cassette tape, memory module, and/or event card b. Power-on display c. Self-test OK d. Monitor display functional e. "Service" message display off f. Battery charging, low battery light off g. Correct time displayed—set with dispatch center		
6. ECG Recorder*		
a. Adequate ECG paper b. Recorder prints		
7. Charge/Display Cycle		
a. Disconnect AC plug—battery backup units b. Attach to simulator c. Detects, charges, and delivers shock for "VF" d. Responds correctly to non-shockable rhythms e. Manual override functional f. Detach from simulator g. Replace cassette tape, module, and/or memory card		
8. Pacemaker*		
a. Pacer output cable intact b. Pacer pads present (set of two) c. Inspect per manufacturer's operational guidelines		
Major problems identified (OUT OF SERVICE)		

Signature: _____   * Applicable only if the unit has this supply or capability

Figure 2.4

Manual Defibrillator Checklist

Manual Defibrillators: Operator's Shift Checklist

Date: _____ Shift: _____ Location: _____
Mfr/Model No.: _____ Serial No. or Facility ID No.: _____

At the beginning of each shift, inspect the unit. Indicate whether all requirements have been met. Note any corrective action taken. Sign the form.

	OK as Found	Corrective Actions/Remarks
1. Defibrillator Unit		
Clean, no spills, clear of objects on top, casing intact		
2. Paddles (including pediatric adapters)*		
a. Clean, not pitted b. Release from housing easily c. If internal paddles are included, verify their availability in a sterile package. Periodically inspect as with external paddles.		
3. Cables/Connectors		
a. Inspect for cracks, broken wire, or damage b. Connectors engage securely		
4. Supplies		
a. Two sets of pads in sealed packages, within expiration date b. Monitoring electrodes c. Alcohol wipes d. Hand towel e. Scissors f. Razor g. Spare ECG paper h. Spare charged battery available i. Cassette tape j. Gel or other conductive medium present and stored properly		
5. Power Supply		

a. Battery-powered units
  (1) Verify fully charged battery in place
  (2) Spare charged battery available
  (3) Follow appropriate battery rotation schedule per manufacturer's recommendations
b. AC/battery backup units
  (1) Plugged into the outlet to maintain battery charge
  (2) Test on battery power and reconnect to line power		

6. Indicators/ECG Display		
a. Power-on display b. Self-test OK c. Monitor display functional d. "Service" message display off e. Battery charging, low battery light off f. Correct time displayed—set with dispatch center		
7. ECG Recorder		
a. Adequate ECG paper b. Recorder prints		
8. Charge/Display Cycle for Paddle or Adhesive Pad Defibrillation		
a. Disconnect AC plug—battery backup units b. Charge to manufacturer's recommended test energy level c. Charge indicators working d. Discharge per manufacturer's instructions e. Reconnect line power		
9. Pacemaker*		
a. Pacer output cable intact b. Pacer pads present (set of two) c. Inspect per manufacturer's operational guidelines		
Major problems identified (OUT OF SERVICE)		

Signature: _____ * Applicable only if the unit has this supply or capability the incidence and severity of the types of problems defibrillator users encounter when suddenly called on to deliver shocks with manual or automated defibrillators, though this remains to be established, ideally by means of a follow-up evaluation of checklist usage. The widespread implementation of early defibrillation so strongly encouraged by the American Heart Association will necessitate a system of frequent and thorough assessment of device readiness if this effort is to achieve maximum benefit and safety. Attending cardiac arrest patients in defibrillator-treatable arrhythmias with improperly assessed devices poses obvious and usually preventable problems. At this time, regular use of the checklists as proposed appears to provide the optimal mechanism for minimizing such problems.

Revised reporting requirements for adverse incidents related to use of defibrillators and other medical devices are now mandated by the Safe Medical Devices Act of 1990, which became effective November 28, 1991. The new requirements are detailed in a proposed rule published in the November 26, 1991, *Federal Register*. Because underreporting was shown to be occurring under the Medical Devices Reporting Regulation of 1984, the new regulation will require healthcare facilities to report deaths and serious injuries or illnesses in which devices such as defibrillators were considered to have been contributing factors. Deaths must be reported to both the FDA and the device manufacturer, while serious injuries or illnesses must be reported to the manufacturer or forwarded to the FDA only if the manufacturer is unknown. The reports must be submitted within 10 working days of the incident. Manufacturers and importers of devices still will be required to report injuries and deaths to the FDA.

Research Initiatives

Defibrillator checklists are being made available for use at a time when the mechanisms for reporting adverse incidents related to use of defibrillators are being strengthened to avoid underreporting. Further research is needed to determine what the outcome of these two events will be, particularly because it will also be a period in which more defibrillators will be placed into service in a wide variety of settings and usage frequencies. Adherence to regular use of these checklists seems especially critical and timely.

Acknowledgment

The assistance of the staff of the FDA Center for Devices and Radiological Health, Kaye F. Chesemore (public health adviser for the Division of Professional Practices), and the Defibrillator Checklist Task Force is gratefully acknowledged.

References

Cummins, R. O., J. P. Ornato, and W. H. Thies, et al. "Improving Survival from Sudden Cardiac Arrest: The 'Chain of Survival' Concept." *Circulation* 83 (1991): 1832-1847.

Cummins, R. O., K. F. Chesemore, and R. D. White, et al. "Defibrillator Failures: Causes and Problems and Recommendations for Improvement." *JAMA* 264 (1990): 101-102.

Emergency Care Research Institute. "Hazard: User Error and Defibrillator Discharge Failures." *Health Devices* 15 (1986): 340-343.

FDA. "Medical Devices; Medical Device, User Facility, Distributor and Manufacturer Reporting, Certification and Registration; Proposed Rule." *Federal Register* 56, no. 228 (1991): 60024-60039.

GAO Report. *Early Warning of Problems is Hampered by Severe Underreporting.* PEMD-87-1.

Kerber, R. E. "Statement on Early Defibrillation from the Emergency Cardiac Care Committee, American Heart Association." *Circulation* 83 (1991): 2233.

March, M. G., and J. J. Crowley. "An Evaluation of Anesthesiologists' Present Checkout Methods and the Validity of the FDA Checklist." *Anesthesiology* 75 (1991): 724-729.

Safe Medical Devices Act of 1990. Public Law No 101-629.

White, R. D., K. F. Chesemore, and the Defibrillator Checklist Task Force. "Charge! FDA Recommendations for Maintaining Defibrillator Readiness. *JEMS* 17 (1992): 70-82.

Source

Reprinted with permission from Annals of Emergency Medicine, *February 1993. At the time of original publication, Roger D. White, MD, was a professor of anesthesiology at the Mayo Clinic in Rochester, Minn. He was also corporate medical director for Gold Cross Ambulance in Rochester.*

Care of Contaminated Equipment and Work Areas

Lynn Zimmerman, Deb Jurewicz, and Mary Neuman

In the United States, over 200 deaths and 9,200 bloodborne infections in healthcare workers are reported each year. It is clear that the most critical area of maintenance and equipment management involves contamination. In this article, adapted from the book Infection Control for Prehospital Care Providers, *2nd ed., the authors describe the proper care and cleaning of any potentially contaminated piece of equipment or work area.*

To MINIMIZE THE RISK of bloodborne infections in healthcare workers, specific actions must be taken for handling and cleaning disposable, non-disposable, and other potentially infectious materials (OPIM). Since distinguishing body fluids in an emergency environment is difficult at best, all body fluids should be considered potentially infectious.

Disposable Equipment and Supplies

Disposable items are to be discarded after single patient use. These items include nasal cannulas, oxygen masks, suction tubes, endotrachea tubes, dressings and bandages, and IV equipment. These items should be placed in an appropriate trash bag or container and disposed of in accordance with company policy.

Contaminated articles should be handled with care using universal precautions to prevent contamination of employee or clean equipment.

Regulated Wastes

Regulated waste is defined by OSHA as

- Any liquid or semi-liquid blood or other potentially infectious material
- Contaminated items that would release blood or OPIM in a liquid or semi-liquid state if compressed
- Items caked with dried blood or OPIM and capable of releasing these materials during handling
- Contaminated sharps
- Pathological and microbiological wastes

Regulated waste must be placed in a biohazard labeled bag or container and disposed of in accordance with local, state, and/or federal EPA regulations. This often means incinerating the waste or sterilizing it before hauling it to an approved landfill. The container for regulated waste must be closeable, constructed to contain all contents and prevent leakage of fluids, and closed properly for removal to a second container that meets all of these requirements.

Needles and sharps pose a unique hazard to the healthcare worker and thus require special handling. Needles and sharps are not to be broken, bent, sheared, or recapped. An exception to this rule is if there is no feasible alternative to recapping and it is required for medical reasons. For instance, if a partial dose is administered from a pre-loaded medication syringe and a second dose is to be given later, recapping of the needle is permitted. However, the needle must be recapped using a one-handed technique or a mechanical device.

Needles and sharps are to be discarded immediately or as soon as feasible in containers that meet OSHA standards.

Needles and sharps containers must be

- Closeable
- Puncture resistant
- Leakproof on sides and bottom
- Labeled or color-coded as a biohazard
- Easily accessible to personnel
- Located close to area of use
- Maintained in an upright position
- Replaced routinely and not allowed to become overfull
- Closed before moving to prevent spillage
- Placed in a secondary container if leakage is possible

Broken glassware is to be cleaned up using a hands-free technique. A broom and dustpan or other similar procedure may be used.

Non-Disposable Items and Work Surfaces

It is an employer's responsibility to ensure a clean and sanitary work environment for employees. In addition, equipment used on patients must be cleaned, disinfected, and in some cases sterilized between patient uses.

Written cleaning schedules and methods of decontamination should be developed with these considerations in mind:

- Location of area to be cleaned
- Type of surface to be cleaned
- Type of soil or debris present
- Tasks or procedures performed or equipment used in the area

Routine cleaning of work and environmental surfaces including cans, bins, pails, shelves, floors and walls of vehicles, benches, and seats should be completed on a regular schedule at least once per shift or day. When no blood or body fluids are present, the surfaces and equipment that do not have contact with patients should be cleaned with an intermediate- or low-level disinfectant. Manufacturer's recommendations should be followed in selecting cleaning and disinfecting solutions and methods for cleaning. Failure to do so can result in damage to surfaces being cleaned.

The CDC has developed recommendations for reprocessing equipment used in the prehospital setting.

For critical equipment, instruments, or devices that penetrate skin or contact normally sterile areas of the body, sterilization is the preferred method of cleaning. Sterilization may be accomplished using steam (autoclave), a gas (ethylene oxide), dry heat, or immersion in an EPA-approved

> It is an employer's responsibility to ensure a clean and sanitary work environment for employees.

chemical "sterilant" for six to 10 hours following manufacturer's instructions. Liquids should only be used on those instruments that cannot be sterilized with heat.

Semi-critical equipment, which includes all reusable instruments or devices that come into contact with mucous membranes, requires high-level disinfection. High-level disinfecting is accomplished by hot water pasteurization (80° to 100°C for 30 minutes, or exposure to an EPA-registered "sterilant" chemical for a period of 20 to 45 minutes per manufacturer's instructions).

Non-critical equipment—instruments, devices, or surfaces that come into contact with intact skin only—that have been contaminated with blood or body fluids need intermediate-level disinfectant. EPA-registered "hospital disinfectant" chemicals with a label claim for tuberculocidal activity or commercially available hard-surface germicides or solutions of 1:100 dilution of bleach are effective for this level of disinfection. However, the selection must be made carefully. The particular item to be cleaned may be adversely affected by the chemical chosen or in some cases may absorb the chemical only to release it later when in contact with a patient. Carefully follow manufacturer's recommendations for both the product to be cleaned and the disinfectant used. Remember also to get all instructions and usage information in writing.

Low-level disinfection is indicated for routine cleaning or removing soil from non-critical equipment, provided there is no blood or body fluid contamination. An EPA-registered "hospital disinfectant" chemical may be used to accomplish this level of cleaning. If blood contamination has occurred, a higher-level disinfection is required.

Environmental surfaces such as floors, walls, ambulance benches or seats, and shelves can be cleaned and disinfected using any agent intended for this purpose.

Prior to sterilizing or disinfecting, all visible debris, including blood or body fluids, must be removed. Failure to do so can result in inadequate disinfection, as many disinfectants/sterilants are ineffective (inactivated) in the presence of organic matter.

After thorough cleaning and disinfecting, most patient care products must be thoroughly rinsed to remove all traces of the chemical sterilant or disinfectant.

While carrying out all cleaning and disinfecting procedures, personnel should wear appropriate personal protective equipment to prevent exposure to contaminants, blood, and body fluids and as protection against the cleaning agent itself. Again, it is very important to follow all manufacturer's instructions when using these products. Employers are required to provide training in the use of these chemicals and to post Material Safety Data Sheets (MSDS) on all chemicals used in the workplace. It is important that personnel know where these sheets are kept and are familiar with their content.

Linens/Contaminated Clothing

If you are with a service that is permitted to leave linens at your receiving hospital, you will need to follow the hospital's policy for handling dirty laundry. Remember, any laundry contaminated with blood or body fluids must be handled following universal precautions and using authorized personal protective equipment. These linens should be placed in specially designated laundry containers per hospital policy.

If you are a service responsible for your own laundry, you will need to develop several procedures.

Table 2.5

Cleaning of Contaminated Articles

Article	Level of Disinfection	Recommended Method	Time for Cleaning/Special Notes
Airways	High level	Sterilant	
Nasopharyngeal	High level	Sterilant	20-45 min MR
Oropharyngeal	High level	Sterilant	20-45 min MR
Backboards			
If blood present	Intermediate level	HD/TB	MR
No blood/body fluids	Low level	HD	MR
Bag/Valve/Mask	High level	Sterilant	20-45 min MR
Bed Pans	High level	Sterilant	20-45 min MR
Bite Blocks	Dispose		EPA rules may apply
B/P Cuffs			
Bladder, tubes, manometer	Low level	HD	MR
If blood/body fluids	Intermediate level	HD/TB	20-45 min MR
Cuff	Laundry	Detergent disinfectant	MR
Bulb Syringe	Dispose		EPA
Cervical Collars			
If blood	Dispose		EPA
No blood	Low level	HD	MR
Cold Packs	Dispose		EPA
Combi Tubes (PTL)	Sterilize or dispose	Sterilant	6-10 hr MR
Cricothyroidotomy Kit	Sterilize	Sterilant	6-10 hr MR
Dressings, Bandages	Dispose		EPA
Drug Boxes/Container			
Metal or plastic			
If blood	Intermediate level	HD/TB	MR
If no blood	Low level	HD	MR
Cloth (soft packs)	Laundry	Wash in water with detergent/disinfectant	MR
Emesis Basin	High level or dispose	Sterilant	20-45 min MR
End Tidal CO2 Detector Units (disposable)	Dispose		EPA
Endotracheal Tubes	Dispose		EPA
Esophageal Obturator Airway			
Masks	High level	Sterilant	20-45 min MR
Tubes	Dispose		EPA
E-Stretcher			
Blood	Intermediate level	HD/TB	MR
No visible blood	Low level or environmental level	HD	MR

Table 2.5 (cont.)

Article	Level of Disinfection	Recommended Method	Time for Cleaning/ Special Notes
External Cardiac Compression and Resuscitation Unit (i.e., Thumper, CardiO$_2$, HLR)			
Airway tubing	High level or dispose	Sterilant	20-45 min MR
Exterior	Intermediate level	HD/TB	MR
Respiratory valves	High level	Sterilant	20-45 min MR
Hot Packs	Dispose		EPA
Intravenous Fluid			
Containers	Dispose		EPA
Tubing	Dispose		EPA
Intravenous Poles			
If blood	Intermediate level	HD/TB	MR
If no blood	Low level	HD	MR
Laryngoscopes			
Blades	High level	Sterilant	20-45 min MR
Handles	High level	Sterilant	20-45 min MR
Linens			
Blankets, cot covers	Laundry	Detergent disinfectant	MR
Pillow cases, sheets	Laundry	Detergent disinfectant	MR
Magill Forceps	High level	Sterilant	20-45 min MR
MAST Trousers			
If blood	Intermediate level	HD/TB	MR
If no blood	Low level	HD	MR
Monitor*, exterior only			
If blood	Intermediate level	HD/TB	MR
Includes patient cable and non-disposable lead wires	Low level	HD	MR
Needles and Syringes			
Non-reusable	Dispose	Sharps container	EPA
Reusable	Sterilize	Sterilant	6-10 hr MR
Other Electronic Equipment* (i.e., IV pumps, Apcors, pulse oximetry units)	**Special precautions with electronic equipment. Choice of cleaning agent and method must follow manufacturer's recommendations. Use of other agents may damage electrical components or pose a hazard to user or patient.*		
End Tidal CO$_2$ Detector Units*			
If blood	Intermediate level	HD/TB	MR
If no blood	Low level	HD	MR
Oxygen Delivery Equipment			
Extension tubing	Dispose		EPA
Face masks	Dispose		EPA
Nasal cannula	Dispose		EPA
Oxygen Flow Meter	Environmental	*Caution: See manufacturer's recommendation to avoid fire hazard or damage to unit.*	
Oxygen Humidifiers	Sterilize or dispose	Sterilant	6-10 hr MR
Oxygen Nebulizers	Sterilize or dispose	Sterilant	6-10 hr MR
Oxygen Powered Positive Pressure Breathing Device (Robertshaw, demand valve, Elders valve, etc.)			
Hose	Varies by product		MR
Masks	High level or dispose	Sterilant	20-45 min MR
Oxygen Regulators	Environmental level	*Caution: See manufacturer's recommendation to avoid fire hazard or damage to unit.*	
Oxygen Tanks	Environmental level	*Caution: See manufacturer's recommendation to avoid fire hazard or damage to unit.*	
Penlights	Dispose		
Pillows	Laundry/dispose	Detergent/disinfectant	EPA
Pocket Masks	High level	Sterilant	20-45 min MR

Table 2.5 (cont.)

Article	Level of Disinfection	Recommended Method	Time for Cleaning/Special Notes
PTL Tubes (Combi tubes)	Sterilize or dispose	Sterilant	6-10 hr MR
Restraints			
Cloth	Laundry	Detergent/disinfectant	
Leather	Scrub with detergent disinfectant		
If blood	Intermediate level	HD/TB	MR
Resuscitators (bag/valve/masks)	High level	HD/TB	20-45 min MR
Safety Pins	Dispose	EPA sharps container	EPA
Sandbags	Intermediate level	HD/TB	MR
	Dispose		EPA
Shears or Scissors			
If blood	Intermediate level	HD/TB	MR
If no blood	Low level	HD	MR
Splints			
Air, metal, wood			
If blood	Intermediate level	HD/TB	MR
If no blood	Low level	HD	MR
Cloth support straps	Laundry	Detergent/disinfectant	MR
Sterile Solutions Once Opened (i.e., eye wash, saline solution for burns, etc.)	Dispose		EPA
Stethoscope			
If blood	Intermediate level	HD/TB	MR
If no blood	Low level	HD	MR
Straps	Laundry	Detergent/disinfectant	MR
Stretcher			
If blood	Intermediate level	HD/TB	MR
If no blood	Low level	HD	MR
Stylets	Sterilize or dispose	Sterilant	6-10 hr MR EPA
Suction units			
Catheters			
Flexible	Dispose		EPA
Tonsil tip (yankhauer)			
Metal	Sterilize	Sterilant	MR
Plastic	Dispose		EPA
Collection unit			
Bag	Dispose		EPA
Bottle	High level	Sterilant	20-45 min MR
Tubing from patient to collection unit	High level or dispose	Sterilant	20-45 min MR EPA
Unit or machine exterior	*Caution: Follow manufacturer's recommendation.*		
If blood	Intermediate level	HD/TB	MR
If no blood	Low level	HD	MR
Thermometers	Sterilize or dispose	Sterilant	6-10 hr MR EPA
Tongue blade	Sterilize or dispose	Sterilant	6-10 hr MR EPA
Urinals	High level or dispose	Sterilant	20-45 min MR EPA

Code:
Sterilant = EPA-registered "sterilant"
HD/TB = EPA-registered "hospital disinfectant" with label claim of tuberculocidal
HD = EPA-registered "hospital disinfectant"
MR = Manufacturer's recommendation

Source

Excerpted from the book, Infection Control For Prehospital Care Providers, *2nd ed. Reprinted with permission from Mercy Ambulance, Grand Rapids, Mich. Copyright © 1993. Lynn Zimmerman is the clinical coordinator for Mercy, Deb Jurewicz is Mercy's quality assurance manager, and Mary Neuman supervises the Communicable Disease Division at St. Mary's Hospital in Grand Rapids, Mich.*

Routine laundry should be placed in a container and returned to the facility for appropriate washing. These linens may be washed in a regular washer using a detergent disinfectant.

Linens and other laundry items (i.e., clothing) that have been contaminated with blood or body fluids must be immediately placed in a designated container and may not be sorted or rinsed at the site of use.

A biohazard-labeled container is required for contaminated linens if people other than those trained specifically in how to handle contaminated linens may come into contact with them and if universal precautions are not followed for all linens.

If only trained persons using universal precautions and familiar with the company's exposure control plan (ECP) have contact with the linens, an alternative labeling system other than the biohazard label may be used.

Contaminated linens may be washed in a regular washer using detergent disinfectant following manufacturer's instructions. Persons handling these linens should be instructed in the company's ECP and wear appropriate personal protective equipment.

If an employee's uniform becomes contaminated with blood or body fluids, it should be changed before responding to the next call and should not be permitted to be taken home by the employee. The uniform should be properly laundered before being returned to the employee.

Care of Contaminated Articles Chart

All articles contaminated by infective material from patients with known or suspected infectious diseases must be decontaminated or disposed of properly. Table 2.5 provides the healthcare worker with guidelines for determining the type and extent of cleaning that must be completed to ensure adequate decontamination.

For further information on selecting clinical disinfectants, refer to the EPA for a listing of registered chemicals by their classification and to APIC guidelines for the selection and use of disinfectants. Also refer to an article by Dr. William Rutala published in *The American Journal of Infection Control*, April 1990, volume 18, no 2. This article more fully describes the use, advantages, and disadvantages of the various chemicals and provides practical advice on the selection of appropriate germicides for your operation.

Effectively Managing Growth

FORECASTING MEANS FUTURIZING the business of an organization, looking ahead and projecting where the owners or board members want the organization to be at some point. Your organization probably has policies in place that codify its philosophy of business. Now it's time to calculate what you want and when you want it, to set specific goals, and to develop methods of getting there. Most important of all is getting there; it's all for naught if you don't.

Forecasting

In an established business, the forecasting process needs to take place once a year, about 90 days prior to the end of one fiscal year or at the beginning of a new one. However, avoid forecasting beyond 18 to 24 months into the future, because of the rapid changes in business and in the economy over the past few years.

In thinking about goal setting, it is necessary to keep in mind eight areas of business focus:

- Market share
- Innovation
- Human resources
- Financial resources
- Physical resources
- Productivity
- Social responsibility
- Profitability

The first step is to make a realistic assessment of where your operation is in each of these eight areas. In every category, managers must know where they've been and where they are now before they can make realistic plans for where they want to go. If the goals of the organization

Setting and Achieving Goals

Eric R. Voth and Ron Myers

Experienced entrepreneurs Eric Voth and Ron Myers provide a step-by-step process for forecasting, strategizing, and achieving goals in an EMS organization. In this article, excerpted from their book, Making the Transition from Employee to Employer, *they describe how to calculate what you want and when you want it.*

Projecting where the business needs to be can be done by planning for a greater percentage than what your company did the year before, or it may be done according to some other need of the business.

are where the manager wants to be in the next two years, forecasting them involves quantifying the objectives and projecting that data into a specific time frame.

At our private ambulance service, department heads are given annual budgets to operate their respective parts of the business. The amount allocated to each budget results from a process in which all the managers take part, so they are fully aware of their department's needs for each of the eight areas of business focus.

In private companies, the lion's share of responsibility for forecasting generally falls to owners because, when they leave behind the Lone Ranger Syndrome—the urge to do everything themselves—they've bought themselves more time to maintain an overview of the business. Although the owner handles most of the task, successful completion of the procedure requires a two-way view. The job of the managers is to get today's work done today, and this week's work done this week. Nevertheless, managers have a valuable perspective to bring to the process.

Projecting where the business needs to be can be done by planning for a greater percentage than what your company did the year before, or it may be done according to some other need of the business. A satisfactory decision about which need should be met cannot be made by guessing or by whim; that's why it's so important to do forecasts based on all eight areas of business focus.

While an owner wants the business to be profitable every year, in a particular year it may be more important to find a new building or buy some capital equipment. That's going to cut into the company's profitability. Or the entrepreneur may want to increase market share, which necessitates devoting large sums of money to advertising and promotion. This may not only limit profitability, it may mean that the company has to forego buying that new piece of equipment or getting the parking lot repaved.

There are always offsetting situations with respect to the eight critical areas of focus, because all of the elements are interactive and mutually reliant. It's difficult to do everything at once, in life as in business. When there is a projected increase or expansion for one of these areas, all of the others will be affected. If the owner decides that increasing social responsibility is a high priority during the coming year, the business may become a little better known, a little more popular, and have a stronger image in the community. However, the cost of accomplishing this goal may diminish financial resources and reduce that year's profits.

Actually, it might be fair to say that a forecast is always needs-driven. Even if the owner decides that the objective is to increase the percentage of what the company grossed last year, the decision is still based on the need perceived by the owner. The choice is not necessarily founded on some macro-economic figures; it's initiated because of the direction the owner wants the business to take that year, a selection established by the owner's understanding of market conditions and situations within the company's environment.

For the owner, it's a matter of setting priorities of accomplishment, often with the guidance of the managers. In a successful setting, management team members can advise the owner about which objectives need to come first. For example, perhaps the business owns a fleet of trucks. Several of them are always in the shop, and in past years the owner's decision was to continue repairing them. This year, the managers may tell the owner that it will be more cost effective to replace the trucks than to repair them.

When owners were employed as managers, they had their fingers on the pulse of these matters on a daily basis. When managers become owners, they have to rely on the data and judgment of others for current information about where the company is and where it needs to go within the eight areas of business focus.

Market Share

An owner's goals with respect to market share depend on what stage in the life cycle the business is in, and what share of the market the company is currently serving. Establishing the company's current market share may be a project in itself, requiring an outside firm to study what the total market is for your company and then what share of it you now have. For example, if you own a retail store in a crowded metropolitan area, it may be very difficult to know what your market share is without extensive research. On the other hand, if you own a mom-and-pop store in the middle of a residential area, your total market, and the share you have of it, may be easier to determine.

Innovation

Making forecasts for innovation means deciding how your company can make the best use of advances in technology, production, administration, research, and development. In addition to knowing where the company is now, it's important to know what innovations are being brought into your industry in any of these areas. Owners can educate themselves about these by reading trade magazines, attending trade shows, and exposing themselves to other realms beyond the confines of their own shop's walls. Having done that, the next step is to decide which innovations are appropriate to bring into the organization over the next year or two.

Owners also have to recognize that innovation is costly, for the item itself, for the necessary start-up time, and for the resistance to change among workers that is often the result of introducing new equipment and procedures. Before taking such a step, an owner might be well advised to look around at what competitors are doing. If your company is already several steps ahead of its rivals, you may decide that it is not cost effective to do anything innovative in a given year. Conversely, the fact that competitors are not doing anything innovative might be just the reason you decide that you can't rest on your laurels.

Whether or not a particular owner thinks his company needs to be

> ### Eight Areas of Business Focus
>
> - Market Share
> - Innovation
> - Human Resources
> - Financial Resources
> - Physical Resources
> - Productivity
> - Social Responsibility
> - Profitability

innovative may relate back to the mission statement. Is the owner's vision to run a forward-looking, cutting-edge company, or to be a basic service provider, dependable but not necessarily imaginative? There's nothing wrong with dependability; some companies choose to reach that stability stage in the growth process and just stay there.

Human Resources

Once a year, the forecasting and planning process needs to visit anything connected with human resources. For example, what is your company's general commitment to consistent, formal employee education—orientation, management training, sales training, and general development of human resources? What is your company's commitment to these issues over the next 12 months?

An owner may decide that the company's employee orientation program must be upgraded, which is going to take a lot of time and effort, or he may decide that there's nothing needed this year to improve that program. You may want to revise your employee handbook/personnel policy manual. If you're affected by a recession, it may be a good time to engage in management training because employees are not as busy with their regular work. On the other hand, you may decide that the recession makes it economically impossible to finance management training this year.

The ever-rising cost of health insurance may motivate an owner to revisit the benefit package the company offers its employees. To save premium dollars, you may want to explore options other than the standard healthcare policy, such as managed care programs, preferred provider groups, wellness programs, or employee assistance programs. You may also decide to decrease the company's expenditures for human resources by ceasing to pay the entire cost for each employee, insisting instead that the health insurance premiums be more equitably shared by the company and the employees.

Financial Resources

Most of the major decisions regarding financial resources will probably be made by the owner and the chief financial officer, using input from the heads of each department of the company. In most businesses, it is left to these two individuals to do the overall planning, to coordinate how all of the departments tie together, and to combine all the discrete components of the business into one financial statement.

Many people are curious about who is privy to the amount of the owner's salary. In our company, there are only three people who see how the whole budget is put together: the two owners and the chief financial officer. In other companies the owners may be reluctant to share "confidential" information with internal people, so only the outside accountant and the owners see the whole budget.

Sometimes a business will need a bank loan for expansion or to institute a new program. In our company, when it is determined that we need to borrow money, the initial contact with the bank is generally made by the chief financial officer. That individual and the company's financial department do the preliminary work, including providing the bank with the data it needs to grant the loan. When it's time to sign the papers, the owners and the bank representative meet to complete the deal. In other words, if the system is working well, the owner doesn't have to come into the process until the end.

The company needs to engage in the ongoing process of building a relationship with the bank and the banker. To further that end, the company should issue monthly or quarterly copies of its financial statements to the bank. Thus, when the company needs a loan, there should be no problem granting it, because the bank has been tracking the business and it already has on file a lot of the necessary information.

Physical Resources

The company's physical resources consist of the buildings, the land, the equipment, and all the other hard assets that can be touched and seen. Planning and forecasting for the next year might include enlarging the shop, adding more locations, purchasing more capital equipment and rolling stock, replacing equipment, or modifying systems such as the telephones or the computers.

In a well-organized company, recommendations about physical resources are often made by the department heads. If a suggestion is costly, teamwork begins to be called into play. The department head making the recommendation contacts the chief financial officer. They discuss what's needed, what it's going to cost, if the company can afford it in this year's budget, or perhaps whether the business can afford only part of it. After conferring with the financial officer and gathering all the appropriate information, the department head requesting the expenditure brings the request to the management team table at planning time.

For example, the department head might recommend that the company build a 500-square-foot addition onto the building to house a compressor. The manager consults with the in-house accountant, the accountant agrees that the project needs to be given priority in the next year, and the manager researches relevant data and brings it to the management team meeting. There, the manager presents the proposal, suggests that the job be bid out to three different builders for construction and three different suppliers for pats, and lays out the dollars and cents figures that the company needs to spend in the next year for this item.

Ideally, owners don't get involved in the process until it's brought to them for approval. Of course, owners may choose to get involved at any point in these negotiations. At our company, however, we've found it's best to give the responsibility to the managers and to grant in their job descriptions written authority to wield it. When the proposal is presented to the owners for final approval, other questions may be raised that the managers have not thought to ask.

The owners may want to know whether additional courses of action have been considered; they may suggest various options to the manager; and they will want to know how this expenditure will affect the seven other areas of business focus. Therefore, the more alternatives the managers can come up with before they make a presentation to the owner, the fewer questions they'll be asked and the more likely they'll be viewed as competent managers.

Productivity

Productivity is the full utilization and coordination of personnel and financial and physical resources for profitable results. The overall judgment about productivity is made by the owner, who must have input from all of the company's managers about the productivity within their own departments.

Social Responsibility

Social responsibility means considering what efforts you will make over the next year to maintain a positive image in your community. If your business grosses more than $1 million or $2 million in sales per year, it's at the stage where it's likely to be noticed, and some effort to be a good corporate neighbor will have to be made.

This aspect of forecasting belongs almost totally to the owner, though managers may be assigned a subordinate role. An owner might decide that the aesthetics of the company's premises are a social responsibility, and may upgrade their appearance, create new landscaping, or do something else to improve the way the business looks from the street. Or the owner might ask if the company has put in place positive environmental practices, such as a recycling program. Whatever method the company chooses to contribute to the good of society, the owner wants to make sure that it's publicly known, and that it gets tied, in a subtle way, to the company's marketing program.

In one city we know of, one of the largest and oldest local funeral homes has created ties to the religious institutions in the community. If a church has more than 500 members, an employee of the funeral home is one of those members. They strategically place their employees into membership in those congregations, because they consider that this activity fulfills their social responsibility to the community. We don't know whether it's socially responsible or marketing savvy!

Profitability

Profitability is also contingent upon several different factors. It may not always be within the control of an owner, particularly if the business is involved in ordering goods and reselling them, or carrying large inventories. In those cases, where the sources of supply may shift radically and prices may go up and down, the profitability factor may fall out of the owner's hands for some period of time, perhaps a year. Thereafter, the owner would readjust to the new reality, and profitability would once again become an item for planning and forecasting.

However, if there are no major disruptions in the business beyond its second or third year—certainly past the business cycle stage of adolescence—the company should be able to gauge its profitability within one or two percentage points. However, occasionally something like a volatile labor issue intervenes, in which case predicting profitability is no easier for the service provider than for the entrepreneur who keeps an inventory of goods.

Strategizing

The approach to be used for achieving what the company has forecasted—the strategy—comes out of the compilation and quantification of the eight core elements. Once the numbers have been determined and the forecast put in writing, goals must be developed to accomplish them.

Providing that an individual's goals match that person's beliefs, and providing also that the objectives are achievable, there are no unreasonable goals, just unreasonable timelines. A recent management survey of people who were having trouble finding jobs tracked a group of individuals who went to a resume preparation company. They were divided into categories by what they anticipated earning at a new job, they were taught to set goals, imagine themselves achieving them, and envision themselves working at new positions.

Within 90 days, individuals in all the categories were working at jobs paying exactly what they'd envisioned. They could have set higher goals with bigger incomes; instead they created a self-contained box. The goals we set must be suitable to the objectives we want to attain, but sometimes we need to step out of the box we've been living in and break through to new heights.

A goal is the desired end result with a timeline. To set goals, we must take a look at what focus area we want to address, and work up a goal planning worksheet for that core element. The manager in charge of the project usually completes the worksheet, brings it to a management meeting for discussion, then keeps it for the review process that will occur down the road.

The goal planning worksheet is a tool designed to help managers state goals in a specific, measurable way (Figure 2.5). It is used as an instrument to walk managers through a formalized process that almost forces them to develop precise objectives, according to a formula that clears away the cobwebs and helps them think clearly.

The goals developed in this way are called "SMART" goals; the acronym stands for objectives that are specific, measurable, attainable, realistic, and tangible. This model helps the owner and managers create practical goals that can be attained and evaluated. On the goal planning

> Once the numbers have been determined and the forecast put in writing, goals must be developed to accomplish them.

Figure 2.5

Goal Planning Worksheet

Today's Date   Focus Area   Final Target Date   Date Accomplished

_____   _____   _____   _____

Goal (S-M-A-R-T: specific, measurable, attainable, realistic, tangible)

_____

_____

_____

Benefits from Achieving this Goal: Personally • Professionally • For the Company

_____

_____

_____

_____

        Obstacles   Solutions

_____

_____

_____

_____

_____

Specific Action Steps: The Agenda for Acting	Target date	Date reviewed	Date completed
1. _____			
2. _____			
3. _____			
4. _____			
5. _____			
6. _____			
7. _____			

Affirmations to Support this Goal: Statements of Positive Self-Talk

_____

_____

_____

worksheet, the SMART acronym might play out like this:

Specific: A specific date.

Measurable: So many customer comment cards; so many dollars; so many units sold.

Attainable: It exists in the marketplace and we can buy it; we can modify programs that we have seen operated in other companies.

Realistic: Have we ever done it before? Has anybody in the industry done it before? Have businesses that do our sales volume done it before?

Tangible: We can see the results by comparing each month's sales volume with last year's, by counting the number of customer response cards received, or by determining how often response times were 10 minutes or less compared with response times last year.

Empiricism means quantifying what we do. We need numbers to run the business effectively and to make appropriate forecasts for its future. We bring that into play here by developing a reasonably easy method of measuring the outcome, without having to install a whole new computer program to do it. If the evaluation aspect of the project is going to take a lot of employee time and effort, we may want to revisit the goal and decide whether it's worth it. It's like the Internal Revenue Service spending $10,000 in salaries to send people out to collect $9,000 in revenue. By not collecting the tax, the government would be further ahead; in fact, it would save $1,000.

We also want the goal to be something that we can accomplish. It shouldn't be so overpowering that we will feel intimidated about trying to reach it. On the other hand, if it's too easily attainable, we may need to review the strategy, perhaps lengthening or shortening the time frame in which we think it can be done.

Overcoming Obstacles to Reap Benefits

After we've set out our goals using the SMART criteria, the next step is to write down the benefits we anticipate from achieving them. These, too, are added to the goal planning worksheet.

The number of goals that might be developed for each of the eight core elements depends on the needs of each area. There might be a total of eight goals, there might be a total of 24, there might be three for some and one for others. No matter how many or how few goals there are, a written benefit statement must be added to each.

The written benefits are statements of support for each goal, so that later in the year the managers can be reminded why the goal was thought to be worthwhile. These advantages make clear what each goal is

One of the advantages of involving the whole management team in goal definition is that it prevents having too many company objectives scheduled for completion at the same time.

intended to provide for the company; sometimes what's evident at the beginning of this process isn't so obvious later, or what's apparent at the end is not clear at the beginning.

After enumerating the benefits anticipated from achieving each goal, we make a list of the obstacles that may prevent their accomplishment. Doing this helps us to focus on possible solutions to each contingency, and as we develop each potential resolution, we convert them into specific action steps.

The entire management team and the owner act as accountability partners for the goals, although implementing the goals is the job of a specific manager or managers. Managers who understand the process work on the goals within their areas of expertise, or within the plan they have put together. The managers who are accountable for the project are each responsible for listing the specific action steps, the target date for having the action step completed, the date it's going to be reviewed, and the date that the action steps were actually completed.

One of the advantages of involving the whole management team in goal definition is that it prevents having too many company objectives scheduled for completion at the same time. That would overwhelm the managers, and tax the company's resources. The management team as a whole should try to stagger the times at which culmination of various projects is expected.

We know about one company in our industry that, as a matter of policy, purchased all of its ambulances at the same time. They would simultaneously buy six or eight or 10 ambulances of a particular model year. As time wore on, they found that these units would all break down with the same problems at the same times. If there was a manufacturing defect that caused a vehicle to malfunction when it reached 20,000 miles, all of the vehicles were down when they hit 20,000 miles. So there's something to be said for alternating the purchase of equipment and supplies. If you want to make a budgetary commitment to purchasing all at once, consider staggering delivery.

Affirmations

After we have gone through the process of creating action steps, we develop statements of positive self-motivation to support the goal. This provides additional incentive for owners and managers to achieve their objectives, although it might be just a restatement of the benefits.

As an example, our objective might be to upgrade the company's computer system. The SMART steps are that, by June 1, 1998, we will have in place a 200-megabyte storage capacity computer, with 15 workstations. This goal is specific, measurable, attainable, realistic, and tangible. One of the benefits of achieving this goal would be consolidation of diverse computer equipment to provide faster service to customers calling in with inquiries about bills.

We might even face some obstacles to accomplishing this objective. First, we don't yet own the equipment and we may need to hire a consultant to evaluate it. Second, there might be a snag to implementing the system after it is installed. Third, some of our employees might resist leaving the machinery they're using now, creating issues about retraining. We will be as prepared as we can be in advance of any potential obstacles if we spend some time at this point projecting several methods of overcoming each one.

Next we develop specific action steps that will take us, point by point, to the goal. We start by asking ourselves what the first thing is that we have to do to reach our objective, and we may decide that it is to bring in a consulting firm that will evaluate and make recommendations about the computer system we contemplate installing.

Affirmations of this process might simply be a restatement of the goal or of its benefits:

- I, Joe Smith, manager of the Data Services Department, choose to have this new computer system implemented by June 1, 1998.
- I feel good about the new computer system that we will have implemented by June 1, 1995, because it will provide faster service to customers calling in with inquiries about bills.

Achieving Goals

When the company's management team has gone through the whole process of evaluating, forecasting, creating goals, setting target dates, and developing statements of affirmation, the management team sets the plan into operation. If things are going along well, target dates are met, and everything's on schedule, then everybody tends to be happy. However, one day you may notice that things seem to have fallen behind and that the results in some areas are falling short.

You don't have to accept a subjective judgment about the situation, because you have it in black and white. You go back to your goal planning worksheet, look at the specific action steps and target dates, and, by the time you get down to step three or four, you see that you were right. You're starting to miss target dates.

Because it's all been put into writing, the manager and the owner are both aware of the problem. At that point, the owner may decide to intervene in the role of a consultant, meeting with the manager to discuss what's preventing the goals from being met. Inevitably, that discussion will include an exploration of what options there are to get back on track, and whether it might be prudent to enlist the help of other people on the management team.

The skill and experience of the entire management team can be tapped to assist with any company project, and a true team effort can be an invaluable resource. The team members might be able to offer insights and come up with alternative solutions that neither the owner nor the manager would have thought of alone.

When the results of these efforts fall short of expectations, there are many ways of changing things around to see if they will work better.

- Put the goal "on hold," and come back to it at a more advantageous time.
- Modify the results you're aiming for by shrinking or increasing the goal.
- Change the time frame in which you want the goal to be accomplished.
- Shuffle resources within the company, including altering other goals to achieve this one.
- Add or subtract people from the project.
- Change project managers to see if rearranging personalities will make a difference in the outcome.
- Provide supplementary funds.
- Wait until some other set of goals has been completed that will facilitate pursuing this one.
- Abandon the goal entirely.

Hold that Goal

Sometimes a goal must be abandoned in the short term, because of immediate circumstances that work against accomplishing it. You may hold onto all the information that you've gathered and put the project on a back burner to be brought up again the next fiscal year or during the next budgeting process. When this happens, with any luck, the company will not have made a large financial commitment, or at least not one whose yield will be lost forever.

There are a lot of reasons why you might abandon a goal, temporarily or permanently, and none of them may suggest that the original intention was faulty. It may be that you bit off more than you could chew at that moment, or that other goals came up unexpectedly that assumed priority. When we put a goal on the back burner, we recognize that the objective itself was not a poor choice, but perhaps the timing was.

Our company needed a larger physical plant to give us more room at our main location. We looked around for other real estate in the neighborhood and we couldn't find any. Finally, we found a parcel of real estate several miles away. We looked it over, called in a contractor, and got his estimate for bringing it up to our specifications. When we had a chance to analyze all of the data, we decided that the purchase price together with the renovation costs were too much for us to pay. We scrapped the entire project.

Fortunately, we were not very far into the project at the time. We were just at the examination stage. We had paid $800 to a real estate appraiser to see if the asking price for the property was fair. We lost that $800 and about six hours of time spent with the contractor going through the building. We would have lost a lot more if we had not understood the wisdom of putting the goal on hold right then, because it wasn't going to be cost effective for us to move. We still think the goal of finding larger premises is an important one for our company, and we intend to pursue it at some future time. We simply couldn't accomplish it at that time and under those conditions.

Cancel that Goal

In another situation, we found our original goal completely changed around by new circumstances. We had begun this project by choosing a goal, going through all the forecasting and planning, beginning the action steps, and meeting some of the target dates. Then the project turned out to be a complete bust.

Several years ago, we acquired a new market area by purchasing a company that had been serving two small communities. When we made the acquisition, we set some profitability standards and goals, but it wasn't long before we found that we couldn't meet them. The business generated by these two small communities was so low that functioning there was costing us money.

We had been providing service to those two areas on a 24-hour-a-day, seven-day-a-week basis. We soon realized that we couldn't continue to do that. When we began cutting back the number of hours that the crews and ambulances were available, the population had an adverse reaction. Negative feeling among the citizenry is never good for business, so we approached community leaders to explain our problem. We said that, if they wanted us to be there all the time, we'd have to be subsidized in some way. We thought we had a pretty good shot at making it happen.

The leadership decided that the community shouldn't subsidize a private ambulance enterprise, so they levied the taxpayers and put the local fire department into the ambulance business. When the fire department became proficient at providing emergency service, we stopped serving the community on a first response basis.

That was acceptable to us because, in some cases, it was taking us 10 or 12 minutes to reach the site of an emergency call. Our internal standard is eight minutes. In fact, an individual can die if the brain lacks oxygen for more than eight minutes. Because the fire department took over this role, and performed it well, we could stop worrying about ways to improve the emergency response time of our own ambulances.

In this case, the change in the community's philosophy prevented us from achieving our initial goal. After the leaders elected to put an emergency ambulance service into the fire department, we felt that we were better off giving up that venture entirely. To have stayed there meant risking a negative public image and the possible liability consequences of long response times to emergency situations. It was not worth doing that for the small amount of business being generated. In essence, we abandoned the goal and the venture all together, but they're happy and we're happy.

Typical Goals

Here's a good example of successful goal setting through the traditional procedure.

Several years ago we decided that our employees needed additional training in customer service. We were good at dealing with consumers and we were proud of our track record, but we felt that we could do better. We wanted to become our own competition and surpass our fine record, so we had to find a way to make all of our employees aware of their daily, vital role in customer service.

Our goal was that, three years from the time the decision was made, we would have implemented a customer service training program for our employees that would be fully operational throughout our home office division. At the time we selected the goal, we were in the middle of one year and about to discuss the planning for the following year. Because it needed a long lead time, this particular goal had as its target 24 months from the beginning of our next fiscal year.

We anticipated a ripple effect of benefits that would be gained by achieving the goal. The first would be better understanding by our employees of the importance of customer service; that benefit would lead to increased customer satisfaction; and that, in turn, would lead to increased business and increased profits.

There were two obstacles to achieving the goal. The first was that we didn't know anyone personally who could do the requisite training, so we were probably going to need an outside consultant. The second was that we were worried about finding someone who was familiar with the customer service needs of our specialized industry; we didn't want to have to "train the trainer" about the subtleties of dealing with consumers of ambulance services. The solution to both problems was to find someone who already knew about our industry, who already had a program developed, and who would teach this material to our people. It seemed like a tall order.

A consultant to ambulance services is a pretty rare commodity. The one we found was one of only two such specialists in the country. He had developed a program specifically to teach employees of ambulance services about customer service, and he had used it with two previous clients. We contacted him for references; we spoke to his previous clients to learn what they had experienced as a result of his work; we committed the dollars for the consultant's fee and the ancillary costs of providing the training; and we hired him to make his presentation.

We developed five specific action steps, each of which had a target date for completion:

- Selecting the consultant

- Briefing our management team about the consultant and his program
- Establishing the starting dates for the training
- Determining how the training would continue after the consultant left
- Deciding how we were going to measure the results

The consultant trained a core group of six or seven people in our company. In effect, his work provided us with on-site instructors who could conduct a continuing training program after the consultant left. They learned brainstorming strategies, classroom training methods, role play techniques, all the methods they needed to be able to teach our other employees the nuances of customer service.

The results have been very positive since we implemented the program several years ago. In the first year our business increased 10 percent, and it increased five percent more the next year, for a total of about 15 percent. We're almost at a saturation point now; we've probably got most of the business in town. We do have one competitor who's limping along, but we're constantly eating into his share of the market.

The program was extremely cost effective. Taking into consideration the hours the employees were in classes, the cost of people to cover for them, the consultant's fee, the materials, and so forth, we paid out close to $150,000. So far, we have earned about $600,000 in increased business, and we expect that to continue in the years ahead. No one else in our market area is implementing a program like this, so, while the planning and goal setting were done in the traditional way, the result was an innovation in our market area.

The Challenging Goal

Sometimes a company chooses a challenging goal, one that is unprecedented for the business, and is able to go through all the steps to accomplish it despite the risks. Our company did that with a situation in the Houston market.

A few years ago, we heard a rumor that a small ambulance service in Baytown, Tex., a city 35 miles east of our Houston office, was going to go out of business. The Baytown company wasn't really a competitor because it didn't serve our market area, but its availability was an opportunity to expand our business in Texas.

As soon as we heard the going-out-of-business rumor, we traveled to Baytown. By the time we got there, the owner had closed the doors, but we managed to get in touch with some of the company's former employees. We asked some questions about their run volume, their sales volume, and the expectations of the community. We liked what we heard.

Our goal in this situation was to increase our market share and, in the long run, our profitability. We were faced with a variety of obstacles:

In an established business, the forecasting process needs to take place once a year and needs to set goals in the business focus areas for the following two years.

We were from a big city with a big city name; we didn't have a local telephone number; we didn't know how the remaining competitor in town would retaliate or what sort of rumors he would spread about our service; and we didn't have a garage location in Baytown. These were some of the difficulties that we had to consider, and they seemed formidable.

We didn't have time to plan how we might overcome obstacles—we had to act immediately. We rented a garage, ordered a local telephone line, assigned a crew, and allocated to the town a vehicle from Houston for 13 hours a day, rather than 24 hours a day as the previous operator had done. Then we hired Baytown personnel and purchased additional ambulances locally. Within 30 days of the decision, we were open in that town. The opening was just a little ahead of our target date.

We've monitored the progress of that division since it opened and have found that it has exceeded expectations in the realm of sales volume and profitability. Of course, this is not an example of a goal that was conscientiously planned just before the start of the new year, after analyzing carefully the eight core elements of business. However, it is an excellent illustration of how the forecasting and goal-setting procedures can be used to seize market opportunities as they arise.

We had many times before followed the goal-setting process in our business. We had developed a great deal of experience in its use, which made our responses to its various steps almost second nature. We had even expanded outside our home base before, so we were not strangers to that procedure. In other words, following the process had seasoned us and enabled us to develop the skills we needed to respond quickly to a spontaneous opportunity.

Conclusion

In an established business, the forecasting process needs to take place once a year—about 90 days prior to the beginning of the next fiscal year—and needs to set goals in the business focus areas for the following two years. To begin with, owners need to know where the company has been in the eight areas in the past and where it is now. Then projections for the eight areas can be made.

It is probably not possible to set costly goals for all eight areas, because everything can't be done at once and all the areas are mutually interactive. Money spent for something in physical resources may diminish profitability in a given year. Priorities must be set by the owner, in consultation with members of the management team.

Strategy is the approach developed to achieve the goals. Goals for each of the eight core elements need to be planned on a goal planning worksheet, which forces managers to go through a fixed chronology of events as follows:

- Perform a realistic assessment of where the business has been and is now in each of the eight areas.

- Forecast where the business is to go during the next two years in each of the eight areas.
- Develop a strategy for achieving where the business will go, and set priorities.
- Complete a goal planning worksheet.
  - Develop SMART goals, ones that are specific, measurable, attainable, realistic, and tangible.
  - Create written statements of benefits to be achieved from the goal.
  - Create a written list of potential obstacles to achieving the goal.
    - Create a written list of possible solutions to the potential obstacles.
    - Create a written list of action steps to overcome the potential obstacles.
  - Create a written list of action steps to achieve the goal.
    - Create target dates for completion of each action step.
    - Select a date of review for each action step.
  - Select completion dates for action steps to achieve the goal.
  - Create written statements of affirmation to support the goal.

Once the goals have been committed to paper, the management team puts the plan into operation. Sometimes action steps fall behind schedule, and it looks like the goal won't be met. When that happens, there are several actions that might be taken.

- Put the goal on hold, and come back to it at a more advantageous time.
- Modify the results you're aiming for by shrinking or increasing the goal.
- Change the time frame in which you want the goal to be accomplished.
- Shuffle resources within the company, including altering other goals to achieve this one.
- Add or subtract people from the project.
- Change project managers or other personnel to see if rearranging personalities will make a difference in the outcome.
- Provide supplementary funds.
- Wait until the completion of some other set of company goals that will make it easier for you to pursue this one.
- Abandon the goal entirely.

Source

Reprinted with permission from Business One Irwin. Copyright © 1993 by Business One Irwin, Homewood, Ill. Adapted from the book, The New Owner: Making the Transition from Employee to Employer. *Eric R. Voth and Ron Myers are co-owners of Physicians & Surgeons (P&S) Ambulance Service in Akron, Ohio. Once managers of the company, they purchased the service in 1971.*

Reference

Meyer, P. J., and C. A. Coonradt. *Organizational Goal Setting—Lesson 1.* Waco, Tex.: Success Motivation, Inc., 1987.

Setting Up a New Operation

Brent H. Dierking
and John K. Rester

Implementing a new operation or division can be one of the most demanding aspects of managing an EMS organization. This article describes the key issues involved when the authors accepted a contract in a county more than 100 miles from their base of operation.

COMPANIES INVOLVED IN MEDICAL transportation frequently explore the prospects of expansion by creating or acquiring new operations in areas of need. The success of any new operation depends on five critical factors: the operation's commitment to providing high-quality patient care; employee services; financial stability; implementation and continuous monitoring of operating systems; and community and government relations.

In addition, effective planning is the key for meeting the many challenges to be faced. Some problems, however, will not be realized until it's too late. In order to remain proactive—instead of reactive—during the start-up process, establishing a transition team is most helpful.

The transition team is generally composed of individuals who are experts in specific operational areas. Their goal is to establish and implement "systems" that will ensure that these five critical factors are built on firm foundations. This team should consist of specialists in the following areas: unit hour utilization, unit hour production, communications, human resources, staff development, purchasing, fleet management, sales, marketing, finance, and administration.

Unit hour utilization is a fundamental component in the success of any operation. It is imperative that research and analysis of past call volume statistics be conducted in order to establish effective system status plans to meet call demands while ensuring appropriate response time reliability.

Once system status plans have been developed and the number of unit hours to meet these plans has been determined, production of these unit hours is necessary. This task requires an array of essential activities: purchasing ambulances and medical supplies/equipment; recruiting and hiring qualified personnel; orientation and ongoing training; fleet management; communications; and medical direction.

Given the specific time constraints that affect every start-up activity, all critical equipment, i.e., ambulances, radios, communications base station, recording equipment, etc., and supplies essential to a timely start-up should be ordered without delay. In addition, essential medical equipment and supplies required by respective local and state government agencies should be ordered. Acquiring the necessary information to ensure prompt licensing or permitting for ambulances that provide emergency and non-emergency transportation services should receive special attention.

The successful start-up of any new operation hinges on the abilities of the transition team to communicate their specific goals and timelines. Time is an essential element to a new operation's overall success. Systems that must be up and running within one to three months risk the potential for more problems than those systems that have been granted additional time for start-up. The crucial role of the transition team is to provide support, within given time allotments, for meeting targeted goals.

Another consideration when selecting this team is who will be the key personnel empowered to manage the new operation? Certainly bench strength from existing operations is an added benefit in the developmental process. New operations that are the result of expansions or acquisitions may be absorbed into existing organizational structures. Some operations, however, may create career path opportunities for existing personnel. No matter what process is used in providing management support, the involvement of those individuals (whether existing or new) who will be responsible for managing the operation is essential.

High-Quality Patient Care

In order for an operation to become successful, there must be a focal point that drives its activities. The ambulance service industry depends on daily interaction with people. Thus, customer service should be recognized as the single most important factor that will either make or break new and existing operations.

Patient care represents a continuum of services from the time a request is received until the patient's account is closed. Care is always expressed in the form of community services, including citizen CPR classes, standbys at local school athletic games, and participation in health fairs, to name just a few.

Many programs have been developed to enhance the prehospital care provider's bedside disposition. Though field personnel demonstrate cognitive and practical abilities to comply with established standards of care, most training programs do not provide thorough training for interactions with pediatric and geriatric patients. Programs that focus on psychological development and interaction are essential. Office personnel should also receive training to enhance their interpersonal skills, including telephone etiquette, conflict resolution, and managing difficult customers.

In fact, not many customer feedback cards describe the customer's satisfaction in terms of how well medical skills were performed. Most describe, in detail, whether or not the dispatcher or ambulance crew was "nice" or "compassionate," or "how quickly the ambulance responded." Successful operations must commit to training their personnel in ongoing customer service strategies. This is especially important when beginning a new operation. As EMS is indeed a service industry, operations must be designed to meet every facet of the customer's needs, whether medical, emotional, or financial.

This concept can be reinforced to the organization's labor force by developing a mission statement that emphasizes the commitment to providing high-quality patient care.

> The successful start-up of any new operation hinges on the abilities of the transition team to communicate their specific goals and timelines.

Employee services must be structured to create a positive work environment that facilitates opportunities for financial stability and personal and professional growth.

Employee Services

Employees are any organization's most important asset. Employee services must be structured to create a positive work environment that facilitates opportunities for financial stability and personal and professional growth.

Employees are recruited and hired based on staffing requirements to meet the operation's system status plan. To ensure that only qualified individuals are selected, it is necessary to establish a hiring process consistent with the Americans with Disabilities Act (ADA). Job descriptions for each position should be written outlining the essential job functions. In so doing, specific pre-employment evaluations may be administered to provide information concerning the applicant's knowledge and abilities to meet the essential job functions with or without reasonable accommodation. These evaluations must be designed to determine cognitive knowledge as well as psychomotor skills.

The selection of qualified applicants must reflect the organization's commitment to an affirmative action plan that facilitates the development of a diversified labor force. If this is not possible during initial start-up, the operation must stand ready to develop and implement diversification strategies to ensure that recruitment opportunities are being made to minorities.

After the job offer, applicants are required to undergo a "post-offer" employment medical evaluation. Individual orientation start dates are established that are dependent on the results of the medical evaluation's confirmation of the applicant's ability to perform the essential job functions, with or without reasonable accommodation.

Recruitment and hiring is just one phase of setting up a new operation. The human resources department should also be involved with the development of employee retention strategies. These may include establishing or upgrading benefits packages, developing employee recognition programs, ensuring timely performance appraisals, and providing employee assistance programs (EAPs).

In conjunction with the hiring process, all new employees must be ensured an adequate orientation, no matter how soon the operation has to start. It should be every organization's commitment to make sure new employees succeed. Thus, thorough didactic and practical sessions must be conducted that enable all employees to learn specific administrative and medical policies and procedures of the organization. They must also be held accountable for performing essential job functions. Many situations during this start-up phase may arise that could preclude providing orientation programs. This area requires perhaps the most attention, not only from a performance perspective, but for liability exposure as well.

Finance and Administration

Certainly, an operation's financial stability should be considered prior to any potential start-up activities. Budgets should be formulated based on the ability of a new operation to take over the new market. Will the new operation hold an exclusive 9-1-1 contract? Will there be competition for non-emergency calls? A determination of what the new market will hold for the new operation is essential.

In addition to market shares, the new operation must evaluate reimbursement issues concerning Medicare and Medicaid. What are the established prevailing rates for the immediate area? When were these rates established? Can these rates be changed?

New operations must be able to identify what cost per transport is required to break even. Once known, base rates can be established and "add-on" charges set.

It should be understood that budgets represent guidelines for monetary expenditures anticipated during the course of given time frames. Budgets should also be developed to handle unanticipated costs. Securing a sound financial base can provide a certain level of security when problems arise. The transition team should be involved in budget preparation to ensure financial accountability.

Billing and collection procedures must also be developed to aid in the timely management of all open patient accounts. By reducing the number of days accounts are maintained in the accounts receivable process, timely collections for generating positive cash flows can be ensured.

New operations must be financially accountable in order to pay their bills accordingly. A new operation that is late paying bills is destined for failure, not only from a financial perspective, but also a public relations vantage point. Employees also expect payroll checks to be generated on time with minimal errors. A well-organized finance department can set the stage for positive company morale that has a direct impact on the entire operation.

The finance and administration offices should also be involved with current and ongoing contract negotiations.

Operating Systems

The overall success of any operation depends on systems that are designed to ensure prompt and efficient customer service. The development of the field operations component involves a complex array of intricate systems that must be readily identified and followed to enable smooth processing of ambulance requests for service. The field operations component may be divided into two categories, unit hour utilization and unit hour production.

Unit Hour Utilization

In setting up a new operation, it is imperative that previous call volume statistics be made available for analysis. In conjunction with the concepts of system status management, this information can help develop a plan for how many ambulances will be required to meet the EMS system's demands at any given time throughout the day. These plans are essential

> The overall success of any operation depends on systems that are designed to ensure prompt and efficient customer service.

for determining response time criteria and identifying the number of field personnel necessary for staffing requirements.

Unit Hour Production

Once the request for ambulances is made, efforts must be taken to ensure unit availability. It is imperative to keep in mind that once a plan is designed, it must be followed in order to work. System status plans depend on keeping ambulances available to the system. Measures must be taken to prevent the loss of unit time. Common causes of lost unit time include

- Personnel clocking in late for duty
- Ambulances not being ready for specified shifts
- Mechanical failures
- Extended hospital downtimes

Operations personnel should anticipate other causes and implement measures to minimize lost time. Lost unit time is a waste of resources that can be easily converted to a dollar amount. Operations should calculate how much time a unit hour costs their service to operate. To determine this figure, apply the following formula:

Determine the average cash amount collected per patient transport. This number will equal X. Then determine what unit hour utilization (UHU) ratio your operation desires. A 0.35 means that for every 2.8 hours worked, one patient will be transported (one hour divided by 0.35 equals 2.8). Thus, cash collected, X, divided by 2.8 hours equals cost per unit hour.

Projected unit hour ratios can also be helpful in determining the number of unit hours necessary for budgetary purposes. Take the number of projected transports for the year and divide that by the UHU desired. This formula will yield the number of unit hours needed for the year to manage the projected number of transports. This same process should be utilized to develop staffing plans on a daily, weekly, and monthly basis.

Operational Policies

Policies and procedures must be developed and implemented to ensure the continual success of the operation, particularly in the areas of communication, response, and patient destination guidelines. Employees must be educated about the standards to which they will be held accountable. Systems should be designed to coach employees if policies and procedures are not followed. Continuous breech of policies may then warrant employee action.

Fleet Management

System status plans have been developed to ensure the availability of ambulances to meet call demands while adhering to either self-imposed or contractual response times. To accomplish this criterion, the plans must be followed without any interference. Any decrease in ambulance availability will offset the plan, causing potential problems in managing call demands and response times.

A comprehensive fleet management program, whether in-house or contracted, if appropriately designed and monitored, can ensure ambulance availability. Programs should be designed to perform preventive maintenance as well as establish procedures for more complex jobs.

By coordinating ambulance availability with adequate staffing to meet call demands, lost unit hours should be kept to a minimum.

Communications

Communications policies and procedures must be identified, developed, and implemented in a cooperative effort with existing public service agencies. Primary 9-1-1 calls are often received by law enforcement agencies. In establishing the new operation, it would be advantageous to have these calls, once determined to be medical in nature, routed to the operation's control center via a secondary public safety answering point (PSAP). Then the operation's system status controllers (SSC), who should be trained in the principles of emergency medical dispatch, can manage the call.

SSCs should also be required to undergo extensive training in radio communications, customer service strategies, and organizational skills.

Community and Government Relations

Relationships established within the operation's service area will help ensure that it is well received within the community. Community programs such as CPR training, first aid events, sponsorships for explorer posts, etc., are expected by citizens and should be made available at little or no charge. "Show and tell" programs for schools and community groups not only inform people about EMS but may also be used as recruitment activities, especially for affirmative action purposes. Community marketing strategies should focus on citizens becoming familiar with the name of their ambulance service provider.

Marketing plans should also be developed to include regularly scheduled visits to government agencies within the service area. Periodic visits with key government officials help to identify potential problems that constituents express. This gives the new operation opportunities to correct potential problems before they become a political issue.

Encourage city, county, state, and national leaders to visit the operation. Until these individuals observe, first hand, how a high-performance EMS system is supposed to operate, there may always be the potential threat for other services to venture into the marketplace. Not only do marketing plans secure one's place within the market, but they also ensure obtaining additional calls, especially in the non-emergency market.

Conclusion

The start-up of any new operation requires precise coordination from all members of the transition team. Particular attention must be focused on two specific areas. First, what market will the new operation try to

Source

Original article. Brent Dierking, BS, REMT-P, is the director of operations for Mobile Medic Ambulance Service, Inc.'s Gulf Coast Division. He has over 14 years of prehospital EMS experience. John K. Rester is the president and CEO for Mobile Medic and a board member for American Medical Response, Inc.

capture? In addition to this question, a thorough knowledge of reimbursement issues concerning emergency versus non-emergency (ALS versus BLS) transports is critical to facilitating revenue generation.

Second, qualified applicants who are hired by the new operation must be provided a complete orientation. Often, there may be a tendency, especially if start-up is required within a few months, to brief employees on the essential components of the orientation program. This type of activity may prove detrimental to the operation in that no matter how prepared one might be considered to be, errors in conforming to policies and procedures will occur. The new operation should avoid these potential liability situations. This situation occurs most often with various driver training programs that ambulance services utilize during the orientation phase.

There is much excitement and activity during any start-up period for a new operation. Be careful to constantly keep your sights on the overall picture and not become wrapped up in minute details. That's the job of the transition team. Also remember, no matter how much time and preparation go into the start-up, something will most likely be overlooked. Don't overreact, but meet these challenges head-on. This type of management will set the stage for people to feel secure that the operation is running smoothly.

Let the management team know it is acceptable to make mistakes. No one is perfect. However, once realized, measures must be taken to ensure that the likelihood of a similar problem arising again is minimal. On the other hand, celebrate your successes. Reinforce positive behavior with praise, not just at the management level, but let it filter throughout the entire organization. Working hard to enhance employee morale and "doing the right thing" will certainly position a new operation on a course for success.

THERE IS AN OLD ADAGE that says, "If your business is not growing, then you are going out of business." The evolution of EMS and the medical transportation industry over the past 25 years has added merit to this idea. Consider the following business practices that have impacted the ambulance industry during this period:

- Pricing controls
- Performance requirements
- Fines, sanctions, and financial penalties
- Decreasing labor supply (in most markets)
- ADA, OSHA, ERISA, KKK, HCFA, etc.
- Expanding clinical protocols
- Organized labor
- Plaintiff proliferation
- CAD and telecommunications technology
- HMOs, PPOs, IPAs, and other group purchasing

This list could go on and on, but the point is obvious . . . an entrepreneur who wants to maintain a competitive position must find ways and means of absorbing the escalating costs of providing high-quality service.

The most common response (once the principal discovers revenues are limited) is to make the business grow in order to spread overhead over a larger service base. In doing so, the organization must maximize a larger share of the existing market or examine additional markets.

While a few firms have been successful in competing for a market through the bidding process, many of those hopeful firms have not only walked away without the contract, but with a somewhat deflated ego to match their deflated balance sheet.

Assuming there must be a better way for business development, the organization may well turn their strategies to acquiring markets via merger or purchase. Unfortunately, there is no guarantee that this type of growth strategy will prove successful. However, following some basic guidelines or protocols may make a big difference in both the process and the outcome of an acquisition.

Logical Candidates

Buying an existing company is not as simple as offering a dollar amount equal to or greater than what the seller needs to retire. Most owners of ambulance companies have put years of heart and soul into their business. The company takes on the semblance of a child. To detach themselves from their company is much like seeing a child leave home or get

Expanding Your Market Through Acquisition

Trace Skeen

The mechanism of acquisition will always be one sure way to expand your organization's EMS market share. Author Trace Skeen's unique background in this industry enables him to speak with authority on the potentials and pitfalls of acquisition.

married. Just as a parent measures the fit of a future son-in-law or daughter-in-law, the business owner measures the "fit" of a suitor for his business.

In many cases, the need to familiarize the principals and to reach an appropriate comfort level may take years. Most owners will want to know that they are entrusting their employees and company reputation to someone who will protect the integrity and well-being of both. Conversely, the seller will undoubtedly believe that the new owner will not be able to match the special intricacies instituted by his management regime.

The Courtship

Where possible, the suitor should establish and upgrade the quality and frequency of the communications with the owners or upper-level management of potential acquisitions. As much as you want to learn about the target company, it is equally important that they learn more about your organization.

During this process, you may discover common ground between the two organizations that may present some cooperative opportunities regardless of an ultimate acquisition outcome. Synergies to be considered might include dispatching, regional training, group purchasing, mutual aid agreements, recruiting referrals, and others.

As tools to increase communication, consider the following:

- Place the target company on your mailing list for company newsletters, press releases, marketing brochures, etc. (This is not as proprietarily difficult as you might think once you realize that competitors end up with all this information anyway.)
- Invite the principal of the target company to join you in a meeting with state health directors or elected officials to discuss a common agenda item.
- Invite the principal into your business to attend an open house, management training course, or other on-site activities.
- Recognize that many barriers can be broken down by seeking advice or problem-solving help from your peer in the target company.

If you are successful in these efforts and exhibit a genuine and sincere interest, the ultimate discussion of acquisition will be more readily received.

Creating an "A" List

During the "courtship" period, two objectives emerge as critical elements. First, build a stronger relationship with the target candidate, and second, establish clear criteria that can be used to measure the "fit." A cautionary note: If the criteria for measurement is not established in advance, there may be an emotional response to the efficacy of an acquisition that does not make sense for either party.

Establish a list of preliminary characteristics that are compatible to your own business strategies. These characteristics might include

- Strong relationship with the community
- Strong relationship with allied health agencies
- Long-term contracts
- Performance-based workforce
- Potential for internal market growth
- Strong management bench strength
- "Friendly" regulatory climate
- Geographical practicability
- Viability of fleet and equipment
- Adequate labor pool
- Flexible rate structures
- Medicare/Medicaid profiles
- Barriers to entry

Not only should you consider compatible characteristics, but "red flag" discoveries should also be evaluated. That is, certain conditions may exist that will make any type of business acquisition prohibitive if they are not reversed. These items might include

- Multiple-provider market with low or no barriers to entry
- Lack of contracts that ensure existing revenues are maintained
- Stagnant or decreasing population base
- Strangulating regulatory environment
- Unstable workforce
- Pricing restraints
- Predatory pricing environment

Once you have compiled the preliminary "A" list and have established a positive relationship, you are prepared to move forward with the offer and subsequent due diligence.

The Offer

The offer can be very stressful for first-time participants. The acquiring party that goes into this process with a very specific and inflexible agenda may quickly discover the meeting to be short-lived. Rather, both parties would do well to maintain flexibility and allow the discussion to examine possibilities that had not been previously contemplated.

A proud father who hears a suitor saying, "I would like to date your daughter," is much less stressed than one who hears "I would like to marry your daughter." The entire image is tempered by the opportunity for the father to negotiate if he doesn't like the terms.

In terms of acquisition, the statement, "I would like to talk to you about a mutually beneficial business relationship," may be much more palatable than "I want to buy you out!" The latter may invoke a defensive response that must be overcome before the discussion can go forward and be productive.

The business relationship may evolve into one of several potential forms. These include

- Mutual aid agreements
- Outsourcing support services
  - Dispatch services
  - Training, et al.
  - A/R management
  - Fleet maintenance
  - Short-term vehicle leasing (i.e., event coverage)
- Merger into a common organization
- Stock purchase (purchase of the corporation)
- Asset purchase (purchase of some or all of the equipment, A/R, market share, etc.)

Mutual aid agreements are the most basic types of business relationships. These agreements may allow both organizations to obtain greater utilization with fewer staffed resources.

Outsourcing support services allows each organization to maintain corporate independence while improving the performance and cost effectiveness of the services noted.

A merger relationship essentially allows for combining services identified in outsourcing but also establishes a more formal and integrated legal structure. While management from both organizations is integrated, management downsizing is ultimately exercised in order to obtain some economy of scale.

The stock purchase maintains the integral structure of the target corporation with all its assets and liabilities. This process requires the greatest level of effort in conducting due diligence since pending and potential litigation remains with the corporation. The buying entity must determine the value of maintaining the corporate structure and name identity versus abandoning the acquired corporation and creating a more substantive surviving organization.

The asset purchase scenario allows for the purchase of all or part of the equipment, accounts receivable, and other selected fixed assets. The liabilities and cash generally remain with the seller.

These various methods are briefly mentioned and are not necessarily the focus here. Interested parties on either side of the negotiation should seek competent expertise from a trusted attorney or other professional party.

Due Diligence

Due diligence is a term that identifies the process of close examination. The appropriate completion of the due diligence process will establish the financial worth of an acquisition and identify the risks and cultural modifications that must be addressed as part of the acquisition plan.

By establishing some protocols prior to initiating the acquisition process, strengths and weaknesses can be assigned a risk factor to the purchase. Acquisition protocols relative to the ambulance industry can be broken down into three key areas:

- Business analysis
- Human resources analysis
- Financial analysis

The various factors within each of these analyses are weighed according to their individual degree of importance (Figure 2.6). The risk is then assigned based on the source data using a scale of 1 to 6, with 1 being low risk or most favorable.

The minimum acceptable range is a "red flag" indicator. That is, any factor that fails to meet this minimum criteria may be considered a reason for terminating the negotiations. The source may take several forms, including the following:

Operational audit. This is an extensive survey that examines policy and procedure manuals, activity data, incident reports, union contracts, financial performance, contracts and agreements for transport services,

---

Figure 2.6

Acquisition Analysis Protocol

BUSINESS ANALYSIS

Business: _____
Contact: _____
Location: _____
Date: _____

Factor	Rel. Wt.	Risk Position	Fx Score	Min. Accpt. Range	Max. Score	Source
Competitive Position	16			>32	96	Operational audit Competitor analysis
Market Size	16			>48	96	Operational audit
Market Share	3			>9	18	Operational audit
Market Stability	3			>9	18	Operational audit
Market Growth	16			>32	96	Historical record
Market Regulation	16			>40	96	Operational audit
Economic Demographics	10			>20	60	Operational audit
Market Dominance	20			>40	120	Operational audit Competitor analysis
Total	100			>230	600	

- Risk to be ranked from 1 to 6 with 1 being low risk position and 6 being high risk position.
- Fx score is a mathematical equation of multiplying the relative weight by the risk position factor.

Figure 2.6 (cont.)

HUMAN RESOURCES ANALYSIS

Business: _____

Contact: _____

Location: _____

Date: _____

Factor	Rel. Wt.	Risk Position	Fx Score	Min. Accpt. Range	Max. Score	Source
Current Staffing	15			>45	90	Operational audit
Total Labor Pool Availability	20			>60	120	Operational audit
H/R Systems in Place	5			>10	30	Operational audit
Compensation and Benefits	20			>40	120	Operational audit
Employee Relations	20			>80	120	Operational audit
Management Depth	10			>30	60	Operational audit
Employment Contracts	5			>10	30	Operational audit
Cultural Modification	5			>10	30	Operational audit
Total	100			>285	600	

FINANCIAL ANALYSIS

Business: _____

Contact: _____

Location: _____

Date: _____

Factor	Rel. Wt.	Risk Position	Fx Score	Min. Accpt. Range	Max. Score	Source
Cash Flow Generation	60			>240	360	Pro forma
Liquidation Value	5			>20	30	Balance sheet
Capital Infusion	20			>50	120	Inspection
Debt Structure	5			>10	30	Balance sheet
Collection Rate	5			>15	30	Balance sheet Cash flow
Revenue Mix	5			>10	30	Operational audit
Total	100			>345	600	

and so forth. Companies that have completed ambulance accreditation through CAAS will have this data readily available for inspection.

Competitor analysis. If a profile on competitors in the market is not on file with the target company, additional research will be necessary to complete appropriate competitor analysis. This source should include a strength and weakness analysis on each competitor, salary and compensation comparisons, key political strengths, contracts and transport agreements with key healthcare agencies, etc.

Historical record. This is usually obtained from promotional brochures, interviews with key principals, and corroborating information from local chambers of commerce.

Pro forma. This is the financial projection that will illustrate the value of the acquisition to your organization following the integration. Caution should be exercised in not understating the expenses associated with integration over the initial 12 to 18 months.

Balance sheet and financial statements. These are the pictures that the accountants will be examining in order to evaluate subtle trends that may not be readily apparent. Corporate tax returns are usually included in this examination.

Obviously, this due diligence process lays open the very heart of a company. A confidentiality agreement is generally signed prior to beginning the due diligence efforts in order to offer some degree of security for the seller. Such confidentiality agreements require the buyer to hold confidential information from unnecessary competitive forces and return the data should the negotiations be terminated.

As they relate to the respective analysis, a few of the factors are worthy of emphasis. The human resource section examines the very important issues of merging two corporate cultures while maintaining productivity levels. Employment policies and compensation packages that

Figure 2.6 (cont.)

ANALYSIS SUMMARY

Business: _____
Contact: _____
Location: _____
Date: _____

Factor	Rel. Wt.	Fx Score	Max. Score	Fx Variance %
Business Factors	0.35		210	
Human Resources	0.20		120	
Financial Factors	0.45		270	
Total	1.00		600	

Source

Original article. D. Trace Skeen is the CEO of Buck Medical Services in Portland, Ore. He is director of the Management Training Institute of the American Ambulance Association.

will be integrated should be carefully considered for compatibility. Preexisting employment contracts with the managers may present a negative liability and should be considered for termination or renegotiation.

When you come to the financial analysis, note the heavy weighing of cash flow generation. Cash flow is the driving force regarding the appropriate outcome for the business relationship. You may well discover that the results of this analysis are no different than the results of your "gut reaction" when you started. However, the analysis will not only establish a blueprint for arriving at a price to pay for the acquisition, but will also provide an impressive package for your banker when the time comes.

Knowing that your organization provides a high-quality service that deserves to be replicated will provide you with the confidence to grow your business.

WITH ALL THE RECENT CONSOLIDATION and doomsaying within the EMS industry, the music from the movie *Jaws* is likely playing a constant refrain in the minds of many smaller EMS providers. The word from the consolidators—those large companies buying up small and mid-size ambulance services—is that health maintenance organizations (HMOs) soon will be purchasing EMS and other "out-of-hospital" services. Because HMOs are for-profit institutions, they will be looking for the least expensive EMS delivery system. The consolidators and others with a stake in the new order assert that cost-effective services can only be produced by large national EMS companies, and smaller companies will be left out in the cold. But will they?

Admittedly, many of the consolidators' contentions are supported by present economic theory. Large companies can take advantage of certain economies of scale not available to smaller organizations. These economies of scale enable them to negotiate lower prices by buying equipment (e.g., ambulances, EKG monitors, and portable suction units), medical supplies, and employee benefit plans in volume and to more efficiently operate essential support services.

Additionally, the existence of multiple operations allows larger organizations to better collect data on patient demographics and socioeconomic characteristics and their relationship to response volumes. This in turn enables company managers to make more accurate predictions regarding operational costs, a required skill in capitated payment environments. Finally, these large organizations are more likely to have the revenue to pay for experienced, competent managers to run their companies.

Being big has its drawbacks, however. Big creates bureaucracy, which, if left unchecked, can slow an organization's response to change, significantly inhibiting organizational flexibility and innovation. Big also exposes the organization to a whole new set of labor relations rules. And big means more layers between top management, field providers, patients, and politicians. This greater isolation between organizational leadership and field providers also can reduce the level of effort field providers put into working for organizational success; big companies tend to be more impersonal and may not engender commitment and loyalty among their employees.

Smaller EMS providers, on the other hand, have their own particular competitive advantages. For instance, they have lower overhead costs associated with stations and garage facilities that may already be paid for or leased at lower rates. They also may have the advantage of historical response data, enhancing their ability to compute a more accurate capitated

Cooperation: An Alternative to Consolidation

Geoffrey Cady

While consolidation sweeps through EMS systems at a rapid pace, there are alternatives for both the public service providers and small to mid-size private ambulance services. The author outlines how various cooperative efforts can use the same economies of scale that make consolidation so appealing.

contract price. And they may be perceived as being more willing to invest in long-term system enhancements and community development, which has the potential to create greater consumer loyalty and confidence.

Finally, strong ties with local government may enable local providers to obtain tax support for system enhancements, resulting in lower operational costs and subsequent lower contract prices to HMOs.

So why has industry consolidation been occurring at such a rapid rate in the past two years? To present a detailed list of all of the factors now influencing the industry is well beyond the scope of this article. However, some of the more prominent forces include current trends in healthcare financing, the provision of a wider spectrum of healthcare services by EMS providers, availability of money from capital markets (stock markets), and the speculation that mandated changes in healthcare financing could provide a windfall of profits for investors.

A September 1993 *Forbes* article provides testimony to this fact. In the article, Paul Verrochi, chief executive officer of one of the new giants on the EMS scene, American Medical Response, is quoted as saying, "If Hillary [Clinton] expands access to healthcare, all Americans will be covered by insurance, and that means all my bills will start getting paid."

Interestingly, the article does not discuss the anticipated downward pressure on revenues that will occur from managed competition in a capitated pricing environment. It does, however, conclude that smaller EMS providers will be unable to compete in the future, suggesting that large EMS providers are positioned to acquire a significant market share with little competition from the smaller agencies.

It would appear, therefore, that there are only two options for smaller EMS providers in the near future. One is to sell, sell, sell, taking the money and company stock and looking for another line of work. The other is to work for somebody else in the EMS business.

Yet, while many people in EMS believe they have no choices beyond those two options, that is not necessarily so. In fact, there are still ways in which spirited entrepreneurs and diehards who want to remain their own bosses, not to mention the thousands of fire department, third-service, nonprofit, hospital-based, volunteer, and other providers that want to remain in EMS without being consolidated, can do so.

What Can You Do?
(Or Business Strategies in Times of Consolidation)

At the November 1993 American Ambulance Association Conference, strategies for working within a consolidated industry were presented for those wanting to continue operating their own businesses. Some of those strategies included developing plans for improving profit margins; actively improving service delivery; developing specialty markets in terms of service delivery methods or geographical coverage (e.g., covering special events or developing exclusive contracts with medical facilities); and increasing barriers to market entry through ordinances, stringent prequalification requirements for requests for proposals (RFPs), or the adoption of certificates of need.

But perhaps the most interesting—and possibly the strongest—recommendation was the development of strategic alliances between large and small EMS providers. Such alliances or cooperative structures could eventually be big players in a new healthcare financing environment.

The following illustrates how such a concept could become reality.

Happy Valley, USA

The relatively remote, green, lush valley of Happy Valley, USA, has a population of approximately two million spread across 18,000 square miles. The valley incorporates a mixture of small to mid-size urban communities (60,000 to 350,000), each surrounded by suburban and rural populations. There are six cities within the region's five counties, scattered at approximately 50-mile intervals along one of the state's major freeways.

Presently, each community has a private EMS provider and, in some cases, a non-transport municipal fire department providing BLS and ALS first response. In three communities, ALS is offered by the private provider only. In the other three, the municipal fire departments supply ALS transport services, with the local private provider furnishing 9-1-1 ALS backup, BLS interfacility transports, ALS critical care transports, and ambulance service to unincorporated parts of the valley. All communities have a BLS/defibrillation first response. In addition to the private and public providers, there are two volunteer squads in two remote regions of the valley and three hospital-based air medical programs.

As national standards have been adopted, the Happy Valley EMS systems have kept pace by employing quality improvement (QI) practices that ensure clinical excellence and response-time reliability, with levels exceeding 90-percent compliance. Each city's population has grown steadily over the years, providing enough fee-for-service revenue to replace capital equipment on a timely basis. Personnel practices have been equitable and have created stable non-union workforces.

The relationship between the private and public providers is amicable, as are the relationships between the regional and local EMS agencies. All of the private providers are active members of the state ambulance association. Since the cities are separated by more than 50 miles, there has been little direct competition between providers for market share outside of their respective cities and counties.

The Passing of the Health Security Act

It is now 1995, and Happy Valley has been defined as a "medical trade area," in which the entire valley is considered one healthcare market to be bid on. The HMOs, which now provide healthcare to valley residents, have decided that the most cost-effective provision of EMS, as well as that of out-of-hospital services, can be accomplished only by

> Alliances between large and small EMS providers could eventually be big players in a new healthcare financing environment.

In essence, a cooperative is a group of independently owned and managed businesses or public agencies that contractually agree to abide by a set of governing rules developed by the membership (themselves) for the purpose of engaging in some economic activity.

contracting with one medical transportation provider. The HMOs develop and release an RFP for the provision of emergency and non-emergency out-of-hospital medical services on a capitated cost basis.

The RFP requires that Happy Valley become an integrated medical transport system with an advanced dispatch center equipped with the latest computer-aided dispatch and automatic vehicle locating technology, direct data transmission capabilities, and medical telecommunications specialists trained to interrogate callers and provide pre-arrival instructions and on-line medical direction. It also requires a first response component, with BLS providers trained to defibrillate; an ALS response and treatment component; transportation to the most appropriate facility; air medical services; a primary healthcare delivery component using physician extender personnel; and a prevention and public education component.

The submitted proposals will be evaluated using methodology that will score each organization's ability to meet or exceed the stated clinical and operational performance requirements on a capitated cost basis.

Looking at the RFP, three large national medical transport companies are confident that they will be the only players in this managed competition. After all, they alone possess the necessary capital resources and management expertise to operate the large regional system in a cost-effective manner. They are also confident that their economies of scale will enable them to offer services at lower capitated rates than the valley's individual services could offer. End of story.

Or is it? Is there a way the smaller EMS organizations can compete effectively against the larger national companies? Is there a business structure and the necessary technology to open future competitions to smaller local competitors? Yes. In what many see as the future of EMS, one possible competitive strategy is for several smaller EMS organizations to form an alliance—or cooperative firm—to achieve the necessary size and economies of scale present in the larger companies.

The Cooperative Vertical Organization

A cooperative vertical organization is defined as "the organized collaboration of a group of legally independent cooperating enterprises that operate in the same economic sphere under a single management." In essence, a cooperative is a group of independently owned and managed businesses or public agencies that contractually agree to abide by a set of governing rules developed by the membership (themselves) for the purpose of engaging in some economic activity. The basic structure and operation of an EMS cooperative would be similar to those of the large EMS companies, creating the possibility of EMS cooperatives competing directly with larger organizations for prehospital services in future medical trade areas.

Examples of cooperatives can be found in a variety of U.S. industries that have been the focus of intense consolidation. These include agriculture (perhaps the most widely known), the grocery and related products industry, hardware, drug and drug sundries, and construction materials. In fact, *Fortune* magazine's 1993 listing of the 500 largest companies based on sales includes seven regional cooperatives, five of which have sales in excess of $1 billion annually.

Cooperatives are far more prevalent outside the United States, however. This is primarily due to the Sherman Act, a U.S. antitrust act passed in 1890 that outlawed certain types of businesses on the premise that they restrain (or reduce) trade or competition. Although the act did not actually outlaw cooperatives, it didn't explicitly state that they were exempt from the law either. Also, while federal protection exists for cooperative business structures, individual states may have statutes that could be interpreted in such a way as to result in legal action. It is therefore important that legal counsel be obtained when developing membership criteria and operational procedures for any cooperative venture.

The economic strength of cooperatives occurs as a result of "vertical integration," in which members' resources are organized to achieve efficient economies of scale—perhaps their most important competitive advantage. Nearly all non-agricultural cooperatives are made up of groups of investor-owned firms, each of which is too small individually to compete with larger companies within the market. Management costs are, in principle, equivalent to the bookkeeping and indirect overhead charges that occur between an investor-owned corporation and its departments or subsidiary corporations.

The vertical integration of activities by cooperatives refers to the efforts of the cooperative to include as a member each producer or service provider involved in the sequence of steps necessary for the production of a product or service. For example, in an emergency medical services system (EMSS), each agency with responsibility for a portion or component of the EMSS would be a member of that system's EMS cooperative; when a caller's request for medical assistance is transferred from the primary service answering point to the medical dispatch center, it would enter the first step in the EMS production process.

Cooperation Within the Cooperative

A cooperative's management team, or its "umbrella" organization, is responsible for coordinating and administering the cooperative framework. It serves in the same capacity as the various corporate functional groups that support large investor-owned enterprises. The management team can comprise different organization members or professional managers and is directed by a board of directors elected by the general membership.

The cooperative membership is free to impose obligations on itself and can empower the directors to set down and enforce—either in the bylaws or on a contractual basis—guidelines for certain business decisions (e.g., ensuring that all agencies use the same logo, participate in

> In an emergency medical services system (EMSS), each agency with responsibility for a portion or component of the EMSS would be a member of that system's EMS cooperative.

meetings, support the cooperative financially, and wear the same uniforms). This approach ensures that the board of directors is occupied, or controlled, by the cooperative membership and that the board's policies are consistently in line with the interests of the membership. In this way—at least theoretically—it is impossible for the management or umbrella organization to dominate or expose the collective assets of the cooperative to non-agreed-upon risks.

Membership Participation

Critical to the inception and potential success of the cooperative is the degree of cooperation—or co-management—granted to its members. Operational policy will have to be developed to address whether members have the opportunity to cooperate in the EMSS only when performing their various business tasks or whether all member organizations can be involved in the planning for and monitoring of all or a portion of the business or system operation.

Possible methods for membership participation could include having a representative on the various boards from each agency responsible for providing services within the EMSS or having a representative on the boards from each of the subsystems (BLS, ALS, primary care, air medical, and public education/prevention).

The level of member involvement would vary according to the needs of each cooperative. Experts in cooperative development indicate that situational factors, such as the expertise of members, time constraints, and the social and political relationships of the membership, will set the stage.

The Happy Valley EMS Cooperative

After receiving a copy of the RFP from the HMO consortium, Happy Valley EMS providers call a meeting of their regional EMS council members to discuss options for addressing the outlined system requirements. Council members also perform an analysis of the possible deployment strategies a national EMS company would employ to meet clinical and response-time requirements.

What they determine is that a national provider would have to install a regional telecommunications and dispatch center; depend on existing county and municipal fire departments to provide first response; lease or rent facilities in each of the valley's cities to serve as crew quarters and warehouse facilities; contract for vehicle maintenance or establish its own vehicle maintenance facility in at least two or three cities; and have an appropriate amount of on-site supervision (i.e., operations manager, field supervisors, training and QI coordinators, utility and maintenance personnel, and clerical support). Billing personnel would not be needed, since the services would be contracted for on a capitated basis.

Other business functions, such as strategic planning, management information systems (MIS), human resource development, and finance, would be located at the company's corporate headquarters.

The Happy Valley providers then perform a competitive analysis, in which they determine that if they combine their resources and work cooperatively, they can achieve the operational economies of scale possessed by the national provider. They further decide that since they already have many of the key elements of the system in place, they can design and operate a system that will meet all performance requirements. Since they already have a regional EMS organization, they use this organization to select a task force to quickly investigate the feasibility of some form of EMS cooperative.

Time is critical to the success of the proposal, so a project approach is used to design and execute the development of the cooperative. Using this approach, the providers formulate a comprehensive master plan to encompass the entire region, taking into consideration human, material, financial, and technical resources, as well as environmental factors that might hinder cooperative development. This approach organizes the cooperative's various subsystems (first responder groups, medical transportation, primary care, etc.) around a clearly defined organizational design.

A project team consisting of professional managers with expert knowledge of each of the EMSS subsystems is then assembled to provide the necessary stimuli and guidance for meeting objectives. The providers also secure the assistance of industry experts with previous experience in organizing cooperatives as a more effective means of gaining consensus on difficult system design issues.

The team's first task is to develop a membership policy. In developing this policy, the team emphasizes the importance of having the members "buy into" the cooperative concept. Additionally, they understand that the different members will have varying levels of commitment to the process.

For the private EMS providers, the cooperative will be the only way of obtaining a reasonable return on invested time and capital, so the team knows it can expect a great deal of interest from this group. The fire departments will have varying levels of commitment. The BLS first responder agencies will continue to provide services for any new provider without loss of personnel, so they will be less committed to the change. The transporting ALS fire department EMS programs, on the other hand, stand to lose both revenues and personnel and, therefore, both administration and labor in those departments have a vested interest in participating in the EMS cooperative.

What this team understands is that defining the level of membership participation in the cooperative's management needs to be addressed early in development; participatory management does not mean that all members will be involved in all types of decision making. Essentially, there are three levels of decision making in which the membership can participate. The first level is the formation of the organization's basic goals, the second is the formulation of strategic options to achieve these goals, and the third is the translation of these strategies into operational policy.

With the framework complete, the project team and the membership set out to detail the efficient deployment of the cooperative's resources.

The Deployment Strategy

One competitive advantage the Happy Valley EMS providers are counting on is that they already have the personnel, equipment, and facilities in place to do the job the RFP requires. Using cooperation instead of competition, they can reduce redundancy within the system by combining these strengths. For example, maintenance, station, and training facilities can be combined and shared, along with other physical plants and equipment. And even greater economies of scale can be gained if the cooperative takes on the responsibility of coordinating vehicle, medical equipment, and supply purchases for the entire region.

However, the majority of resources needed to provide prehospital and out-of-hospital services are already in existence and require little in the way of capital investment, except for one area: The valley has no central dispatch. Since the system needs to meet the medical needs of a wide range of possible patients (i.e., everything from colds and sore throats to cardiac arrests to routine transports between medical facilities and homes), a new method for allocating resources is needed.

The cooperative determines that requests for any type of medical care should go through a telecommunications center. In addition to customer convenience, this approach offers many economies of scale. Also, funding for the necessary modifications to the center can be obtained through loans secured by cooperative member assets or performance bonds.

The telecommunications center, or medical access point, will be the hub of the regional EMS system, responsible for coordinating the region's entire medical care resources. The rationale behind this approach is to eliminate the need for customers or patients to differentiate between an emergency and non-emergency medical condition and to enable the cooperative to have greater control over health resource utilization.

Having a single medical access point also removes the need for duplicate communications centers—one for emergency and one for non-emergency calls—and it reduces the public's confusion as to whom to call for what type of medical complaint. Additionally, the telecommunications center staff will be able to schedule routine visits to primary care physicians, schedule interfacility transports, and call taxis as necessary.

The center can also serve as the on-line medical control component for a host of out-of-hospital services and can be responsible for monitoring regional trauma centers and hospitals, so hospitals can be activated or deactivated according to system demands. Therefore, the center is the most logical entity for coordinating cooperative efforts between multiple prehospital and out-of-hospital services. As the information processing

Figure 2.7

A Comparison of the Organization of Capital, Plant/Equipment, and Personnel for the EMS Cooperative and EMS Corporation

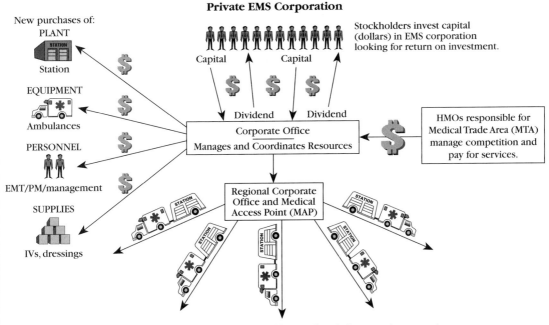

Private EMS Corporation

New purchases of:

PLANT
Station

EQUIPMENT
Ambulances

PERSONNEL
EMT/PM/management

SUPPLIES
IVs, dressings

Stockholders invest capital (dollars) in EMS corporation looking for return on investment.

Capital · Capital

Dividend · Dividend

Corporate Office
Manages and Coordinates Resources

HMOs responsible for Medical Trade Area (MTA) manage competition and pay for services.

Regional Corporate Office and Medical Access Point (MAP)

EMS corporation sets up new stations/offices with ambulances and personnel.

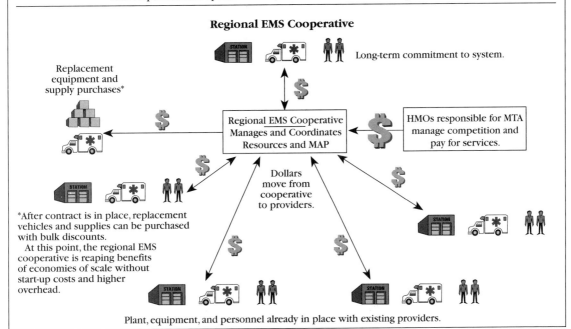

Regional EMS Cooperative

Long-term commitment to system.

Replacement equipment and supply purchases*

Regional EMS Cooperative Manages and Coordinates Resources and MAP

HMOs responsible for MTA manage competition and pay for services.

Dollars move from cooperative to providers.

*After contract is in place, replacement vehicles and supplies can be purchased with bulk discounts.
At this point, the regional EMS cooperative is reaping benefits of economies of scale without start-up costs and higher overhead.

Plant, equipment, and personnel already in place with existing providers.

center for the medical resources of an entire region, it also has the ability to capture extensive data on system performance and operation and is the most logical place to operate and house the enormous MIS necessary to efficiently manage the cooperative's resources.

After several meetings of the cooperative's board of directors, a medical resource deployment plan capable of meeting the requirements of the RFP is approved. Having completed and agreed on the plan, the members of the cooperative go back to their organizations and begin developing cost estimates for providing services in their individual response areas.

The first responder fire departments estimate the marginal costs their organizations will incur as a direct result of providing first responder services. The private ambulance services develop cost estimates based on the previous year's response and patient transport volume. They find, however, that developing estimates for providing primary healthcare services is much more difficult than estimating emergency service, since historical use rates are not readily available. In this case, the private providers, who will be responsible for providing these services, decide to include a contingency clause in the contract that allows them to renegotiate their fees as more cost and use-rate data are obtained.

Once all members of the cooperative submit detailed financial quotes regarding their costs, the membership appoints another task force to review each of the financial quotes to determine if any operational redundancies have been missed in the system design phase that could be eliminated through resource sharing (e.g., vehicle maintenance, equipment retrieval and cleaning, both durable and disposable equipment purchases, and retraining). Using the total capitated-cost estimates developed by each of the EMS system components, they submit their final bid.

To be continued. . . .

Conclusion

While an EMS cooperative as described here has yet to evolve, the ability of cooperatives to effectively use economies of scale through group purchasing and information sharing is a viable strategy when competing with large, private organizations for both emergency and non-emergency out-of-hospital services.

As members of cooperatives that combine resources and data and compete for and win regional contracts, smaller EMS providers can provide medical care in the post-healthcare reform environment. If these smaller EMS companies lack the necessary management skills to pull such cooperative efforts together, larger management companies can be enlisted to perform information management and coordination functions on a fee-for-service basis.

Small local providers may be in a better position—with the appropriate data management—to estimate per capita costs than outside competing providers. They may also possess stronger, more cooperative relationships with local fire departments, which will continue to be part of the EMS system as first responders. Additionally, the coordinated, independent operation of subsystems nurtures an air of innovation and employee loyalty not found in larger, more bureaucratic organizations.

Ultimately, though, the successful creation and operation of EMS cooperatives depend on the ability of their members to act cooperatively and for the good of the whole instead of the individual. In closing, there exists one truly compelling reason for cooperation, which Benjamin Franklin summed up best when he said, "We must all hang together, or assuredly we shall all hang separately!" It was true then, and so it is now.

Source

Reprinted with permission from JEMS, *April 1994. Geoffrey Cady, a former paramedic, is the research director of* Jems *Communications' Emergency Care Information Center.*

References

Darlin, D. "Hillary to the Rescue?" *Forbes* 152, no. 6 (1993).

Dulfer, E., and W. Hamm. *Cooperatives: In the Clash Between Member Participation, Organisational Development and Bureaucratic Tendencies.* London: Quiller Press, 1985.

Fitch, J. "Prospectus on the Consolidation Movement." Paper presented at the American Ambulance Association's Annual Conference, Orlando, Fla., November 1993.

Heflebower, R. B. *Cooperatives and Mutuals in the Market System.* Madison, Wis.: University of Wisconsin Press, 1980.

Risk Management and Loss Control

Improving EMS Workplace Safety

Jay Fitch, PhD, and Roy L. Manns

Managers often overlook the importance of injury prevention and loss-control programs. Employees are at risk; uncounted careers are ended early due to accidents that should have been avoided. The authors point out that effective safety programs must include the continuous support of both management and labor.

Safety and loss-control programs are misunderstood by EMS leaders and workers alike. Even the word *safety* is indistinct and has to be modified with the phrase *loss control* to have clearer meaning in EMS. Frequently, safety and loss-control programs are a hollow response to OSHA inspection threats or some other distant regulatory or contractual requirement. To be effective, these programs must be supported by both management and labor and become part of the organizational culture.

Like the sudden onset of a patient's cardiac symptoms, organizational warning signs for a safety crisis are usually present, waiting to be recognized and acted upon. And, like cardiac problems, when prevention fails, early detection and excellent treatment can make a difference.

A variety of strategies and rationalizations are used by organizations regarding safety. Some designate a person to be in charge of safety. These organizations create a safety manual and conduct an awareness training session or two and then congratulate themselves on their fine program. Others make a very short-term commitment. They develop a reasonable program but expect it to solve the issues in an unrealistically short period. And, still others treat safety issues like a yo-yo dieter trying to lose weight. That is, their commitment goes up and down like a yo-yo. They profess to be concerned about safety but only act on this concern as a knee-jerk reaction to a particular incident or loss. None of these approaches yields long-term success.

Risk reduction for a cardiac patient centers on making long-term changes in behaviors that reduce risk factors. Cardiologists tell us that motivated patients committed to changing their lifestyles have the best opportunity for reducing the risk of cardiac arrest and living a fulfilling life. The same is true regarding an organization's approach to safety and loss control.

Changing behavior starts at the top. Unless and until top management accepts the need to change its own behavior and implement strategies to change behaviors at multiple levels within the organization, attitudes rarely change. Even the best safety manager makes little progress without top management commitment.

Once the commitment has been made, what next? Several fundamental steps should not be overlooked. They include developing a benchmark against which progress can be measured, determining a program and how that program should be delivered, and, finally, rewarding desired behaviors.

Benchmarking Existing and Desired Performances

Simply put, benchmarking means objectively determining where the organization is compared to other organizations and where it desires to be in the future. Benchmarking can be accomplished using internal or external resources, but it should not be overlooked. Benchmarking is an important first step, because safety is considered a "soft" program. The costs of failing to provide a safe workplace are hidden to the casual observer. Benchmarking provides a starting point and helps the organization see the positive (financial) impact of the program.

There are several strategies for accomplishing the safety program benchmarks. They include developing a baseline of experience from other organizations that have excellent programs, conducting inspections, observations, and audits, and having employees complete a detailed safety questionnaire, which can be cross-tabulated by position, number of safety-related incidents, and the length of employment.

Developing and Delivering a Program

The program consists of concepts, plans, and activities to address safety issues within the organization. Developing a policy statement for the program is an excellent starting point. The policy statement should frame the goals, methods, direction, and processes to be used to accomplish the organization's objectives. The policy statement is a working guide and should be adjusted as required.

There are many areas of emphasis that must be addressed by an effective safety and loss-control program. They include

- OSHA compliance
- Vehicle operations training
- HAZMAT
- HAZCOM
- Lifting and patient handling
- Ergonomics
- Bloodborne and airborne pathogens
- Infectious disease and waste
- Accident avoidance
- Accident investigation

- Employee selection
- Medical control and QI programs

Programs should take a proactive rather than a reactive approach. Written safety manuals, while a good reflection of the organization's commitment to a well-defined safety program, do not constitute the program itself. The program must be developed as an educational tool rather than as a stone to be thrown.

A number of resources are available for developing your own program. The American Ambulance Association developed a loss-control manual for its members a number of years ago. Public sector agencies may find an experienced loss-control engineer or risk manager within another department. Both public and private agencies may also be able to draw upon and modify successful programs of local industries.

Developing a clear plan with measurable objectives is a must. Developing a detailed line-item budget necessary to accomplish the safety objectives is also crucial to the program's success. Objectives should be quantified in a manner that fairly represents the cost avoidance advantages instead of solely relying on cost savings to demonstrate the program's value.

Providing adequate staff resources is another key element. Does the organization require a full-time or part-time manager, or can the function be handled by committee? There is no one right answer to this important question.

Few medical transportation organizations can afford a professionally trained or experienced safety manager from another industry. Often, EMS safety managers are assigned collateral duties. Safety becomes one of many competing priorities. When this occurs, the safety manager's success is usually limited to putting out an endless series of fires. As soon as one unsafe condition is corrected, another is recognized and the manager is caught in a continuous cycle of dealing with problems and accidents. The provision of staff resources to accomplish the goals is one of the true tests of management's commitment to the program.

In many respects, the safety manager often becomes an advisor, or internal consultant, to each of the other departments or divisions. In this model, the department head—not the safety manager—has the ultimate responsibility for safety within his area. This can be an effective approach as long as the chief, owner, or director works with the safety manager to establish reasonable goals for each department and then holds the departments accountable for their performance. In this role, the safety manager may be involved with training, providing department heads guidance on new procedures and equipment, and advising them on how to deal with specific identified hazards.

Regardless of how the safety function is staffed, one of the goals must be to broaden the base of awareness and commitment within the organization. Employee safety committees or task groups may be a helpful mechanism for accomplishing this need. Cross-departmental representation and specific numbers of members from each employee classification may be helpful. There have been recent legal cases regarding the use of employee committees so it may be appropriate to check with the organization's labor attorney on the best structure mechanism.

Rewarding the Positive Behavior

Medical transportation organizations and many other entities or industries fail to make the connection that they are constantly reinforcing employee behavior by their corporate actions. This includes passively reinforcing negative behaviors by not adequately monitoring and correcting them, and—more importantly—not positively rewarding the desired behavior. Some managers take the attitude that "it's part of their job and I shouldn't have to reward them for it." A more enlightened approach is an awareness of human nature—employees will focus on those things that the manager's actions (not words) tell them are important.

A number of employee attitudes and behavior patterns involving safety exist. Employee motivators may be primarily negative or positive. Negative motivators—or the desire to avoid negative consequences—include the avoidance of infectious diseases, injuries, or discipline. Positive motivators may include peer recognition, recognition by management, and financial rewards.

Peer recognition takes many forms, including positive individual comments, peers seeking advice and counsel about safety matters, and suggestions to supervisors by peers regarding the work on safety issues being done by the individual.

Recognition by management can be as simple as the director or manager pulling the employee aside to tell him how much his involvement in the safety task group or contribution to making the workplace safer is appreciated. Formal certificates, plaques, and community-wide recognition are additional possibilities.

Positive financial rewards may be most effectively used to reinforce peer pressure to develop a safe workplace. Occasionally, financial rewards have been used as a gainsharing tool with supervisory staff to share a loss-control cost avoidance pool of dollars. While financial incentives may provide short-term reinforcement, they should be mixed with other forms of recognition for maximum effectiveness.

Recognition and rewards must be multi-focused and must occur at multiple levels within the organization if each level is to support the others' change of behavior.

Conclusion

Changing one's lifestyle to reduce the risk of heart disease is a life-long process that starts with making a commitment to get started. Likewise, effective safety and loss-control programs for EMS organizations are neither simple nor easy to implement. But with commitment and hard work, these programs can be accomplished.

Source

Original article. Jay Fitch, PhD, is the president of Fitch & Associates, Inc. Roy L. Manns is an EMS safety consultant in Glendale, Ariz., specializing in training programs. He has over 20 years of experience in prehospital care.

Improving safety and loss control requires the commitment of both leadership and labor. The organization must have clear benchmarks of current and desired performance. A sound plan and method for both delivering and monitoring the program have to be developed. These efforts must be coupled with rewards for positive behavior.

A final note—safety and loss-control programs are not expense items. Instead, EMS administrators should consider them cost avoidance mechanisms. More than that, however, effective safety and loss-control programs offer the opportunity to save individuals both inside and outside the EMS organization from unnecessary pain and suffering. Achieving that goal supports the fundamental premise for most EMS organizations' existence.

Making the Future Safe

Bill Leonard

Risk management and loss-control programs are cost-effective mechanisms for improving patient care. In this article, noted EMS safety expert Bill Leonard points out key steps for stacking the odds in the system's favor.

FOR THE PAST 25 YEARS, EMS managers have focused on improving training and equipment for high-performance EMS. In retrospect, however, we have probably neglected the most important element—safety.

On average over the past 10 years, 26 fatal EMS vehicle accidents have occurred annually in the United States. This is based on a recent review of statistics prepared by the National Highway Traffic Safety Administration and its Fatal Accident Reporting System. In those 26 fatal accidents, 10 EMT/paramedics and 31 civilians have died annually.

Obviously, agency managers have their work cut out for them. To best meet the needs of their respective agencies, managers need to know what form EMS will take in the next 10 years. By identifying industry trends, EMS managers will be better equipped to lead their agencies safely into the next century. What follows are trends and predictions the savvy manager may find helpful in this task.

Insurance

A review by the AZStar Center for Safety & Risk Management in Phoenix found that EMS vehicles are involved in some type of motor vehicle incident every 85,000 traveled miles. This is equivalent to 15,000 accidents per year, 41 accidents per day, or one EMS vehicle accident every 1.7 hours. As the number of fatal accidents increases, auto liability and general liability rates will rise accordingly.

To help keep insurance costs down, EMS managers should consider the following:

- Re-evaluate management's attitude toward loss control and safety. A 100-percent commitment to a safety program is essential in the overall protection of employees.
- Commit money to the safety program. An effective safety and loss-control program can dramatically increase an agency's bottom-line profitability and reduce the expense of providing service. A successful safety program, however, needs adequate funding to succeed.
- Authorize safety managers to solve problems and take corrective action without forcing them to wade through many levels of management. Safety managers will learn how the agency's insurance policy is structured and what they can do to lower costs. By being keenly aware of loss ratios and severity and frequency of claims, safety managers will be better able to make improvements.

Rewriting Procedures

In the coming years, the Occupational Safety and Health Administration will more actively enforce its guidelines, rules, and regulations pertaining to EMS. As a result of OSHA's involvement in EMS, agencies will need to modify their policies and procedures.

Procedures should be rewritten with a detailed description of the sequence of activities necessary for the achievement of a particular goal, that is, who does what and when. The new policies and procedures will serve as a training tool for new employees and can be used as a defense in the event legal action is taken against a service.

Quality Assurance

EMS systems will re-evaluate their patient quality assurance programs to encompass total system QA, not just patient care alone. Total system QA includes how agencies recruit, hire, and fire employees. Companies will concentrate on improving orientation, continuing education, and total service, not just patient care. Upgrading dispatching systems and procedures, practicing preventive maintenance of vehicles and biomedical equipment, and documenting these actions will be concerns as well.

Pre-Employment Testing

Agencies will need to rethink their hiring policies and begin using pre-employment profile testing. Pre-employment testing will be able to identify drivers who are safety conscious; determine applicant attitudes toward safety and working in a safe environment, toward company policies and procedures, and toward state driving laws; recognize the ability to accept constructive criticism from management; and determine if applicants are likely to be long-term employees.

Medical examinations for EMS drivers will more closely resemble those given to airline pilots. Baseline strength testing for prevention of back injuries and other soft tissue and skeletal injuries may be implemented. In addition, more in-depth eye examinations will be administered to document depth perception, peripheral vision, and color blindness problems. Standardized pre-employment skill testing will evaluate an applicant's ability to use patient-handling equipment in addition to determining the applicant's patient skills.

Technology

During the '90s, more emphasis has been placed on crew safety in the patient compartment such as the development of a safety restraint system to protect the EMT while rendering patient care. This type of restraint system allows responders to move about the vehicle and still remain protected in an accident.

In the driver's compartment, a heads-up display system will increase driver safety. Drivers will be able to see the functions of the vehicle, give voice commands to the vehicle, and speak on the communications system without having to move knobs or push buttons.

Probably by the late '90s, ambulances in the United States will be equipped with radar-directed collision avoidance systems. The system will be able to bring the vehicle to a stop anytime it gets in a hazardous situation by observing approaching obstacles or unavoidable collisions before the vehicle reaches the hazard area. This technology alone will have a dramatic impact on the industry. It is presently being tested by the National Trucking Association.

Along with the new technology and redesign of the ambulance chassis, a whole new training program will be developed for the modern EMS vehicle operator/driver. Low-force driving will be a key training goal.

Driver Training

In 1986, more than 60 percent of all ambulance accidents throughout the United States occurred in intersections. With risk management and the training of safety managers and operator/driver instructors, intersection accidents were reduced to 50 percent in 1988, 36 percent in 1989, and only 27 percent in 1990. Training has been a key factor in bringing about these changes.

With proper education, EMTs have learned it is mandatory to stop at an intersection before proceeding through it. The most effective procedure mandates the insured come to a complete stop at all controlled intersections and make eye contact with all drivers before entering the intersection on an emergency run.

Another effective policy follows that if there are any vacant lanes, such as left turn lanes, a secondary stop must be made before crossing that lane. One other factor that has been important in the reduction of intersection accidents is the correct use of the siren and educating responders how the "yelp" mode is to be used for their protection and safety.

In this decade we will finally stop high-speed training of EMS drivers in the pursuit-type driving techniques that are used in police work. This type of training is uncalled for in high-performance EMS. The safe delivery of the system to the patient by well-trained caregivers and the safe transport of that patient to definitive medical care are what EMS needs to accomplish to create a safe work environment.

Low-force driving emphasizes the driver and driving awareness, systematic eye movement, constant rate acceleration, use of compression in stopping, smooth braking, the four-second following rule, knowledge of the rear-tire stopping distances, 10-second lane changing rule, rear- and side-space cushions, backing with ground guides, and safely loading and unloading the patient.

All this will be necessary since the gross vehicle weight ratings of

Source

Reprinted with permission from Emergency, *December 1991. At the time of original publication, Bill Leonard was the executive vice president of the AZStar Center for Safety & Risk Management in Phoenix.*

modern EMS vehicles are increasing rather than decreasing. We now have vehicles available to EMS systems that are approaching 23,000 GVRW. EMTs will need to master new driving techniques to compensate for the changes in vehicle weight. This new training will use on-board computers to monitor the driver and the operation of the vehicle and its mechanical systems.

From the Top Down

Safety, loss control, risk management, claims reduction, and reducing unnecessary injury to the workforce start at the top. The modern manager in a high-performance EMS system will endorse the safety and loss-control program and communicate his involvement to the staff. When the manager does not give total commitment and hold the safety manager accountable for the program, the system will falter and, in all probability, will not succeed.

EMS in the '90s will realize loss control and safety must be an attitude within the system and should be as important to management as patient care and bottom-line profit.

Pre-Employment Back Injury Screening: The Employer's Crystal Ball

Casey Terribilini, DC, and Kate Dernocoeur, EMT-P

Failing to evaluate and test prospective employees for previous injuries can be costly for everyone. Specific criteria must be followed for testing to be meaningful. The changing legal criteria must also be closely followed.

THE SELECTING AND HIRING of emergency care personnel is in an exciting stage of EMS evolution. Rather than using the "p-squared" approach (Got a patch? Got a pulse? You're hired!), many employers are turning toward a more objective, predictive, and fair process: pre-employment screening. Using a properly designed screening process can save savvy EMS managers considerable time, effort, and money. While pre-employment screening allows employers to determine whether a worker is medically fit for employment, preplacement screening allows for appropriate job assignments once someone has been hired.

Screening is best described as the use of various tools to determine whether job applicants are at risk of incurring occupational injuries and illnesses. Such tools may include a medical history interview, low-back X-ray, laboratory tests, strength and flexibility tests, and a variety of other procedures. These processes can help eliminate much—or most—of the crystal ball guesswork regarding an applicant's suitability for a particular job. The result? For the employee, the result is minimization of the physical and financial hardships that injuries can cause. For the employer, the result is the reduction of the economic costs of absenteeism, turnover, disability claims, work compensation, and lost productivity.

The importance of EMS pre-employment back health screening is obvious: Field personnel face many physically grueling challenges, particularly lifting, and subsequent back injury can plague an individual for months or even years. Indeed, any health problem is disruptive to everyone on the team.

The concept of medical screening is not new. For more than 80 years, many industries have employed "factory surgeons" to determine whether applicants and employees are free of disease or other work-limiting ailments. In one of the earliest recorded programs (begun in 1909), Harry Mock, MD, conducted physical examinations at Sears, Roebuck and Co. to identify individuals with tuberculosis.

Although appropriate hiring efforts are an excellent idea, poorly designed screening programs can backfire; a major problem is the potential for discrimination. Certain clearly inappropriate medical procedures being used by some EMS systems lack due regard for the legal, ethical, moral, social, and economic consequences of their use, issues that affect the usability of nearly all pre-employment processes.

As a rule of thumb, when evaluating a program for use in preplacement testing, the EMS manager should examine five areas of concern: safety, reliability, job-relatedness, practicality, and predictiveness.

Each is outlined by the *National Institute of Occupational Safety and Health (NIOSH) Work Practices Guide.*

Safety of administration. The test for physical performance should be safe to administer; risk of injury to the person being tested should not outweigh the value of the data gained. Similarly, the test procedure should not set specific goals for the individual being tested; anything that might encourage the individual to perform beyond a personally safe and comfortable level should be avoided. For example, in some systems, the test given to newly hired personnel is to lift a heavily loaded stretcher and place it in the ambulance—without the benefit of training in proper lifting principles.

Reliability. There is great variation among tests in providing reliable, measurable, and reproducible results, but data that are unreliable in any way are unusable. For example, having someone do 10 pull-ups does not yield the same information as if you conducted a computerized, measured test of the same musculature on a CYBEX or similar machine.

Job-relatedness. If the task used to test the applicant is not job-related, the process cannot be considered valid. This aspect of screening is critical for maintaining compliance with the Equal Employment Opportunity Commission (EEOC) guidelines and preventing discriminatory action suits. For example, in 1978, one of the authors of this article simply had to weigh 150 pounds to "pass" the test for employment at one EMS agency. More appropriate in prehospital care is a test that is related to lifting heavy weights at various levels.

Practicality. The selection procedure's usefulness to the employer will partly be based on the practicality of its development and implementation. The employer needs to consider the following as up-front expenses: the cost of job analysis, protocol design, testing of those personnel already in a specific position (known as "incumbent testing"), and the necessary validation studies. In essence, testing procedures should be quick and simple to deliver, and training those who will administer the tests should not require excessive time or resources.

Predictiveness. Finally—and most importantly—the screening procedure should be able to accurately predict the risk of future illness, injury, and performance. This phase requires a careful comparison of test results to injury and performance data obtained from other tested populations, as set forth by the Department of Labor under the unified guidelines on employee-selection procedures as part of the Civil Rights Act of 1978.

In October 1986, the Occupational Safety and Health Administration requested public comments to help develop guidelines for preventing lifting injuries. The resulting guidelines recommended ergonomic redesign, strength testing of new and existing workers, training of employees so they could utilize proper lifting techniques, and physical conditioning or stretching programs. OSHA aimed to reduce the incidence of on-the-job injuries, particularly back injuries, which would also decrease morbidity and the high cost of medical treatment.

Back injury is very expensive, with costs divided into direct and indirect costs. Direct costs include the cost of medical care and compensation for lost wages, while indirect costs include personal suffering, loss of production, and employee turnover.

One of the most comprehensive estimates of back care cost was done in 1984: three surveys conducted by the National Center for Health Statistics demonstrated that nearly $16 billion was spent in direct medical costs alone during that year. In 1980, Liberty Mutual Insurance Co. reported that it spent almost $1 million *each working day* on compensable back pain. And at that time, Liberty Mutual represented only approximately nine percent of the insured workers' compensation market.

In an unpublished survey of a dozen companies conducted by one of the authors of this article, back injury was found to be the leading cause of early medical or physical retirement in the EMS industry. According to another study, the direct costs per case of back pain ranged from $3,500 to $5,800. Of particular interest in the latter study: Only 25 percent of the injuries were responsible for 93 percent of the costs. If that 25 percent of employees could be properly placed or screened out of high-risk environments, substantial amounts of money could be redirected toward better uses.

In terms of indirect costs, the sums attributable to back pain are enormous. According to the National Safety Council, workers' compensation costs for injury identification and medical care represent only a fraction of the total costs of occupational injuries. Some of the obvious indirect costs are

- Wages paid to other workers during the time the injured person's work is interrupted
- Wages paid to the injured worker between the time of the injury and when workers' compensation payments begin (usually known as the "waiting period")
- Wages paid to the injured worker's supervisor for time spent assisting the injured, investigating the incident, preparing reports, and training a replacement employee
- The cost of full wages to a replacement worker during the learning period, when job output is less
- Wages paid to clerks and others to prepare and process compensation application forms

There is no question that the cost of back pain within the EMS industry is very high. At an average of up to $6,000 per claim, even one injury per year can dramatically affect the bottom line of any organization's profits.

Developing a Screening Process

The development and implementation of a screening program need to be carefully approached to ensure that it is effective and meets legal standards. Four basic steps are critical to a good program: identification

---

Direct costs of back injury include the cost of medical care and compensation for lost wages, while indirect costs include personal suffering, loss of production, and employee turnover.

Four basic steps are critical to a good program: identification of high-risk jobs, a complete job analysis, test design (to know which testing "tools" to use), and validation of the process.

of high-risk jobs, a complete job analysis, test design (to know which testing "tools" to use), and validation of the process.

When examining existing screening programs, the most complete ones appear to require three elements: a comprehensive medical history, a thorough physical examination, and strength and flexibility testing. Once data are gathered, the results can be used in two ways. First, the results help determine whether an individual can safely perform in a particular job with its unique physical requirements. Second, the results can be used to design a precautionary exercise prescription for those approved for a particular job.

Medical History

The main purpose of taking a complete medical history is to identify high-risk individuals in terms of the potential for future injuries, particularly to the back. Because recurrent episodes of low-back pain appear to be part of the nature of back problems, a vital key is to determine whether there is a history of such problems.

A recent literature search performed in preparation for this article yielded more than 25 articles that clearly support the fact that a history of low-back pain increases the risk of future problems. One cross-sectional survey conducted in 1985 included 558 male and 583 female back pain patients. In the year following examination, there was a significantly increased occurrence of back pain in subjects with many previous episodes of low-back pain; many days of lost work due to low-back pain; short intervals between episodes of low-back pain; and an aggravated course of low-back pain, or reinjury, prior to complete recovery from an episode of back pain.

Not only is prior history relevant to the identification of high-risk individuals, but severity of low-back pain also has strong predictive value. In 1981, one study determined that a history of more than three previous episodes of low-back pain was ominous, as new episodes were found to be both longer and more severe. Beware, however, that cases of low-back pain that involve fractures, usually due to accidents such as falls, motor vehicle accidents, etc., may not reliably predict recurrences. Although it may seem paradoxical, fractures often allow injured workers to return to work sooner than do moderately severe sprains and strains of the back.

All of the studies researched for this article suggest that a complete and accurate medical history is a useful part of the pre-employment process. But additional research shows that simply obtaining a medical history is not enough to reduce back injury rates. A more comprehensive approach is clearly indicated, thus the need for physical examination and strength and flexibility testing.

Physical Examination

The purpose of physical screening is to detect signs of dysfunction that indicate an increased risk of future back pain. Five physical signs have significant predictive value, especially in patients with any history of low-back pain: a restriction of pain-free, straight leg raise, which indicates tight hip and thigh muscles; an inability to sit up from a supine position, indicating trunk flexor weakness; pain or weakness during the hip-flexion test; back pain during lumbar extension; and low-back pain with straight leg raise, indicating tight hamstring muscles. When more than one of these signs is present, there is an even greater risk of recurrence.

An assessment of general physical fitness should be part of a thorough physical exam. One fitness study of Los Angeles firefighters looked at flexibility, lifting strength, and cardiovascular status and found that the most fit experienced the least back pain. Similar findings were reported by David Imrie, MD, (co-developer of the "Back Power" program for the National Safety Council) in a 1983 study of Toronto paramedics.

Although there are no direct lab screening tests for low-back pain, lab tests can be a valuable tool in assessing an applicant's *general* health. Many employees, however, rely heavily on X-rays to assess the lumbar spine of applicants. Yet the value of low-back X-rays is debatable. In fact, many sources question the ability of such X-rays to predict the at-risk back.

In 1977, the American Occupational Medical Association, the American College of Radiology, and the American Academy of Orthopaedic Surgeons joined in a conference to evaluate the efficacy of low-back X-rays. They concluded that their use as a sole criterion for selecting workers was not justified and that workers should be protected from the unnecessary radiation exposure of such examinations. And a 1982 study that summarized 11 papers on 40,017 subjects who had received pre-employment low-back X-rays concluded that the screening techniques had a very low sensitivity and low specificity for predicting low-back pain.

While a single lumbosacral X-ray probably does not carry a significant health risk, repeated radiographs can result in considerable radiation exposure. It has been shown that low-back X-rays are the single largest contributor to gonadal irradiation in the United States, increasing the risk of radiation-caused diseases by as much as 25 percent. Therefore, low-back X-rays should always be considered a potential health risk, and any unnecessary use should be discouraged.

Strength and Flexibility Testing

The use of pre-employment strength and flexibility testing has met with considerable enthusiasm in the past decade. The obvious goal is to ensure that only people with sufficient strength to perform a job safely will be assigned to that job.

There are many different types of strength tests, but each must meet the criteria of safety, reliability, job-relatedness, practicality, and predictive fairness. The EEOC has set clear guidelines regarding the use of such testing procedures. To be considered legal and non-discriminatory, tests must clearly be job-related and must actually measure the predictiveness of the applicant's ability to safely perform the necessary tasks associated with that job.

Caution must also be taken to carefully match the capabilities of the person being tested with the job requirements. This is usually best accomplished through careful job analysis, which is a detailed discovery process that lists exactly what a person does on the job, how often, in what environmental circumstances, etc. In EMS, for example, a job analysis would include statements about lifting a certain number of pounds a certain number of times per day and traveling some distance with that load in all types of weather over variable and often uneven surfaces.

Strength testing is usually divided into two broad categories: functional strength and muscular strength. Functional strength describes the applicant's ability to exert lifting, pushing, and pulling forces in any position he chooses. In other words, applicants can use their bodies in whatever way they wish to accomplish the requested exertion. A typical EMS functional strength test is the physical agility test so commonly used by fire and police agencies. Conversely, muscular strength testing typically uses machines that require the applicant to use force in a dynamic, or isokinetic, manner; these machines are usually available only through clinics or doctors' offices.

Clearly, the physical agility test—which is one of several forms of functional testing—is the most job-related strength test for EMS, as positions encountered during patient handling can be closely simulated. Additionally, the test administrator can see how applicants use their bodies for each activity.

Functional testing does have several disadvantages, however. One primary issue is safety. For example, many patients are victims of poorly designed—even dangerous—physical agility tests. Also, because applicants can use their bodies in any way they choose to perform the task, it is extremely difficult to isolate areas of muscle weakness. This hampers development of a rehabilitation program for each individual. Furthermore, the extreme subjectivity of the results makes this type of testing a target for allegations of discrimination.

There are several machines that test functional strength. Such machines are typically isometric testers; the applicant exerts force in a given posture against fixed resistance. The results are then compared to the job requirements, which have been established through careful job analysis. A commonly used isometric tester is the floor-mounted dynamometer—much like an upside-down produce scale—against which the applicant pulls with as much strength as possible. Isometric tests are considered safe, reproducible, and simple to administer. They are also recognized by the *NIOSH Work Practices Guide for Manual Lifting.*

However, isometric testing has recently been criticized for several reasons. First, isometric tests study body motion in only one geometric plane, whereas actual human motion normally cuts across three planes. Second, they test only one position devoid of joint movement, not allowing for the changes that take place in posture, joint loading, and muscular length tension ratios that make up 82 percent to 84 percent of body movement. Thus, while isometric testing may be an excellent starting point for research and comparison of other test protocols, it is not thoroughly predictive, job-related, or reliable.

Muscular strength testing—also called dynamic or isokinetic testing— allows the measurement of forces exerted on the body throughout all ranges of motion. Such testing involves being strapped to a computerized machine that precisely measures muscular strength in a range of motion.

Isokinetic testing of trunk muscles began in the 1970s and has led to the development of reproducible normal values for various muscle groups. Unlike isometric testing, isokinetic testing uses strength-to-body weight, rate of muscle contraction, and flexion/extension ratios. Extensive sample bases have been developed, and it appears that these scores remain constant across a broad population of normal subjects.

More importantly for this discussion, people with low-back dysfunction deviate from these normal values in a predictable and reproducible manner. Research has indicated that abnormal trunk flexor/extensor ratios exist in some otherwise asymptomatic people, indicating that potential back problems may be noted before the onset of symptoms. The usefulness of these tests as predictors of future injuries is therefore encouraging.

Isokinetic testing is now demonstrating predictable patterns among back-injured individuals. Furthermore, baseline information obtained during pre-employment assessments using isokinetic testing are proving useful in quantifying the amount of post-injury limitation. This helps guide the rehabilitation process prior to releasing the patient back to preinjury duty status. Another benefit of isokinetic testing is the possibility of weeding out those pretending to be injured from those with actual injuries, as those who attempt to limit their efforts are easy to identify and can thus be eliminated from the compensation pool.

The largest obstacle encountered with dynamic muscle testing is the cost of equipment. For many companies, the answer is to contract with clinics, hospitals, and sophisticated testing centers that use such equipment.

Flexibility is typically evaluated as part of the physical examination process. Areas usually tested are the legs, trunk, and shoulder girdle. This can be too subjective for employment decisions, but it is beneficial for employee education and encouragement toward self-motivated improvement in physical condition.

Conclusion

It is important to note that implementation of a well-designed back screening program does not exonerate the employer from the responsibility of providing a safe, well-designed workplace or from making reasonable accommodations and prudent placement decisions for high-risk applicants. Also, preplacement selection procedures should not be considered a means for disqualifying high-risk applicants. Rather, they are a

Source

Reprinted with permission from JEMS, *October 1991. Casey Terribilini is a doctor of chiropractic with 12 years of experience as a paramedic. Kate Dernocoeur is a writer and paramedic and a frequent contributor to* JEMS. *She is the author of* Streetsense *and co-author of* Principles of Emergency Medical Dispatch.

tool for making responsible and appropriate job assessments and assignments. The task of testing and developing the protocols for proper screening lies with responsible companies that are willing to make the effort. Such companies understand the importance of working with the medical community to abandon archaic employee testing formats.

Selecting and hiring of EMS personnel is at an important stage of evolution. Control measures can be costly, but they are usually less costly than continuing to pay for low-back pain. An investment in the workplace to prevent back pain is a wise business decision. And, more importantly, given the wide variety of hazards that face the EMS provider, pre-employment screening can protect susceptible workers from unnecessary injury.

References

Andersson, G. B. J., and T. R. Jehmann. "Worker Selection." Paper presented at the Occupational Low Back Pain Conference, Hilton Head, S.C., October 1988.

Bierring-Sorensen, F. "Physical Measurements as Risk Indicators for Low-Back Trouble Over a One-Year Period." *Spine* 9 (1984): 106-119.

Cady, L., et al. "Strength and Fitness and Subsequent Back Injuries in Firefighters." *Journal of Occupational Medicine* 21 (1979): 269-272.

Gould, J. A., and G. J. Davies. *Orthopaedic and Sports Physical Therapy.* St. Louis: The C.V. Mosby Co., 1985.

Holbrook, T. L., et al. *The Frequency of Occurrence, Impact and Cost of Selected Musculoskeletal Conditions in the United States.* Park Ridge, Ill.: American Academy of Orthopaedic Surgeons, 1984.

Joseph, R. "Use and Effectiveness of Low Back Radiographs in Screening in Occupational Medicine." *Journal of Occupational Medicine* 773 (1983).

Lloyd, D. C. R. F., and J. D. G. Troup. "Recurrent Back Pain and its Prediction." *J Soc Occup Med.* 33 (1983): 66-74.

Mayer, T. G., et al. "Measurement of Isometric and Multispeed Isokinetic Strength of Lumbar Spine Musculature Using a Prototype CYBEX Testing Device in Normal Subjects and Patients." Presented at the International Society for the Study of the Lumbar Spine, Montreal, 1984.

McIntyre, D. R., and J. A. Sawhill. Unpublished data, May 1984.

National Research Council Advisory Committee on Biological Effects of Ionizing Radiation. "The Effects on Populations of Exposure to Low Levels of Ionizing Radiation." *Proc Natl Acad Sci USA.* 55 (1972)

Pederson, P. A. "Prognostic Indicators in Low Back Pain." *Journal of the Royal College of General Practitioners* 31 (1981): 209-216.

Pope, M. H., et al. *Occupational Low Back Pain.* New York: Praeger Publishing, 1984.

Snook, S. H. "The Costs of Back Pain in Industry." *Spine: State of the Art Reviews* 2 (1987): 1-5.

Snook, S. H., R. A. Campanelli, and J. W. Hart. "A Study of Three Preventive Approaches to Low Back Pain." *Journal of Occupational Medicine* 20 (1978): 478-481.

U.S. Department of Health and Human Services. *NIOSH Work Practices Guide for Manual Lifting.* Cincinnati: U.S. Department of Health and Human Services, 1981.

THE DEPARTMENT OF LABOR has published an amendment to the Occupational Safety and Health Act (OSHA), which describes requirements for employers of employees who have occupational exposure to bloodborne pathogens.

Enforcement of this rule rests with federal OSHA officers or, in states that have state plans, with state OSHA officers. Federal OSHA applies to most employers except municipal employers. In states with state plans, the rule applies to municipal employees as well. This article should be used as a guide to assist in complying with the rule, but employers must review and be familiar with the standard for requirements that apply to their own settings.

Background

OSHA issued the bloodborne standard to provide protection to 5.6 million workers and to prevent 200 deaths and 9,200 bloodborne infections annually.

While the risk for occupational transmission of HIV is rare, the lethal nature of the infection requires that every precaution be taken to prevent exposure. Infection with hepatitis B or C from occupational exposure occurs more readily than infection with HIV.

Employers are required to develop exposure control plans that will eliminate or minimize occupational exposure to bloodborne pathogens.

Exposure Control Plan

The bloodborne pathogen rule requires employers to establish a written exposure control plan designed to eliminate or minimize employee exposure.

The plan must contain at least the following:

- Exposure determination, which shall contain
  - A list of all job classifications in which all employees in those job classifications have occupational exposure
  - A list of job classifications in which some employees have occupational exposure
  - A list of tasks and procedures performed by employees in the second classification above in which occupational exposure occurs
- The schedule and method of implementation for
  - Methods of compliance

The Bloodborne Pathogen Standard: A Summary

Lynn Zimmerman, Deb Jurewicz, and Mary Neuman

The amendment to the Occupational Safety and Health Act, which describes employers' requirements for exposure to bloodborne pathogens, changed the way all services do business. In this excerpt from their book, the authors review the standard, describe ways to set up an exposure control plan, and outline procedures to follow on a daily basis.

Definitions

For purposes of this article, the following definitions apply.

Assistant Secretary—the Assistant Secretary of Labor for Occupational Safety and Health, or designated representative.

Blood—human blood, human blood components, and products made from human blood.

Bloodborne pathogens—pathogenic microorganisms that are present in human blood and can cause disease in humans. These pathogens include, but are not limited to, hepatitis B virus (HBV) and human immunodeficiency virus (HIV).

Clinical laboratory—a workplace where diagnostic or other screening procedures are performed on blood and other potentially infectious materials.

Contaminated—the presence or the reasonably anticipated presence of blood or other potentially infectious materials on an item or surface.

Contaminated laundry—laundry that has been soiled with blood or other potentially infectious materials or laundry that may contain sharps.

Contaminated sharps—any contaminated object that can penetrate the skin including, but not limited to, needles, scalpels, broken glass, broken capillary tubes, and exposed ends of dental wires.

Decontamination—the use of physical or chemical means to remove, inactivate, or destroy bloodborne pathogens on a surface or item to the point where they are no longer capable of transmitting infectious particles and the surface or item is rendered safe for handling, use, or disposal.

Director—the Director of the National Institute for Occupational Safety and Health, U.S. Department of Health and Human Services, or designated representative.

Engineering controls—controls (e.g., sharps disposal containers, self-sheathing needles) that isolate or remove the bloodborne pathogens hazard from the workplace.

- Hepatitis B vaccination and post-exposure evaluation and follow-up
- Communications of hazards to employees
- Record-keeping of the standard
- Procedure for evaluation of circumstances surrounding exposure incidents

A copy of the plan must be accessible to employees. The plan must be reviewed and updated at least annually and whenever necessary to reflect new or changed tasks or procedures or new employee positions with occupational exposure.

Methods of Compliance

Universal Precautions

Universal precautions must be observed to prevent contact with blood or other potentially infectious materials (OPIM). When differentiation of body fluids is difficult, such as in emergency situations or uncontrolled environments, all body fluids should be considered infectious.

Engineering and Work Practice Controls

Engineering and work practice controls must be instituted that eliminate or reduce employee exposure. If occupational exposure still exists after instituting these controls, personal protective equipment should be used.

Examples of engineering and work practice controls that should be implemented in the prehospital environment include the following:

- Handwashing facilities must be readily accessible to employees, i.e., in station or garage area, separate from areas where food is prepared, stored, or consumed.
- When handwashing facilities are not feasible, antiseptic towelettes or antiseptic hand cleansers with towels may be substituted.
- The handwashing policy should ensure that employees wash their hands, and any other skin, with soap and water immediately after contact with blood/body fluids and immediately after removal of personal protective equipment (PPE).
- Contaminated needles and other sharps cannot be bent, recapped, or removed unless no other alternative is available and it is medically required. Any recapping or removal of a needle

must be done mechanically or using only one hand. Breaking or shearing of needles is prohibited.

- Reusable sharps must be placed in a puncture-resistant container until processed.
- All sharps containers (disposable and reusable) must
  - Be puncture-resistant
  - Be labeled or color-coded
  - Be leakproof on sides and bottom
  - Prevent or forbid removal by hand
- Eating, drinking, smoking, applying cosmetics or lib balm, and handling contact lenses are prohibited in work areas where there is a reasonable likelihood of occupational exposure. This includes the patient compartment of the ambulance. The cab of the ambulance can be maintained as a clean area provided that
  - The separating partition between the cab and patient compartment is closed at any time occupational exposure may occur
  - All personal protective equipment or contaminated clothing/items are removed prior to entering the cab
  - Hands are washed prior to entering the cab
- Food and drink shall not be stored in refrigerators, freezers, shelves, cabinets, or on countertops or bench tops where blood or OPIM are present.
- Procedures involving blood or OPIM shall be performed in a manner that minimizes spraying, splashing, aerosolizing, or spattering.
- Mouth suctioning/pipetting is forbidden.
- Containers for blood or OPIM must be leakproof, labeled or color-coded, placed in a second container if the outside becomes contaminated, and puncture-resistant if applicable.
- Equipment must be decontaminated prior to shipping or servicing. If unable to be decontaminated, it must be appropriately labeled as a biohazard, and this information must be conveyed to the receiving person or company to ensure appropriate precautions are taken.

Personal Protective Equipment

The employer is responsible for providing personal protective equipment to all employees where there is occupa-

Exposure incident—a specific eye, mouth, other mucous membrane, non-intact skin, or parenteral contact with blood or other potentially infectious materials that results from the performance of an employee's duties.

Handwashing facilities—a facility providing an adequate supply of running potable water, soap, and single-use towels or hot air drying machines.

Licensed healthcare professional—a person whose legally permitted scope of practice allows him to independently perform the activities required for hepatitis B vaccination and post-exposure evaluation and follow-up.

HBV—hepatitis B virus.

HIV—human immunodeficiency virus.

Occupational exposure—reasonably anticipated skin, eye, mucous membrane, or parenteral contact with blood or other potentially infectious materials that may result from the performance of an employee's duties.

Other potentially infectious materials (OPIM)—

- The following human body fluids: semen, synovial fluid, pleural fluid, pericardial fluid, peritoneal fluid, amniotic fluid, saliva in dental procedures, any body fluid that is visibly contaminated with blood, and all body fluids in situations where it is difficult or impossible to differentiate between body fluids
- Any unfixed tissue or organ (other than intact skin) from a human (living or dead)
- HIV-containing cell or tissue cultures, organ cultures, HIV- or HBV-containing culture medium or other solutions, and blood, organs, or other tissues from experimental animals infected with HIV or HBV

Parenteral—piercing mucous membranes or the skin barrier through such events as needle sticks, human bites, cuts, and abrasions.

Personal protective equipment (PPE)—specialized clothing or equipment worn by an employee for protection against a hazard. General work clothes (e.g., uniforms, pants, shirts, or blouses) not intended to function as protection against a hazard are not considered to be personal protective equipment.

Production facility—a facility engaged in industrial-scale, large-volume, or high-concentration production of HIV or HBV.

Regulated waste—liquid or semi-liquid blood or other potentially infectious materials; contaminated items that would release blood or other potentially infectious materials in a liquid or semi-liquid state if compressed; items that are caked with dried blood or other potentially infectious materials and are capable of releasing these materials during handling; contaminated sharps; and pathological and microbiological wastes containing blood or other potentially infectious materials.

Research laboratory—a laboratory producing or using research-laboratory-scale amounts of HIV or HBV. Research laboratories may produce high concentrations of HIV or HBV but not in the volume found in production facilities.

Source individual—any individual, living or dead, whose blood or other potentially infectious materials may be a source of occupational exposure to employees. Examples include, but are not limited to, hospital and clinic patients; clients in institutions for the developmentally disabled; trauma victims; clients of drugs and alcohol treatment facilities; residents of hospices and nursing homes; human remains; and individuals who donate or sell blood or blood components.

Sterilize—the use of a physical or chemical procedure to destroy all microbial life including highly resistant bacterial endospores.

Universal precautions—an approach to infection control. According to the concept of universal precautions, all human blood and certain human body fluids are treated as if known to be infectious for HIV, HBV, and other bloodborne pathogens.

Work practice controls—controls that reduce the likelihood of exposure by altering the manner in which a task is performed (e.g., prohibiting recapping of needles by a two-handed technique).

tional exposure. This equipment should include but is not limited to

- Gloves, disposable, single-use
- Gloves, utility, to prevent injuries during extrication or when working in other hazardous environments where broken glass or sharps may be present
- Gowns or other protective outerwear
- Face shields or masks and eye protection
- Mouthpieces, resuscitation bags, pocket masks, or other ventilation device
- Surgical caps or hoods and/or shoe covers or boots when gross contamination can reasonably be anticipated

It is the employer's responsibility to ensure personal protective equipment is

- Provided at no cost to employees
- Appropriate (prevents blood or OPIM from reaching employees' clothing, skin, or mucous membrane)
- Used appropriately by employees
- Readily accessible in appropriate sizes; when necessary, alternative products are made available to meet needs of employees with allergies to selected gloves
- Cleaned, laundered, and/or disposed of at no cost to employees
- Repaired and replaced at no cost to employees
- Removed immediately or as soon as possible if penetrated by blood or OPIM
- Removed prior to leaving the work area

Housekeeping

Cleaning

Employers must ensure that the work site is maintained in a clean and sanitary condition. A written schedule for cleaning and the methods of decontamination must be developed based on

- Location within facility
- Type of surface to be cleaned
- Type of soil present
- Tasks or procedure being performed

The schedule shall include

- Cleaning and decontamination after contact with blood or OPIM spills

- Cleaning after completion of procedures
- Cleaning immediately or as soon as feasible after blood or OPIM spills
- Cleaning at end of work shift if surface may be contaminated
- Cleaning of bins, cans, and pails that may become contaminated with blood and OPIM
- Hands-free picking up of broken glassware

Regulated Waste

Contaminated sharps must be discarded immediately or as soon as feasible and placed in containers that are

- Closeable
- Puncture-resistant
- Leakproof
- Labeled or color-coded
- Easily accessible and located as close as possible to the area where sharps are used
- Maintained upright throughout use
- Replaced routinely and not permitted to become overfull
- Closed prior to moving to prevent spillage
- Placed in a secondary container if leakage is possible
- Not opened, emptied, or cleaned manually, if reusable

Other regulated waste should be placed in containers that are

- Closeable
- Constructed to contain all contents and prevent leakage
- Labeled or color-coded
- Closed prior to moving
- Placed in a secondary container if outside becomes contaminated

Disposal of all regulated waste must be in accordance with applicable federal, state, or local regulations.

Laundry

Contaminated linens must be

- Handled as little as possible
- Bagged at site of use and not sorted or rinsed at location of use
- Placed and transported in bags or containers that are labeled or color-coded
- Placed in a leakproof container if soak-through is possible
- Handled by trained employees wearing appropriate PPE
- Placed in biohazard-labeled containers if shipping off site to a laundry that does not utilize universal precautions

Hepatitis B Vaccination and Post-Exposure Evaluation and Follow-Up

Employers must make available to all employees who have occupational exposure a hepatitis B vaccine, a post-exposure evaluation, and follow-up for exposure incidents. The vaccine, evaluation, and follow-up must be

- At no cost to employees
- Made available at a reasonable time and place
- Performed by or under the direction of a physician or other licensed healthcare professional
- Provided in accordance with current U.S. Public Health Service recommendations

In addition,

- Lab tests must be conducted by an accredited lab and at no cost to employees
- A healthcare professional's written opinion of evaluation must be made available to the employee within 15 days of evaluation

Hepatitis B vaccination must be given to all employees with occupational exposure

- After receiving required training and within 10 days of initial assignment to the job
- Unless previously vaccinated
- Unless antibody positive by lab test
- Unless contraindicated for medical reasons
- Unless an employee refuses and a declination statement is signed

---

Figure 2.8

Hepatitis B Vaccine Declination (Mandatory)

I understand that, due to my occupational exposure to blood or other potentially infectious materials, I may be at risk of acquiring hepatitis B virus (HBV) infection. I have been given the opportunity to be vaccinated with hepatitis B vaccine at no charge to myself. However, I decline hepatitis B vaccination at this time. I understand that by declining this vaccine, I continue to be at risk of acquiring hepatitis B, a serious disease. If, in the future, I continue to have occupational exposure to blood or other potentially infectious materials and I want to be vaccinated with hepatitis B vaccine, I can receive the vaccination service at no charge to me.

_____   _____

Employee Signature   Date

_____   _____

Witness   Date

Booster shots are given if recommended by the U.S. Public Health Service.

Post-Exposure Evaluations and Follow-Up

When an exposure incident occurs, the employer will make immediately available confidential medical evaluation and follow-up including at least the following steps:

- Documentation of route and circumstances surrounding the exposure
- Identification and testing of the source individual as permitted by law and provision of the results of testing to the employee; the employee will be informed of disclosure laws and regulations regarding the identity and infectious status of the source individual
- Collecting and testing of employee's blood for HBV and HIV status; if the employee initially refuses testing but allows blood draw, blood will be held for up to 90 days to allow the employee to elect to have the test done
- Post-exposure prophylaxis when medically indicated following U.S. Public Health Service recommendations
- Counseling
- Evaluation of reported illnesses

The employer is required to provide the following information to the healthcare professional (person selected to provide post-exposure evaluation).

- Copy of the regulation
- Description of the exposed employee's job duties as related to the exposure incident
- Documentation of route and circumstances of exposure
- Results of source individual's blood tests, if known
- All relevant medical records of the employee

The employer is responsible for obtaining and providing the employee with a copy of the evaluating healthcare professional's written opinion within 15 days of evaluation.

Communication of Hazards to Employees

Labels and Signs

Employers are required to provide warning labels on regulated waste containers and other containers of blood or OPIM. Labels should be fluorescent orange or orange-red and include a biohazard symbol and legend. Red bags or red containers may be substituted for labels.

Training

Employers must ensure that all employees with occupational exposure have participated in a training program that is

- At no cost to employees
- During working hours
- Provided at the time of initial assignment to tasks where exposure may occur
- Offered at least annually thereafter and whenever new tasks are introduced or changes in plan occur
- Provided by a person who is knowledgeable about the subject matter as it relates to the particular workplace
- Appropriate in vocabulary and content to the educational level, literacy level, and language of employees

The training program should minimally contain

- Accessible copy of the standard
- Explanation of the standard's contents
- Explanation of epidemiology and symptoms of bloodborne disease
- Explanation of modes of transmission of bloodborne pathogens
- Explanation of the exposure control plan and how to obtain a copy
- Explanation of how to recognize tasks that may cause an exposure incident
- Explanation, use, and limitations of engineering controls, work practice controls, and personal protective equipment to prevent exposures
- Information on type, proper use, location, removal, handling, decontamination, and disposal of PPE
- Explanation of the basis for selection of PPE
- Information on the hepatitis B vaccine
- Information on the actions to take and the person to notify in case of an exposure incident
- Information on post-exposure evaluation and follow-up
- Explanation of labels and signs
- Opportunity for interactive questions and answers with person conducting training

Record-Keeping

Medical Records

The employer is required to establish and maintain accurate, confidential medical records for each employee with occupational exposure, which include

- Name and social security number
- The employee's hepatitis B vaccine status including dates received and records relative to the employee's ability to receive the vaccine
- Signed declination, if applicable

- Copies of all results of exams, medical testing, and follow-up as required
- The employer's copy of the healthcare professional's written opinion after evaluating the exposure incident
- A copy of the information given to the healthcare professional at the time of the exposure incident

These records must be kept for the duration of employment plus 30 years.

Training Records

Employers are required to maintain training records that include

- Dates of training sessions
- Contents or summary of training sessions
- Names and qualifications of persons conducting the training
- Names and job titles of all persons attending

These records shall be maintained for three years.

In addition to developing and writing an exposure control plan, employers will want to conduct monitoring and surveillance to ensure the plan is working and employees are knowledgeable in its content and application. Records documenting monitoring of the plan should be maintained.

When monitoring identifies areas where the plan is not working or there is non-compliance, an action plan to correct the deficiency should be undertaken.

The exposure control plan described in this article may be a part of a company's larger infection control plan or health and safety program. However, it must be easily identifiable within the larger plan and must be able to stand on its own as a separate document in the event an employee requests a copy for review.

Source

Excerpted from the book Infection Control for Prehospital Care Providers, *2nd ed. Reprinted with permission from Mercy Ambulance, Grand Rapids, Mich. Copyright © 1993.*

Operational Training Issues

Keeping the Spark Alive: Five Strategies for Motivating the Adult Learner

Richard A. Cherry, MEd, NREMT-P

Adults learn differently than youths. Veteran EMS instructor Richard Cherry shares five strategies for improving the learning process and increasing the success potential for adult students.

SPORTS EXPERTS AGREE THAT TALENT among athletes is virtually equal at the professional level; what separates the players is that spark of passion and the coach's ability to coax it out. Just as each coach has his own motivational style, so should every EMS instructor. Although there is no quantitative evidence linking motivation and adult learning, it is generally assumed that when there is no motivation to learn, there will be no learning.

Motivating a student can make the learning process exciting and enjoyable for the student *and* the instructor. Students who leave an educational experience with a good feeling about what they have learned are more likely to pursue that interest than the unmotivated student is. They are also more inclined to use what they have learned, and ideally, they become lifelong learners.

Research consistently shows that the most popular type of education among adults is vocational and practical. Being highly pragmatic learners, adults have a strong need to apply what they have learned and to be competent in that application. They strive to understand and master skills and tend to be more motivated when they are effectively learning something they value.

People are always motivated to do something. The aim of EMS instructors should be to get students motivated to learn what instructors want them to learn. Every instructor needs a motivational strategy that is incorporated into the course objectives and lesson plans. Failing to plan for motivation can result in a situation in which students do not learn. This article outlines five basic strategies for motivating students and for keeping them motivated.

Strategy 1—Help Students Develop a Positive Attitude

When motivating adults, it is important to help them develop positive attitudes toward the instructor, the subject matter, and the learning process itself. Since learning will be partly attributable to the instructor, it can be assumed that students will more readily accept instruction when they genuinely like and respect the teacher. Would you buy an appliance from a salesperson you dislike? Would you accept a gift from someone you don't respect?

When introducing yourself at the first session, briefly describe who you are and where you are from. Welcome the group to your program and let them know you appreciate the opportunity to teach them. This will begin to break down any barriers that may exist between student and instructor. It is important to get off to a "hot" start; this first impression will have a lasting impact. The beginning of any new learning experience is critical in terms of determining how the students will respond to your teaching strategies. Present yourself as strong, sincere, confident, enthusiastic, interesting, and non-threatening. Once formed, that first impression will strongly affect your students' attitudes and will be very difficult to change later on.

Adult learners come from a variety of educational backgrounds and experiences, some of which may have been unsuccessful. A critical motivational strategy at the start of any adult learning program is to set the tone for success. Indicate to the students that it is your intention to help them improve their competency through this new training experience. Vince Lombardi, former head coach of the Green Bay Packers, believed that the difference between a great coach and a mediocre coach was that the great coach foresaw what the end result should be and conveyed that vision to his players. Set clear standards of excellence by indicating how competence will be evaluated. When a clear picture of the criteria for success and failure is drawn, your students will become partners in the learning process, often charting their own educational course. Always explain the reasons for requirements and the relevancy of assignments. Tell them they will be held accountable for their own progress, and stick to that promise.

Throughout the course, you will convey your attitudes through non-verbal as well as verbal communication. Therefore, if you have a negative attitude, so will your students; they will follow your lead. Be certain that the attitudes you model are the attitudes you want your EMTs to have.

Some adults may be skeptical about the training program. Many of your students will have been out of the classroom for a number of years and may be apprehensive about their ability to learn new "tricks." Design the first class session so that all components, policies, and procedures are clearly outlined and understood by the students. Stress that everyone will learn, but it may take more time and greater effort for some.

Few adults realize how much effort an EMS learning experience will require. As long as they know what is expected of them, self-motivation is the key to their learning success. Let your students know you will be helping them increase their competence. Encourage them through

> When motivating adults, it is important to help them develop positive attitudes toward the instructor, the subject matter, and the learning process itself.

Maslow's Hierarchy of Human Needs

- Physiological
- Security
- Belonging
- Esteem
- Self-Fulfillment

the early stages of the course and minimize their mistakes. Show your confidence in their ability to learn from their mistakes. Make yourself available for remedial training and attribute success with effort. Showing students the results of their efforts is an extremely powerful self-motivational strategy.

Finally, make a contract with the students that describes what you expect from them and what they can expect from you. Your part of the contract should be a pledge to provide quality instruction, prompt feedback on their progress, and concrete evidence that their efforts will make a difference.

Experience as a foreign language instructor taught me the importance of proper student motivation. I would have the students first master a few basic expressions. Inevitably, they would leave the room feeling successful, confident that they could learn a new language, excited about the learning process, and motivated to learn more. Always leave them hungering for more.

Strategy 2—Understand and Satisfy Needs

In *Motivation and Personality*, Abraham Maslow outlined five basic human needs. Knowledge of each of these needs is essential to understanding what motivates your students to want to learn. Your students will progress to the next step only if the previous need is satisfied. It is your job to satisfy these needs.

Physiological Need

Physiological need is the need for food, water, fresh air, warmth, and rest. Climate control is a key, but often forgotten, element in the classroom. A freezing, sweltering, or suffocating student cannot concentrate, no matter how noble the cause. A full bladder also makes it difficult to think about much else. Strategically timed breaks, sufficient ventilation, and adequate bathroom facilities can enhance learning activities. The key is watching for restlessness on the students' part. The restless student is a nonproductive student. Avoid the tendency to cram more information into the last few minutes before a break. A good rule of thumb is 30 minutes of break time for every three hours of instruction.

Security

Security is feeling safe and free from fear and anxiety. Everyone needs to feel secure within his or her environment. In the classroom, this translates into program stability. Your students should feel secure within the structure of the program. By all means, vary the presentation of learning materials throughout the course, but don't change the basic framework of the program, such as starting times, assignments, tests, feedback, and homework. Also, knowing how they will be evaluated, what is expected of them, what constitutes success and failure, the criteria for dismissal, and any other structural components of the course will allow students to relax and concentrate on learning rather than worrying about what will happen next. Disciplinary action must be enforced consistently and fairly. An orderly and organized learning environment is the goal.

Finally, introduce the unfamiliar through the familiar, and always try to build on what your students already know; relate each new topic to one previously learned. Repetition is the essence of learning. The more you incorporate repetition and previously learned concepts into new learning, the more quickly students will assimilate the new knowledge and the longer it will be retained. This will also help alleviate anxiety about final exams and the students' ability to apply newly learned skills.

Belonging

The need to belong is a need for affection and appreciation. Every instructor should take advantage of students' desire to belong, to have an identity within a group, to feel respected, and to receive genuine affection from peers. Everyone wants to feel that they belong to something special. Isn't your program something special? If you don't think it is, maybe you should consider a career change. You must believe it first and then inject your students with that feeling. Kirk Gibson, Los Angeles Dodger and 1988 World Series hero, claimed that he felt like he had been a Dodger all his life. This was quite a statement, considering he had just completed his first year with the team. No one can dispute the motivational power of Dodger manager Tommy Lasorda, who inspired a super-team effort with a group of average baseball players.

Esteem

Esteem means the need for recognition. Adult learners want to raise their performance level. They enter into a training program to increase their ability to function within a career objective. They seek the self-esteem and self-respect that comes with competence, confidence, mastery, and achievement. Instructors should use this idea as a motivational strategy to nurture students toward competence. You cannot overlook the fact that adults also seek recognition from outside the group. The need for fame, appreciation, and prestige within the community is evidenced by the "patch and badge syndrome." Although carried to extremes at times, this is a strong motivational tool.

Self-Fulfillment

Self-fulfillment is the need to reach full potential. When all previous needs have been satisfied, the learner can strive for self-fulfillment and experience full potential. The motivating instructor will challenge students to extend their boundaries and strive for excellence.

Strategy 3—Be a Stimulating Instructor

The great leaders of modern history shared a single trait: All were outstanding, inspirational, and motivational public speakers. Although it seems that some people are born with this talent, the art of public speak-

rules

ing can be developed. The following are some suggestions that can help you improve as a motivational speaker.

- Know your subject well. Be an expert. Whatever it takes to prepare your lesson plan, do it. Your credibility is at stake, and that is something an instructor cannot afford to jeopardize.
- Believe in the importance of your subject. Your sincerity will show through right away. Remember, if you do not believe in your topic, why should your students? Here's a hint: It's all in the eyes.
- Be enthusiastic about your subject. Be excited about what you are teaching. Enthusiasm is contagious. What is your "enthusiasm quotient"? Check Table 2.6 to find out.
- Consider the learner's perspective. It is what the students learn—not what you teach—that counts. Tailor all presentations to the learner's level of understanding.
- Keep the students involved. Passive learning is the least

Table 2.6

Determining Your Enthusiasm Quotient

Category	Low	Medium	High
Voice	No variation, monotone, same volume	Some change in pitch and volume	Effective and frequent variations in pitch and volume
Pace	Constantly slow or fast, no variation, no pauses	Some change of pace, occasional pauses	Effective and appropriate variations in pace, good use of pauses
Clarity	Mumbling, inaudible, inarticulate, poor pronunciation	Reasonably clear and understandable, mostly audible	Fluent, clear, articulate, good pronunciation
Eyes	Dull, lifeless, boring, no eye contact with audience, motionless	Fairly lively, some eye contact, some expression	Alert, alive, sparkling, expressive, eye contact maintained with audience
Gestures	Rigid, does not move arms, hands hidden	Some arm/hand movement used to emphasize words	Open, sweeping movements, hands and fingers flexible
Body Movement	Seldom moves from spot, paces nervously	Moves freely, slowly, steadily, flexibly	Appropriate physical movement, energetic, natural, unpredictable
Overall Energy Level	Lethargic, sluggish, appears inactive	Appears energetic, demonstrative sometimes, mostly an even keel	Exuberant, high degree of energy and vitality, highly demonstrative

retained of all learning experiences. Try to incorporate active participation as often as possible. Discussions, question and answer sessions, and problem-solving activities all force students to actively engage in the learning process.

- Use street experience liberally. Instructors who have expertise, experience, and the ability to entertain an audience are indeed a rare breed. Relate theory to practical application as often as possible, but be careful not to overdo it.
- Provide variety. Keep the class interested by presenting learning materials in different ways. Appeal to as many senses as possible, and be inventive.
- Connect new learning with past experiences. Give students something to hang onto. Past learning is like a life raft: Once students learn to swim with the new information, they won't need help. In the beginning, however, your assistance is essential.
- State objectives clearly. Inform the class of your intentions, present the material, and then summarize what you imparted. Let them know where you're headed and, after you've arrived, remind them how you got there.
- Never apologize. Whenever you feel the urge to apologize for the subject matter, the length of the session, or your expertise in the topic, *don't*. Apologies are an admission of weakness that deflate both you and the students.

Strategy 4—Help Learners Attach a Value to What They Are Learning

Emotions are always present during adult learning and are an important influence on learner motivation. The emotional atmosphere in the classroom comes from a variety of sources. The student will be influenced by his own personal disposition, the group's general mood, the instructor, and the learning exercise. It is your job to maintain a pleasant atmosphere. A hostile, negative environment is not conducive to learning. Don't, however, confuse a pleasant atmosphere with that of a coffee club. A professional, serious, yet enjoyable learning environment is the goal.

Once your students have attached a value to learning, they are more apt to store the information into long-term memory. If it is useful, it will be learned. Try to deal with the human perspective in each topic. This is easy to do in EMS courses. After all, victims are real people, not just injury types. Your students should realize that their ultimate goal is to care for human life. If they assign a humanistic value to each injury and condition they study, it will have a dramatic effect on their learning.

Encourage a collaborative atmosphere among students. Field personnel should consider themselves part of a total team effort in EMS that begins in the classroom. Use team problem-solving exercises, rotating each

> A professional, serious, yet enjoyable learning environment is the goal.

Competence breeds confidence and self-motivation.

student as leader. Including personal emotions and value association in each lesson will enhance adult learner motivation.

Strategy 5—Build Competence and Confidence

Finally, make every attempt to build the learners' competence and show them how they are improving. Competence breeds confidence and self-motivation. Don't you feel good when you've done something well? Everyone does. Let the students see for themselves what a good job they are doing, and watch their self-motivation improve. Allow your students to progress through a series of successful events en route to the end result. Pride in accomplishment may be the ultimate motivational strategy.

Giving effective feedback is the key to maximizing positive growth and minimizing student and instructor frustration. Adults are very goal-oriented and are prepared to accept the responsibility for their own development. If they are left to navigate through fog, however, their destination will often deviate from the expected goal. It is your responsibility to outline the training program's goals and objectives and to provide students with timely, non-judgmental feedback on their progress. Not every instructor feels comfortable giving students feedback, especially if that feedback is negative, so here are some tips.

- Keep feedback informational, not personal. Focus on what they did, not who they are. Avoid personal remarks that may destroy personal integrity and self-esteem. If they know you genuinely like and respect who they are, they will accept your criticism more openly.
- Base feedback on performance standards. Distribute performance standards beforehand so that everyone knows what is expected of them, and then base your evaluation on those standards.
- Make evaluations quantitative. Use a scoring device based on the performance standards. Numbers and letters indicating a grade will help students definitively gauge their progress. Avoid ambiguous evaluations.
- Identify corrective measures. Give students guidance and direction for self-remediation. Show them how to improve their performance; this is precisely why they are there.
- Give feedback promptly. It does little good to reprimand a pet two days after misbehavior. Likewise, student mistakes and errors should be corrected quickly. Grade and return assignments, quizzes, and exams promptly.
- Give feedback often. Don't let students wonder how they are doing. Seeing their progress is a powerful motivational device. Show them how they have improved as often as possible, and give them a reason to continue to progress.
- Keep evaluations positive. Talk in terms of how to perform

correctly. Avoid belaboring mistakes. Learners are very vulnerable to negative input and can be permanently impaired by heavy-handed criticism.

Conducting a successful training program is directly related to the instructor's ability to motivate his students. This is not rocket science, just common sense. If you are successful in properly motivating your students, the rewards will not only be more skillful graduates and knowledgeable field providers, but also people who are turned on to learning and will probably continue their education long after your program has ended. Imagine refresher students who are motivated to learn. A fantasy? No! A motivating instructor can accomplish this by keeping that spark alive.

References

Bloom, B. S., et al. *Taxonomy of Educational Objectives.* New York: David McKay Co. Inc., 1956.

Cherry, R. A. "A Course on Training: When Experience Alone Isn't Enough." *JEMS* 13, no. 9 (1988).

Gephart, W. J. "Teacher Enthusiasm." *Practical Application of Research* 3, no. 4 (1981).

Herzberg, F. "One More Time: How Do You Motivate Employees?" *Harvard Business Review* 5 (1987).

Maslow, A. H. *Motivation and Personality.* New York: Harper and Row, 1970.

McCullough, W. J. *Hold Your Audience.* Englewood Cliffs, N.J.: Prentice-Hall Inc., 1978.

McLagan, P. A. *Helping Others to Learn: Designing Programs for Adults.* Washington: American Society for Training and Development, 1983.

O'Brien, M. *Vince: A Personal Biography of Vince Lombardi.* New York: William Morrow and Co. Inc., 1987.

Peters, T. J., and R. H. Waterman. *In Search of Excellence.* New York: Warner Books, 1982.

Wlodkowski, R. J. *Enhancing Adult Motivation to Learn.* San Francisco: Jossey-Bass Publishers, 1986.

Source

Reprinted with permission from JEMS, *March 1990. Richard A. Cherry, NREMT-P, is the director of paramedic training at the State University of New York Health Science Center in Syracuse, N.Y. He holds a master's degree in education and has over 20 years of teaching experience.*

A Practical Approach to Paramedic Precepting

Michael Giannini,
EMT-P

*Giving paramedic
students an opportunity
to work side by side with
experienced field
personnel has become a
standard part of the
paramedic curriculum.
To be effective, field
internships need to be
well structured. This
article describes criteria
for preceptors and
outlines key components
for a successful program.*

MANY PARAMEDIC TRAINING PROGRAMS throughout the United States use a curriculum that encompasses three separate, increasingly advanced phases of education. These phases are didactic, or classroom, instruction; clinical, or hospital, instruction; and field, or ambulance, instruction.

These different aspects of training allow the student to gradually increase his knowledge and skills as he progresses through the program. The didactic sessions provide the basic information and skills necessary to become a paramedic, while the clinical phase refines those skills in the controlled environment of a hospital. After the student has successfully demonstrated his ability to care for patients in the hospital setting, he progresses to providing care in the field.

The field training phase, or internship, should allow the student to apply and refine the knowledge and skills learned in the classroom and the hospital. It should enable him to learn field-specific techniques for patient care and prepare for the safe practice of prehospital medicine. By understanding these goals and undertaking a plan to achieve them, the program developers can provide students with every opportunity for success.

Before the field phase of a paramedic training program can begin, the program administrators must develop a detailed plan outlining how this phase is to be accomplished. The program director, in close association with the program staff, should draw upon input from all available resources—practicing paramedics, students, and directors of other training programs—in developing this plan. The ideas can then be used to outline a program that will satisfy both local and state training regulations. Once developed, the field training program should be detailed in a handbook and explained to students and instructors during separate introductory workshops. Student workshops focus on the internship, while preceptor workshops are geared more toward the process of adult learning.

Basic Internship Requirements

The first requirement of a successful internship program is a qualified preceptor. Paramedics become involved in precepting in a variety of ways; some volunteer, and others are recommended by their superiors.

A well-qualified preceptor possesses many attributes. He is recognized by his peers as an excellent clinician, has good teaching skills, and is knowledgeable about field medicine. Indeed, paramedics who do not have these abilities may be unable to effectively precept an intern. To ensure that students receive the best training possible, some states, such as California, require that paramedic preceptors have at least two years of field experience. And many paramedic training programs require that the preceptor attend a workshop that teaches him about the adult learning process.

The preceptor must also be motivated; he must be willing to give 100 percent of his work time and energy to train the intern. He must realize that he is, in effect, taking on a second job that will last a minimum of two months. Not only will he be responsible for rendering patient care in the field but also for educating the intern. A paramedic who is ambivalent about precepting or who is called upon by his employer to take on a student against his will is doing a disservice to the student. A truly motivated preceptor will request that a student be placed with him.

Another requirement of a successful internship program is support among those involved in field care, including the preceptor's partner and employer. His partner must be willing to accept the additional stresses associated with the presence of an intern on the prehospital care team. Living conditions may be more cramped, detailed critiques of calls are frequent, and stress levels may be high.

Support must also come from the preceptor's employer. At the very least, the employer must approve the intern's participation in delivering patient care and in representing the agency. In a broader sense, the employer should not demand too much of the preceptor during this period; the same individual should not continually be asked to train students. Much time and energy is required to do the job well, and even the best preceptor needs a break from the rigors of training.

Before the Internship

Before the intern begins his field training, he should receive basic information, such as what the internship consists of and what standards he must meet in order to successfully complete the program. This material can be outlined both verbally and in an orientation handbook, which should incorporate the thoughts and needs of the preceptors themselves. Some of the preceptors should be brought into the classroom to discuss what the interns can expect once they begin their field training.

A suitable location for the field training must then be chosen by the program administrator, preceptor, company/agency, or all three. One consideration that must be taken into account in this selection process is the amount of potential patient contacts the intern may have. Whenever possible, care should be taken to avoid placing a student in an area that has a low call volume. The more patients an intern sees, the greater the likelihood of seeing a variety of medical conditions.

It is also beneficial for students to intern in the county or system where they will eventually work. Being familiar with the inner workings of an area can be very helpful for the newly qualified paramedic. However, this may mean that the student will intern with a prospective em-

> A truly motivated preceptor will request that a student be placed with him.

ployer, which could be problematic. For example, preceptors may be encouraged by their employers to pass a borderline student in order to bring manning levels up and reduce overtime expenditures. On the other hand, these employers may now have a vested interest in this potential employee and be motivated to develop the best paramedic they can. The result largely depends on the underlying philosophy of the organization.

Students should avoid doing their internship with a preceptor who is a friend, as this may not only compromise the internship but the friendship as well. Many paramedic programs are limited in the number of EMS providers and preceptors available in a given area, however, making such considerations unfeasible.

Once a suitable location and preceptor have been matched to a student, the training program staff should review the purpose and goals of the internship with that preceptor and his supervisor to clarify the instructor's role. The student's academic progress should also be discussed at this point, including his strong and weak areas. This gives the preceptor a basis from which to develop a plan that will serve to improve the performance of the intern and achieve the ultimate goals of the internship.

The next step is for the preceptor to meet with the student; if a face-to-face meeting is not possible, a lengthy telephone conversation will suffice. At this time, the preceptor and student should exchange information about their EMS backgrounds and review the goals of the internship and their respective expectations. The preceptor should inform the student of exactly what is expected of him, including the time he is to arrive at the station, where he is to park, what he is to wear, how meals are arranged, and what he is expected to do on calls. The preceptor should also supply the intern with a copy of local county protocols, which will allow him to better function on the scene and interact with hospital personnel.

The Internship

On the first day of the internship, the student should receive information from the preceptor regarding the crew's daily routine. He should be told what his responsibilities are in checking the equipment, cleaning duties, and paperwork. This information should be supplemented with a written document that the intern can refer to on an as-needed basis.

The intern should not be asked to do more than his share of non-medical work. He is not, after all, a clean-up boy, "gofer," or slave, but a student.

The first day should also include a tour of the service area—both the good and bad parts of town. Visit the fire stations, and introduce the intern to the first responders with whom he will be working. Drive by the hospitals and base station if possible, and let him meet the nurses and doctors. Give him a feeling for what the area and its people are like.

In terms of patient care, the intern's first day should be limited to observation. Set an example for him to follow by allowing him to see how you care for patients.

The first day is also a good time to explore the intern's knowledge base. A good way to accomplish this is by quizzing him orally. It is important to begin by asking basic EMT questions, which will allow him to build his confidence and reduce his anxiety. (Think how you would feel if your medical director began by bombarding you with tough questions.) This session will give you a good idea of how much material your intern has been able to absorb in his training so far. This type of oral quizzing should be done each day during the internship to keep the student's knowledge base at a high level.

The second and remaining days of the internship should be spent as productively as possible. Allow the intern to assume the role of paramedic (under preceptor supervision), including caring for the patient, reporting patient information to his partner and/or the base station, completing required paperwork, and performing whatever other functions the preceptor would normally do. Allow him to become completely immersed in the role.

The preceptor's job, on the other hand, is to supervise the intern's actions. He must be sure that the services delivered to the patient meet his agency's standard of care. There may be a time when the intern's patient care is inadequate. When this occurs, the preceptor must coach, guide, or help the student as necessary while avoiding the temptation to take over the call and assume the role of caregiver. The preceptor should only assume control if the intern's behavior significantly affects patient care.

Telling the intern to step back and watch contributes to a negative perception of his own performance. Learning reinforced by success is far preferable to, and more productive than, learning motivated by failure. Generally, the preceptor must be able to sit back and let the student care for the patient. Make mental or written notes of the good and bad aspects of the intern's performance during any calls. Refer to and discuss these notes with the intern during the critique, which should follow each run as soon as possible.

The critique of the call can be very stressful for all concerned, as mistakes will inevitably be made. These must be pointed out, however, so that improvements can be made. The best way to reduce stress and make the critique a beneficial experience is to conduct it in a positive manner. While returning to the station after the call, for example, ask the intern what he thinks went well with the call. Add to his list the positive aspects that you noted as you observed his performance, and praise him for these things. Next, ask the intern what he thinks his weak areas were. Express concern about his legitimate weaknesses while suggesting ideas for improvement. Because of the earlier positive feedback given to him, he will be more receptive to criticism.

The preceptor should remember that there may be a number of correct ways to accomplish a certain task and that the student should not necessarily be expected to perform it the preceptor's way. It is also important to remember that the student should not be expected to perform as well as an experienced paramedic. He should, however, complete his tasks in a safe, competent, and consistent manner.

Another important part of the critique process is documentation. The student's performance level should be well documented as he progresses through his field internship. After each shift, the preceptor should document the intern's performance in a variety of areas, such as assessment techniques and technical and communication skills. This is best accomplished through the use of a printed evaluation form that covers all aspects of patient care. The student should be given the opportunity to read the comments made by the preceptor and initial that he has done so. Allowing the student to read his evaluations ensures that there is no breakdown in communication regarding his performance level.

Once the internship is under way, a clinical coordinator or other representative from the training program should visit the station to monitor the intern's progress, which is easily done by reviewing the preceptor's evaluation forms. During this meeting, the coordinator, preceptor, and student can discuss the student's progress, and goals can be set to deal with any deficiencies. (If at any time during the internship the preceptor or the student feels that a major problem exists, however, the program representative should be contacted immediately.) The number of visits required varies from program to program. No more than four visits is typically needed unless the student has severe problems.

A good way to deal with an intern's deficiencies in patient care is to direct him to practice the desired technique on simulated patients. Simulations of emergency situations can be used to review just about any problem area, and they provide an effective but low-key way to learn. The student can make mistakes without harming actual patients. Simulations are also an excellent way to make use of spare time when calls are not being run.

Problems and Solutions

Even under the best of circumstances, problems may arise during the internship. One of the more common difficulties that may occur is a personality conflict between the preceptor and the student. Imagine that, after two or three shifts, the preceptor and the student are at such odds with one another that they cannot even agree to disagree! Such a scenario can occur when expectations are not met and there is a breakdown in communication. For example, the preceptor may expect the intern to act or perform a certain way, perhaps the way that he did in his internship. If this happens and the preceptor fails to communicate his wishes, problems will inevitably result.

The intern may similarly have expectations that are not fulfilled. To avoid this problem, the intern should start out with valid and realistic ideas of what to expect from the preceptor. If a problem does come up, he should talk about it. Neither the intern nor the preceptor should be afraid to call upon the program representative to help smooth things out. Chances are that he has dealt with problematic situations before.

Another common problem can occur when the preceptor and his partner give conflicting information to the student, for example, concerning the delivery of patient care. Who is the student to believe? Both ideas may be correct. However, if it is apparent that someone is wrong, consult an acceptable reference, such as a textbook, physician, instructor, or another paramedic.

Ideally, as the field internship draws to a close, the student will have learned a great deal about how to practice prehospital medicine in the field. The conclusion of the internship can also present the paramedic with the opportunity to learn something about his abilities as a preceptor. Soon after the last shift, the intern should be asked to evaluate the paramedic's performance as a preceptor. Was he a good role model and teacher? Did he influence the student in a positive manner? What did he excel in? What areas need improvement? And, should he be asked to precept again? This feedback will serve to improve the internship process in the future.

The end of the internship also gives the preceptor one more chance to reward the student with positive feedback. Toward the end of the intern's last shift, make an effort to surprise him with a gift, such as a cake or some other congratulatory item. I was really surprised when the Vacaville, Calif., Fire Department brought out a huge cake on the last day of my paramedic internship. At that moment, I felt like I finally belonged to an elite group of very special people.

Conclusion

The field internship is the final and most critical phase of training for the paramedic student. Successful completion is determined by meeting the goals that are outlined at the beginning of the internship to both the student and the preceptor. By following a set plan to achieve these goals, the student will have the best opportunity to graduate from the training program and make a significant contribution to the lives of others.

Source
Reprinted with permission from JEMS, *August 1991. Michael Giannini, EMT-P, has been active in EMS for 16 years.*

Acknowledgment
The author would like to thank all of the paramedic students whom he has had the pleasure to precept.

References
California Code of Regulations. Title 22. Social Security. Division 9. Prehospital Emergency Medical Services. Sec. 10014.
Hilgard, E. R. *Theories of Learning.* New York: Appleton-Century-Crofts, 1956.
Rehmar, S. *Stanford-Foothill Prehospital Care Program.* Preceptor workshop, 1989.
"State and Province Survey." *Emergency Medical Services* 11 (1989): 201–231.

Building the Ultimate Instructor

Richard A. Cherry, MEd, NREMT-P

How many of you have listened to (or given) boring, poorly planned lectures? Great instructors are not born—instructional skills must be learned and practiced. This article presents 25 ideas for self-improvement that instructors should review before presenting their next lecture.

I\n 1991, *JEMS* FEATURED a two-part article by Mike Taigman and Kate Dernocoeur on kaisen, the Japanese philosophy that encourages life satisfaction through personal and professional growth. Kaisen is a never-ending process of making small, incremental improvements in one's life. The great American poet Henry David Thoreau could have been describing kaisen when he wrote, "I know of no more encouraging fact than the unquestionable ability of man to elevate his life by a conscious effort."

If there was ever a group of people who could use kaisen in their lives, it's EMS instructors and training officers. In the rapidly changing world of prehospital emergency medicine, instructors who do not keep up with advances become obsolete—even dangerous. It's like trying to walk up a down escalator: Either you keep moving upward, or you end up at the bottom. But by improving just one aspect of your teaching each year, you will make great strides. It's never too late to identify your weaknesses and make a conscious effort to strive for continual improvement in those areas.

The ultimate EMS instructor would have the up-to-date medical knowledge and top-notch clinical expertise of Dr. Ronald Stewart, the EMS field experience of Thom Dick, the adult education skills of Dale Carnegie, the dynamic and inspirational public speaking qualities of Billy Graham, the motivational powers of Vince Lombardi, the leadership confidence of Ret. Army Gen. Norman Schwartzkopf, the compassion and dedication of Mother Theresa, and the personal commitment to excellence of Jim Page. I'm reasonably certain that the only person who had all of these qualities was born under a bright star and had gifts brought to him by wise men. The important point is to make the personal commitment to become the best you can be in all of these areas.

Turning your professional life into an endless quest for perfection is bound to bring with it a measure of success. John Wooden, former University of California, Los Angeles, basketball coach, defined success as "peace of mind, which is a direct result of self-satisfaction in knowing you did your best to become the best that you are capable of becoming." It is the journey—not the goal—that enriches our lives.

Why bother? Once again in the words of Henry David Thoreau, "If one advances confidently in the direction of his dreams and endeavors to live the life which he has imagined, he will meet with a success unexpected in common hours."

The following are 25 tips for self-improvement that will help you become an ultimate instructor. Give them a try.

Develop a Positive Attitude

The essence of kaisen is adopting a positive attitude about everything you do. According to this philosophy, attitude is the most important thing you can develop in your life. While ability determines capability, attitude determines performance. You may only have been given certain abilities, but how close you come to realizing your full potential is directly determined by your attitude. Rather than dwelling on your shortcomings and deficiencies, make the commitment to improve them.

Former Green Bay Packers head coach Vince Lombardi once said, "Making the effort to be perfect is what life is all about. If you will not settle for anything less than the best, you will be amazed at what you can do with your lives." You don't have to be a sports fan to appreciate the tremendous difference attitude—a "can-do" versus a "can't-do" attitude—makes. It's not always the best athlete or team that wins, but the one that wants it more. With the proper attitude, you can accomplish great things.

Be Better Prepared

Many instructors teach concepts they do not fully understand themselves. For example, teachers with a limited medical background find it difficult to explain complex physiological phenomena or adequately answer students' questions. Confidence in the classroom comes from being prepared, from having a thorough understanding of the subject matter and the clinical experience to relate it to real-life emergency medical situations.

Increase your medical knowledge by enrolling in a class offered at a local college with an allied health curriculum. Courses in anatomy and physiology, pharmacology, pathophysiology, and medical physics, among others, can substantially increase your basic understanding of what you teach. A number of specialized certification courses, such as basic trauma life support (BTLS), advanced trauma life support (ATLS), advanced cardiac life support (ACLS), pediatric advanced life support (PALS), and prehospital trauma life support (PHTLS) focus on specific subject areas. Identify your weaknesses, and make the effort to get smarter.

Stay Current

Reading current medical literature is an excellent way to be prepared. There are three types of journals with which to familiarize yourself. Peer-reviewed medical journals, such as *Annals of Emergency Medicine, Journal of Emergency Medicine, American Journal of Emergency Medicine,* and *Prehospital and Disaster Medicine,* publish original research articles. They provide the sound clinical data that support the current practice of emergency medicine.

Medical educational journals and newsletters, such as *Topics in Emergency Medicine, Emergency Medicine Clinics, ACLS Alert, Emergency Reports,* and *Prehospital Care Reports,* present topics of current interest and provide an excellent source of information when developing lesson plans.

And EMS trade journals, such as *JEMS, Rescue, Emergency Medical Services,* and *Emergency,* provide news articles and features on the latest trends in EMS. In addition, a monthly video magazine, *Emergency Medical Update,* presents major incident news coverage, subject lessons, and helpful field hints.

Developing a library is an excellent individual or organizational project. Cataloging a variety of resources by specific topics will provide ready handouts for students and background research material for yourself.

Attend Staff Lectures

Although most EMS agencies sponsor continuing education classes, it would benefit EMS instructors to attend the lecture series that most teaching hospitals' academic departments provide for their medical staff. These lectures are given by experienced clinicians and are geared toward the less-experienced staff members (e.g., medical students, interns, residents, and fellows). Ask permission to attend these informative sessions (perhaps your physician medical director can help you) and learn how practicing clinicians think.

An excellent example is emergency department (ED) lectures. Because emergency physicians see a great number of patients in a short time, they must conduct assessments and formulate diagnoses quickly. Often, they do so by developing specialized decision trees, mnemonics, and algorithms. Their lectures are filled with pearls of wisdom you will never find in medical textbooks.

Whenever I inject these types of items into my lectures, I find it makes my class more interesting, it helps my students learn more, and, most of all, it increases their motivation to learn.

Get Clinical Experience

The adult student learns what is relevant. Teachers with extensive book knowledge but little clinical experience (hospital or street) are ineffective because they cannot relate the classroom lectures to what happens in real situations.

If you have a limited clinical background, make arrangements to spend time in a hospital, ideally in the ED, surgery, labor and delivery suites, psychiatric units, and intensive care units. Find a staff member who is willing to act as your personal preceptor, and then learn as much as you can for as long as you can. If your EMS background is limited, spend time with experienced field crews to learn the practical, realistic side of street medicine. Don't just accept your limitations as such; do something about them. Prepare yourself by getting the necessary clinical experience in the hospital or field.

Learn to Teach

EMS instructors typically do not have educational backgrounds. They are excellent field providers who were chosen to teach based on their outstanding clinical records. They seem ready to teach, but are they prepared? Ask an unemployed person if he is ready to take a million-dollar executive position, and he'll say yes. But would he be prepared?

If you have no formal educational background, enroll in courses at a local college that offers a teaching curriculum. Take the same courses that future teachers take, such as principles of adult education, lesson planning, educational psychology, tests and measurements, and teaching methods, which provide a solid foundation for teaching. Also, many state and local EMS systems offer instructor training programs that follow the U.S. Department of Transportation EMS Instructor Training Program curriculum. If you want to teach, learn your craft.

Create the Perfect Lesson Plan

Communicating with your peers is an entertaining and interesting way to learn new ideas and broaden your educational horizons. Teachers in Japan and China spend considerable time constructing lessons and sharing learning materials with each other in search of the perfect way to teach their particular subjects. They call it "polishing the stone." What better way to grow as an instructor than to engage in teaching and learning activities with your peers? Join an existing EMS instructors' organization, start your own, or just informally get together with other instructors.

Creating lesson plans is an important part of a teacher's overall responsibility. Just as a contractor requires an exact plan to build a house, the lesson plan is the blueprint for learning. It is the essential first step in teaching any class. Develop an insatiable appetite for constructing the perfect lesson plan. Try to discover the best way to teach cardiovascular anatomy or pediatric intubation. Like our Japanese and Chinese counterparts, polish the stone until it shines with brilliance.

Build Pyramids of Understanding

Human beings are inherently not good at processing large amounts of new information. Just as experienced house builders first lay a solid foundation, effective instructors must first establish a base of previous knowledge in their students. New material is then presented in a logical sequence and added to this existing framework of knowledge and experience until a higher level of learning has been constructed.

This is a continual process. Always reinforce previous learning by relating new material to it. At the end of a lesson, check for understanding by having your students summarize the subject. If this seems simple, it is. Remember, teaching is mostly common sense. The ancient Egyptian pyramids are still standing because each new block of granite was placed on an existing framework of blocks. Review your curriculum, and design ways to build your own pyramids of understanding.

Teach to Both Brains

There are vast differences in the ways individual students learn. If you are left-brain dominant (i.e., analytical, deductive, rational, and logical), you probably use left-brain teaching techniques. Some of your students may, however, be right-brain dominant (i.e., imaginative, symbolic, artistic, and emotional) and require a different approach. Therefore, it is important to teach to both sides of the brain.

For example, when teaching about pneumothorax, describe the mechanism of injury, pathophysiology, signs and symptoms, and field treatment, which will appeal to the left-brain learners. In addition, use photos, drawings, and case histories, which will appeal to the right-brain learners.

Left-brain learners need the structure of lists and analytical data, while right-brain learners need to visualize the process. Both groups learn well—just differently. A good mix of logically presented data and field accounts ensures that you will satisfy all of your students' learning needs and will make the class more interesting. Everyone loves a good story. Real life is an excellent teaching tool, and experienced instructors use it to the greatest advantage.

Be a Coach

Make an effort to provide your students with timely feedback on their progress. They appreciate it, and it will help them avoid repeating mistakes. Correct and return quizzes, homework, and exams by the next class session. Let your students know they can count on a prompt, objective evaluation. Make yourself available for extra help, and always outline a plan for correcting deficiencies. Show them the way to success.

This also applies to practical skills. Practice in itself does not make perfect, as anyone with a 10-year-old learning to play the trumpet will tell you. Only perfect practice makes perfect. Be a coach, and guide your students through psychomotor skill sessions by using the stop-start-continue method: Have them stop doing it the wrong way, start doing it the right way, and continue doing it that way.

Instill a Passion for Learning

An instructor must establish a pleasant learning environment. A boot camp is as unproductive as a country club; an instructor should be neither intimidating nor a pal. Rather, an instructor should encourage a climate of mutual respect in which he is seen as the senior colleague. It is a basic principle of adult education that the instructor lead and inspire. If you can ignite your students with a spark of passion for learning more about the

---

Teacher Evaluations

Students Like Teachers Who

- Demonstrate genuine concern for their problems
- Exhibit a high degree of enthusiasm
- Make them think
- Challenge them
- Are patient
- Have a pleasant disposition
- Are kind and considerate
- Have high expectations of them
- Are open-minded to suggestions
- Are cooperative and flexible
- Can correct without being insulting
- Are well prepared and proficient in the subject
- Have a sense of humor
- Deliver fair and impartial treatment
- Encourage questions
- Are "real" people

human body and emergency medicine, the flame may continue to burn long after they leave your program.

This may be the most important thing we can accomplish as EMS instructors. Method is just as important as content—it's the drawing out, not the pumping in, that marks a great teacher. Average teachers have the knowledge. Good teachers have the knowledge and can relay the information. Great teachers instill a passion for learning.

Evaluate Your Performance

Solicit an honest course evaluation at the end of your program, and analyze the responses. Make a checklist based on the data to use for future course evaluations. Remember, it's what the students think that's important.

Designing a reliable evaluation tool is a crucial part of any continuous quality improvement program. But unless you are willing to take a critical look at evaluation results, you will never identify or remedy the areas that need improvement. Just as the customer defines quality in service, the student defines quality in education.

The "Teacher Evaluations" boxes list the most common responses about teachers that I receive from students. The most striking observation is that most of the responses are people/personal-oriented, not subject-oriented. Just as patients focus more on customer service than the ambulance crew's technical expertise, students focus more on the instructor's interpersonal skills than on his knowledge of the subject.

Teach People, Not Subjects

Successful coaches agree that while the Xs and Os are important, what wins championships is dealing effectively with the players. In the same way, how an instructor deals with adult learners has a tremendous impact on the success of the instruction.

More than 20 years of teaching has taught me that the way you interact with your students is a crucial component of your teaching style and their ultimate learning experience. Required reading for any teacher is *How to Win Friends and Influence People* by the great American educator Dale Carnegie. The next five points will expand on this concept of just how an instructor can improve his interaction with students.

Be Hard to Please

I believe that the average person, if given the opportunity, will take the path of least resistance. Also, we try the hardest to please those who are the hardest to please. Up to a point, anxiety can increase learning. While the breaking point varies with each student, it is important for instructors to establish an anxiety level that demands a consistently high level of achievement.

Teacher Evaluations

Students Dislike Teachers Who

- Are disorganized and unprepared
- Read from text and notes
- Deliver monotone lectures
- Test on irrelevant material
- Intimidate them
- Sit while lecturing
- Appear disinterested and bored
- Are unsure of material
- Frequently cancel class
- Use only passive learning activities
- Lack variety in teaching methods
- Hate the subject
- Go off on tangents
- Conduct business during class
- Ask questions but don't allow students to answer them

When you squeeze an orange, you get what's inside: orange juice. Only by applying pressure to your students will you—and they—find out what they are actually capable of doing. People really don't know what they can do until they try, and it's your job to make sure your students try. By holding them more accountable, you are telling them that you refuse to accept anything less than a commitment to excellence.

Be Accountable

Accountability is a two-way street. If you expect excellence from your students, they should be able to expect the same from you. Be a positive role model for them. When asked why he always played hard, even in exhibition games, former New York Yankee Joe DiMaggio answered that there might be someone in the stadium who had never seen him play before. He always gave 100 percent because he held himself to a higher standard than the average baseball player.

As EMS instructors, we must hold ourselves to a higher standard. Don't demand anything of your students that you are not willing to commit to yourself. Actions that demonstrate commitment to such qualities as punctuality, dependability, and reliability speak louder than words. Always be on time! When you are late, you are in essence showing your students that you do not respect them and that you believe your time is more valuable than theirs. Respect begets respect. Always come to class prepared, and avoid the temptation to "wing it" just because you've taught the same lesson for 10 years.

Expect Nothing But the Best

It's clear to me that when I have high expectations of my students, they do better. Every year, I allow my students to establish the minimum passing grade for the course. In this way, they participate in their future evaluation by determining what the minimum quality performance for the class will be. An interesting thing happens every year: The students always set the mark higher than I would have. Does this indicate that we don't expect enough from our students? Are they willing to give more than we expect? We want to be the best, to excel, and to be a part of something special. Show your students a picture of a popular Olympic champion, and emphasize that all the money in the world cannot buy a gold medal. You get it the old-fashioned way: You earn it.

Make your students believe that what they are trying to achieve is something special and that achieving it will take hard work, dedication, and intense desire. No effort is more worthy of this commitment than providing emergency medical services to people in need.

Use Positive Reinforcement

"Nothing succeeds like success" is a time-worn phrase, but its application to education is still valid. Without overdoing it, reward early accomplishment. If you want to change a student's behavior (e.g., tardiness, poor performance, or bad attitude), positive reinforcement is much more effective than negative reinforcement.

Notice your students doing something right, and reinforce their behavior with an appreciative word. If one student is always late for class, ignore him rather than reinforce his negative behavior. The first time he arrives on time, however, show that you noticed. Tell him immediately that you are pleased that he arrived on time and that it demonstrates a renewed attitude on his part in making a commitment to excellence. Then, look him straight in the eye, and tell him that you are proud of him for making that commitment. If he believes you are sincere, you've got him.

Given properly, positive reinforcement can work miracles. And it's fun to outsmart your students.

Challenge Them to Be Great

Every year, on the first night of class, I ask my students: "Who wants to be a great paramedic? Stand up!" Naturally, they all stand up. Now they have made a public commitment of excellence to themselves, me, their classmates, and their future patients. Later, when they complain about lengthy reading assignments and strenuous labs, I remind them that I'm only helping them do what they want—become great paramedics.

Greatness is in the heart and mind. I had one student who earned a "C" for her performance in a particular skills lab. When she asked me about it, she said she thought she had done pretty well. I agreed that she had done well for an average student, but for the excellent student I believed she could be, she only had done average. I asked her if she wanted me to change the grade to an "A." She replied, "I'll take the 'C.'" From then on, I knew she would become a great paramedic, and she did.

View Teaching as a Performing Art

In this high-tech age, it is important to be not only informative, but to be entertaining and inspirational as well. Just as performers concentrate on perfecting their skills, try to improve your classroom presentation techniques. After they have mastered the mechanics of their roles, great performers add their own special touches of emotion and creativity, raising their roles to higher levels of excellence. You can raise the level of your performance capabilities by practicing the final six tips.

Look Them in the Eye

Make eye contact with every student as many times as possible during each class session. By doing this, you tell each person in the class that you are talking to him. Eye-to-eye contact is the most direct, emotional, and powerful way to communicate. People who attend Billy Graham crusades often report that at least once during his sermon, Graham's eyes looked directly into theirs. This is remarkable, considering he usually speaks to audiences in excess of 50,000 people.

Your eyes should be alert, alive, and expressive. They are the windows to your soul, and your sincerity and enthusiasm show through clearly. Many speakers tend to favor one side of the room over the other. If you catch yourself looking at one side the majority of the time, make a conscious effort to turn to the other side. Don't leave half of the class feeling neglected.

Speak With Your Body

Non-verbal language speaks louder than words. While your words say one thing, your facial expressions and body language can say something entirely different. Who and what you are speaks loudly. Students watch for patterns in your most minute actions and are wise enough to distrust words that in any way mismatch your deeds.

Match your physical behavior with your words. How can you spread enthusiasm if you stand lifelessly in front of the room? While I don't recommend jumping around as though you just won the lottery, be energetic. Vary your style by using planned, deliberate, controlled movements at appropriate times. Take command of the stage. Words and information are simply not enough; bring the subject to life by becoming a more enthusiastic speaker. Often, it's not what we say that counts, but what students see and hear.

Use the Power of the Pulpit

Do not underestimate the power of speech. Throughout history, all major world leaders from Churchill to Hitler have been dynamic, powerful public speakers. Studies in communication suggest that form is more important than substance and that much of a listener's focus is on attitude, not on the actual words spoken. How you say something may have more impact than what you say. Experienced speakers change the tone, pitch, and volume of their voices to express the intent of their words and add dramatic effect.

Do you sound like a priest reciting his daily prayers or a hot dog vendor at Yankee Stadium? Are you a slow, methodical, monotone speaker, or do you bark your words like an auctioneer? If done consistently, these all are ineffective communication techniques. But by varying your style, you can make a tremendous impact with your words. Radio personality Paul Harvey's 30-minute reports are filled with peaks, valleys, and dramatic pauses. In this way, Harvey effectively emphasizes particular points. Just as Texas Ranger Nolan Ryan keeps batters off balance by varying the speed of his pitches from a 95-mph fastball to a much slower change-up, you can keep students alert by varying your speaking style.

Inject Life Into Your Lectures

Anything that can be learned can be learned in an enjoyable manner. Just as hot spice added to a basic recipe makes it more tantalizing and definitely demands attention, case histories, anecdotes, and humorous stories relating to your specific lesson provide hot spice to a lecture. Adding some hot spice to your lesson every 10 minutes adds frequent emotional lifts and helps maintain student interest.

My favorite story involves a baseball player who suffered severe memory loss following an on-field collision with another player. Not only did he lose his abilities to read and write, but he could not differentiate between his mother and any other female, which must have made for some very interesting interludes. I tell this story whenever I teach about the brain. It reinforces the concept of brain anatomy and physiology while adding humor and human interest to the lesson.

Over time, you can collect a number of hot spice items to enliven your classroom lectures. Alert, stimulated students learn more and will appreciate your efforts to make learning more enjoyable.

Believe in Your Subject

In his book *Hold Your Audience*, William McCullough writes, "It is not enough to know your subject, you must believe in it. Many men have become famous because of their sincerity; because they believed wholeheartedly in the cause they were supporting." Successful salespeople believe in what they sell. Why should your students learn what you are teaching? Sell them on its relevance, and allow them to attach a value to what they are learning. Since they will often adopt your value system, you must believe in the importance of what you teach. If you don't, why are you teaching it?

Be Excited About Teaching

Good teaching is the art of getting average students to do superior work. Are you eager and excited about teaching? If not, rethink your commitment to EMS education. An instructor's enthusiasm for the subject is infectious. Exuberance and a high degree of energy and vitality demonstrate a high level of enthusiasm and will stimulate your students. During my student-teaching days in college, my supervising instructor once told me, "If you aren't fired with enthusiasm, you will be fired with enthusiasm."

Getting Started

What are your weaknesses? Successful dieters say the best way to get started on a diet is to stand naked in front of a mirror (without holding in your stomach) for an honest evaluation. Likewise, instructors need to remove any obstacles that prevent an honest evaluation of their teach-

Source

Reprinted with permission from JEMS, *October 1992.*

ing. Be self-critical, and make small improvements in those areas that need it most. Be patient. As any weekend golfer can tell you, improvement comes slowly.

Think back to your most memorable teachers. Didn't they possess a unique combination of knowledge and personality? Didn't they demonstrate dedication and commitment, along with a tremendous desire to be successful? Make a personal commitment to emulate them.

A wise old French teacher once told me that when you are making a success of something, it's not work—it's a way of life. You enjoy yourself because you are making your contribution to the world. I understand now what she meant. She was describing kaisen.

References

Carnegie, D. *How to Win Friends and Influence People.* New York: Pocket Books, 1976.

Dernocoeur, K., and M. Taigman. "Kaisen: Continuous Improvement Is a Lifelong Challenge." *JEMS* 16, no. 1 (1991).

Dernocoeur, K., and M. Taigman. "Kaisen: EMS as Theater of the Streets." *JEMS* 16, no. 3 (1991).

Massar, I., ed. *The Illustrated World of Henry David Thoreau.* New York: Grosset & Dunlap, 1974.

McCullough, W. J. *Hold Your Audience.* Englewood Cliffs, N.J.: Prentice Hall Inc., 1978.

O'Brien, M. *Vince: A Personal Biography of Vince Lombardi.* New York: William Morrow and Co. Inc., 1987.

Stigler, J. W., and H. W. Stevenson. "How Asian Teachers Polish Each Lesson to Perfection." *American Educator* (Spring 1991).

Wooden, J. *They Call Me Coach.* Waco, Tex.: Word Inc., 1972.

FETN Dishes Out Training

Katy Benson

Providing high-quality training in a cost-effective manner is an issue that every EMS administrator must face. Satellite broadcasting is an emerging resource that can provide continuing education to EMS professionals.

DEDICATED EMS PROVIDERS go to great lengths to get the best possible training. The profession would be sorely troubled if not for the hundreds of hours its members spend in continuing education and the hundreds of miles they travel to distant training centers. But zapping into outer space—isn't that too much to ask?

No, not when the Fire & Emergency Television Network (FETN) does the traveling and the receiving stations need only say, "Beam me up." FETN joins video and interactive laser videodiscs to create the new generation of training media used by EMS providers.

Satellite broadcasting is hardly new, of course, but FETN is one of a scant handful of satellite broadcasts devoted to EMS, fire, and rescue programming. And, so far, it is the only one to do so on a national subscription basis. Produced by Westcott Communications in Dallas, FETN offers a sleek, entertaining, and effective tool for enhancing an agency's training program.

FETN

Westcott enters the emergency and fire arena with a nearly spotless record in business satellite television. It is the creator of networks for law enforcement and the automotive industry, and a similar network aimed at in-house security, which evolved into a successful videotape training program. In 1990, Westcott shouldered fire and EMS as well when it acquired American Heat Video Productions, a provider of subscription videotapes for fire, rescue, and EMS. FETN continues to provide *American Heat* and *Pulse*, although FETN sales are undermining the videos' success.

FETN tested its programming during the summer of 1991 and began weekday operations in September of that year. It broadcasts six hours of news and training segments each day, with programs repeated throughout the day and week to accommodate different time zones and on-duty shifts.

The core, *Turnout*, looks like a morning show, with two co-hosts presenting a series of short segments directed at volunteers, firefighters, fire management, in-house fire departments, rescue teams, paramedics, and EMTs. *Turnout* is produced twice weekly, with each show repeated seven times.

The half-hour show specifically for EMS is *E-Med*; it repeats two times daily for a week. Last year it covered such topics as crush syndrome, smoke inhalation, intraosseous infusion, and burnout among prehospital care providers.

The Need for Satellite Training

The desire for this kind of product appears to be escalating. Several trends in EMS, fire, and rescue operations suggest why.

Emergency agencies face public demand for increasingly sophisticated equipment and procedures. In addition, they are taking on new, diverse situations such as hazardous materials incidents.

"The fire service is really stretched, as is EMS," said Mark Lockhart, director of paramedic education for St. John's Mercy Medical Center in St. Louis. He is president of the National Association of EMTs, which endorsed FETN's programming in the fall of 1991. "It's not possible, especially for the smaller [departments], to cover everything there is to do. This [FETN programming] is filling a void."

EMS professionals, too, are products of a high-tech society and yearn for information in easily digestible bites. Dennis Murphy, division chief of the Springfield, Ore., Department of Fire and Life Safety, described the appeal of satellite training, "We're used to TV bringing us a world where they can do anything. The mind says, 'Let's be entertained.'

"With the spoken word, maybe 10 percent is retained," he said. "But with [visual] media, we have the experience of going right along with a hazmat situation or a big fire."

Finally, there is budget hysteria. Many FETN subscribers feel the installation charge of $750 plus a sliding-scale monthly fee of $188 to $488 beats the cost of other forms of education. "We get a whole slew of training for a month for the cost of one videotape," claimed Chief John R. Turner, Jr., of the West Odessa, Tex., Volunteer Fire Department.

Praise and Criticism

Ironically, cost is a factor that both supporters and critics of FETN cite in their respective arguments. The network's closest competitors, the federal Emergency Education Network (EENET) and Virginia's Emergency Medical Services Satellite Training (EMSAT), are government funded and cost nothing for the viewer. Although their programming differs significantly, both focus on emergency and EMS issues.

EMS providers who subscribe to FETN, on the other hand, receive little more than half an hour of emergency medical programming a week, along with three hours of fire-related programming. Special reports address various topics. FETN's mix reflects a figure of 60 percent of EMS handled by fire or combined-service departments. Still, agencies looking strictly for EMS education are apt to feel slighted.

Sandy Hartley is one EMS training coordinator who is unhappy with FETN's programming ratio. Last year, Hartley, a paramedic with the third-service Escambia County EMS in Florida, shared subscription costs with the county fire department. FETN provided "no worthy training" in EMS, Hartley claims, adding that what was available was too basic and too brief to help her department.

"I told FETN that any department willing to pay $6,000 a year for a training tool probably is not one that needs bandaging and splinting information. We want new avenues, new information," Hartley said.

"Some of it, yes, is pretty basic," countered Dennis Godfrey, director of Caribou County, Idaho, Emergency Service and Public Safety. "But we're trying to get away from basics, and that's not always good."

When Godfrey accepted the volunteer department's only paid staff position in spring of 1991, he found that the three EMT units had been operating with little direction. They had received no hazmat training, despite their proximity to chemical plants, phosphate mining operations, and major truck and railroad routes. Godfrey is using FETN's EMS segments to review the basics and its special reports, such as the one on hazardous materials, to introduce new skills.

Speaking in favor of FETN's cost effectiveness, the network's director of training and education, Ken Hines, points to the comparative cost of sending a department of 20 paramedics to a seminar. The instructors with whom FETN contracts are nationally respected EMS and rescue trainers, found through affiliations with Parkland Memorial Hospital in Dallas, Southwest Medical Center, the NAEMT and other sources. As NAEMT's Lockhart says, watching FETN is "like attending a national conference, but without all the expense."

Moving Forward

In any case, FETN appears ready to bulk up its EMS programming. Hines envisions adding broadcast days to the week and program hours to the day. Additional EMS coverage could come also in the *Turnout* briefs. He hears requests for more material on subjects such as hazardous materials and high-rise and first responder emergencies.

The NAEMT endorsement indicates its sincerity in building the EMS connection. "It's our hope we can work with them in expanding their EMS programming," said Lockhart. "They are fulfilling a need in the fire service—I hope they can do the same in EMS." NAEMT gives technical and editorial input to the programming staff.

In a recent move, FETN has formed an affiliation with the University of Texas Southwestern Medical Center at Dallas to offer continuing education units based on *E-Med* segments. Knowledge assessment provided by FETN to instructors allows an EMT to earn up to 26 CEUs a year.

FETN has also added program innovations. It is now using the Internal Fire Service Training Association manual sections as a basis for a series of half-hour shows. The satellite training serves as a visual adjunct to the IFSTA training manual, according to Hines.

How a Show Is Created

Hines described how his staff plans and implements EMS segments, as well as the changes and additions waiting in the wings.

FETN appears ready to bulk up its EMS programming. There are requests for more material on subjects such as hazardous materials and high-rise and first responder emergencies.

Individual EMS
instructors are
encouraged to
follow up with
supervised practice,
adapting it to fit
that department's
procedures and
equipment.

The weekly *E-Med* program is sketched out two months ahead. The staff meets to decide on timely topics with appeal to both basic and advanced life support providers. That balance between routine and unusual is the first criteria, says Hines. Then he approaches his resources to find qualified instructors to present nationally accepted standards.

Lectures are usually on-the-scene walk-throughs. "We're a how-to network," Hines said. "We look right at the camera and talk with the audience. We're striving to make them feel like they're there." Nevertheless, the inherent limitation of canned training is that it's "all didactic, not hands on," he says.

Individual EMS instructors are encouraged to follow up with supervised practice, adapting it to fit that department's procedures and equipment. FETN has developed a trainer's guidebook and performance objectives that help instructors present knowledge related to broadcast segments. In addition, "competency checklists" are mailed to instructors each month with the program guide; they aid in evaluating hands-on performance of a technique taught during a show.

Once Hines has the right instructor, along with two backups, an FETN talent coordinator arranges the topic and filing schedule with the instructor. Staff film crews are used on location for training segments. News updates come from regional ABC news bureaus, allowing FETN to respond immediately to breaking events in fire, EMS, and rescue.

Making the Best Use of FETN

Lockhart praises FETN's quality of work, from the physical facilities to the enthusiasm of the staff for its product. "They are totally committed to their mission, to provide quality fire and emergency education," he said.

Users, too, extol the benefits of FETN's programming. Turner, of West Odessa's fire and rescue volunteer department, runs a training program that incorporates manual instruction and satellite programs with his department's local slant. "FETN gives us the overall tactics," he said. "Then we adapt it to how we can use it here."

Like the majority of chiefs contacted, Turner tapes the shows for distribution to his volunteer staff to watch as they are able. He gives them a quiz after watching and applies passing credits toward training completion. Watching a professional do a procedure gives his volunteers an edge when they reach the hands-on practice, he believes.

Eventually, he will have a good-sized library of tapes to use during classroom training. After just two months of being hooked up to FETN, Turner says, it had already altered the training curriculum. When he sees an upcoming segment that will correspond to reading material, he assigns the reading to be done by the date the segment airs. In addition, he started an officer-training night to coincide with FETN's *Fire Company* management program.

Turner appreciates that FETN is "geared to the little guys as well as the big guys." Indeed, 75 percent of the network's subscribers are small or volunteer agencies, according to FETN Vice President and General Manager Steve Almer. But even the programming that pertains to larger departments is useful to small ones, Turner thinks. He wants his volunteers to see what they might encounter someday. "It gets their wheels clicking," he explained. "They think, 'what if that happens here?' They start asking questions where they didn't before."

Murphy of the Springfield safety center finds subtle rewards in getting "that global experience we wouldn't get as a small department." As the local first-response team in a hazmat incident, his department plays a secondary, defensive role to the regional team in neighboring Eugene, Ore. After watching FETN's hazmat series, Murphy says, his people realize how crucial their secondary role is. It has boosted morale and motivated the department to sharpen its skills.

Springfield's training officer edits tapes of all the programs so that instruction reflects how Springfield operates. For example, Murphy says, a segment filmed in Memphis, Tenn., might explain a way to treat air packs; Springfield, however, uses a different brand that requires different treatment. "We don't want our people to think we've changed our procedure," Turner said, "so we'll edit it or point out the difference in class."

FETN emphasizes that its programs are strictly supplementary to existing training in any department. It tries to reflect widely accepted standards; yet its acknowledged strength is as a purveyor of new information and in kick-starting discussions. Ricky Davidson, chairman of the EMS section of the International Association of Fire Chiefs, says FETN has "just tapped the potential."

"It's not an answer to solving all the training problems across the country. It doesn't address local requirements, practice drills, or variant methods," he said. "But it has the potential of being very useful in keeping emergency services abreast of the latest techniques and events."

In the quest for accessible, effective, and high-quality EMS education, FETN may discover that the sky is the limit.

Source

Reprinted with permission from Emergency, *August 1992. Katy Benson is a freelance writer in San Diego.*

Marketing

The Press: Our Overlooked Ally

Jerry L. Durnbaugh

EMS administrators often have a negative visceral reaction to dealing with the press. Most have had at least one tabloid or 60 Minutes-style interview experience during their careers. Author Jerry Durnbaugh tells why moving beyond adversarial relationships with the press can offer many positive opportunities.

The newspaper business is the only enterprise in the world where a man is supposed to become an expert on any conceivable subject between one o'clock in the afternoon and a 6 P.M. deadline.
—Robert S. Bird

ADMINISTRATORS FROM A NUMBER of area public service organizations in a medium-size Northeastern city were meeting to work on a disaster plan. The group, which included many members of the local EMS council, was trying to decide which agencies should be involved.

"What about the media?" one service chief asked.

"Oh, we'll call them just before our disaster drill," said the chairman, "and tell them what we want."

The problems of public relations and the resulting poor public concept of EMS are common.

"The trouble is, the public doesn't know what we're trying to do," the chairman complained. "It doesn't have any concept of what EMS is all about. You never see anything about EMS in the paper."

Someone suggested inviting reporters to all council meetings to the horror of council members.

"We can't do that," insisted the chairman. "Our bylaws state that all meetings are private. We deal with medical issues, you know, and we certainly wouldn't want our financial condition to become public knowledge."

In another situation, an EMT was driving the ambulance back to the base for restocking after handling a dramatic multi-victim auto accident.

"Boy, did I tell off that TV cameraman," he declared to his partner. "They make me so mad. They always turn up with their lights and gear while we are trying to extricate people and save lives. One photographer tried to take my picture when I was getting the long board, and I almost had a cop arrest her."

The same EMT was complaining about the coverage of the event on the six o'clock news later in the day.

"Can't they get anything right?" muttered the EMT. "Look at that! She only got me from the back."

"And she didn't even mention the service's name," noted the manager. "Oh, and don't forget to tell the next shift to be sure to clip the story and picture out of the paper for the company scrapbook."

The above samples are certainly not isolated incidents. They happen every day in the EMS community and are representative of the way that a large share of those in the EMS industry view and deal with the press.

Public Perception of EMS

Yes, by and large, the public *is* ignorant of EMS. But the cause of this ignorance is neither the public nor the media. Of all the public service agencies, none has done a poorer job of dealing with the media than EMS. The only image the public receives of EMS—aside from the individual who actually uses the service—is whatever image is presented by the media. Unfortunately, this image is often erroneous.

There are some very fine services whose excellence goes largely unreported, and hence unrecognized. On the other hand, some services with stellar local reputations are in reality a danger to the sick and injured.

While there are exceptions, the public in general appears to perceive EMS in light of its administrative structure: Proprietary services are bad, municipal services are good, and volunteers are at the top of the heap. Judgments are often colored by local pride. The myths of quality may well be propagated by the media because the media are ignorant of the factors by which a successful or substandard EMS system can be evaluated. The fault lies not with the media but with ourselves.

And it is hurting.

Money alone does not guarantee a good EMS system, but it takes money to operate any system, even a poor one. That money is getting harder and harder to come by. Budgetary considerations are reducing reimbursement schedules. Municipalities are in financial crunches as taxpayer revolts trim what used to be sacrosanct accounts. And people are complaining of the high charges for ambulance service; charges are as high as a $375 base rate for an emergency call.

Less affected, perhaps, are the volunteers who generally enjoy strong local support and can count on fund drives and fried fish dinners to make up operating deficits or to acquire new equipment. But even some superb volunteer companies are in financial difficulty.

It is going to take an informed public to decide which services deserve support and then come up with the cash to operate them.

The public's view of our industry is shaped through media coverage. Good public relations isn't just a matter of image; it is essential to our very survival.

Improving Media Relations

Two main considerations should be taken into account when trying

> The public's view of our industry is shaped through media coverage. Good public relations isn't just a matter of image; it is essential to our very survival.

Involving the media in the official planning stages not only ensures a professional media plan, but provides the opportunity to "educate" the media in the role of EMS and to build a reserve of good will with those who analyze and report our activities.

to improve media relations:

- The media are not our enemies.
- Rather than sit back and wait for our image to improve, we must take the initiative to see that we have an open dialogue with the media and that the media's knowledge of our industry is accurate and up-to-date.

When the media are after a story, they will get that story whether we cooperate or not. If the information obtained from other sources is inaccurate, if we stonewall and refuse to make ourselves available, if we succeed in alienating the media instead of cultivating their friendship, that is our responsibility.

Let's start with that disaster planning situation described earlier.

The media participate in disasters in three ways, so their participation in planning is absolutely essential:

First, in any disaster situation, the scene and participating agencies are going to be inundated with media representatives. Electronic and print reporters, as well as cameramen, will flock to the scene like nails drawn to a magnet. A disaster plan must make provisions for meeting the logistic needs of the press. While they have no desire to interfere with rescue operations, they have an important job to do and may inadvertently become a nuisance if no arrangements are available to meet their needs.

Second, any disaster is a highly confusing situation with rampant rumors, misinformation, and lack of information. No journalist wants erroneous information, but he is working on a tight schedule and has questions that need to be answered promptly. In our planning, it is up to us to develop a mechanism whereby up-to-date and accurate information can be collected quickly and made available for the media. No journalist will operate by censorship or handouts. Official agencies must recognize they are not the only sources of information and they cannot control the information obtained or used by the media. For official information to be believed and used, it is absolutely essential that there be no attempt to launder, cover up, alter, or distort information in an effort to minimize—or inflate—the scope of the disaster or the role of the agencies involved. There must be credibility. If an agency is caught in a lie or a distortion, its credibility with the media is destroyed, and the negative repercussions will live long after the disaster. Providing timely, accurate information when needed will generate good will, which can never be bought with money.

And third, as public service agencies, we have all the latest high-technology communications equipment and communications networks. Still, we have absolutely no way of getting official, important, and necessary information and directives out to the public. In time of disaster, a great deal of information must be given to the public. Some of this may be essential to survival. The only way we can disseminate this information is through the facilities of the media. Therefore, our relationship with the media *must* be good.

Acknowledging these points, the best technique for dealing with the media comes from the media themselves. Involving the media in the official planning stages not only ensures a professional media plan, but provides the opportunity to "educate" the media in the role of EMS and to build a reserve of good will with those who analyze and report our activities.

What is true for disaster planning is no less true for our regular, routine (and less spectacular) activities. In fact, it may be even more important.

The Media at EMS Meetings

An EMS council or body that excludes the press from its deliberations is a system that is setting itself up for a possible public confrontation.

The natural inclination of the press, when excluded, is to wonder what an organization is trying to conceal. Reporters will then search out information elsewhere. If a reporter feels strongly enough about it, he may well dig around until he has uncovered a skeleton—real or imagined—in the EMS closet.

An invitation to the press to cover EMS activities and discussions carries with it an element of risk. An agency may become involved in a discussion of items it would rather keep to itself. It is suicidal, however, to attempt to cover up or censor the media's account of an incident or meeting. Not only will such an approach destroy credibility, it will encourage the reporter to seek the information from other sources. That information may well be untrue and may ultimately be much more damaging than an open account from the agency.

We have no right to tell a reporter what or how to write, or tell a photographer which pictures to take. EMS events do not always occur in positive terms, and we should not duck the negative ones.

If the public, whom we ultimately ask for support, is to judge us accurately and fairly, it must know the bad as well as the good.

This doesn't mean we are obligated to hang out our dirty linen, it merely means we don't duck the embarrassing and tough questions. Our credibility with the media will then be strengthened, and their respect will grow. No ethical reporter will go out of his way to put down an individual or organization he respects. But he won't cover up for it, either. If we lie, whitewash, pressure, or otherwise attempt to control what is written about us, we deserve the resulting bad press.

EMS and Media—Day-to-Day

So far we have talked about dealing with the press on a high level, the rarefied atmosphere of policy set by top management. But the bulk of contact with the media does not take place there. Rather, it is the day-to-day, on-the-scene contact between the beat reporter and the EMT.

Many EMTs, because they may have some power to order people around, will use that power to make life difficult for a reporter or photographer who is only trying to do his job. That same EMT will be the first to complain about any inaccuracies or poor coverage that his own acts may have caused.

Care of the patient must never be compromised, but press requests at the scene that are legal and in no way detrimental should be complied with if at all possible.

It would be foolhardy to say that reporters and photographers never interfere with the work of an EMT at the scene. But such instances are rare. In 37 years—18 of them on both sides of the camera—I have never been interfered with, nor inconvenienced by, media representatives at the scene, and to the best of my knowledge, I have never interfered with care or rescue operations being rendered by others while still getting in very close to obtain dramatic photographs.

An incident such as a multiple vehicle accident or a fire is a public event; the reporter or photographer has just as much right to be there as does the EMT. In general, anything that can be legally witnessed can be photographed for non-commercial purposes. (Whether one feels that the photograph is in good taste or not is immaterial. That decision can only be made by the photographer and his editor.)

Care of the patient must never be compromised, but press requests at the scene that are legal and in no way detrimental should be complied with if at all possible.

Medical details are, of course, privileged information, and requests for this type of information cannot be honored without the patient's permission. For some public agencies, however, this information becomes a matter of public record when recorded on an official run form. Laws on this vary from state to state, but withholding information that is public does nothing but create enemies in the press, which is what we are trying to prevent.

In the event a media representative at the scene is truly a problem, the first obligation is to the patient. The scene is not the place to get into a pushing or shouting match with a reporter or photographer. Protect the patient first. If that means having a policeman physically remove an unruly photographer from your ambulance, do it. But be certain you are legally in the right and that such action is absolutely necessary. If you feel the newsman's conduct and actions are really out of line, discuss it with your supervisor *after* the incident. It's then up to the supervisor, not the EMT, to make an official complaint to the newsman's editor.

I assure you, the editor will take the complaint seriously if it is legitimate. He is just as interested in the public image conveyed by his employees as we are.

Initiate Contact With the Media

One need not wait for an incident to have contact with the press. You can, and should, initiate your own stories.

Both electronic and print media are always on the lookout for good and positive stories. It is only a myth that reporters are only interested in negative ones.

Bad stories are easy to come by: Police are involved in a high-speed chase of a stolen car filled with teenagers. The 15-year-old driver loses control of the car on a patch of ice. It flips and is hit by the police cruiser. Three are dead and six are injured, and the scanner goes off in every newsroom in town. Three TV crews and four still photographers are on the scene by the time the second ambulance arrives.

Of course, it is news.

The public has a right to know what happened, how the public service agencies responded, whether the chase was justified, what social pressures led to this tragedy, and how EMS handled it.

Good stories are harder to come by.

There is no scanner announcing a good deed done by an ordinary citizen. There are no crowds observing daily humanitarian acts of kindness. Editors are always on the lookout for these stories, contrary to what many people believe. These stories usually develop because somebody contacted a reporter.

A lot of good things happen in EMS, but the public will never know about them if the media don't know, and editors will never find out if we don't tell them. If our service receives an award for saving a life, we can't blame the press for the lack of coverage when no one has notified them. No one else will do it for us, so we need to take the initiative.

Taking the initiative, though, doesn't mean that the editor will always agree that we have a story. He doesn't run stories to please us; he runs them for his readers or viewership. He's in a much better position to judge the item's newsworthiness; that's why he is the editor. What may appear to be a good story to us may be seen by him as self-serving publicity puff. Or maybe it's really an advertisement disguised as a news story, and that's an anathema to any editor.

But don't be discouraged if he doesn't pick up on a particular story. The editor appreciates the fact that you thought about him, and he'll remember it. Maybe you'll connect on your next tip. If so, everyone benefits: The editor has a good and positive story, the image of your service is enhanced, and the public has learned more about the EMS system. As a secondary benefit, your credibility with the media is being developed. The more stories you provide, the stronger your link to the media.

Perhaps it is even more important to take the initiative in contacting the media when one of those negative or embarrassing stories develops. Don't duck the issue. Your credibility will leap forward, and, at the least, the public will get the chance to hear or read your side of the story.

On a major story, the press conference approach can be used, not because it is a good approach, but because it may be the most practical in some circumstances. Most editors prefer exclusivity, but pass good stories around anyway. Don't play favorites. You can't have too many friends in the media.

This approach is not buying off the media, just good public relations.

If you are open, honest, and above board, you will establish a number of contacts in the media, and you will have built a bridge of credibility before you have to use it.

Remember, the media are not your enemies. They are the best allies EMS can have.

Source

Reprinted with permission from JEMS, *August 1987. Jerry L. Durnbaugh is a journalist with 42 years of experience. He has been involved with prehospital emergency care for 26 years.*

Courting the Media: How to Gain the Upper Hand

Janet E. Smith, EMT-I

Using the media to tell the EMS story is a skill that enhances an administrator's success. Janet Smith is widely known for developing highly effective media presentations. In this article, she explains key roles and helpful steps for "getting the word out."

SITTING IN THE SPACIOUS LOBBY of the Sheraton Hotel in Baltimore after a two-day meeting on EMS public education and information, I noticed something strange. Across from the lobby was an open-air cocktail lounge. Two televisions flanked the long bar, where about 10 people sat; a few other people sat at tables. Every eye was glued to the TV sets, including the bartender's. No one ordered a drink, no one spoke. They simply watched. I was curious as to what sports event or news expose had them so mesmerized. It was *Rescue: 911.*

The promos for *Rescue: 911* point out that many lives have been saved by people who have used the lifesaving techniques they learn by watching the program. The emergency responses portrayed every week in *Rescue: 911, On Response,* and *9-1-1 Emergency* showcase the noble, caring, and professional expertise of those who practice field medicine. Many of the programs' viewers have never been a patient or a bystander at a medical emergency. By watching these programs, the viewers may well be learning all they will know about EMS until they have to call us.

A good local media relations program can help balance the sensationalism of EMS by entertainment and reality programming with news stories that let the people in your community know that you have anticipated their EMS needs and that you are trained, equipped, and ready to respond to any call for help.

Everyone Has a Role

Administrator

In order to establish a positive working relationship with local media, it is critical to cultivate a rapport with health reporters, assignment editors, and news directors of TV stations, as well as with the city editor's desk at local newspapers and radio stations. While you can't expect the news media to be a cheerleader for you, you can expect to be treated fairly (especially if a good relationship already exists). If you are from a small town or rural area with no local television, it might be necessary to create your own media in the form of a company newsletter designed to reach a broad audience.

EMS administrators must recognize the importance of good media relations and dedicate time, training dollars, and human resources to conducting a comprehensive media relations campaign.

Public Information Officer

A public information officer should be designated and trained to design and implement a public information program so the media will recognize the organization as a credible information source. The PIO and the public relations director (in some cases these individuals may be the same person) should focus on educational and informational news stories as well. The PIO should be dependable, accurate, sensitive to deadlines, honest, and sensible. He should have 24-hour access to the CEO of the company and be ready to respond to any crisis involving the organization in a timely manner.

Communications Center

The communications centers for EMS organizations are hubs for newsworthy incidents and stories. They should be integrally involved in the media relations plan. The PIO should be initially contacted by the communications center early in the emergency when newsworthy events occur so that media contacts can be made. (To ensure a good working relationship, the PIO should establish contacts with the local media before an incident takes place.) The communications center should be prepared to offer the location of the incident, the number of patients involved, the type of injury, and patient destinations.

Field Paramedic

The field paramedic should not be asked to participate in media interviews at the emergency scene. He should tell the media that the PIO will be available to answer any questions regarding the incident. The field paramedic and EMT play a vital role, however, in those news stories generated by the company specifically for the purposes of educating the public about EMS. Paramedics and EMTs should be briefed about the story before the interview. They should be coached as to how to keep interviews positive and then allowed to demonstrate their knowledge and expertise.

Getting Started

If you work for an ambulance service and put "Next Week Is EMS Week" posters all over town, that's advertising. If you put the posters on an ambulance and parade through town, that's promoting EMS. If you have the ambulance paramedics and EMTs visit a recovering victim of cardiac arrest at a hospital, that's a publicity event. If you can get the patient to testify to the value of EMS, that's public relations. And, if you can get the local newspaper to publish the story on page one, that's effective media relations.

Public relations and marketing will play a significant role in the future of EMS. It is through a comprehensive community relations plan that we can bolster the image and reputation of our individual organizations and of the EMS industry as a whole.

A prehospital care organization's community image and reputation depend on its ability to be visible in positive ways. Unfortunately, if we only depend on the limited audience of past users of service, patients,

> Public relations and marketing will play a significant role in the future of EMS.

and bystanders, our ability to communicate with all our potential customers becomes limited.

Publicity

To boost publicity for your organization, try these ideas:

- Send an editor a personal letter about new developments in your organization. This novel format can spark enthusiasm where the traditional news release may appear dull and routine.
- Take a stand on an issue. There are many EMS issues that are hot topics or are just emerging. Position your CEO as an industry leader by promoting a position on a relevant issue.
- Give reporters a free sample of your services. Media ride-alongs or photo essay opportunities are popular with the media. Offer ride-alongs to coincide with EMS Week or other related EMS events.
- Provide color photos for magazines. They add impact to the story and increase its chance for placement.

Writing for the Media

Knowing the rules of the written word and following them are essential to success in working with the media. The reason is simple: The media deal in words. You have to have more than a good story. Your grammar, punctuation, and style play a key role in effectively communicating the story as well. These books can help polish your writing style:

- *American Usage and Style: The Consensus*, by Roy H. Copperud. Van Nostrand Reinhold Co., 135 Southwest 50th Street, New York, N.Y. 10020.
- *How to Write, Speak and Think More Effectively*, by Roudolf Flesch. New American Library, 1633 Broadway, New York, N.Y. 10019.

Writing a Press Release

A simple way to get your message across is with a press release. If your release is clear and well organized, the chances of it being used are greatly increased.

Follow the inverted pyramid style (most important information first), and be sure to include all the facts accurately. The first paragraph should capture and hold the reader's attention. Put the least important information at the end. Take the time to include the names of all people involved. Don't forget the times, places, and dates. A news release should also be presented in an objective manner, avoiding a self-serving tone or exaggerations. Short sentences and paragraphs containing colorful quotes from your agency's personnel make a release easy to understand and

---

Getting the Good Word Out About EMS

- Get to know the media on a friendly basis.
- Position yourself as a news source, not as a news subject (such as when someone criticizes your company or employees).
- Be sensitive to deadlines.
- Don't ask reporters not to publish articles if an interview goes badly.
- Don't ask for approval of a story before it is printed.
- Tell the truth—or nothing.
- Don't go off the record.
- Always return reporters' phone calls.
- Don't expect to bat 1,000.
- Be human. Stilted interviews often lead to boring news stories—be passionate about your role in EMS.

interesting to read. Don't forget to include the name and telephone number of a contact person for more information.

Press releases should be double-spaced, typed on only one side of each page, and limited to two pages (three at the most). Include the word *more* at the bottom of each page except the last; the last page should end in "30" or "###."

The TV Interview

The media and EMS organizations have a mutualistic relationship. It's important to orchestrate and maintain a positive relationship. However, that doesn't give free reign to the media when they want to interview you. You do have to keep them informed, but you also have rights of your own.

As an interviewee, you have the right to know who is interviewing you and whom they represent. After all, the legitimacy of the news organization is as important as the news. Additionally, when being interviewed, it's fine for you to request personal space. If microphones and lights are being thrust in your face, just let the reporter know this is distracting, and he will usually accommodate your request for more space and less glare.

EMS news is often unpredictable. But just because a meeting may be hastily arranged doesn't mean that you and the reporter can't go over some ground rules. If you're not both in total agreement about the tone and what is going to be asked, the interview will not be a positive experience for either of you. Always try to be courteous, but don't misconstrue leniency for courtesy.

If both you and the reporter have agreed that "off-the record" comments will be deleted, you have a right to have that request honored. However, the better rule-of-thumb would be to avoid making off-the-record comments altogether.

Another right you have as an interviewee is the "reasonable time" right. After the important questions have been addressed, don't hesitate to break the interview off. Dragging an interview on after the salient points have been discussed not only wastes time but allows an opportunity for the reporter to ask hypothetical and irrelevant questions.

Good media relations and aggressive strategies to maximize positive media representation are key to any effective communications effort. Visibility in non-medical areas like community service projects and community education initiatives is also a crucial strategy in getting the word out about the good people who work in EMS. By doing a good job and getting credit for it with the help of positive media relations, we can position ourselves in our communities as being vital to the well-being of every citizen.

Source

Reprinted with permission from Emergency, *April 1992. At the time of original publication, Janet Smith was a partner in the public relations and EMS consulting firm On Assignment. She is a former marketing director for Mercy Medical Services in Las Vegas, as well as a past chairperson of the industry image committee for the American Ambulance Association.*

Marketing EMS: Responding to the Marketplace

Michael A. Delaney, MHSL, and Keith Pipes, MHSL

Learning to communicate effectively to a multitude of audiences is central to the success of any marketing program for public and private services. This article profiles how to respond to the marketplace and create a marketing mission.

MARKETERS, MUCH LIKE EMS RESPONDERS, use certain tools and techniques to reach their objectives.

Whether it involves a large corporation or a small regional business, the essence of marketing is determining one's audience, assessing the needs and attitudes of the audience, and then designing one's product or service to match the audience. The key here is to shape the organization's goals to meet the various needs of its various audiences. But does EMS have an audience? The answer is yes—several.

Audiences with common needs who can use your services in a particular way are known as "market segments." Some market segments are easy to define. Acute care hospitals, convalescent facilities, outpatient radiology centers, and walk-in clinics might represent segments attractive to ambulance services. Local EMS authorities might define private ambulance firms, fire departments, emergency departments, and the taxpayer as their primary market segments—those groups to whom one's organization addresses its services—also known as "target audiences."

All too often, when the time comes to communicate to these market segments, organizations fail to recognize that each of these segments is a different audience. They forget that good communicators always consider the listener before they define the message. The same people who would not dream of approaching every extrication rescue in an identical manner are quite content to use the same tools and the same approach to communicate to different audiences. Such information as the opening of a new station, the addition of a non-urgent transfer service, the passage of new regulations, the need for qualified candidates for the new system status management course, or the announcement of a subscription service program is presented to the segment without regard to the attitude or beliefs of the audience.

EMS can borrow the tools of the marketer and devise unique and effective ways to speak to its audiences. It is in this way that EMS professionals can communicate their message to maximize the desired effect.

Understanding the Target Audience

Generally, most audiences want to know the personal benefits associated with the message. For example, an announcement regarding the availability of a new subscription ambulance program should include what it is, who is eligible, how one can enroll, and *why they should*. The last point—perhaps the most critical—is typically omitted from the message.

Features are listed without promoting the *benefits* of the service or program being discussed.

For instance, subscription ambulance services are sold on the basis of a cost savings: no unexpected, large ambulance bill at the time of service. But what if the majority of your audience is not compelled by that argument? Maybe they think their health and lifestyle habits adequately protect them from the need for EMS (that all-too-common denial). Perhaps they view the cost as unnecessary. In this case, the service could avoid wasting precious dollars by focusing on a message that holds stronger appeal for this audience.

This awareness of the target audience—pinpointing what is important or desirable to them—is crucial to the success of any communication. Marketers often go to great lengths to discover these factors, through market research, demographics, and psychographics. The researchers consider age, sex, education, and income *before* they begin to design a communication. They want to know whether the audience is predominantly yuppies, baby boomers, white or blue collar, or retired, or possesses other characteristics that determine how people make their purchases. Remember, know your target audience and communicate information of specific interest to them. The imaginary service used in this example might consider which appeal to use based on which audience motivation is most prevalent.

In our scenario, other reasons to subscribe to an ambulance service should be considered as a topic of the message. Possibilities include the benefits of expanded services, a greater availability to the needy, the advantages of upgrading equipment and training, etc. The actual topic would be determined by audience factors through research.

Motivating the Audience

Audience behavior is the next step. Once knowledge and attitude factors are defined, you can concentrate on motivating the audience. Occasionally, only basic information is necessary to motivate people (here, to subscribe to a particular ambulance service). But if the target audience is not quite sure that the service is right for them, then information that lessens perceived risk can be employed. For instance, testimonials, guarantees, success stories, length of time in service, and certification data all suggest reliability and help create a favorable response.

The message should provide a stimulus for people to act. The action can be anything you wish—to learn more about CPR, support your local EMS system, attend a fundraiser, or vote for laws to protect rescuers and their families. Whatever the message, the stimulus must be believable to the audience.

Turn to the Specialists

So now that you know a little about marketing, how can you go about implementing this new information? Unfortunately, just as with

Source

Reprinted with permission from JEMS, *April 1987. At the time of original publication, Michael A. Delaney was vice president of an advertising agency in Fresno, Calif. He has experience as a paramedic and an ALS instructor-trainer. Keith E. Pipes was the public information/education coordinator for the Central California EMS Agency.*

extrication training, a little bit of knowledge can be dangerous. Technical undertakings are best left to the specialists. A professional advertising agency or marketing consultancy is often the best resource to guide the program or campaign. By looking at the desired objectives, professionals can create a plan that combines marketing tools, advertising opportunities, and public relations efforts that best suit your budget.

By developing a successful strategic plan with key people in your group and then engaging professional services to become involved where appropriate, the EMS leader can make significant progress toward better communication with his audiences. And most marketers will agree that to know how to communicate with one's audience is to know one's audience better. When you really are in touch with your audience, you can *serve* them much better as well.

A Marketing Response Checklist

Perform an Inventory

What does your organization do? What does it do well? What don't you do well? Where does demand for certain services come from? Who does what in your organization? How is your service or organization perceived by your audiences? How do the audiences access your services? Does your catalog of resources—human, capital, and financial—appear adequate for the marketplace and its challenges?

Assess Your Response Zone

What obstacles are you likely to face? Do you have to overcome apathy, disbelief, or a competitor's service? Are alternatives to your service perceived as stronger? Is there a chance for you to provide a needed service better than the alternative? How will you respond to your market? Newspaper, direct mail, or magazine? What's the most cost-efficient approach to reach your identified market segments? How have others tried? Which route was successful and why?

Alert Your Team

Does everyone in your organization know what the plan is? Do they know what services you provide? Has everyone been briefed on goals and objectives?

Do they know the hidden dangers in your marketplace response zone? Have you sought their advice and input as you developed your strategic plan? Are your people a well-informed, cohesive team, prepared to respond to market demand?

Respond to the Challenge

With your fingers on the pulse of the marketplace, can you be proactive? Will you detect shifts in consumer demand and respond before the competition? Will you work now to convey an image that fights the out-of-town megaservice before they move in? Will you develop marketing tools (yes, advertising) that are so distinctive, so commanding, so professional that they can get your team into that most difficult to reach of all places—your audience's minds?

Debrief the Response

Do you critique past marketing missions periodically? How well does your response plan work? Does it still reflect the resources of the team? Were past efforts successful? Were objectives accomplished on time, on budget? Are new response plans formulated to respond to new challenges? How can you update and improve your marketing response plan?

MUCH HAS BEEN WRITTEN about clinical excellence in recent years, and sophisticated mechanisms exist in many EMS systems to ensure that patients receive quality medical care. But patients can receive quality medical care and, at the same time, be "mistreated." This scenario has the net effect of killing the customer relationship even though the patient may survive.

Clinical excellence is a cornerstone of every medical transportation service. However, clinical excellence alone will not sustain an organization's growth. Another important building block is making sure the customer's experience with the organization is as favorable as possible. This is important, not just from the point of view of the patient on the stretcher, but also during dispatch, billing, and every other point at which a customer—or potential customer—comes into contact with the organization.

EMS can learn a lot from other industries. For example, Jan Carlzon, president of Scandinavian Airlines System, used a customer service philosophy to turn an $8 million loss into a $71 million profit. Profits have climbed consistently since Carlzon achieved his goal of redirecting the airline's mission toward service so that customers would see the difference between SAS and other airlines and keep coming back.

Who Is the Customer?

SAS learned that the person flying was not the only customer. Customers also included family members, travel agents, tour representatives, and others who influenced the traveler's decision about which airline to use.

Unfortunately, EMS personnel often view the patient as the only customer. This limited view results in a failure to be attentive to the other customers, including the patient's family, discharge planners, emergency department nurses, hospital floor nurses, nursing home personnel, nursing directors, and fire and police personnel. These individuals are all customers in that they can influence the decision of which service to call. Each of these customers has a different need that can and should be met. It is our responsibility to make sure the services we provide are user friendly.

Public agencies and private services that provide the only service in town sometimes fall into the trap of thinking, "People here can't really choose a service, so this stuff doesn't apply to me." Not so. Increasingly, public services are realizing that they have as many "customers" as private services, including elected officials and managers throughout their local government structure.

How to Avoid Killing the Customer Relationship

Jay Fitch, PhD

The best form of marketing? Positive word-of-mouth accounts of a customer's EMS experience. This article defines who the real customer is and promotes the improvement of customer service.

Killing Customer Relationships

I recently made a long-distance telephone call to schedule transportation to the hospital for an elderly aunt. The person who answered the phone was abrupt. It sounded like things were busy, and I was put on hold several times during the call.

"It is impossible for us to handle her in the next hour unless it's an emergency," he said. "You should have called earlier in the day." It was as if he expected me to feel sorry for the organization because they were busy and had not planned adequate resources to handle the situation.

That experience was in sharp contrast to what happened when I immediately called their competitor—who was equally busy. The person who answered the phone was helpful and understanding. Imagine my surprise when, less than 45 minutes later, someone called me to say that my aunt was at the hospital and resting comfortably.

Which service do you think I called to take her home? The long-distance callback is standard policy for this service when relatives are calling from out of town. They realized the patient was not the only customer and that I, the other customer, needed to be reassured that everything was handled smoothly.

In addition to surly and harried dispatch personnel, dirty units and unkempt personnel also kill relationships with customers. Most social workers, discharge planners, and others responsible for making ambulance arrangements genuinely care for their patients. They would not knowingly make arrangements with an ambulance service that provided substandard service. Some discharge planners even stop by the ED loading area to check the back of a vehicle and see just how clean and well equipped it is. One planner told me about walking alongside a unit and hearing a crew talking about "that old puss bag." Not a good impression.

Failing to make the patient feel pampered and personally important is a common error of many services. Sometimes it's easy to forget that our job is to provide a service and that, once a patient's medical needs are met, we must care for the total person. Although the patient may not be the only customer, our treatment of that person undoubtedly influences how others, including first responders and bystanders, perceive the service.

Failing to recognize or solve the problems of the non-patient customer can also kill customer relationships. For example, response times are often considered critical on emergency assignments. However, successful medical transportation companies have learned that response times are also important in non-emergency patient movements. In these situations, the hospital is another customer.

One example of solving the other customer's problem involved a fire department first responder unit that was having trouble getting supplies, such as cervical collars, back from a hospital. This required sending an engine across town, out of its district, to retrieve materials from the hospital.

An alert EMT suggested that the responding ambulance service resupply first responders with all items used on patients. The service added these items to the patient's invoice and solved the problem with their customer, the fire department.

Making billing procedures as confusing to our clients as Medicare makes them for us is another effective way to kill customer relationships. Do we expect customers to run through our organizational maze to get insurance reimbursements processed? Put yourself in the customer's shoes and imagine someone dispassionately telling you, "I'm sorry, but you'll have to talk to Susie; she handles our Medicare accounts. No, she's not here right now. Why don't you call back this afternoon?"

We should aim to make billing third parties as easy as possible. To meet this goal, the service does not necessarily have to accept assignment. It does mean, however, committing staff to working with patients and others to help resolve the billing process, which is often confusing.

Preventing Unnecessary "Deaths"

All members of the organization have to realize their responsibility for one of the "moments" in the service cycle that make up the customer's total experience with the organization. Carlzon's book, *Moments of Truth*, describes how each interaction a customer has with an SAS employee may be the moment that decides whether the organization will succeed or fail. For airlines, those moments include booking reservations, checking luggage, boarding, in-flight meals, landing, and retrieving luggage.

Ambulance services also have points in the service cycle that represent moments of truth. Consider all the different interaction points your service has on each assignment.

The Service First program, developed by Fitch & Associates Inc. of Kansas City, Mo., has applied this concept to emergency medical services. The program is designed to teach personnel to recognize the needs and expectations of different customers and assume responsibility for the quality of service delivered.

There are five major phases of the service cycle emphasized in the Service First program. Each phase has a number of moments that can be positive or negative.

Call reception. This may be the first point of customer contact. What types of needs do different customers have that can be met at this moment?

Interactions on scene. How is the patient greeted? Are others on the scene treated respectfully and cheerfully? Does the crew move briskly or sluggishly?

Involvement en route. Do crew members engage the patient in meaningful conversation when appropriate, or do they stoically perform their duties in a clinically excellent but service-deficient manner? What about driving skills? Simple courtesies extended by the driver

Source

Reprinted with permission from JEMS, *September 1989.*

will go into the mental report card that your customer keeps on your organization.

Interactions at the destination. What are the patient's and the other customers' needs at this point in the cycle? Are field personnel in touch with how to meet those needs and leave a positive impression?

Post-assignment contacts. Billing and collection personnel sometimes think that the entire business exists just so they can keep track of the books. This is often the point where we turn a cold shoulder to a customer needing our help. What things can the organization do at this point to improve the customer's experience?

Customer relationships are difficult to manage. We interact with patients and other customers at stressful times. To avoid killing the customer relationship during any of the moments of truth, we must become more aware of each point at which the service interacts with a customer and use each one to create a lasting, positive impression.

Not every experience is going to come out right. But if each customer's needs and expectations are understood, the service will score consistently high marks on as many moments as possible.

Interactions with customers usually take place far from management's view. EMS leaders must manage these interactions indirectly by creating customer-oriented organizations, customer-friendly systems, and work environments that support the ideal of putting service first.

Case 2

When Turf Wars Prevail

This case is a real-life example of how EMS operational needs can be overlooked as different agencies fight for turf within a community. This major EMS system was consumed by the energy spent on "who's in charge," rather than on the components necessary to provide excellent, cost-effective service to its citizens. The name of the community has been changed to Middleburg to protect the responsible parties.

System Background and Organization

Middleburg lies in the largest county in the state. The region is populated by less than half a million people and is relatively stable. The EMS system is a county administrative oversight agency established in the mid-1970s. It contracts with five separate municipalities for emergency service. Fourteen fire departments provide first response service, and eight fire departments transport. In addition, five private firms provide non-emergency services. The total system transports almost 50,000 patients per year to nine area hospitals.

The contract between the county and the municipalities contains few performance standards, and county supervision is minimal. Fear and distrust among agencies is common. At times, meetings on system issues degenerate to little more than shouting matches.

System Components

The Communications Center

The primary access point for emergency medical assistance is through the 9-1-1 phone number. Calls from throughout the county are answered at the 9-1-1 communications center in Middleburg. The 9-1-1 personnel are not trained in medical dispatch, but procedurally question callers in detail and enter information into the database. This public safety answering point (PSAP) then notifies EMS communications and the first responder agency of an assignment via computer. In some areas of the county, the information is transmitted to the county sheriff's communication center, which then notifies the first responder agency's dispatch. The system design and procedures require that calling parties be asked detailed medical questions. The 9-1-1 answering procedures consume valuable time and often aggravate callers when the same questions are repeated by the EMS communications center. Typically, information is transmitted to other agencies via computer.

The EMS communications center provides a "live" call-screening function for calls referred by the 9-1-1 center. This center provides direct dispatch service for some squads and medical channel assignment for all units in the county.

Personnel assigned to the communications center complete a locally developed medical dispatch training program, which is not consistent with current nationally accepted standards. Little in-service education or recertification, and few retrospective medical audits have been provided for these personnel in recent years. Supervision of the EMS communications function has become highly specialized in the past seven to 10 years, but the county system has not kept pace.

EMS communications phone lines and radio transmissions are recorded and kept on file for approximately 90 days. Neither first responder nor private service communications are part of this recorded data. The communications center receives approximately 36,000 requests for EMS per year, resulting in 17,500 annual dispatches. Other private provider communications centers handle the remaining dispatches. A minimum of two operators are on duty at all times with the capability to staff three console positions.

Many services within the county are not pleased with 9-1-1 and routinely instruct callers to dial their seven-digit number direct for emergency assistance. Assignments entering the system this way are then reported to the communications center as they are independently dispatched. There is no way to verify the actual call reception or the possible delays for patients entering the EMS system in this manner.

Figure 2.9 illustrates the flow of information and the multiple patient care handoffs that often occur in this system.

First Responders

The various fire departments located in the county provide medical first responder resources. Medical first responders are trained and have supplies to stabilize and provide initial treatment to patients prior to the arrival of the ambulance. The level of training for these agencies varies from basic first responder (similar to first aid training) to EMT-A to EMT-P. There currently is no state-enabling legislation to permit (non-EMT) first responders to defibrillate.

Procedures for first response vary widely throughout the county. Some departments send fire engines, others use mini-pumpers, and still others use paramedic-equipped ambulances as first response units. First responders are sent to almost all medical emergencies. In many instances, these personnel are sent to check out the problem and determine if a paramedic unit is needed. This practice has significantly delayed care in some instances and has resulted in inappropriate decisions being made by non-paramedic personnel. First response to all emergencies significantly impacts the resources available for fire suppression in some communities, particularly in suburban departments.

Response Times

The county contractors and first responders report their response time performance in terms of the average time it takes for units to arrive on the scene after they are dispatched. There are no current measurements of, or standards for, first responder or ambulance response time performance on a countywide basis. No ongoing external measurement or response time monitoring occurs. Key response time components are not measured either.

Measured on an eight-minute/90-percent-compliance fractile basis, the system complies 60.4 percent of the time. From the patient's perspective, response times and transport times are elongated due to the handoffs between caregivers and the secondary response times. This occurs for most patients.

Deployment, Transport Policy, and Utilization

The county agency uses a fixed deployment strategy. In other words, ambulances are located at specific locations rather than in gen-

Middleburg EMS System Flow of Information and Handoffs

Figure 2.9

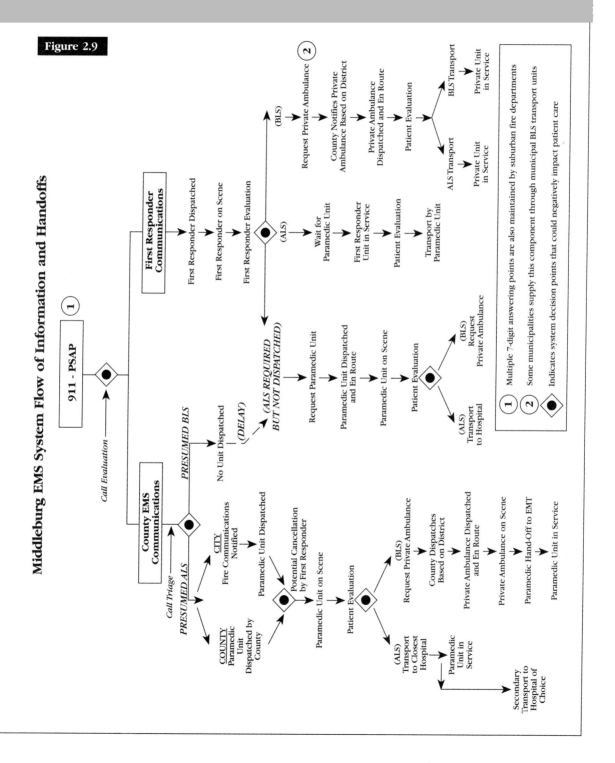

eral areas. They are staffed on a 24-hour basis. Although paramedics report being overworked, the system-wide unit hour utilization is 0.09.

The communications center does not track or control the location of units within the county. Therefore, it is impossible for the center to routinely move and relocate available units for better area coverage.

County policy requires that EMS units transport emergency patients to the closest hospital despite the fact that almost all hospitals are within a 15-minute transport time. Patients are often transferred to their hospital of choice by private services following evaluation. Non-emergent patients are referred to private ambulances. In areas with no private service, municipal BLS units handle transport.

Medical Direction

Medical direction for county units is provided by the Board of Medical Control. It is an advisory group to the system's medical director. This group includes representatives of the hospitals in the community. Each member is board certified in emergency medicine. There is no local legislative mandate that governs this group's functions.

Some first responder agencies and private services have their own medical control physicians. There is no formal requirement for these individuals to be involved with the county's board or to follow established guidelines.

Area hospitals provide radio communication between advanced life support personnel and physicians during an incident. In practice, a nurse relays most instructions. Written standing orders, procedures a field medic may undertake before contacting a base hospital physician, exist but are not presented in a ready reference format. Physicians are not required to have any base station physician training. Medics give inconsistent radio assess-

ments. Generally, radio communication is more of a reporting function to satisfy procedures rather than a strong tool for interactive medical control.

Retrospective analysis occurs on an anecdotal basis rather than on a systemic one, a frustrating process for the medical director. Patient care patterns exist that demonstrate inconsistency in the clinical performance of field personnel. The care given is provider- and hospital-specific.

Each provider agency follows its own set of review procedures. Generous latitude in interpretation and oversight is allowed between hospitals and the paramedics. Medical policies must be communicated through a number of administrative levels within each operation. Medical direction has been hampered by the lack of legal authority to control all medical aspects of the system and by the lack of cooperation of non-county services.

Case Questions

1. Describe the different ways a call screening system similar to the one used in Middleburg negatively impacts patient outcome?
2. What system decision points in Figure 2.9 could be eliminated without changing the system design?
3. What actions could you take to facilitate improvements with this system if you were the county administrator? A fire chief responsible for first response? A private ambulance owner?
4. How is the medical director's authority limited in this system? What mechanisms could be employed to improve quality assurance processes?
5. Outline major litigation and risk management concerns regarding EMS operations as described in this case.

Part Three

Financial Issues

Adversity is often the window of opportunity for change. Few people or organizations want to change when there is prosperity and peace. Major changes are often precipitated by adversity.

—Leif Anderson

Prosperity has eluded many EMS organizations in recent years. Instead, financial adversity has created major opportunities for change. Shrinking tax resources, coupled with expanding service demands, have squeezed the life out of some systems while prompting others to find new ways to accomplish more with fewer resources.

Whether your organization is financially prosperous or suffering from financial adversity, the articles in Part Three will help you develop skills necessary to be effective. Specific sections address understanding your costs and budgets, dealing with the billing and collection process, managing financial issues at home and work, and identifying funding alternatives.

—Jay Fitch

Part Three Contents

Understanding System Costs and the Budget Process

The Cost of Excellence

Edward A. Rose,
BS, MBA

As the saying goes, "There is no free lunch." In this article, EMS administrator Ed Rose describes two ways of paying for quality in EMS, and why the obvious way may not be the best way.

WE JUST FINISHED OUR ANNUAL budget ritual and found that our employee incentives in Richmond, Va., had worked exceedingly well. These incentives encouraged our field and communications personnel to advance to paramedic-level training and certification from more basic levels.

The employee mix of emergency medical technicians, cardiac technicians, and paramedics was far different than we had anticipated. Because it was skewed in favor of more paramedic personnel, we wound up with a $108,000 problem for our fiscal year '93-'94—more salary than budget. When we had worked out our proposal for Richmond three years earlier, we had made certain assumptions about employee certification and related compensation. We were wrong, but in a way our "mistake" should have yielded a higher quality of care to the patient. Our staff is almost all advanced life support-trained now and care should be better, right? Well, the jury is still out, and that question won't be answered in this article. Yet we tend to believe that higher-trained individuals yield better care.

In his book *Quality is Free*, well-known quality expert Philip B. Crosby asserts, "Quality is free. It's not a gift, but it is free. What cost money are the unquality things—all the actions that involve not doing jobs right the first time." Crosby goes on to ask that if you don't measure quality, how can you know whether it is free or not? Our organization measures quality in terms of processes and outcomes. It is part of everyone's job to find ways to fund quality.

Measuring Quality

One point not in dispute was that our cost to achieve what we perceived as quality was not free. So we confronted the age-old argument of trying to balance quality and cost.

Many people in our industry will suggest that you can't really measure quality until you measure specific outcomes. Some outcomes may include

- Percent of patients who have a return of spontaneous circulation (ROSC) in the prehospital setting
- Percent of success in endotracheal intubation
- Percent of success in intravenous sticks
- Effectiveness in delivering prehospital care in eight minutes or less with at least 90-percent reliability

It is important that quality be determined by a standard measure in every EMS system. That measure is set by the medical community and the system's medical director, whose license the system operates under.

While outcome research is still under way, we can all recognize the characteristics of quality based on our own experiences. The profile of a quality EMS organization is one that

- Continuously pursues clinical excellence
- Is held to and meets the system's standards of care
- Meets and exceeds the measures of response time performance and reliability

Sources of Funds

Even before the research is in, we must all pursue quality and excellence. But we also need to find ways to finance it. Just discussing costs would not be very helpful. We must also talk about where money comes from to fund a business, and thus fund quality.

In a privately owned ambulance service, there are only four sources of funds.

- Shareholder funds—money the owner puts in directly
- Loans—from the bank or an uncle
- Retained earnings—the difference between income and expenses (the plan works best when you have more income than expenses)
- Depreciation—recognizes that equipment costs can be accelerated for tax purposes, and thus considered an expense without the corresponding use of cash (the accountants will scream at this explanation)

Funding Quality by Cutting Expenses

Now back to the conflict between quality being free and our $108,000 problem. It was clear that we were heading in the direction toward quality at a much more rapid pace than we first estimated.

Rather than slow down our progress, or even run from it, we sought to find ways to fund it. The only real options to fund the difference were decisions about whether to increase rates or decrease operating costs. As we will discuss later in this article, an increase in rates is almost always the most inefficient means of raising money, so we chose to look toward reducing expenses.

First and foremost, labor expenses are the largest single cost item in our business. We examined shifts and productivity to determine if the company was as efficient as other companies were in similar circumstances. This is called benchmarking. You may find that your colleague's service is more efficient, boasting a better unit hour utilization (UHU) rate than your firm. If that's true, look at what a small improvement could mean in your organization. If a company has a unit hour utilization ratio of, say 0.33 (approximately three hours of coverage per patient transport), what would be the economic benefit of improving productivity to 0.40? This is an easier statement to make than the results are to produce. But the math is very instructive.

For example, if the marginal cost of a unit hour is $40 (remember, we are only adding unit hours, not overhead, new units, etc.) and we are spending three hours of coverage per patient transport, the marginal cost per patient would be $120. Compare that with a 0.40 UHU, or 2.5 hours per patient transport, and your marginal cost would amount to $100 per patient—a labor savings of $20 per patient. Remember that a better unit hour utilization can be realized by more accurately matching patterns staffing to meet variable demand. Your firm may find it easier to maintain five 24-hour units, even though you know that demand is not constant. You must examine these areas thoroughly if you are trying to free up funds to support quality.

While we looked at labor costs first, there are other costs to review, including equipment replacement and upgrade, vehicle replacement and upgrade, and scheduling. We were surprised when we assessed our current monitor/defibrillator and found we could upgrade to a new model with more state-of-the-art technology and save money. How? While the residual value (trade-in) was high, the repair and maintenance costs on this same unit were also high. We also needed to retrofit the existing units for continuing service. In addition, the vendor was anxious to complete a sale. Thus, we parlayed a low cost of capital less than the prime rate, low cost of service covered under a service agreement for the life of the product, and discounts for quantity into a net annual savings and an

Table 3.1

Defibrillator Assessment

Item	CF	6% Factor	Present Value
Buy new defibrillator	($8,000)	1	($8,000)
Salvage old defibrillator	$2,000	1	$2,000
Annual operating costs	($500)	3.4651	($1,733)
Value in four years	$3,000	0.79	$2,370
Present value of net cash flows			($5,363)
Keep defibrillator (now five years old)			
Refurbish now	($3,000)	1	($3,000)
Annual operating costs	($800)	3.4651	($2,772)
Value in four years	$500	0.79	$395
Present value of net cash flows			($5,377)

improvement in our clinical capability. See Table 3.1 for the economic explanation.

While the savings ($14) are very small, the example does illustrate a point about how current technology can, in fact, be less costly than old equipment. This same approach is used to determine if a company would be better off financially by holding onto aging ambulances or trading them in. You can also determine where in this continuum the costs to keep an aging fleet become greater. The same assessment can be made comparing Type II and Type III ambulances. The accountants refer to this type of cost matrix as the Least Cost Approach.

These are a few ways to fund the $108,000 payroll deficiency. Or you could add new equipment and technologies, and increase benefits and salaries. Now review the wisdom of raising rates.

Increasing Rates

Understand that the results of rate increases, while easier to implement than cost savings, diminish as the rates go higher. For instance, depending on your payer mix (the number of Medicaid, Medicare, and private pay patients), a price increase of $10 may only result in revenue from the private pay patient, as your collection from Medicare and Medicaid may be capped. So, you have huge bills drawing in only a fraction of the money needed.

A municipality recently approached our service and wanted to lower its subsidy payments. The company was able to demonstrate that for every $10 of increased rates, only 20 percent of the total charges were collectible. This, would result in a collection effort that yielded $2 for every $10 billed to patients.

You will not be successful in upgrading your organization if you only look at charging more for services. The most powerful dollars for clinical excellence are those currently in your possession. Evaluate your internal cost controls before seeking external funding from patients or municipalities. If you don't control your own costs, there are many people out there who will make these management decisions for you.

Source

Original article. Ed Rose is the chief operating officer of Mercy Services, Inc., in Grand Rapids, Mich., a subsidiary of Laidlaw Medical Transportation, Inc.

References

Brigham, E. F., and L. C. Gapenski. *Intermediate Financial Management*. 2nd ed. Chicago: The Dryden Press, 1987.

Crosby, P. B. *Quality Is Free*. New York: Mentor, 1980.

Public/Private Partnership Committee, American Ambulance Association. *AAA Contracting Guidelines*. Sacramento, Calif.: American Ambulance Association, 1994.

The EMS Subsidy/Price Tradeoff

Jack Stout

There is a complex relationship between the amount of subsidy and the fees charged for services. In this article from 1988, which the author has updated for this publication, former EMS consultant Jack Stout describes a method communities can use when comparing the mix of fees and subsidies.

DURING A COFFEE BREAK, someone asked the question, "What is the most practical tip you can give us—something we can take back home and use right away?" I was conducting a management workshop for members of the Michigan Ambulance Association, probably boring them to death with the endless details that distinguish high-performance EMS systems from run-of-the-mill operations. The question was a good one. The answer is the subject of this article—the best management "trick of the trade" I've stumbled across this year.

In the past, I've struggled with trying to explain to elected officials the relationship between EMS subsidies and EMS prices. On first thought, the solution seems simple—when subsidies go down, prices go up. And, in general, that's true. The difficulty comes in trying to explain how a given price structure will actually be affected by a change in level of local tax support. Until a few months ago, I had never quite succeeded in developing an easily understood way of displaying the subsidy/price tradeoff. Now I've got it, and you can use it, too.

Why It's So Important

There are two good reasons to regularly remind local elected officials and the local press of the relationship between EMS subsidies and EMS prices. The first is to protect against unfair and uninformed criticism. For example, during recent mayoral elections in a city served by one of our industry's most cost-effective EMS systems, a candidate suggested the public would benefit by a government takeover of EMS operations. With government takeover and an annual subsidy of only $2 million, user fees could be lowered by 50 percent, according to the candidate.

The numbers weren't wrong. They should, however, have raised another question. Since the privately operated system was receiving no subsidy at all, and its entire annual budget (funded from fee-for-service income) was only $2.5 million, shouldn't a $2 million subsidy injection produce considerably more than a 50-percent drop in user fees? The truth is that a $2 million subsidy of the privately operated system would produce approximately an *85-percent reduction in rates,* not the 50 percent promised for the government takeover. Put another way, $2 million in subsidy plus 50 percent of the current system's fee-for-service income would fund new system costs three-quarters of a million dollars *higher* than the total cost of the privately operated system. For what purpose would the windfall funding be used?

The privately operated, all-ALS, full-service system had been operating for years at levels of productivity nearly triple those typical of government-operated services. The quality of clinical performance and response-time reliability was literally second to none on the national scale, with well-above-average wages and benefits. The system was clearly a public service bargain, but its managers had neglected to periodically make clear that its rates were high because the subsidy was low—not because the system was inefficient.

In EMS systems serving multiple jurisdictions, offering a range of subsidy/price options to each jurisdiction eliminates the need for uniform subsidy levels among participating jurisdictions. That is, affluent communities able to afford high subsidy levels can opt for a higher subsidy/price ratio. At the same time and within the same EMS system, less affluent communities can obtain identical service simply by selecting a lower subsidy/price ratio. Neither jurisdiction is subsidizing the other, but both communities benefit from the improved economies of scale by creating a single larger system.

> In EMS systems serving multiple jurisdictions, offering a range of subsidy/price options to each jurisdiction eliminates the need for uniform subsidy levels among participating jurisdictions.

Presenting the Choices

For years I've tried to display these relationships and to present the funding policy options by a variety of methods, none completely satisfactory. The solution came when I was working on converting the MedStar system in Fort Worth, Tex., into what will eventually become a countywide system.

Our firm originally developed the MedStar system to serve the city of Fort Worth. After its first two years of operation, a favorable editorial in the Fort Worth *Star-Telegram* called for the expansion of MedStar to a countywide service area. (In addition to the city of Fort Worth, the MedStar system currently serves nine neighboring municipalities.)

To facilitate multi-jurisdictional financing, the decision was made to convert the system from the "failsafe franchise model" to the more flexible and more stable "public utility model" structure. However, the problem of displaying the subsidy/price tradeoff again reared its head; annual subsidies among the various jurisdictions ranged from zero to just over $3 per capita per year. We had to find a better way to display and explain the funding choices available under the expanded MedStar system. The "uniform subsidy/price option schedule" furnished the solution.

To establish the expanded system, we converted Fort Worth's Ambulance Authority into a multi-jurisdictional legal entity by way of an "interlocal cooperation agreement." (Every state has passed some form of an interlocal cooperation act allowing these local partnerships.) Next, we converted the business structure to a public utility model form and developed a "uniform EMS ordinance" to ensure uniform quality of care throughout the MedStar service area.

The final step was to offer opportunity for membership to the various jurisdictions. To join the MedStar system, each local government had to approve the interlocal cooperation agreement, adopt the uniform EMS ordinance, and choose a funding method from the uniform subsidy price/ option schedule.

For example, the city of Fort Worth currently chooses to subsidize ambulance service at the rate of $4.15 per capita per year, while the other nine participating municipalities provide subsidy at the rate of $3 per capita per year. The line shown on the subsidy/price tradeoff chart (Figure 3.1) identifies every combination of subsidy level and user-fee charge that is capable of generating the $10,153,888 needed to fund the MedStar operation. So long as every jurisdiction chooses a combination of subsidy and price that rests on the subsidy/price tradeoff line, MedStar will be financially stable, and no jurisdiction will be inadvertently subsidizing (via excessive user fees or tax contributions) services rendered in another jurisdiction.

Thus, to avoid cross-jurisdictional subsidization of services, MedStar's total average bill for transports originating within the city of Fort Worth (currently subsidizing at $4.15 per capita per year) should be $485.91. Given the quality of service provided by MedStar, the comparatively low Medicare reimbursement rates in the region (because the Medicare "prevailing rate" in Texas is dominated by an unusually high percentage of heavily subsidized government providers billing at rates far below their costs, MedStar's "allowable charge" is well below the actual cost of the most efficient providers), a Medicaid program limited in both eligibility and payment, and a high percentage of medically indigent patients, MedStar's current subsidy/price tradeoff line is extremely competitive.

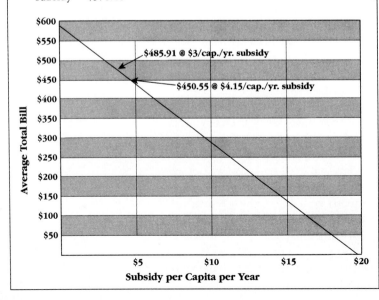

Figure 3.1

MedStar's Subsidy/Price Tradeoff—1994

Level of service: All-ALS full-service with 90-percent eight-minute standard on life-threatening calls; all advanced certifications required; dispatch by EMD/SSM-trained paramedics

Service area population (exclusive) = 539,933

Number of cities served = 10

Annual patient transport volume = 43,581

Total annual cost of ambulance services (including depreciation) = $10,153,888

Actual cost per patient transport = $233

Collection rate (unadjusted for contractual allowances, but including membership sales) = 40.3 percent

Average bill reduction per $1 subsidy per capita = $30.75

Per-capita subsidy required to fund annual system costs at zero user fees = $18.80

Total average bill required to fund total system costs at zero subsidy = $578.16

$485.91 @ $3/cap./yr. subsidy

$450.55 @ $4.15/cap./yr. subsidy

Average Total Bill

Subsidy per Capita per Year

Building Your Own Subsidy/Price Schedule

The subsidy/price matrix is the same for every system. However, where the option line actually appears on the matrix and the option line's slope depend on several factors. If your system is small, you may not enjoy the economies of scale that occur in larger systems. If that is the case, the entire option line may be elevated (i.e., more expensive across the board). On the other hand, in larger systems, better economies of scale should allow the option line to be lower (i.e., cheaper).

Lower standards of care or less stringent response time standards should obviously result in a drop in the subsidy/price option line. Less capable management and less efficient production strategies (e.g., multi-tiered systems and other forms of specialized production strategy) will, of course, raise the option line. For many heavily subsidized urban systems using specialized production strategies, the zero-subsidy rate will easily approach $1,500 per patient transport.

Potential collection rates affect the slope of the option line. That is,

---

Figure 3.2

Formula for Finding Maximum Average Bill at Zero Subsidy

Line 1. Current total average bill = Gross user-fee revenues billed ÷ Total patient transports
Line 2. Net revenues from user fees = Gross user-fee revenues bill x Collection rate percentage (unadjusted for contractual allowances, etc.)
Line 3. Per capita subsidy required to reduce user fees to zero = (Net revenues from user fees + Current total subsidy) ÷ Primary service area population
Line 4. Value of user-fee reduction per $1 subsidy per capita per year = Current total average bill ÷ (Line 3 - Current subsidy per capita per year)
Line 5. Maximum average bill at zero subsidy = Line 4 x Line 3

To plot subsidy/price tradeoff line on chart, proceed as follows:
(subsidy/price tradeoff line slopes from upper left to lower right, forming a right triangle)

Max. Average Bill

Local Tax Subsidy per Capita per Year

Step 1. Plot Line 3 result on the horizontal axis.
Step 2. Plot Line 5 result on the vertical axis.
Step 3. Connect the two points to create the subsidy/price tradeoff line.

Check for accuracy: Plot the intersection of the current total average bill and the current per capita per year local tax subsidy. It should be on the subsidy/price tradeoff line.

at higher levels of subsidy, losses from uncollectibles have little influence on user-fee structures. As the percentage of funding from subsidy increases, collection potential increasingly impacts the option line slope. For example, at a 50-percent unadjusted collection rate, for every $1 drop in level of subsidy, $2 must be generated in additional fee-for-service billing. In contrast, at an unadjusted collection rate of 70 percent, the required increase in receivables generated is only $1.43 for each subsidy dollar lost. Thus, the optional line slope is easier to climb where collection rates are better.

Many factors affect collection potential, e.g., prevailing Medicare rates, Medicaid payment levels and eligibility policies, the local economy, and the effectiveness with which accounts receivable is managed. In the Fort Worth area, collection potential is well below average; thus, the option line slope is comparatively steep. Fort Worth's local economy is depressed by the decline in oil prices and related factors, and a provision in the Texas Constitution makes bad debt collection particularly difficult. Thus, in most EMS markets, less slope is required than in MedStar's environment. (For example, the subsidy/price option line for the ambulance system we developed for Pinellas County, Fla., enjoys a gentle slope, starting at about $210 at the zero-subsidy level.)

Warning!

When applying this method in the real world of rate regulation, four dangers should be avoided.

Cash flow lag. For several reasons, a reduction in subsidy produces an instant reduction in cash receipts, but the corresponding increase in user fees generates a painfully slow increase in monthly net revenues that will not realize its full dollar value for approximately 18 months. For example, Medicare reimbursement is limited to the provider's "customary" charge over a 12-month period ending more than six months ago. Thus, the effective date of a subsidy reduction should not be less than nine months—and preferably 12 months—after the effective date of the corresponding rate adjustment.

Collection elasticity of prices. The medium-range (i.e., one to three years) collection rate on the incremental portion of a rate increase will always be less than the historical collection rate related to the original charge. For example, if the historical collection rate on a $400 average bill has been 60 percent (unadjusted), it would be unrealistic to expect that a $100 increase will produce a $60 increase in cash. There is not space here to describe the process used to estimate incremental collection rates over time, except to say that failure to adjust for this factor may result in serious financial problems, which will only become apparent several months after the opportunity to correct such problems without subsidy has passed. (Viewed on a short-run basis, the subsidy/price tradeoff line is actually a curved line whose slope looks something like a ski jump with its top at the left of the chart.)

Get real Where faulty system designs and/or poor management create economically inefficient operations, the adjusted zero-subsidy user-fee level routinely exceeds $1,500. As one might expect, financial life support for these systems is universally sustained by annual injections of local tax support in the range of $10 to $20 per capita per year and more. Such systems obviously cannot be made self-sufficient simply by adjusting the price to the zero-subsidy level. Someone is bound to notice.

Negative subsidy. Where an ambulance service provider is required to furnish training services or replacement supplies for first responders, or required to pay a franchise fee or license fee as a condition of the award of market rights, the horizontal axis of the subsidy/price tradeoff should be extended to the left, i.e., beyond the intersection of the vertical axis. Such arrangements may violate federal anti-kickback laws and regulations, with possible felony implications for both government officials and the contractor involved. To the extent such arrangements are legal, their financial effect should be reflected on the subsidy/price chart.

Comparisons Are Revealing

Now that you understand the relationship between EMS subsidies and EMS prices, you might wish to develop a subsidy/price option schedule for your own paramedic service. Remember to base calculations only on frequency of patient transport—not calls. But be prepared for a shock, and keep the shredder handy.

Source

Reprinted with permission from JEMS, *August 1988. Jack Stout is an advisor to the Business Council at Med Trans. For 25 years, he was president of The Fourth Party, an EMS consulting firm that designs and implements EMS systems.*

The EMS Budget Process

Rodney Dreifuss, MPA, EMT

Underestimating expenses and overestimating revenues can significantly shorten the professional life expectancy of an EMS administrator. This article reviews budget basics and outlines the budgeting process used in a major U.S. city to illustrate how budgeting can be both a planning and a control mechanism.

F REQUENTLY I AM ASKED the question, "What is the hardest part of your job?" When I respond that the most challenging aspect of being an EMS manager—and what gives me the most headaches—is the personnel management of EMTs and paramedics, most people are surprised. Inevitably, the next question is, "What about the budget?" I usually respond, "It's really not that bad."

This article provides an overview of the budget process, fixed and variable costs, and ways to justify your budget. It is intended for those EMS professionals who feel a shiver up their spine when asked to participate in the budgeting process.

Budget Basics

A budget is a financial action plan that results in the appropriate planning and control of an EMS system. It is the framework for objectives, plans, and policies for the department. A budget provides a reference for evaluating financial performance and, when used properly, can be a tool for cost control and financial awareness. The EMS manager must continually monitor the budget in order to prevent inappropriate variances.

Budgeting develops goals and objectives that are realistic and obtainable in relation to an EMS department's expenditures and revenues. However, without a financial commitment from the governing body and administration, a budget is just a piece of paper.

The budget is most often prepared for a one-year period, which is referred to as the budget year or fiscal year. Many organizations use a calendar fiscal year, but often a fiscal year begins and ends in the middle of a calendar year, such as July 1, 1992, through June 30, 1993. This would be referred to as FY 92/93.

There are different types of budgets or budget philosophies. The most common type is a line-item or objective-based budget, which is an offshoot of the management by objectives (MBO) philosophy of business management. The line-item budget is developed in relation to the department's operational and financial objectives and predicted revenues and expenditures based on previous years. Each financial component of a department is assigned a budget number or function and is allocated funding predetermined through the budgeting process. These components are often broken down into broad categories such as personnel or employee costs, other-than-personnel costs (OTPC), and fixed payments.

Program budgeting is similar to line-item/objective-based budgeting, but the budgeting components are grouped into programs. For example, an emergency medical service would have an emergency response program that would include costs for the EMTs and paramedics, medical supplies and equipment, fuel for the vehicles, and other costs directly related to emergency responses. Another program would be administration, which would include costs for the management, support, and training staffs, office supplies, training material, rent payments or mortgages, leases on office equipment, and insurance. Other programs in an EMS program budget might be communications and support/ancillary services.

Zero-based budgeting is a budgeting philosophy not commonly used in the healthcare field. A zero-based budget does not consider expenses until the very end of the budget process. In zero-based budgeting, objectives are based on the level or quality of service that the organization will strive to achieve in the next fiscal year. Each department prepares a "decision package" that defines each current or proposed function or activity. The decision package identifies resources and personnel needed to perform the activity and reviews the benefits of the function, but does *not* include required funding. The agency administrators then review the decision packages from the various departments and prioritize each proposed activity for the next fiscal year. When prioritizing is complete, funding is allocated. For those functions deemed low priority, funding may not be available. Zero-based budgeting takes a lot of effort and is often difficult and time-consuming to implement.

The Budgeting Process

The following budgeting process review will examine the most common type of budget used in emergency medical services, the line-item budget. Obviously, the budget process will vary from service to service depending on the type of EMS provider. For instance, tax-supported municipal services often do not include the "indirect" costs that a private service may incur, i.e., rent, utilities, insurance (vehicle and professional), facilities maintenance, depreciation/amortization, entertainment, taxes, professional services (legal, accounting, payroll), printing, etc.

In a municipal EMS, many of these services are paid for or provided by the municipality. When assessing the monetary responsibility delegated to a public sector EMS manager, an additional 15 percent of the operating budget typically must be calculated for these indirect costs. This is because it is the EMS administration's role to ensure that the services and funding provided by the municipality are used appropriately. For example, here is the FY 92/93 St. Louis EMS budget:

Operating budget	$4,815,571
Indirect costs	722,336
EMS billing department budget	350,000
Capital budget	200,000
TOTAL	**$6,087,907**

Besides financial information, the EMS manager needs to review call volume, salary benefits, and maintenance costs when preparing a budget.

Because many EMS systems are not publicly funded, the budget process will be reviewed in a generic manner.

Budget requests or proposals are prepared by using previous experiences while also developing objectives for the future. Besides financial information, the EMS manager needs to review call volume, salary benefits, and maintenance costs when preparing a budget. The heart of the budget process is the budget request or proposal. The approved or modified budget request will eventually become your annual budget. Usually, a separate budget request/proposal is prepared for the operating and capital budgets.

The operating budget consists of all expenses and revenues required for the efficient (profitable) operation of the service. The operating budget includes personnel costs, all supplies and materials, contractual services, and payments (leases, rent, etc.). The four components of an operating budget proposal are

- A review of previous fiscal year expenses and revenues
- Current fiscal year appropriation
- The anticipated expenses for the coming fiscal year
- Incoming revenue predictions

The capital budget is an itemized listing of the major equipment purchases anticipated for the next fiscal year. Capital equipment is often financed instead of paid for outright. It usually depreciates over a predetermined life expectancy. The annual capital budget is generally separate from the operating budget because capital purchases are not repetitive and often very expensive. Included in an EMS capital budget would be rolling stock, medical equipment (portable monitors/defibrillators, pulse oxymeters, etc.), two-way radio equipment, and office equipment. Many departments have a five-year capital projection that includes the annual replacement of ambulances and other rolling stock.

Fixed and Variable Costs

When preparing a budget, all expenses, fixed and variable, must be included. Fixed costs can be divided into committed fixed costs and discretionary fixed costs. Committed fixed costs are those that will exist even if the service ceases operations. These costs would be related to long-term debt payments, certain lease payments, mandated employee pensions, and funds due on non-cancelable contracts. Discretionary fixed costs are costs that the service has chosen to become fixed costs. They can be reduced, increased, or even eliminated. Examples of discretionary fixed costs are payroll, insurance, non-mandated fringe benefits, and cancelable leases.

Variable expenses are more easily controlled by the EMS manager in relation to the quantity and quality of service. Variable expenses include medical supplies, overtime compensation, motor vehicle repairs, etc. While in theory a cost may be variable in the EMS world, in actuality many expenses are constant, or even increase, from year to year. Examples of these so-called variable costs are vehicle maintenance and vehicle repairs. While the EMS manager has control over the servicing and parts purchases for vehicles, keeping the ambulances mechanically sound and in adherence to standards is a necessary and ongoing requirement.

When preparing an EMS budget, as with almost any budget in a service industry, the most expensive line items will be those related to personnel costs. These include salaries, employer-paid medical insurance and benefits, worker's compensation/disability, and overtime. Personnel costs in municipal services range from 70 to 80 percent of the operating budget. Therefore, when developing a budget proposal, anticipating changes in the personnel management of the organization is imperative. Such changes include cost-of-living increases and salary increases based on performance. Other considerations include additions, deletions, and promotions in the organizational table based on departmental activity and efficient human resource allocation.

The remainder of the operating budget, the other-than-personnel costs or OTPC, has a much smaller impact on the bottom line of your proposed operating budget. Remember that major purchases such as vehicles, expensive medical equipment, and office equipment are included in a separate capital budget. In services where call volume, staffing patterns, and OTPC expenses remain basically unchanged from year to year, your budget, nevertheless will increase. This increase is mostly due to personnel expenses related to cost-of-living or merit raises and increases in employer-provided benefits.

Regarding benefits, an EMS manager should add 20 to 30 percent to each full time employee's (FTE) annual salary to approximately calculate employer-sponsored benefits. Because personnel costs are such a large portion of an EMS budget, a separate, itemized table of organization is usually included as a supplement to a budget request. This itemized personnel roster includes each title or job classification within the service, the number of employees in each job classification, and the resulting expected expenses. Benefits can be calculated in this section, but it is usually easier to itemize benefits separately under a specific account designation, i.e., worker's compensation, life insurance, etc.

When an EMS manager is told to keep expenses at the same bottom line as the previous year, it actually means a reduction of one or more departmental components because of annual increases in personnel costs and probable increases in OTPC accounts. When revenue predictions are down, EMS managers must often develop an operating budget reduced by a predetermined amount or percentage.

In the event an EMS manager is asked to actually reduce expenditures from the previous year, there most likely will be a resulting decrease in the level of service, which may include layoffs or unfilled vacancies through attrition. Decreases in the level of service due to reduced funding for the overall system is almost always a direct effect of reduced staffing. Because personnel costs are the largest single line item of the operating budget, reducing personnel services is really the only

> When preparing an EMS budget, as with almost any budget in a service industry, the most expensive line items will be those related to personnel costs.

effective means of significantly reducing expenses. OTPC can also be reduced. However, most OTPC accounts are essential for the service operations and can only be marginally cut. Remember, OTPC is only about 20 percent of your EMS operating budget.

Contingency Plans

Inevitably, the EMS manager will be requested to prepare contingency plans outlining proposed budget reduction initiatives and the resulting effects on the level of service. These plans are usually based on reduced personnel deployment and must take into account scheduling options and how many FTEs are required to staff an ambulance or rescue unit. The manager should also calculate anticipated vacation time, holidays, scheduled days off, and sick time. For organizations using an eight-hour shift on five days a week, approximately 10.5 FTEs are required per unit to operate 24 hours a day for seven days a week. On a 12-hour shift (42-hour workweek), nine employees per unit are required.

These staffing contingencies must be presented when plans to reduce the EMS operating budget are not approved. The increase in the number of calls per unit when personnel reductions are made must also be considered. An EMS manager is often asked to predict changes in response times when staffing has been altered. This calculation is only a guess. Conversely, when the EMS manager wants to increase field deployment in the budget request/proposal, the number of new FTEs must be calculated in proportion to the increased unit hours.

The final item in a budget request is an organized breakdown of all components within an EMS. Each component is given a designation (account number) and past expenditures are reviewed for each account for the last one or two budget years. The current allocated funds and the fund requests for the upcoming fiscal year are also listed. The table of organization is usually displayed on a supplemental report outlining past, current, and expected expenditures for each employee within the department. Projected expenditures must, of course, be calculated on current and anticipated revenues.

The EMS manager assesses cash flow and revenues through the review of revenue reports generated on a monthly or quarterly basis. In the EMS field, the greatest source of operating revenue is the revenue from patients received through EMS billing. Other sources include fees from contractual agreements and "stand-by" charges for prehospital services. All other revenue is considered non-operating revenue.

One non-operating revenue source is the subsidy from an ambulance taxing district or jurisdiction through which the department is partially or completely funded (tax based). Other non-operating revenues may include interest from savings and investments, fees collected from training programs, fundraising income, donations, bequeaths, grants, and money obtained from the selling of equipment.

Revenue sources have account designations (or numbers) similar to expenses, i.e., private pay, Medicare, Medicaid, private insurance, stadium or shopping mall contracts, late payment charges, etc. When revenues are included in a budget proposal, the proposal may resemble a balance sheet.

Municipal EMS systems often have a rather awkward system of revenue collection. The municipal system may be allocated a certain dollar amount per year to operate the EMS system. Funds collected through patient billing are deposited into the municipality's general revenue account and do not go back into the EMS accounts. Most incoming revenue of all types is placed in this general revenue account. For instance, if your ambulance is involved in an accident and a settlement is made, the check from the insurance company does not go into the EMS vehicle repair account, but rather into general revenue—bureaucracy at its best. Therefore, managers of municipal services are often less cognizant of collected revenues than managers of private services.

Justifying the Budget Proposal

When the budget request is complete, the EMS manager is often required to justify the budget proposal before a committee with fiscal authority over the EMS.

In tight budget periods, it is common for an EMS to reduce the level of service because of inadequate funding. This is particularly true in many large cities where poor revenues have forced reductions in services. However, it is often politically unacceptable to lay off public safety workers. To close a firehouse or to lay off police officers or paramedics usually results in a great community outcry. Therefore, when a reduction in the table of organization must occur, it is usually accomplished through attrition: Paramedics and EMTs who resign, retire, or are terminated do not get replaced. Sometimes the position just remains vacant until more fruitful financial times; in other instances, the position is erased from the organizational table.

Once your budget request/proposal is approved, you are set for another year. Most organizations will generate a biweekly or monthly flow sheet or financial report reviewing each account, the amount appropriated, the available balance, the percentage of remaining appropriation, and, for that fiscal-year period, the expected percentage of the funds under ideal conditions. These flow sheets are a great tool for the EMS manager to review and use to make adjustments during the fiscal year.

Many systems allow the transfer of funds from one account to another in the event one account is low and there are excess funds in a different account. These flow sheets must be referred to regularly because they represent your predictions versus current reality. The flow sheets identify areas of over- and underspending and flag potential financial problems for the manager's intervention.

All of the flow sheets, your worksheets, and justification proposals

Source

Original article. At the time of writing, Rodney Dreifuss was chief of the St. Louis Emergency Medical Service. He also worked for New York City EMS for 12 years as an EMT, paramedic, supervisor, and administrator.

should be filed and referred to throughout the fiscal year. When budget time comes again, you will need to take those files out and review the budgeting from the previous year. Then, creating a new budget really won't be *that* bad.

References

Beck, D., *Basic Hospital Financial Management.* 2nd ed. Gaithersburg, Md.: Aspen Publication, 1984.

Fitch, J., et al. *EMS Management: Beyond the Street.* 2nd ed. Carlsbad, Calif.: Jems Communications, 1993.

Newkirk, W., and R. Linden. *Managing Emergency Medical Services: Principles and Practices.* Reston Publishing Co., 1984.

Stoner, J., and E. R. Freeman. *Management.* 4th ed. Los Angeles: Prentice Hall, Inc., 1989.

Understanding EMS Costs: Buying Smart

Richard A. Keller

Financial pressures continue to increase. Achieving greater purchasing effectiveness is one mechanism for giving taxpayers and users the best value for the dollars they've invested in their EMS system.

ALL EMERGENCY ORGANIZATIONS are being affected by the lethargic performance of the U.S. economy. Local governments are feeling the effects of "trickle-down" economics as the federal government provides less money to the states. The states, in turn, are reducing the money allocated to local jurisdictions, which are then faced with the challenge of meeting their citizens' expectations for increased services with fewer available dollars.

To survive these tough times, public and private organizations alike must strive for greater efficiency. Reducing expenses is a typical response to less money, and the first target is often the money spent to acquire capital equipment and supplies.

Those responsible for purchasing equipment and supplies for their departments must buy smart. The goal is to reduce expenditures while maintaining adequate equipment and supplies for your personnel to do their jobs. Thus, you need to lower expenditures for capital equipment, reduce the cost of inventories, and manage supply purchases.

Capital Equipment

Capital equipment is defined as those items that cost a significant amount of money (more than $500) and are expected to last a number of years. Examples include vehicles, computers, furniture, and defibrillators.

Many organizations react to a lack of money by curtailing capital purchases. This is often only a short-term solution that will hurt the service in the future. For example, a delay in the purchase of a badly needed new vehicle will result in increased maintenance costs on the old vehicle and a higher purchase price for the new vehicle in future years. This cost-cutting tactic should be avoided if possible.

The following questions need to be answered before deciding what items to purchase.

Do we need this item to meet our mission, or is it a luxury that would not significantly increase the department's performance? In fiscally tight times, the cost of new supervisory cars, delivery trucks, or passenger vans may be luxuries that can be avoided. At the same time, the replacement of an eight-year-old rescue truck with 150,000 miles may be essential for the service to meet its response obligations.

Have we developed specifications for a top-of-the-line vehicle with all of the possible options, or have we defined a basic vehicle with the minimum amount of extras needed to do the job? Many organizations have a tendency to develop specifications that attempt to respond to all possible desires and potential situations that might arise. For example,

Specifications should be generic enough to allow multiple vendors to respond to a request for bids. This ensures the forces of competition will provide the organization with the most beneficial price and product.

developing specifications for a four-wheel-drive ambulance, capable of transporting four supine patients, with an abundance of chrome and stainless steel might result in a highly appealing vehicle for the service, but it may not be cost justifiable. If the service projects the need for four-wheel drive only three days a year and only two of 100 patient encounters result in multiple patient transports, the money for these "extras" may be better spent elsewhere. The focus of specifying a vehicle or any other large purchase should be function, not desires or visual appeal.

On the other hand, are the specifications so limited that only one vendor can provide the item? Personal preference and brand loyalty result in buyers purchasing a specific product first. They then write specifications so that only that item from a particular manufacturer can comply. While this may result in the selection of the desired manufacturer's item, it will preclude the benefits of the competitive bid process. A company that knows it is the only one that can supply requested items has no incentive to competitively price its product.

Specifications should be generic enough to allow multiple vendors to respond to a request for bids. This ensures the forces of competition will provide the organization with the most beneficial price and product.

Inventory Reduction

Many organizations have extensive inventories of supplies and parts, and many have found it is possible and beneficial to reduce the amount of money tied up in this inventory. Freeing this money allows it to be used for other purposes without impairing the organization's ability to meet its responsibilities. Automobile manufacturers have almost universally moved to "just-in-time" deliveries of parts in order to reduce the amount of money tied up in inventory. This simply means that supplies and parts are not delivered until they are needed. This strategy can also be used in emergency organizations.

A thorough analysis of usage is needed in order to reduce the number of days an item needs to be available in house. Many organizations buy a number of items in bulk because of the price break. This may result in increased costs of warehousing, waste, expiration, loss, and encumbered money, which exceed any savings realized by the initial purchase. Reducing the amount of cleaning and medical supplies, vehicle parts, forms, and computer supplies may be a wise move for cost containment.

This process requires renegotiation with vendors and the possible use of alternative suppliers, including local firms or hospitals, to ensure necessary supplies and equipment will be available when needed. At the same time, the quantity of supplies and equipment stored in house will be reduced.

Inventory Control

Many organizations experience significant loss of equipment and supplies through damage, waste, and theft. In tight financial times, it is extremely important for services to develop strict inventory control procedures to eliminate these losses. Asset tracking is an ongoing process that takes time and effort but is well worth the commitment. The monitoring of supply usage is also important and should ensure that all supplies are used in support of the organization's mission. Numerous inventory control monitoring systems have been developed to facilitate tracking and reordering of supplies and equipment.

Equipment deserves special attention. If money is not going to be readily available to replace equipment, it is extremely important to maintain current equipment. A routine equipment preventive maintenance program should be in place for all items used. Each item should be regularly inspected, cleaned, tested, and repaired. These inspections and repairs should be documented. Many items have a preventive maintenance schedule provided by the manufacturer that offers a basis for a sophisticated in-house program. Huge savings are possible by extending the useful life of equipment. For example, if an $8,000 defibrillator has an expected useful life of five years and that life can be extended one year through diligent preventive maintenance and routine care, the organization would in effect save $1,600 ($8,000 divided by five years). If this type of preventive maintenance program enjoyed similar success with all the service's vehicles and equipment, a significant amount of money could be saved or freed for other important purchases.

> Equipment deserves special attention. A routine equipment preventive maintenance program should be in place for all items used.

Supply Purchases

Periodically, an organization should rebid all supply and equipment items to ensure the service continues to secure the best available price. Many organizations have a tendency toward inertia in their relationships with suppliers. Initially, an organization will let for bid a number of supply items. The best bid is selected, and supplies are ordered from that vendor. As long as the supplier's service is perceived as satisfactory, there may not be any impetus to re-evaluate the price. It is easier to reorder from a current vendor than it is to go through the bid process again. Although the supplier offered the best price initially, that may not be true after several years without competitive bidding. Remember, the easiest process usually does not result in the best price.

Two other strategies that can reduce the cost of supplies are negotiation and group purchasing arrangements. Many buyers believe the catalog or list price is not subject to negotiation, particularly with small orders. This is often not the case. Many vendors have the latitude to discount or reduce prices, particularly when faced with the loss of an account. Suppliers face the same economic realities as buyers, and pressure is placed on salespeople to maintain and expand sales. It is much easier, and less expensive, for sales personnel to maintain an existing account than it is to capture a new account.

Source

Reprinted with permission from Emergency, *November 1992. Richard A. Keller is a partner at Fitch & Associates, Inc. He is nationally known for his work in EMS system operations, reimbursement, and design. He is a principal author of the book* EMS Management: Beyond the Street, *2nd ed.*

Industry associations, fleet operators, state or local government purchasing departments, hospitals, and other groups are possible sources for expanding a single organization's buying power. More favorable pricing can be achieved when multiple buyers join together to purchase in bulk. This provides the advantage of bulk buying discounts without extensive funds being tied up in inventories. Investigation of possible group arrangements could reveal previously untapped opportunities.

Buying smart has never been more important. If organizational buyers would expand their efforts and be more innovative in purchasing strategies for their service, organizations might find that adequate funds are available, not only for the bare essentials but for some of the items needed for improvements. This can only be accomplished by focusing the efforts and attention of the entire organization on buying only what is necessary to do the job, and then only when prices have been determined to be the best that can be achieved.

Billing, Collections, and Third-Party Payers

RECENTLY THE OWNERS OF SEVERAL private ambulance companies have been prosecuted, convicted, and imprisoned for violating Medicare or Medicaid regulations. In addition, the tremendous civil monetary penalties levied in these cases have driven the companies out of business.

In the rush to reduce budget deficits by billing Medicare (and other third-party payers) for ambulance service, many public officials also are overlooking Medicare rules and regulations and the steep penalties (civil and criminal) they could face from violating these rules.

Conversations with local EMS and fire department officials, billing agents, and city and county attorneys have uncovered the fact that although the public agencies may bill Medicare, many of them are not aware of the rules—or the penalties—involved. Although these rules apply to both Medicare and Medicaid, this discussion will focus on Medicare so as not to confuse the issue. Reference will be made to Medicaid as needed.

It must be understood that no public officials or agencies are immune from criminal prosecution if Medicare is billed improperly. Nor are they exempt from civil monetary penalties and sanctions. In addition to subjecting public officials to criminal penalties, ignorance of the rules can severely damage the financial well-being of the communities such officials serve.

Criminal Penalties

Section 1128B of the Social Security Act makes it a felony—punishable by up to $25,000 in fines, five years in jail, or both—to violate any of the provisions involved. These provisions include making false statements or misrepresenting material facts in billing, receiving payment in return for referring patients, or receiving payment in return for ordering or arranging any services. This is known as illegal remuneration. Violation of any of these statutes can result in criminal penalties.

Warning: Improper Medicare Billing May Be Hazardous to Your Fiscal Health

David M. Werfel, Esq.

Reimbursement consultant David Werfel knows the ins and outs of Medicare. In this article, he outlines 10 specific Medicare violations that could send the unsuspecting EMS leader "directly to jail—without collecting $200."

One example of a false statement is an insurance claim for transportation when the service rendered was only a response—even with treatment at the scene. (If a patient is not transported, Medicare does not pay for the response, nor does it cover treatment at the scene.) It is considered fraud or a false statement when a non-covered service (e.g., response or treatment) is billed as a covered service.

An example of illegal remuneration is a situation in which a public official or agency receives payment from the provider of a service (e.g., a private ambulance company) in return for referring patients to that company, granting it a particular contract, or arranging for patients to be transported by that company.

While these violations cover only one statute, the federal government has many such statutes it can use for criminal prosecutions. For example, companies can be—and have been—prosecuted for Medicare violations under the mail fraud statute. In those cases, agencies didn't have to receive payment from Medicare to be prosecuted. All they had to do was file a false claim.

Civil Penalties

The conditions under which civil penalties can be imposed are well documented. For instance, section 1128A of the Social Security Act states the following:

> Any person (including an organization, agency, or other entity) that presents or causes to be presented to an officer, employee, or agent of the United States, or of any department or agency thereof, or of any state agency . . . a claim that the Secretary determines is for a medical or other item or service that the person knows or should know was not provided as claimed, or is for a medical or other item or service and the person knows or should know the claim is false or fraudulent, or presents or causes to be presented to any person a request for payment which is in violation of the terms of [an assignment agreement or a participation agreement] shall be subject, *in addition to any other penalties* . . . to a civil money penalty of not more than $2,000 *for each item or service.* In addition, such a person shall be subject to an assessment of not more than *twice the amount claimed* for each such item or service in lieu of damages. . . . In addition, the Secretary may make a determination in the same proceeding to exclude the person from participation in the programs. . . . [Emphasis added.]

"Any person (including an organization, agency, or other entity)" includes state, county, and local governments. In fact, when the initial regulations concerning the anti-kickback statute of the act were issued in 1983, they stated:

> Because state, county, and municipal institutions are among providers of services in these programs, they are within the ambit of the statute. Public entities may also be among those persons

receiving grant funds from a state. . . . Nothing in the statute or legislative history provides a rationale for excluding those entities or their agents and employees from the scope of the plain meaning of the statute. Hence we have clarified the proposed definition of "Person" [in the regulation] . . . by adding the words "public or private" following the word "entity."

In sum, violations of these laws are subject to civil monetary penalties of $2,000 for each *item* incorrectly billed, plus an assessment of double the amount billed for the incorrect item. In other words, if the agency bills incorrectly for a base rate and mileage for three miles for a total of $500, the total fines and assessments could be $5,000 for that one claim ($2,000 for the base rate, $2,000 for the mileage, and $500 multiplied by two for the assessment).

Also, an agency that is billing incorrectly is probably doing so consistently, which can create incredible financial burdens if the billing problems have been occurring for some time. The federal government can actually go back six years to calculate the civil money penalties related to Medicare fraud. Thus, the amounts penalized can be staggering.

For example, assume that an agency has only 500 claims at issue, with each claim involving only two line items (e.g., base rate and mileage). If each claim is for $400, the total in fines and assessments could equal $2.4 million (500 [2 x $2,000] + $400 [2 x 500]). But 500 claims is a small number considering how many Medicare and Medicaid claims a service submits each month.

The question then arises as to why the federal government goes after cities and counties rather than private companies. The truth is, it goes after both, but cities, counties, and other local government entities have deeper pockets. In addition, members of Congress have raised questions regarding multiple dipping by local governments (e.g., billing Medicare plus being 100-percent tax-subsidized plus receiving block grants plus receiving money from taxes for enhanced 9-1-1 systems).

With Congress looking to cut costs, such matters are receiving increased attention. In fact, questions have been raised as to whether public agencies are even entitled to receive payment from Medicare and Medicaid and, if so, whether the amount of tax subsidization should be taken into consideration when Medicare and Medicaid benefits are paid.

Meanwhile, public officials and fire department administrators—and, of course, private ambulance service owners—can protect themselves and the governments, departments, or companies they represent by avoiding the following practices, all of which violate Medicare rules:

- Routinely waiving Medicare coinsurance payments and deductibles
- Creating subscription or membership agreements that do not meet Medicare requirements (Annual fees must collectively equal or exceed the amounts not billed for co-insurance and deductibles.)

An agency that is billing incorrectly is probably doing so consistently, which can create incredible financial burdens if the billing problems have been occurring for some time.

- Using subscription agreements stating that residents are members merely because they pay taxes (If that was true, there would be no legal obligation for residents—or Medicare—to pay anything.)
- Billing Medicare under transportation code A0220 when the patient is not transported (Responses to the scene and treatment at the scene are not covered. Since A0220 is a transportation code, billing under A0220 when the agency does not transport is fraud.)
- Signing contracts that require the transporting entity to pay the city, county, or other government agency a fee based on the number of referrals given or even in return for getting the contract (The anti-kickback statute makes the recipient of such payments and the party making the payments equally guilty. Examples include contracts—even requests for proposals—stating that the contractor must pay a certain amount per patient, a percentage of net or gross earnings, or a fee to serve a certain zone.)
- Billing Medicare but not other third-party payers
- Billing Medicare for more than the amount billed to other patients or their insurers (Common examples are situations in which cities bill Medicare but do not bill patients without insurance, in which they bill Medicare a higher fee than they bill patients without insurance, or in which they bill Medicare but do not bill residents for co-insurance.)
- Illegally billing patients after accepting assignment (Some agencies will accept assignment on some claims but not on others. Once an agency agrees to accept assignment, it cannot bill a patient for anything except co-insurance, deductibles, and noncovered services. In other words, it cannot bill for the amounts that Medicare does not pay.)
- Billing patients for more than is allowed when the agency has agreed to be a participating provider (Many cities sign up to be participating suppliers of Medicare-covered services but do not understand what that means. Thus, they often violate the terms by billing patients for the difference between their actual bills and their Medicare-allowed amount when they are not allowed to do so. Participating means accepting assignment on all claims for covered services.)
- Failure to provide patients with advance written notice when certain noncovered services are provided (Failure to provide patients with this information, when required, violates several provisions that may subject the agency to various penalties and sanctions.)

In addition, many other infractions (e.g., failure to provide access to records, employment of sanctioned individuals—those previously convicted or suspended due to Medicare fraud—without federal government notification, self-referrals, and excess charges) can lead to criminal prosecution, substantial civil monetary penalties, and other sanctions.

This point was made rather convincingly in 1991, when subpoenas were served on seven private ambulance companies and nine cities and towns in Massachusetts. These subpoenas required the agencies to provide tens of thousands of records covering all elements of the provided service, including financial and contractual agreements, going back to 1987.

Prior to the subpoenas, the Region One inspector general (IG) of the U.S. Department of Health and Human Services had written a letter, dated July 16, 1991, advising private ambulance companies and municipalities in New England that contracts in which cities and towns are paid for referring emergency calls to private ambulance companies are illegal.

His letter acknowledged that this type of relationship is attractive to cities and towns looking for alternative sources of revenue to supplement their rapidly dwindling state aid. But, he wrote, "a legal review of these types of relationships . . . where the contracts call for the ambulance companies to provide a lump-sum reimbursement to the towns at the start of the arrangements, or a per-patient referral payment at the time of service, [has determined that] both the municipalities and the ambulance companies would be in violation of the anti-kickback statute of the Social Security Act (42 U.S.C. 1320a-7b)."

Additionally, the IG wrote, "It has also come to our attention that some cities and towns have entered into contracts with ambulance companies requiring that the ambulance companies waive co-insurance and deductibles in order to get the contracts as a means of keeping the citizens out of the municipalities happy by not having to pay the co-insurance or deductibles. . . . We want to use criminal prosecutions and sanctions only as a last resort . . . on the theory that a number of participants may not be aware that they are in violation of the anti-kickback statute. If, however, it becomes evident that cities and towns . . . continue these practices . . . we will investigate such cases and refer them for criminal prosecution."

Following delivery of the subpoenas, a November 27, 1991, *Boston Globe* story reported that federal investigators were looking into "allegations that municipal ambulance services are being illegally billed to Medicare. . . . In some cases, the municipalities . . . may be violating federal regulations by entering into agreements that allow . . . bill[ing] Medicare . . . for ambulance rides that are provided without charge to other residents."

"The town has been ambushed," a selectman of one town was quoted as saying in the *Boston Globe* on December 19, 1991. Apparently, this town's contract *allowed* the 20-percent Medicare co-insurance to be waived. Town counsel had even looked at the contract prior to its being signed and provided an opinion that it was legal.

The names of the agencies involved in this case have been intentionally omitted to avoid embarrassing anyone. The main point of this

Source

Reprinted with permission from JEMS, *March 1993. David M. Werfel, Esq., is the Medicare consultant for the American Ambulance Association. He is a former prosecutor, as well as a former director of program security for Blue Cross/Blue Shield in New York.*

case is that if public entities are going to bill Medicare (or even have a billing agency bill for them) and do so incorrectly, the department is liable for criminal prosecution, civil monetary penalties, and sanctions.

While those who serve as legal counsel for cities, counties, and states are typically well versed in law, the fact of the matter is that they are often unfamiliar with Medicare laws and regulations. What is legal in many areas of the business world (e.g., payment of sales commissions and discounts to an independent contractor) may not be legal in the Medicare arena. Thus, government officials may have to implore their legal counsel to study these laws and regulations in depth.

This is not to say that public agencies should stop providing EMS or stop billing when it is appropriate. What is suggested is that agencies know what they are doing. Otherwise, the deficit they are trying to close may widen substantially.

Also, remember that the federal government desperately needs to close its budget deficit. One area that is receiving tremendous attention in this effort is the Medicare/Medicaid budget. Consequently, many federal agencies—including the Federal Bureau of Investigation—have targeted the healthcare field for prosecution of offenders to deter abusive practices and to collect substantial amounts in penalties. In this effort, local, county, and state governments are not exempt from criminal prosecution or civil penalties.

The best advice, then? Both public and private officials that bill Medicare better know the rules.

References

42 U.S.C. 1320a-7a.
42 U.S.C. 1320a-7b.
Preamble to regulations. 48 *Federal Register* 38827. 26 August 1983.

The ABCs of EMS Billing and Collection

Richard A. Keller

Effective third-party reimbursement depends on the systems and procedures used in the business office. In this article, EMS consultant Rick Keller explains how to enhance the business office's billing and collection performance.

MANY PUBLIC AND PRIVATE EMS managers have had to assume the role of financial overseer for their organizations. The success of an EMS operation, whether fire department, other government, hospital, or private, is rapidly becoming dependent on the collection of revenues for the services delivered. This article reviews the billing and collection process through a step-by-step examination of all necessary functions.

Each step of the process is essential in every organization. How well each organization develops and accomplishes these procedures determines its billing and collection effectiveness.

The billing and collection process is divided into five different stages: collecting source data, preparing the data, managing the accounts, closing the accounts, and exception track processing.

Collection of Source Data

Before a bill can be processed or an insurance claim prepared, adequate information must be collected from three potential sources: the communications center, previous patient records, and the crews themselves. Of these, the data collected by the field personnel is the most important source for starting the billing and collection cycle.

Poor documentation by field personnel is the most common problem office workers encounter. This information is essential for accurately and appropriately collecting revenues. An organization should create work standards that describe the acceptable performance level for the field collection of information. For example, there should be complete and accurate documentation for 95 percent of patient encounters delivered at the end of the shift. Paperwork should be delivered on 100 percent of the crew's dispatches at the end of the shift.

This type of work standard sets the expectations for field personnel. While it is unrealistic to expect that information will be available on all patients, in reality the information required is usually available either from the patient, the patient's family, or the hospital admissions staff.

In addition to work standards, all documentation should be legible and spelled correctly. The number of organizations that accept patient care reports that can't be read—and with misspelled words—is amazing. They often brush it off as a characteristic of field personnel, but this perception should be rapidly corrected. Patient care documentation must be legible. There is no room for misspelled words in patient care reports that could ultimately become legal documents.

The communications center is often a neglected part of the billing

The process of collecting the source data, reconciling the patient care reports with the dispatches, and checking for completeness and accuracy should be completed within 24 to 36 hours after service is rendered.

and collection process. The center may not even be under the control of the EMS service. Key information from the communications center can reconcile paperwork from the field and can include information collected from the caller.

Many patients are repeat customers. This is a third potential source of patient information. These patients should be quickly identified to enhance information being collected in the field or through the communications center.

The second step when collecting source data is the reconciliation and collation process. This activity simply matches the dispatches of each crew with the paperwork they submit at the end of the shift. A weakness seen in many services is the lack of documentation provided by field personnel. Organizations often don't even know that the paperwork is missing until days or weeks after the event. The longer paperwork is missing, the more difficult it is to reconstruct.

The work standard in this situation is straightforward: All dispatches should be matched with the paperwork at the end of the shift. At this time, assess the completeness and accuracy of the documentation. Any omissions or inaccuracies should be noted, and paperwork should be rerouted back to operations for completion.

The process of collecting the source data, reconciling the patient care reports with the dispatches, and checking for completeness and accuracy should be completed within 24 to 36 hours after service is rendered.

Preparation of Data

A number of steps are required to prepare the data for filing insurance claims or generating invoices. The first step is coding and verification. This process verifies the accuracy of the information received from the field, the communications center, and previous patient records. It also identifies the treatment provided, the conditions or reasons that the ambulance was called, and any available diagnostic information.

This is also the first step in the clinical quality improvement process. Treatments are identified and comparisons made with the patient care report and the supplies and equipment used.

Many services will code the information to facilitate data entry. It is very important that accurate coding and description is available on each patient transport. Data entry is the next step. It is necessary to enter the appropriate patient, clinical, and billing information, either into a computerized billing and collection system or into a manual system. An example of a work standard for data entry would be the following: Patient and transaction information for 75 patients is entered during each eight-hour shift with 95-percent reliability.

Reconciliation, posting, and distribution of accounts occur next. In these steps, information entered into the billing system is compared and verified for accuracy. The charges are posted to the accounting system, and the accounts are distributed among the staff for further handling. These are the final steps prior to preparing an invoice for filing insurance claims.

An invoice should be generated for all patients other than those on Medicaid. The invoice is sent to the responsible party, preferably with the organization's billing and collection policies. Questions like the following should be answered on the invoice form:

- Does the organization expect payment prior to processing by the insurance company?
- How can the patients receive assistance in filing insurance claims?
- How long before payment can be expected?

Many organizations will then file assigned Medicare and insurance claims for the patient, who can authorize the organization to collect directly from the third party. Or, unassigned claims may be filed where the patient will be the recipient of the funds.

The first invoices and insurance claims should be mailed within 72 hours from the time of service. Quick information processing, prompt insurance claims filing, and invoice mailing have the greatest positive impact on collection rates.

> Quick information processing, prompt insurance claims filing, and invoice mailing have the greatest positive impact on collection rates.

Account Management

Management of the accounts receivable workload can be allocated by specialization or by a simple alphabetical division of accounts. There are pros and cons to each method. Which method you choose will largely be determined by the workload, the number of specialized payers, and the complexity of the accounting processes.

For example, one person may be in charge of filing all Medicare for every patient transported, another may specialize in Medicaid, and a third person may specialize in commercial insurance. Each account is managed differently depending on the payer type. Certain activities need to be described in a schedule for Medicare patients, while another set of activities should be directed at the private pay accounts. A separate comprehensive schedule should be developed for each payer type. The major payer types are Medicare, Medicaid, Medicare *and* Medicaid, commercial insurance, auto accidents, worker's compensation, contracts, commercial insurance, managed care, and private pay. The account manager responsible for a specific account should follow the payer schedules. Systemization and follow-up are the keys to success in the collection of EMS revenue.

Account Closing

The final outcome of accounts is their closing. A positive closing of an account generates revenue to the service. The best way to close accounts is by payment in full. Once full payment is received, the account is closed, and it no longer remains on the books in accounts receivable.

There are a number of other ways that accounts may be closed. For example, the organization may take assignment on Medicare. Once the Medicare payment has been received, it will be necessary to write off any contractual allowance and bill the 20-percent co-insurance amount to the patient. After the patient pays the 20 percent, the account will be closed. On the other hand, once payment is received from Medicaid, the remainder of the bill is written off to the Medicaid contractual allowance. At that time, the account will be closed. Other ways that accounts can be closed are if they are written off to charity or bad debt or if they are turned over to an outside collection agency.

The performance standard of the account specialist should be based on closing the appropriate number of accounts. If a service does 100 transports a day, the billing and collection department should close at least 100 accounts per day. If not, they will be continually building a backlog and falling behind in the process. The collection rate and the amount of money coming into the organization will suffer. If 30 percent of the accounts are Medicare, then the account specialist handling Medicare should expect to close at least 33 Medicare accounts, on average, per day. Instead of focusing on the amount of money collected by individuals working within the billing and collection department, the organization should focus on the number of accounts closed.

Payments are processed in the account closing procedure. If the payment is paid in full, it is closed. If not, other steps need to be taken, including collection activities, rerouting back to the account management for billing of secondary insurance, or possibly refiling insurance claims.

Inactive accounts should be reviewed after a specified period of time. A decision must then be made whether they should be returned to account specialists for further work, turned over for collection, written off to bad debt or charity, or assigned for legal action. All of these steps will ultimately result in the appropriate closing of the accounts.

Exception Track Processing

One feature that many billing and collection offices neglect is that of exception track processing. The premise behind exception track processing is that clean claims are paid quickly. Therefore, the office should make every effort to process those clean accounts promptly in order to receive payment as soon as possible. This prevents an account that has inadequate or incorrect information from slowing down the entire processing flow. These problem accounts are routed to the exception track.

The best and brightest personnel should be assigned to exception track activities. These personnel should be skilled at investigation and quality control monitoring. Creative thinkers are needed who can determine the best way to collect information or provide additional support to facilitate payment.

Exception track processing should include items such as returned mail with incorrect or incomplete addresses. More importantly, complaints received regarding billing and collection should be processed through the exception track. This allows for some quality control efforts to take place within the organization and will facilitate correction of problematic or incorrect activities.

Typically, accounts should not remain active for more than 120 days. If the account has not been paid at that time, it is unlikely that further activity will result in the collection of much revenue. The best step to take at this time is either to write off the accounts, if it is determined that they are probably uncollectible, or to turn the accounts over to an outside collection agency. This frees personnel to focus on more current accounts where collection potential is higher.

Conclusion

Regardless of the type of organization, it is necessary to recover as much revenue as possible from third-party payers and outside sources in order to support EMS activities. The organizations that develop a comprehensive and high-quality collection program will be able to capture the essential costs of providing emergency medical services.

Source
Original article.

Dealing With Third-Party Payers

Richard A. Keller

Significant system revenues are controlled by Medicare and other third-party payers. Although guided by strict rules, people make interpretations and decisions about how guidelines are implemented. Relationships can be a major factor in these decisions. This article describes methods you can use to enhance relationships with third-party payers.

THERE ARE MORE THAN 1,200 possible payers for emergency medical services. Each payer has established its own set of rules and criteria for processing reimbursement claims. It is impossible for any one person to identify all of the policies that need to be followed for each individual payer, but each service should devise a comprehensive strategy for developing payer relationships.

Surprisingly, many billing and collection departments classify their relationships with third-party payers as adversarial, particularly with regard to Medicaid and Medicare claims processors. If you are asking someone for money, it would make sense to develop a positive relationship with the person responsible for determining payment.

A number of specific strategies can be developed within an organization to enhance third-party payer relationships. These include developing personal contacts, establishing internal policies and procedures based on payer requirements, training personnel within the office to deal with one set of payers, and most important, reversing the internal perception that the organization is a client of the payer. This customer service reversal will go a long way toward enhancing dealings with third-party payers. The ultimate result will be faster and more effective payment of claims.

The Payer Is the Client

Customer service representatives should be trained to serve payers as customers. They should go out of their way to meet and exceed the customers' expectations and make sure that all interactions with the customers are positive.

Customer service representatives must be well informed in order to respond effectively to the payers. Inquiries regarding transport, equipment, and supplies are just the tip of the iceberg. Customer service representatives should be knowledgeable in the following areas as well:

- Distinguishing among levels of service
- State and county assistance programs
- Insurance benefits and specific requirements of all major payers
- Current changes and additions to reimbursement programs
- Assisting patients in dealing with third-party payers
- Quick tracking of new and existing accounts
- Field personnel documentation
- Early identification of potential litigious circumstances

Levels of service. The level of service provided to a patient helps determine the charges and reimbursement levels, particularly wheelchair versus ambulance transportation and advanced life support (ALS) versus basic life support (BLS). Customer service representatives must understand what situations and patient conditions distinguish the appropriate level of service and be able to communicate how a specific patient transport met the criteria for the level of service indicated on the insurance claim or invoice.

Government assistance programs. Government assistance programs are complex and confusing, especially to the patients. A proficient customer service representative can help patients understand the process, their eligibility, and benefits. Early recognition that a patient may qualify for government assistance and facilitation of the application process can result in reimbursement for a trip that otherwise might have gone unpaid.

Helping patients with third-party payers. Assisting individuals with their insurance companies will facilitate rapid payment for ambulance services. Each payer may have unique requirements, forms, and procedures to follow. The customer service representative should be able to provide the patient with appropriate forms, addresses, contacts, and assistance with these payers. The customer service representative should be aware of changes and additions to payer requirements, and have a comprehensive knowledge of the benefits and procedures used by various third-party reimbursers.

Access to account information. In order for customer service representatives to respond effectively to inquiries from patients and payers, they must be able to rapidly locate pertinent information about specific transports, account activity, and filed claims. A system must be in place so that all pertinent information is readily accessible for processing information requests and answering specific questions about the transport, billing, and collection activities.

Understanding field documentation. Essential information is provided in the patient care report completed by field personnel. Customer service representatives would be at a significant disadvantage if they did not understand these field reports. They should understand commonly used definitions, patient condition and diagnostic information, treatment delivered, and supplies used on the assignment.

Identifying potential problems. The customer service representative is often the first person to become aware of a potential problem with an account or event. Callers who express dissatisfaction with the service or who ask questions regarding why certain procedures were or were not completed could be indications of potential litigious situations. The handling of complaints and the early identification of potential problems are important functions of the customer service representative. Appropriate management personnel should be informed so immediate action can be taken to ameliorate the problem.

To treat all payers similarly will not result in quick and efficient processing of your reimbursement claims. A schedule for each payer type, and sometimes each specific payer, needs to be developed in order to enhance rapid claims processing within the payer's organization.

Enhancing Payer Relationships

The organization should undertake specific activities to enhance payer relations. These could include visits to the third-party payer's headquarters to understand the unique needs and constraints within the payer's processing system. These visits will also begin to develop personal relationships between your personnel and the personnel at the insurance company responsible for processing your claims. In many cases, inviting claims processors from the insurance companies to your location is also a good idea, so they can understand the challenges your organization faces when developing reimbursement claims.

Specialization leads to consistency. One or a few individuals within your organization dealing with a few individuals at the payer organizations will facilitate positive communications. For example, one person may be responsible for following Medicare claims. That person can develop a personal relationship with an individual at the third-party carrier location and will know who to contact if a problem arises. In the same way, if difficulties arise, the claim's processor at the Medicare carrier will also know whom to contact within your organization to resolve any issues. Even though one person may have primary responsibility for a specific payer, others within the office should be cross-trained to provide backup or coverage in the event of illness, vacation, or resignation.

The procedures, policies, forms, and schedules vary for each potential payer. To treat all payers similarly will not result in quick and efficient processing of your reimbursement claims. A schedule for each payer type, and sometimes each specific payer, needs to be developed in order to enhance rapid claims processing within the payer's organization.

In addition, specific procedures and sometimes specific claim forms need to be used to facilitate claims processing. It is much easier to deal with unique payer requirements on the front end than it is to respond to ongoing requests for additional information 30 to 60 days down the road. It may seem cumbersome and time-consuming to have to develop these customized procedures and schedules for each payer, but cost savings in the long run include quicker turnaround of payments, reduction in duplicate handling of the same account, and a reduction in the number of denials.

Specific schedules should be developed for all potential payer types. There should be a unique schedule of activity for each of the following:

- Medicare
- Medicaid
- Medicare and Medicaid
- Commercial insurance companies (some insurance companies may require their own schedule, e.g., Blue Cross/Blue Shield)
- Auto insurance
- Champus
- Managed care payers (i.e., HMOs and PPOs)

- Hospitals
- Government contracts (e.g., V.A., county indigent, psychiatric transports)
- Private pay
- Indigent
- Facility contracts (e.g., hospitals and nursing homes)
- Membership program participants
- Accounts pending because of legal action
- Bankruptcies
- Special processing (for accounts not included in other categories that occur infrequently)

Source

Original article.

Changes on the Horizon

Ambulance service organizations need to prepare for changes in the billing and collection process. There is a significant trend toward increasing the number of individuals who are covered by managed care health plans. One result is that more ambulance services are contracting with organizations on a capitated rate instead of fee-for-service. Capitation is a process by which insurance companies pay ambulance companies for services on a monthly basis based on the number of members of the health plan. This flat fee is designed to cover all medical transportation needs to the members and is not based on the actual number of ambulance trips provided to the plan's members.

A lot of momentum is also developing to create a universal claim form for all insurance companies. This would greatly facilitate the work in the billing and collection office and reduce confusion for patients.

Health reform initiatives may dramatically change the procedures used by ambulance services for reimbursement for services. It is still too early to determine the full impact, but changes will result in reduced paperwork and a significant decrease in the number of potential payers. Instead of 1,200, there may be only a dozen or so potential payers for each ambulance service.

The most important lesson to learn in dealing with third-party payers is to not antagonize those whose job it is to pay you money, and to develop positive and friendly relationships in order to facilitate your work. The question to ask representatives from third-party payers is, "What can I do to make your job easier?" Responding to their answers will create a more productive and customer-oriented department within your organization. The net results will be a reduction in the days outstanding of your accounts receivable and ultimately a decline in the number of claim denials and refilings.

Preparing for Capitated Payment and Integrated Delivery Systems

Don Jones, JD, MBA

Are you ready for capitated reimbursement and integrated service delivery models? Author Don Jones describes why this form of payment and organizational structure will be preferred, with or without healthcare reform. More importantly, he describes how you can best prepare your service for this environment.

MANY HEALTHCARE EXPERTS EXPECT prospective capitated reimbursement (a fixed payment received before services are rendered and for which the provider is at financial risk) to became the primary method of reimbursement—with or without healthcare reform. In fact, capitation appears inevitable in the future of EMS nationwide, replacing fee-for-service, discounted fee-for-service, flat rate, and other payment schemes.

Medicare-risk HMO plans—such as FHP's Senior Plan, PacifiCare's Secure Horizons, and HealthNet's Seniority Plus—are the fastest growing segment of many HMOs and provide an excellent indication of the federal government's direction.

Although it is unclear whether capitation will emerge as the dominant EMS reimbursement system in rural areas (due to the potential lack of competing health plans), there are working examples of rural providers operating in capitated payment environments. In Arizona, for example, all Medicaid recipients are already in managed care plans. California has enrolled 300,000 Medicaid (MediCal) recipients in HMOs and plans to have the state's entire Medicaid population in managed care by 1996. And at least 30 other states are working on plans to capitate Medicaid payments.

To date, managed care has gained a foothold in some parts of the United States much faster than in others. In many areas, managed care has had little impact thus far. In others, such as Seattle, Chicago, and Albany, N.Y., managed care now encompasses between 10 percent and 30 percent of the market. In a few areas, such as urban California, Boston, and Portland, Ore., HMOs have already enrolled at least 50 percent of the medically insured population. And in Minneapolis, virtually all healthcare providers have become part of integrated healthcare networks. Eventually, all medical marketplaces will likely look like Minneapolis.

Effects of Capitated Healthcare

When preparing for the world of capitated healthcare, EMS providers should consider that, once they contract to be paid on a capitated basis, they no longer operate as profit or revenue centers. Instead, all aspects of the providers' operations will be looked on as cost centers. This will be one of the most challenging philosophical shifts for EMS providers. It will also mean large changes for EMS organizations.

Accounts receivable costs and problems will be significantly reduced, eliminating the need for large billing and collection departments. In their place will be vastly more intricate cost-accounting systems and actuarial, data collection, and statistical reporting packages for analysis—creating the need for statisticians, actuaries, and managed care contracting specialists.

To focus on the needs of managed care buyers, contracting and pricing functions will gain importance relative to field operations. EMS management will have to learn to market services to managed care organizations and large employers.

Any organization that undertakes a capitated payment agreement will also need a utilization review department. Expenses will be examined from a cost-reduction perspective rather than from a revenue-enhancement perspective. Furthermore, the revenue enhancers now used by many EMS organizations—such as additional charges for mileage, supplies, and medications—will become obsolete. Organizations will need to develop in-house expertise in defining medically necessary and "appropriate" service levels. Providers wanting to purchase expensive equipment will have to prove it will improve patient outcome. Even the definition of what constitutes an emergency will come under strict scrutiny.

There are some changes you can make now to prepare your organization for a capitated payment environment.

- Reduce costs to the bone—but don't skimp on quality. "Highest quality, lowest cost" will become the motto of any provider selling service to managed care organizations.
- Plan to accept financial risk.
- Maintain a sharp lookout for new value-added services to offer managed care organizations. Figure out how to price these services and structure your fees to include them.
- Examine the scope of practice you provide. EMTs and paramedics are likely to need expanded training and certification or licensing in the future, since managed care interests will push primary care services as an essential part of the services provided.
- Move quickly to work with managed care under any arrangement possible. Also target large employer groups that self-insure.
- Prepare your staff to spearhead your managed care effort. If you have no idea how to get involved with managed care, affiliate with someone who does, or hire experts from a managed care organization or large physician group. Retain experienced healthcare counsel to advise you on the complexities and variations of managed care contracts.
- Develop in-house systems to study, analyze, and report on utilization, medical appropriateness, and costs. Remember, most EMS software systems on the market today do not begin to address our industry's future concerns.
- Finally, educate your staff to anticipate and respond to the changes expected when managed care dominates EMS.

Integrated delivery systems, or health-care provider networks that offer one-stop shopping to healthcare payers, are rapidly becoming important players in the managed care environment.

The Rise of Integrated Delivery Organizations

Integrated delivery systems, or healthcare provider networks that offer one-stop shopping to healthcare payers, are rapidly becoming important players in the managed care environment. Whereas health maintenance organizations (HMOs) and preferred provider organizations (PPOs) sell healthcare plans to employers, integrated healthcare organizations (IHOs) actually provide healthcare.

Most IHOs offer physicians, acute care hospital services, outpatient surgery, urgent care centers, and other medical services from a single source. Some advanced IHOs even offer skilled nursing facilities, birthing centers, hospice programs, durable medical equipment, home healthcare, and ambulance services.

Examples of IHOs include the Henry Ford system in Detroit and, in California, Health Dimensions of Santa Clara County, Mercy HealthCare and Sutter Health of Sacramento, and Sharp HealthCare and Scripps Health, both in San Diego.

When choosing a healthcare plan, employers generally must analyze the choices offered by HMO and PPO delivery networks. Such a network typically includes lists of physicians, hospitals, and ancillary healthcare providers (often including ambulance services) that have individually negotiated reimbursement agreements with the HMO or PPO.

Putting together a comprehensive provider list is a time-consuming, expensive process, which can involve dozens of contract negotiators and thousands of attorney hours. As a result, each list and contract is generally unique.

But with the one-stop shopping convenience offered by an IHO, an entire array of healthcare services delivered by a large pool of professionals and facilities can be contracted for in a single negotiation process. In some communities, health plans can provide geographically diverse, comprehensive services through a single contract with just one IHO. The efficiency of this contracting process, combined with the competitive service pricing an IHO is able to offer when all healthcare dollars are bundled to a single entity, is rapidly changing the relationships between traditional healthcare providers.

Hospitals are merging or acquiring their competitors. Physicians are abandoning small practices for large multi-specialty group practices. Many physicians are selling their practices to hospitals or hospital-sponsored foundations. These entities then manage the physicians' practices, provide support staff (nurses, technicians, office personnel), and perform the contracting services necessary to compete for managed care payer contracts. The physicians in turn contract to provide professional services for a period of time (10- to 20-year contracts are not unusual).

But IHOs are not so easily explained by the above descriptions. Some healthcare insurers and HMOs are also IHOs. The Kaiser Permanente HMO, with over nine million members, provides healthcare services through its own network of hospitals, clinics, and physicians operating out of facilities it owns. FHP, the nation's fourth largest HMO, owns and operates a network of Southern California hospitals and physician practices and owns its own ambulance service. Traditional indemnity insurers Aetna and Prudential are rapidly purchasing physician practices—primarily in the southeastern United States. Cigna, another traditional indemnity insurer, already owns a Southern California network of hospitals, clinics, and multi-specialty group practices.

On the other hand, some IHOs—such as San Diego-based Sharp HealthCare—are beginning to offer their own HMO plans.

And the managed care trend continues to grow in various ways. In Minnesota, for example, insurers and providers are beginning to link together. And many California counties are considering whether to form their own HMOs or contract with commercially available plans for MediCal-eligible recipients.

Ambulance services are not immune to these changes. Many IHOs, such as Sharp HealthCare in San Diego are starting to operate network ambulance services through management contracts with local ambulance services.

It is important to note that these changes in traditional healthcare delivery mechanisms are occurring without healthcare reform legislation. They are the result of economic pressures asserted by healthcare buyers (employers and government) and insurers (traditional indemnity firms, HMOs, and PPOs).

At what stage is your community in the development of integrated delivery systems? By looking closely at all the players in your area, you can see what to expect in the future and position your organization accordingly.

Source

Reprinted with permission from EMS Insider, *March and April 1994. Don Jones, JD, MBA, is vice president for strategic business development for MedTrans, the healthcare services division of Laidlaw, Inc.*

Managing Personal and Professional Financial Matters

1994 EMS Salary Survey

Richard A. Keller
and Edward I.
Weinberg

*For the past seven years,
Fitch & Associates has
collaborated with* JEMS
*magazine to conduct
the annual EMS salary
survey. This article
analyzes 1994's trends
in compensation and
benefits.*

As CONSOLIDATIONS, MERGERS, AND ACQUISITIONS of ambulance companies continue to make news, as the public versus private provider debate rages on, and as ambulance companies interface with the ever-increasing number of healthcare alliances and networks, EMS providers will only be able to survive by offering high-quality service in a cost-effective manner.

The tremendous growth in the managed care arena will have, by most accounts, an even greater influence on medical transportation. As the method of reimbursement shifts from fee-for-service to capitation, ambulance companies will seek contracts with managed care plans to transport their members for a preset fee. However, these contracts will be performance based, with the providers responsible for meeting very specific quality standards. Ambulance providers will be managing with an eye toward maximizing their productivity while still providing high-quality patient care. Only the most imaginative and industrious providers will succeed in this new environment.

Thus, in today's challenging healthcare environment, medical transportation services must implement strategies to acquire and retain highly motivated workforces that are willing to work hard, expand their capabilities, and deliver higher levels of quality care while meeting stiffer performance standards. Since personnel costs consume the majority of an organization's budget, information provided in this salary survey is designed to assist managers in plotting their organizations' futures from financial and human affairs standpoints. The survey covers a variety of salary and salary-related topics, from annual compensation to standard benefits.

The Survey

As in the past, a consistent sample of providers responded to a standardized questionnaire that elicited information regarding salaries and benefits for their respective services. It should be noted this survey is designed to identify and monitor annual changes in the same sample year after year, so trends can be tracked over time. It is not intended to simply highlight data in a single year.

The number and percentage of respondents by provider type are listed in Table 3.2. Specifically, the number and type are the following: 10 private, for-profit providers; 24 fire departments with cross-trained personnel; five fire departments with separate EMS staff; 12 hospital-based providers; 19 other public entities (including counties, districts, and law enforcement); and eight nonprofit non-government organizations, for a total sample of 80 EMS providers.

Four regions are represented in the survey: Northeast, Southeast, Central, and West. The geographic distribution of respondents can be seen in Table 3.3. Table 3.4 indicates that more than two-thirds of the respondents (67.5 percent) serve communities with populations between 100,000 and 1 million people; in 1993, only 61.7 percent served such large communities.

Table 3.2 Respondents by Provider Type		
Provider	Respondents	Percent
Private for Profit	10	12.5%
Public		
Fire Department, Cross-Trained	24	30.0%
Fire Department, Separate	5	6.25%
Other Public*	19	23.75%
Nonprofit	8	10.0%
Hospital	12	15.0%
Other	2	2.5%
Total	**80**	**100%**

*Incorporates third services, such as city, county, and police agencies.
Percentages are rounded off to the nearest whole number.

Annual Compensation

The annual salary for each job category by provider-type classification demonstrates without exception that every job category in the fire department had a higher salary than other provider types. Overall, the private and fire department providers offer higher salaries than the nonprofit and hospital-based services.

Table 3.5 reports changes in compensation in nine positions and updates the seven-year comparison. On average, there was an increase of 4.6 percent, with executive directors, division supervisors, and intermediate EMTs exceeding that mean increase. The smallest increase was for administrative directors at 3.3 percent.

Table 3.6 shows annual compensation for each position according to region. Com-

Table 3.3 Geographic Distribution of Respondents		
Region	Respondents	Percentage
Northeast (Connecticut, Maine, Massachusetts, New Hampshire, Delaware, New Jersey, New York, Pennsylvania, Rhode Island, Vermont, Michigan)	**10**	**12.5%**
West (Alaska, Arizona, California, Hawaii, Idaho, Nevada, New Mexico, Oregon, Utah, Washington, Colorado, Texas, Montana, Wyoming)	**30**	**37.5%**
Central (North Dakota, South Dakota, Nebraska, Kansas, Oklahoma, Ohio, Minnesota, Iowa, Missouri, Illinois, Wisconsin, Indiana)	**20**	**25.0%**
Southeast (Florida, Georgia, Alabama, Mississippi, Arkansas, Tennessee, North Carolina, South Carolina, Kentucky, Virginia, West Virginia, Louisiana, Maryland)	**20**	**25.0%**
Total	**80**	**100%**

Table 3.4		
Respondents by Population Served		
Population Range	**Respondents**	**Percent**
Less than 20,000	5	6.25%
20,000 to 49,999	5	6.25%
50,000 to 99,999	16	20.0%
100,000 to 249,999	29	36.25%
250,000 to 999,999	22	27.5%
Greater than 1,000,000	3	3.75%
Total	**80**	**100%**

pared with last year's survey, the Northeast experienced a downturn in average salaries this year with the exception of executive directors, operations managers, and EMT-basics (dispatchers and first responders also showed negligible increases at a few hundred dollars each). The West, however, saw salaries increase from last year's survey, some by several thousand dollars. The overall mean showed increases in most of the job categories.

Emergency response volume and service area populations have little impact on compensation levels. Low-volume services (fewer than 2,000) have compensation levels comparable to those of larger-volume services. The same holds true whether services provide care for regions of 20,000 or 100,000 with salary levels being fairly consistent.

Age and Tenure

Data describing the age, number of years in the organization, and number of hours worked per week for each of the 14 job categories in the seven provider classifications offer a profile of each position. The compensation data can then match individuals with a particular salary picture.

The data show that, in general, the private paramedic is 30 years old, has been with his service for four and a half years, and works approximately 50 hours per week. The typical firefighter/paramedic is 33 years old, has been with the department for more than 11 years, and works slightly more than 51 hours per week.

The hourly wage comparison of paramedics and EMT-basics over a seven-year period is presented in Table 3.7. As in the past, the average hourly wage is computed by dividing mean annual salaries by 52 weeks and then again by the average number of hours worked per week. Wages for paramedics continue to increase, as evidenced by the data. Hourly wages for EMT-basics also show increases, although at a smaller rate than that for paramedics.

Table 3.5				
Changes in Compensation from 1987 to 1994				
Position	**1994**	**1987**	**Percent Change**	**Avg. Annual Percent Increase**
Executive Director	$61,564	$45,050	+36.7%	5.2%
Administrative Director	$48,453	$39,330	+23.2%	3.3%
Operations Manager	$49,102	$37,030	+32.6%	4.7%
Div/Ops Supervisor	$45,360	$33,420	+35.7%	5.1%
Field Supervisor	$36,203	$28,470	+27.2%	3.9%
Paramedic	$31,058	$24,100	+28.9%	4.1%
EMT-I	$27,196	$19,840	+37.1%	5.3%
EMT-Basic	$25,234	$18,710	+34.9%	5.0%
Dispatcher	$25,900	$19,740	+31.2%	4.5%
Average			**+31.9%**	**4.6%**

Table 3.6

Annual Compensation by Region

Region	Executive Director	Admin. Director	Operations Manager	Div/Ops Supervisor	Field Supervisor	Paramedic	EMT-Intermediate
Northeast	$54,667	$38,000	$38,450	$33,663	$31,900	$28,602	$22,666
West	$61,107	$59,672	$54,992	$50,978	$38,976	$35,611	$33,525
Central	$62,220	$41,100	$44,763	$42,265	$34,785	$27,587	$19,486
Southeast	$63,032	$47,424	$51,162	$42,863	$36,096	$30,300	$26,357
Mean Salary*	$61,564	$48,453	$49,102	$45,360	$36,203	$31,058	$27,196

Region	EMT-Basic	First Responder	Dispatcher	Medical Director	Training Dir/Officer	Public Info/ Ed. Officer	QA/QI Officer
Northeast	$25,300	$33,200	$22,806	$21,000	$34,582	N/A	$33,000
West	$31,478	N/A	$28,643	$27,833	$45,175	$47,489	$43,908
Central	$22,397	$27,370	$26,213	$17,200	$41,163	$38,985	$31,539
Southeast	$21,740	$30,622	$24,225	$22,000	$39,866	$35,479	$36,058
Mean Salary*	$25,234	$30,454	$25,900	$23,329	$41,507	$41,078	$37,091

*Mean salary of all respondents combined.

Employee Benefits

Employee benefits are an extremely important component of a person's compensation package and are factored into the "cost" of an employee to a company. Table 3.8 lists those benefits for which the employer is responsible in some fashion.

It is clear from the table that essential benefits related to the health and welfare of the employee are provided for most of the respondents. Benefits provided for more than 70 percent of the respondents are employee major medical insurance, life insurance, retirement or pension plans, liability insurance, and employee assistance programs (which include various forms of counseling services). Other benefits provided to the employee include uniform allowance, tuition reimbursement, and conference attendance.

To varying degrees, employers provide additional health and economic benefits, including disability insurance, profit sharing, and financial incentive programs. It should be noted, however, that profit sharing is found only in the private sector.

Paid time off is an important aspect of an employee's job and economic remuneration. Although not reported in a table, on average, after one year, employees earn 97 hours of vacation time; after two years, 110 hours are earned; 144 hours are earned after five years; and 171 hours are earned after 10 years of service. The typical employee receives nine paid holidays and almost 14 days paid for sick time.

Table 3.7

Changes in Hourly Wages from 1987 to 1994

Provider Type	Paramedic			EMT-Basic		
	1994	1987	% Change	1994	1987	% Change
Private	$10.23	$7.31	+39.9%	$5.97	$5.66	+5.5%
Public						
Fire Department	$14.51	$10.81	+34.2%	$12.00	$9.80	+22.4%
Other Public*	$11.55	$8.46	+36.5%	$10.45	$7.17	+45.7%
Hospital	$10.91	$7.78	+40.2%	$7.60	$6.61	+15.0%
Mean**	**$11.80**	**$9.16**	**+28.8%**	**$9.01**	**$7.37**	**+22.2%**

*Includes third service, such as city, county, and police agencies.
**Mean of all respondents combined.

Table 3.8

Benefits Provided by Respondents

Benefits	1994	1993
Major Medical—Employee	96.3%	97.9%
Life Insurance	95.1%	93.8%
Retirement or Pension Plan	90.0%	88.7%
Uniform Allowance	90.0%	87.6%
Tuition Reimbursement, EMS Only	88.8%	79.4%
Paid Seminars and Conferences	85.1%	78.4%
Liability Insurance	83.8%	85.6%
Employee Assistance Plan	78.8%	77.3%
Dental Insurance	76.3%	82.5%
Major Medical—Family	76.3%	73.2%
Long-Term Disability	68.8%	52.6%
Short-Term Disability	61.3%	58.8%
Educational Incentives, Non-EMS Courses	55.0%	53.6%
Optical Insurance	42.6%	46.4%
Shift Differential	30.1%	24.7%
Meal Allowance	23.8%	26.8%
Financial Incentive Programs	18.8%	15.5%
Profit Sharing	7.5%	10.3%

Additional Data

Another key element in this analysis is a description of the level of care provided by the respondents. More than 98 percent of the respondents reported that they provide ALS care, and of that group, almost 80 percent send a paramedic on all emergency calls. For non-emergency calls, the percentage sending paramedics declines, with slightly more than 50 percent doing so. In addition, more than 50 percent of those responding stated that they use EMT-intermediates in their service.

When queried as to whether ambulances are staffed by personnel with less training than an EMT, 95 percent of the respondents responded no. In fact, almost 60 percent staff their ambulances with two paramedics, and an additional 30 percent have at least one paramedic on the ambulance. BLS ambulances are used by slightly over one-third of the services responding to the survey, and 40 percent of these stated that BLS units are dispatched to some emergencies. Two-thirds of the sample indicated that early defibrillation programs are in place in their communities using EMTs and first responders. However, contrary to last year's survey, in which more than 50 percent of those services without an early defibrillation program indicated they would implement one in the next 18 months, only 30 percent of this year's respondents propose to do so.

In addition, approximately 85 percent of the respondents indicated that they normally provide transportation from the scene, and more than 75 percent stated they would not allow another service to transport the patient if they had already begun to provide ALS care at the scene.

Approximately 70 percent, or 56 of the 80 respondents, indicated that they have both strength and flexibility testing for new hires, as well as physical fitness standards for new employees (Table 3.9).

Forty-five percent of the respondents indicated that their employees are unionized. This is an increase of 10 percent over last year's results, in which only 35 percent of the respondents reported that their employees were unionized.

Approximately 93 percent of the services use a medical director/advisor, and 67 percent fund this position. Only 21 percent of the services have this medical director on a full-time basis. However, in 66 percent of the services, the medical director does have the authority to independently discipline or restrict the activity of field personnel.

Conclusion

This year's salary survey continues the tracking of information garnered over the past seven years. It is designed as a guide and has demonstrated the fluctuation of salaries in the various provider organizations. However, as changes in sample size, demographics, and other variables influence these results, reliance on the absolute numbers in this report would be misleading. Therefore, it should be placed in context with other industry information when making decisions regarding compensation levels.

Source

Richard A. Keller is a partner at Fitch & Associates, Inc. Edward I. Weinberg, MA, MPH, is a senior associate at Fitch & Associates, Inc., and a former CEO for a hospital consortium specializing in air medical transportation, education, and research.

Table 3.9

Fitness Standards

| Type of Service | New Hires | | | | | | Current Employees | | |
| | Strength Test | | | Fitness Standards | | | Fitness Standards | | |
	Yes	No	Total	Yes	No	Total	Yes	No	Total
Private for Profit	6	4	10	5	5	10	2	8	10
Public									
Fire Department, Combined	26	3	29	27	2	29	11	18	29
Fire Department, Cross-Trained	23	1	24	22	2	24	10	14	24
Fire Department, Separate	3	2	5	5	0	5	1	4	5
Other Public	14	5	19	11	8	19	2	16	18
Nonprofit	6	2	8	6	2	8	2	10	12
Hospital	3	9	12	5	7	12	2	6	8
Other	1	1	2	1	1	2	0	0	0
Total	**56**	**24**	**80**	**55**	**25**	**80**	**19**	**58**	**77***

*Three did not respond to this question.

Personal Financial Planning— Eight Steps to Security

Paul W. Ewing

Getting out of the paycheck-to-paycheck rut is a challenge for EMS workers, regardless of how much they make. Real commitment is required to honestly evaluate lifestyle issues, plan resources, and then stick to the plan. This lighthearted article provides eight steps for improving your financial outlook.

WHILE A CAREER IN THE EMERGENCY medical services can be financially rewarding over time, the rewards develop slowly and incrementally. As a result, many fail to recognize the importance of establishing financial behaviors that will enable them to retain some of their earnings for financial security. Many people incrementally increase their spending and borrow against the future. But if you save and invest today, you will save (and make) more dollars tomorrow.

The Ant and the Grasshopper

The fable of the ant and the grasshopper teaches the virtues of thrift. It shows how diligent pursuit can provide the reward of security, but at the price of enjoying life. It seems an inescapable choice. Do I spend for today or save for tomorrow? Do I live "pig happy" or "Socrates sad"? Is it less filling or does it taste great? Today, the grasshopper uses some secrets in order to avoid making these choices. Simply put, we want it all.

This article describes eight ways to increase your financial lot in life and move toward financial security. I challenge you to put at least five of them to work within the next 30 days. Start at least one today and one before this week is out. At the end of the 30 days, you can consider yourself a neo-grasshopper.

The life of a grasshopper is a thrilling, music-filled adventure, full of carefree days. It is difficult to be carefree when you are in debt and have no hope for financial security. It is hard to swallow an expensive meal at a fine restaurant when you sit down to eat and realize all your credit cards are past their spending limits. Grasshoppers would never make decisions that would allow the things they own to own them. Perhaps you know someone like that. They just had to have an expensive new car, even though they could barely afford it. Now they have to eat macaroni and cheese and work overtime just to make the payments. We are surrounded with the stimuli to urge us to spend up to, if not beyond, our capacity. Only we can make the choice.

In the last decade, grasshoppers have come out of the haze and have seen a need to take charge of their carefree ways by taking control of their finances. The following are eight of their very best secrets to help you on your way.

Eight Steps to Financial Security

Establish a reward for successful results. This is the most crucial of the eight secrets. Decide what specific reward you are going to give yourself for sticking with your plan. Visualize this reward, write it down, draw a picture, and set a date. This is not about what you must do without; this is about how much more you can have by making good, intentional choices.

Today is the day to kick the credit card debt. This is a war—"operation credit storm." You should not stop until you pay your balance in full every month. First, you must stop indiscriminate use, and you must make the cards inaccessible. Then you must inflict heavy collateral damage by reallocating other resources to eliminate any high balance. Any balance remaining will be managed as follows: The balance will be calculated and divided by six; seven payments of that amount will be made in the seven months that follow. This formula must be followed no matter what. If you cannot retire that amount in seven months, you are headed for financial meltdown. Keep track of any credit charges from this day forward. Subtract the amount of each charge directly from your checkbook to ensure that you have adequate funds to pay the bill in full each month from now on.

Let's decide who's the boss here. If your car or home is too expensive, it's time to take that money-soaking crocodile to task. Some people think they can justify having non-deductible consumer debt and these extravagances, but you now know better. You cannot allow the things you own to own you. Your next investment is going to be in a want ad. Garage sale, anyone?

Identify the two most expensive, self-indulgent items that you spend money on—one of them has to go. If you just can't part with it, at least you can cut the expenditure in half. Perhaps reinstating this privilege will be your reward for being successful.

Do something to make some money beyond what you are doing now. You may want to mow lawns, rake leaves, or walk the neighbor's dog. Everyone has some talent that can be both interesting and fun, but it must be for pay. And that pay must be allocated to debt reduction, building cash reserves, or investing. You can allow yourself to be a capitalistic money-monger in pursuit of not only money, but the sense of accomplishment that comes from earning money—not just to live on, but to use to get ahead.

Put together your own team. Find a like-minded soul you can share ideas with who will help you stay on track. Your team may include a professional financial planner or advisor, but you should stay in control of your decisions. Many in the financial services field are only equipped to deal with the insurance side of the process or they may only recently have entered the investment area. You will soon outgrow them, and you may find some of their counsel conflicts with your objective to build a growing nest egg. Find an advisor who is investment-oriented first, yet capable of advising you on insurance matters in proper perspective. You should develop a game plan. Decide what amount of reserves are appropriate for you between liquid accounts and available credit. Having credit available for emergency needs or so you can take advantage of a genuine bargain opportunity is not evil or taboo. Carrying a credit card balance is.

Try to own your car outright next time. Do some math on this one. First, decide how much longer you will want to keep your jalopy. Then, project what it will be worth when you dispose of it. Next calculate what you will still owe. Take the difference between what it's worth and what you will owe, plus the cost of your next car, as your funding target. Now you know how much you will need and how long you have to save up for it. Divide the amount needed by the number of months until you need it. That equals the amount of money you need to set aside each month for the outright purchase of your next car. If you cannot afford to do this on your next car, perhaps you can make it a goal for the following acquisition—or reassess how much of a car you need to be driving. This is a great example of how you can begin to have interest paid to you instead of paying interest (non-deductible) to someone else.

Learn how to be an investor. You'll need to learn what risk is, how economics can impact different investment performances, and where you can find reliable information to make decisions. When you retire, the quality of your lifestyle will depend on your ability to manage your money. Many new clients come to me with the expectation that I can help them grow their nest egg into a sizable amount when they retire. I challenge them to become actively involved and to develop their investment acumen. Not only will they have more to work with, they will know how to earn a greater income from their portfolio. It is not rocket science to say that investors with a 10-percent yield can have twice the income than if the bank just pays them five percent on the same funds.

Stick to your chosen strategies for another 30 days and they will become a new behavior. These new behaviors will help you obtain financial freedom. Just 60 days from now, you can be a Socrates-happy, more filling, full-fledged grasshopper that can afford to have great taste. Good luck.

Cash for Caliber: EMS and the Pay-by-Merit System

Joe Rudd and John Hitchens

Compensation plans are changing. Annual seniority raises are giving way to performance-based compensation systems. This article describes the path taken by one county EMS system in moving to a pay-by-merit system.

FEW PEOPLE WOULD DISAGREE with the concept that employees who work harder should be paid more. After all, material reward for accomplishment is the American way. Why, then, is the pay-by-merit concept—compensation based on individual accomplishment—so controversial in EMS?

Pay by merit is not a new concept. In small businesses and organizations in which the owner or director has personal contact with each employee, it is a fair and reasonable way to determine an employee's monetary worth. Under such a system, employees who work hard for the organization, who are not excessively absent or tardy, and who uphold the philosophies of the organization when in contact with the public receive greater monetary compensation than those who take a less serious view of their duties.

The most common compensation system, however, is one in which hard work is not rewarded; everyone—whether a diligent laborer or not—receives the same pay raises based on longevity rather than productivity. This is sometimes referred to as the "heartbeat method," i.e., if your heart beats the requisite number of times, you receive an automatic pay raise equal to that of your fellow employees whose hearts beat at the same rate.

This system, based on length of service rather than quality of performance, has been adopted by most organizations for one simple reason: It is easy to administer. It is also preferred by some employees because people are rarely fired except in cases of blatant misconduct. It is very easy for people to disappear into this type of system and never be heard from again—except on payday.

Challenges of a Pay-by-Merit System

Large businesses and organizations have experienced numerous difficulties when attempting to implement pay-by-merit systems. The foremost problem is that employees lack confidence in such a system. Many reasons are given for this lack of confidence, but they can be summarized in the following statements:

- Employees don't fully understand what is expected of them by supervisors.
- Employees don't trust supervisors to administer the program fairly.

This distrust may not necessarily be the supervisors' fault. In a Gallup poll, 80 percent of the American workers surveyed believed that they fit

Job performance in EMS is not easily measured. Because supervisors rarely accompany employees on emergency calls in the field, supervisors are reduced to relying on infrequent feedback from patients and other EMTs.

into the upper 20 percent of the workforce in their companies with regard to quality, productivity, and company loyalty.

Obviously, these perceptions cannot be true. It is easy, then, to recognize the difficult situation faced by supervisors who must explain to the individuals in the other 60 percent of the workforce why their ratings do not match their self-perceptions. Add to that the time and expense necessary to administer a pay-by-merit program, and it is immediately apparent why more organizations don't put one into practice.

But is the pay-by-tenure, or longevity system, which can encourage waste and inefficiency, really saving these organizations money in the long run?

A Research Project

This is the question that in 1986 launched a research project undertaken by John Hitchens, director of Whitfield EMS in Dalton, Ga. Hitchens joined an EMS system that had just initiated a pay-by-merit system that still had many problems. He researched the available literature and found that, although studies had been published concerning the pros and cons of merit pay, none of them related specifically to EMS. In fact, the vast majority of research on the subject was geared toward the teaching profession.

So Hitchens began his own research. Using basic EMTs in the Whitfield County EMS organization, he began a year-long project studying job descriptions and past annual review scores.

EMTs were selected at random by employee number to take part in the project. Each person was then interviewed and polled on his views concerning the system as it existed and how it could be improved. The sample group raised several legitimate concerns and suggestions.

First, job performance in EMS is not easily measured. Because supervisors rarely accompany employees on emergency calls in the field, supervisors are reduced to relying on infrequent feedback from patients and other EMTs, which may not correspond with the way the employee views his own skills and work habits.

Second, the group determined that too much emphasis was being placed on administrative concerns. Rating an employee on productivity, using criteria such as the number of patients transported and the amount of equipment and supplies used on each patient, does not yield accurate information about the EMT's performance, as he has limited control over the number or severity of calls to which he responds. In fact, an employee wishing to favorably influence his evaluation could be guilty of overtreating patients and, thereby, raising costs for unnecessary treatment.

A third concern was that employees did not understand what constituted an "above-average" performance standard. For instance, if the standard was "maintains a clean vehicle," most employees felt that washing their vehicles once a day was sufficient to obtain an "exceeds standard" rating. The administration, however, may construe such a rating to mean that, in addition to washing the vehicle whenever necessary, other efforts should be extended, such as waxing the vehicle, blackening the tires, or occasionally shampooing the interior and carpet.

A final concern of the group addressed the semantics of the review. Many objected to the terminology used, such as "average" or "performance expected at all times without exception."

After the poll was completed and the answers tabulated, Hitchens found that, while 80 percent of the employees agreed in principle with pay by merit, only 70 percent felt that supervisors had the ability to give fair and impartial evaluations. This appeared to stem less from a lack of confidence in the supervisors' ability to manage and more from a lack of confidence in their ability to judge employee performance based on limited contact with crew members.

Another interesting fact emerged from this study: The concerns raised by the EMS employees were identical to those raised by teachers in similar studies. Apparently, EMS is similar to other professions in which unsupervised work is performed and then measured.

In those teaching organizations in which pay by merit was tried and abandoned as unworkable, the main reason for the failure was a lack of means by which to measure actual accomplishments. In those organizations in which the pay-by-merit system succeeded, a means of measurement existed that was as objective as possible based on tangible evidence.

In some cases, employees were actually asked to evaluate themselves and were told that, if they could qualify all scores, the evaluations would be approved as the employees wrote them. This took the evaluation process out of the realm of the employer and made it an agreement between the supervisor and the employee—a joint effort that was fair to both.

Creating an Effective Pay-by-Merit System

After evaluating the results of the EMS study, Hitchens was faced with the decision of whether to continue the pay-by-merit system, change it to a tenure-only program, or combine the two. He chose the most difficult of the three options: to continue with and improve the existing pay-by-merit system.

In doing so, Hitchen's first action was to rewrite the performance evaluation criteria, giving specific examples of what constituted average, below-average, and above-average performance. For instance, in the category "wears uniform in a professional manner," the standard had been "maintains a neat and clean appearance." This was changed so that the rating "exceeds standard" was only given to those employees who, in addition to wearing a clean uniform every day as expected, went the extra length in bringing a backup uniform and changing at midshift or if the uniform became soiled.

By making each criterion clear to both the employee and the supervisor, much of the subjectivity of the evaluation was eliminated. The result

> The concerns raised by the EMS employees were identical to those raised by teachers in similar studies.

Examples of Revised Wording to Differentiate "Standard" from "Exceeds Standard" Ratings

Original: Operates vehicle in a safe manner
Revised: Emergency Vehicle Operator's Course-qualified or
Member of accident review board committee or
No accident or incident for three consecutive years

Original: Maintains ambulance and equipment
Revised: Waxes vehicle regularly or
Initiates repairs or
Improves vehicle (installs consoles or modifications)

Original: Maintains current training standards or level
Revised: Nationally registered or
Shows instructor potential on ACLS course score or
Teaches EMT/paramedic classes

Original: Maintains professional appearance
Revised: Two uniforms are maintained during 24-hour shifts or
Serves on uniform-standardization committee

Original: Performs patient care permitted by protocol
Revised: Works with medical director to develop new
protocols or
Tests new equipment/procedures and writes
documentation to support their use

was that, when the same employees were polled again, there was an increase in the employees' trust of the supervisors' abilities to judge their performance.

Hitchens augmented these revisions to the performance criteria with a program that included human resources and supervisory training for all administrative personnel, an improved quality assurance system, tuition reimbursement for additional training, and in-services to acquaint employees with the mechanics of the new evaluation system.

As a result of these efforts, there was an increase in employee understanding of the program and willingness to participate. After the process was revised, 79 percent agreed not only with the concept, but with the actual method by which evaluations were conducted.

Tips for Pay-by-Merit Success

The following is some advice for establishing or revising a pay-by-merit system.

If your current review criteria are not understood by the majority of employees, rewrite them. The employees' understanding of the system and willingness to participate in it are crucial for success.

Supervisors must be adequately trained on the system before being responsible for administering it. A supervisor who does not understand the system could seriously detract from the integrity of the program.

For the first year, use review criteria only as an example of what is expected and continue with across-the-board uniform pay increases for all employees. Do not attach monetary values to scores until the system has been in place long enough to be completely understood by all. A review of actual evaluations with supervisors explaining their reasons for above- and below-standard scores remains the best way for any system to adopt reasonable standards.

Allow employees adequate input in the performance evaluation. Both the supervisor and employee should be flexible enough to change a score if the situation so dictates. The willingness to compromise enhances employee confidence in the system.

Continue to improve the quality of review standards by studying the success and failure of past standards. Standards should be written in such a way that they encourage a system-wide rise in compliance. What an employee does one year to get an "exceeds standard" rating may only be considered a "meets standard" rating at the next review if there has been significant company-wide improvement in that standard. However, management should recognize that the standards should be acceptable and understood by employees, and upgrading standards should not be perceived as a punitive measure. This allows a company to improve standards based on actual performance rather than the ideals or unrealistic expectations forced by an administration.

Keep employees advised of their shortcomings between reviews. Don't suddenly spring a year's worth of problems on them at the review. Give each employee a chance to improve during the year, and consider any improvements at the time of the review.

Don't fall into the trap of overrating all employees. Keep standards difficult enough to attain so that most employees fall into the "meets standard" category. If higher scores are too easy to get, a "halo effect" is created that removes the incentive to improve. It also does an injustice to those employees who go to greater lengths in such ways as serving on task forces, obtaining instructor licenses, or taking on extra projects.

Always remember that, while job descriptions, standards, and evaluation forms are important, they are only "tools" for facilitating discussion. Do not let the instrument become more important than the original concept of why the performance appraisal is important.

In the book *In Search of Excellence*, author Tom Peters summarizes the key ingredients of America's best-run companies:

> The essence of excellence is the thousand concrete, minute-to-minute actions performed by everyone in an organization to keep the company on its course. Excellent companies are brilliant on just a few basics: behaving with courtesy toward customers, providing innovative services, and, above all, gaining the commitment, ingenuity, and energy of all employees.

The pay-by-merit system has allowed Whitfield EMS to bring its management and street personnel closer together in their attitudes toward employee compensation by providing a sounding board for concerns from both sides. This, in turn, has led to a new commitment to the community it serves.

Source

Reprinted with permission from JEMS, *January 1991. Joe Rudd, RN, has been involved with law enforcement and EMS for over 20 years. John Hitchens is the director for Whitfield EMS and has 23 years of experience in prehospital emergency care.*

References

Balterman, R. "Merit Pay? No." *National Association of Elementary Schools* 52, no. 5.

Gallup, G. H. "Fifteenth Annual Gallup Poll on Public's Attitudes Toward Public Schools." *Phi Delta Kappa* 65, no. 1 (1983).

Rist, M. "Most Teachers Endorse the Merit Pay Concept." *American School Board Journal* (September 1983).

Establishing an Ideal Relationship With Your Accountant

Joseph Palmer, CPA

Accountants often speak in an intimidating financial lingo. Perhaps for that reason, few EMS managers ask the right questions when choosing an accountant. This article outlines important accountant selection criteria, standard services you should expect to receive, and how to evaluate fees.

IN WORKING WITH AMBULANCE SERVICES for a number of years, I have observed the following about CPAs and owners:

- Most CPAs do not understand Medicare and Medicaid, or the fundamentals of operating an ambulance company.
- Most owners do not understand their own financial statements and the accrual basis of accounting.
- Neither CPAs nor owners take a proactive stance to gain knowledge about something they do not understand.

Simply, we fail to communicate with each other because we do not have the time or we are embarrassed by the fact that we do not understand what the other does. We fail to recognize the importance of understanding each other, or we perceive that the lack of understanding is "just the way it is." If you and your accountant are willing to work together, then your accountant can become a more effective advisor. This article explains how you should choose and use your accountant to your greatest advantage.

Choosing Your Accountant

The selection of your accountant should be based on predetermined criteria and the interview process. Your criteria may include the following:

- How many of the CPA's current clients are similar to your size (revenues) and ownership structure
- The CPA's general knowledge of Medicare and Medicaid practices
- How much attention the CPA is willing to pay to you versus other clients
- The CPA's willingness to make a commitment to learn your business without charging you
- The CPA's willingness to make a commitment to teach you how to read and interpret the financial statements produced for you
- The CPA's experience in areas important to you, such as loan negotiations, computer networks, or hardware and software, the CPA's presentation skills, and the CPA's leadership position within the community
- The degree of the CPA firm's typical analytical summary of financial statements showing historic trends and comparative ratio analyses
- The CPA's knowledge of the ambulance industry

In most communities, there should be three or more CPA firms that you can choose from to match your selection criteria. Depending on your organization's size, you need to look for a CPA firm with three or more partners. You should control the interviewing process in order to obtain responses to each of your predetermined questions. Attention should be given to the other firm members and their roles in working with you. In most cases, you should select the firm that you gained the highest "comfort" level with during the interview process. Personalities are extremely important, along with the total support the selected firm can offer you.

Whether you are in search of a CPA firm or questioning what your current CPA is doing for you, the following is a list of services you should be receiving:

- Quarterly meetings to review the interim financial statements and business plans or issues
- Prepared year-end financial statements to be reviewed with you within 90 days after the close of the year
- Proactive tax advice for the corporation and key officers/stockholders
- Assistance in obtaining loans
- Assistance in suggesting hardware and software for your accounting, receivables, and spreadsheet analysis needs
- Assistance in developing a business plan and strategy
- Assistance in potential growth through expansion or acquisition
- Assistance in understanding, interpreting, and using the financial statements
- Networking opportunities
- Operational audit reviews to point out potential revenue enhancement or cost reduction opportunities
- Proactive steps taken to learn more about your business and industry

What Role You Should Play

The CPA should take the lead in establishing the boundaries of the relationship. However, to make it work, you must be a willing participant. Listed below are some ways you can maximize the benefits you receive from this relationship.

- Hire experienced and competent bookkeepers or accountants to provide reliable, internally generated financial statements.
- Clearly define the roles, duties, and responsibilities of your accounting staff and the CPA firm.
- Communicate your plans with your CPA prior to implementation to avoid detrimental tax or financial consequences.
- Use your CPA as a sounding board. Although probably not

Source

Original article. Joseph E. Palmer, CPA, MBA, is the director of Management Consulting Services at Heinick, Apple & Company. He has over 26 years of consulting, industrial, and public accounting experience.

totally familiar with the ambulance industry, your CPA's years of experience with similar issues could be invaluable to you.
- Challenge your CPA to be proactive in dealing with those business issues you may not be as knowledgeable in.

What About Fees?

Truly, you pay for what you get. This doesn't mean that you need to engage the lowest priced CPA firm or accept the lowest bid to gain value. It means that you must define the level of service you need and expect. If you have competent accountants and financially astute personnel, it will not be necessary for you to pay firm fees based on high levels of professional staffing for services you do not need. If you only need reviewed or audited financials, then placing your services for bid with qualified firms is probably the right approach. On the other hand, if you plan to rely on your accounting firm to provide more than financial statements, you may be better off engaging a firm that has the capability to provide the services you need now and, potentially, the services you will need in the future, as long as its fees are reasonable.

You should request that your CPA draft an engagement letter describing the services to be provided and the fees to be charged. Based upon the engagement letter, you can approve or change the scope of the services to suit your budget. You should always ask your CPA what services can be performed in house to help reduce charges.

The Relationship

The relationship should be what you want it to be: one that grows into a professional bounding relationship, if this is consistent with your desires. Professional bounding means that the CPA is looking out for your business and personal best interests. A relationship develops where the CPA anticipates your needs and desires and offers proactive advice.

If you or your CPA becomes dissatisfied, either party should feel free to confront the other without fear of destroying the relationship. Instead, try to strengthen this important relationship through conflict resolution.

Alternative Funding Methods

Defining Membership Program Potential

Christine M. Zalar, RN, MA

A number of groundwork activities are necessary before a membership program can be put in place. The author stresses that the potential for a membership program should be evaluated through a three-phase process that identifies the risks and rewards.

MEMBERSHIP PROGRAMS HAVE PROVIDED an alternative means of generating revenue for air and ground medical transportation services. However, the service must quantify the risk factors of a membership program, which can convert the anticipated "additional revenue" to a costly proposition.

Prospective feasibility research, or quantifying the impact of a membership program, is complex. It requires three distinct phases:

- Assessment of the service's current market penetration and its financial and operational performance
- Qualitative research that includes data gathered through focus groups representative of the target membership population, key medical transportation influencers, and the service's management personnel
- Quantifiable research, generally through development of a survey instrument for telephone administration by an independent market research organization

The survey data should be entered into a computer to allow for multiple statistical evaluations and cross-tabulations of the internal and external factors influencing the market. Finally, the data from each phase of research should be correlated to define the projected outcomes and risks before implementing a membership program for the service.

The first step in any membership program is to prospectively define the anticipated outcomes for the program. The outcomes should stem from the primary reason for offering the membership program. Primary motivators may be the need for additional revenue or the competition from another service in the same market.

Once the program goals have been established, a comprehensive analysis of the membership program potential, specifically for meeting the established goals, should be conducted. The analysis must, at a minimum, quantify the impact on the service's market penetration, financial performance, and operations.

Market Penetration

A number of baseline data indicators need to be measured, including public perception of the service, such as unassisted name recall and credibility; perception of key healthcare influencers regarding the service; public access to healthcare services; and public cost awareness and price sensitivity. The quantifiable outcomes of these factors will determine the market's perception of need for such a service, the likelihood of using the service, and at what price they would purchase a membership. In assessing the demographics of the potential members, the market should be analyzed according to age, income, and insurance coverage mix.

Financial Parameters

Many services have established a price for their potential membership program based on "what other services charge." Experience has proven this to be a dangerous assumption. The price structure that the public will buy differs in every market, not only in terms of the actual price, but more importantly, in terms of who will buy a membership at what price. The key is to isolate the target membership group, and gather the pertinent data that identifies their cost sensitivity. A typical mistake is lowering the price of the membership because more people can afford the lower cost. The result is generally more members, but the payer mix of these members can represent a significantly larger group of self payers.

After it has been determined who will buy the membership, compare their payer profile with the current profile of your service. Note the collections performance in each of the payer classes. The variance is important in determining whether a membership program should continue to be pursued.

Finally, the expenses of offering the program should be projected. Carefully quantify all the associated expenses and the impact of managing the membership program. The number of projected members will define the ability of your existing resources to manage the program. Too often, program resource requirements are projected too low, resulting in expenses over budget, particularly in the second year when volunteerism may begin to wane and the initial excitement of program implementation is over.

Operational Impact

Member utilization, which is typically higher than that of the general public, may impact current basing and deployment strategies. Part of the feasibility research should project member utilization of the service. Then the service must answer this question: Can the membership be served with existing transportation resources? The answer begins with plotting membership penetration per household in each zone or community of the service area and correlating this with ambulance and aircraft base locations.

The analysis of the membership program must be conducted in light of the service intended to be offered. For example, a membership program currently in place providing ground transportation services may not translate to a successful air membership program within the same markets. Factors, including different user profiles and payer mix for each transportation segment and the cost of providing the service (air versus ground), require re-analysis for the air membership potential. Simply increasing current membership price that "extends" membership to include helicopter service may be risky given the market's price sensitivity and the customers' perception regarding their likelihood to use air service. The extension of a current membership service may also have a negative impact on market penetration, resulting in an overall decrease in member participation.

Membership programs represent a supplemental funding concept for ground and air medical programs. But, without adequate preplanning and research, the benefits may fail to materialize.

Source
Reprinted with permission from Management Focus, *Fall 1991. Christine M. Zalar is a partner at Fitch & Associates, Inc. She is widely recognized as one of the nation's leading experts on air medical and hospital-based EMS/medical transportation systems. She is also a principal author of the book* EMS Management: Beyond the Street, *2nd ed.*

Public Sector Ambulance Membership

Dennis Murphy

Public sector agencies are searching for innovative funding sources. In this article, Fire Chief Dennis Murphy shares his experiences implementing the FireMed ambulance membership program in Eugene and Springfield, Ore.

SOMETIMES I FEEL MORE LIKE a scientist in a research and development laboratory than an EMS division chief in a fire department. In a recent phone conversation with *JEMS* Publisher Jim Page, he told me how pleased he was at the progress in his FireMed ambulance membership program, and I couldn't help but be pleased myself.

FireMed is one of a number of recent developments from the "laboratory" in Eugene and Springfield, Ore., that have been field tested successfully in other locations. Because public ambulance providers in three locations are preparing to begin FireMed programs in the next six months and 13 others are in various stages of research and development, I thought it was time to share the good news: Well-run ambulance memberships are allowing public sector providers to offer better service at a lower price per call while actually increasing net income.

Ambulance Membership

Ambulance membership, also known as subscription service, is not a new concept. Its roots date back as far as 1939. What is new is the availability of a fully developed public ambulance membership program that can be successfully transplanted in other areas when managed properly. In fact, if plans now being finalized are successfully executed, these programs will eventually serve the largest geographic area in the nation under a common membership agreement. And participating jurisdictions will be able to offer consumers significant advantages over non-participants. Let's take a look at what ambulance membership is all about.

For the purposes of this article, ambulance membership is defined as the prepayment of uninsured portions of an ambulance bill through a standardized annual membership fee. Operating a membership program requires a thorough understanding of four primary aspects: planning and policy, financial management, public relations and marketing, and field operations.

Planning and Policy

The most important preliminary consideration in ambulance membership is the planning process. It consists of three phases: research and development, implementation, and evaluation. It is during the research and development stage that providers will determine if membership will work for them, and if so, how well.

The first task in research and development involves determining whether ambulance membership is legal in your state. Check with the state insurance commissioner's office. If there are still unanswered questions, it is best to have an attorney get a written opinion. If your path is blocked at this point, enabling legislation may be the only answer. Legislation may take considerable time and effort. Once you've decided that membership is worth the effort, make certain the proper political support is available before proceeding.

Next, develop a "revenue calculator." The calculator will list pertinent facts such as current population, percent of annual ambulance utilization per population, and number of households in the service area. Determine patients transported, average dollar amount billed, average amount collected, and average amount paid by insurance companies on a per-patient basis. Select an amount to charge per household (somewhere between $35 and $50 would be a good starting point based on what others currently charge), and add it to the list. For the purpose of estimation, calculate member utilization rates at double the non-member rate (current operators will substantiate this). Then calculate the number of households and population that would be represented if one percent of the households joined an ambulance membership.

Make two columns and compare non-members with members. (Don't forget to subtract member population and households from current figures before comparing, and remember that insurance payment is the only additional money collected on member billings.) Make a second set of columns for comparing revenue per 1,000 population of non-members versus members. The example in Table 3.10 will make calculations easier. If figures for the revenue calculator are not available, help will be required for accurate calculation. Estimates are possible without having all the facts, but they are less accurate and harder to perform. As in the example, there very likely will be a substantial increase in revenue for the member population. However, before deciding that membership would be a great idea, remember that costs related to administration, marketing, and increased patient workload have yet to be calculated.

Now it's time to mix policy decision into the planning process. Before proceeding, make a list of benefits that each member will receive. This list will determine to a large extent the overhead cost of the program, the way it is marketed, and how successfully, so give it serious thought. Even though slight changes may be made before actually beginning, what is offered later should be substantially the same as the original concept.

Initially, it is best to offer what other membership services have found to be successful. If it flourishes, changes may be made carefully from year to year. Although there are exceptions from one service to the next, the standard fare includes emer-

Common Terms Used in Ambulance Membership

Application—A document that sets forth the terms under which a membership is sold. The provider's promise of service and the member's obligations are included. Also referred to as an agreement or contract. The member is required to sign the document. Contains pertinent information on the member and others listed on the application, including insurance information and billing authorization.

Campaign—Intensive period of public information and education during which membership programs are marketed. Usually lasts less than 90 days. Includes commercial advertising, public service announcements, and group presentations.

Enrollment Period—The only period of time each year when new memberships and renewal of previous year's members are allowed. Operated simultaneously with the campaign.

Household—Residential address where member, spouse, and all unmarried children under a given age are covered under a single membership.

Member—Any person properly enrolled in a membership program and entitled to benefits as set forth in the application. Sometimes also referred to as a subscriber.

Membership—Prepayment of uninsured portions of an ambulance bill through an annual fee. Service is subject to terms described in the application. May include one or more persons living at a single residential address. Sometimes also referred to as a subscription.

Reciprocity Agreement—Written agreement between two or more membership services to honor the other's memberships. The service that cares for the patient bills the insurance.

gency ambulance service, and physician-authorized, medically necessary, non-emergency ambulance service. Benefits are offered only from any point within the service area to another point in the area via ground ambulance. The ambulance provider has the right to bill and collect whatever insurance benefits are available for the member. All uninsured portions are covered by the membership, regardless of how often service may be required. In the case of a provider that offers only emergency service, the membership would include only that service. As an option, emergency-only providers may subcontract with a non-emergency provider and include this benefit in the cost of the program. Benefits are normally limited to member, spouse, and unmarried children under a specific age, when all live at the same address. Make certain that policy decisions are backed by sound reasoning and have been found to be legally correct, then make them very clear in public relations and marketing efforts.

Since the increase in revenue per thousand members and the benefits list have been determined, a professional opinion survey can help ascertain how many thousands may be expected to join the membership. Hire a professional firm to handle the task. Personnel who are too close to the problem may have difficulty being objective and, in many cases, may not have the skills required to perform the survey economically. The survey firm will need help in designing a survey instrument that asks the right questions. In order to get the required information, the questions must include the proposed consumer cost and benefit description.

Provided that preliminary findings are positive, the next task is to establish clearly defined goals and objectives, assign duties, and create a timeline for completion. Whether the primary goal is to hire additional personnel, add needed equipment, increase consumer satisfaction with the price of care, or some combination of these or other goals, it should include something that citizens, elected officials, media, and employees can support. Decide how much money it will take to reach the goal and establish a

Table 3.10

Ambulance Membership Revenue Calculator Example for City of Centerville

(Population 100,000; 50,000 Households)
1 Percent of Households Have Enrolled

General Information

	Non-Members	Members
Population	99,000	1,000
Households	49,500	500
Persons per Household	2.0	2.0
Fee per Household	0	$40
Patients Transported	4,950	100
Utilization Rate	5%	10%
Billing per Patient	$300	$300
Insurance per Patient	$150	$150
Collected per Patient	$200	$150

Annual Revenue Comparison per 1,000 Persons

	Non-Members	Members
Population	1,000	1,000
Utilization Rate	5%	10% *
Patients Transported	50	100
Collections per Patient	$200	$150
User-Fee Revenue	$10,000	$15,000
Number of Households	500	500
Fee per Household	0	$40
Membership Fee Revenue	0	$20,000
Total Revenue	$10,000	$35,000

* Members have a minimum of double the normal utilization rate.

target for reaching that goal. The goal must become a shared vision in order for it to work. But be conservative—the goal, in effect, becomes a campaign promise. If the target is reached, the promised effect must be delivered to avoid a credibility gap.

Consideration must also be given to logistics related to workforce and workspace. Prudent managers will make use of all existing workspace and workforce before considering additions. If the first year's membership is successful, plan carefully for additions in future years to avoid excessive overhead costs. Reassigning duties of key personnel for the short duration of the campaign and hiring temporary assistance from clerical services contractors will help. Borrowing or renting additional workspace and furniture on a short-term basis is recommended.

Budget is the next important consideration. The primary hurdle will be the source of start-up revenue. This is akin to obtaining a bank loan to begin a private business, and risk is involved. Provided that research and development is of high quality, a recognized need is being met, and budget and revenue projections are conservative, a convincing argument can usually be made. Provide for all personnel, materials and services, and capital items directly related to increased costs. This should include both administrative and field operations budget increases. Even if there is some ability to absorb added workload, categories related to patient transports, such as fuel, vehicle maintenance, overtime, and related benefits, must be calculated. Add an appropriate sum for loan payback as well as a reserve contingency fund in case demand or expenses exceed reasonable assumptions.

The implementation phase of the planning process consists of completing plans for financial, public relations and marketing, and field operations activities necessary to support the program and the execution of these plans following a prescribed outline for assignment of duties and timelines. These activities will be discussed in detail later.

The evaluation phase includes planning for and executing a data collection system. Provide for the collection of every type of information necessary to make adjustments in future years and to determine the true impact of membership on the organization. Include a debriefing process for office and field personnel. Find out what worked well and what could have been done better. As soon as possible, include a mechanism such as a questionnaire or hotline to get feedback from your members, too.

Financial Management

Management of the fiscal well-being of membership services requires an understanding of the forces at work. Whenever a member uses the ambulance, the provider bills the member's insurance company at the regular non-member rate and accepts this reimbursement as satisfying the bill, regardless of the amount. Any balance left unpaid is covered by the membership. Since there are no prerequisites for members to have a certain

Annual membership fees must cover all overhead expenses of administration and marketing and must relate directly to ambulance rates in a way that will cause the consumer to be interested in buying.

level of insurance, reimbursements range from zero for the uninsured to as much as 100 percent, depending on the type of policy and the nature of the illness or injury. Because of the tendency of membership programs to attract large numbers of Medicare-aged people, a high number of members will have insurance. The lowest income groups who are typically the least insured will often receive welfare medical assistance and will not join the program. Obviously, community income and unemployment levels vary and this factor should be figured into overall results.

The relationship between consumer and provider is altered in a membership service. Service is delivered to the consumer but sold exclusively to third-party payers, almost always at a reimbursement rate less than the full retail price. However, since consumers do not pay directly for the cost of the service, they are more likely to use the service when they need it. As a result, utilization goes up and the insurance company becomes a sort of wholesale purchasing agent for the consumer. The provider does more business at a lower price per run, and as long as the principles behind volume business and efficiency of operation are applied, the consumer gets a bargain and the provider makes more money.

The proper structuring of ambulance rates to maximize insurance reimbursements is very important for a successful membership. Since all of the business on behalf of members is done with third-party payers, fees not covered become a direct loss. Medicare and private insurance carriers have recognized fee structures for which rates must be designed. Rates should be high enough to cover all new operational expenses. If rates are kept artificially low by tax subsidies, higher utilization is not good news. Even though more user-fee revenue will be generated, each new call will mean a loss in the form of an increase in subsidy costs. Proper rate design means that subsidies, if any, will not increase and may even be decreased or eliminated. Officials should be less reluctant to authorize higher rates if given a good explanation of how membership finances work.

Annual membership fees must cover all overhead expenses of administration and marketing and must relate directly to ambulance rates in a way that will cause the consumer to be interested in buying. Specifically, the ambulance rate for non-members must be six to 10 times higher than the membership fee, or the rational consumer will not consider joining. If the area to be served has a history of high ambulance rates, the membership is very likely to be welcomed by the public as the solution of a problem. On the other hand, if the area has a history of low rates and suddenly rates are raised, even with a membership as a safety valve, it will require high-level political support and an intensive public information campaign to explain the reasons for the changes.

An efficient ambulance billing system is the backbone of the financial management of membership service. Billing personnel are responsible for collecting from third-party payers on behalf of members who have assigned their ambulance benefits to the provider. As the number of transports goes up, so does the workload of the billing department. A well-designed billing system can use such tools as electronic claims processing to work smarter, not harder. The results are more claims processed at a quicker rate, with the same number of employees. Improved quantity and quality of billing services will depend on a requirement that each member fill out an application with pertinent billing data and sign an assignment of insurance benefits prior to being allowed to enroll. The billing system may also be used to encourage non-members to enroll by emphasizing the benefits of membership in written and verbal contacts with people responsible for paying ambulance bills.

A final word about financial management: Be wary of those who seem most interested in the financial outcome of a successful membership campaign, especially if they had nothing to do with the success. You may find that suddenly virtually everyone wants a piece of the pie before it's even done cooking. Go back to the original goals and objectives. If those who are now asking for a piece of the pie are found in the goals, by all means serve it—they probably deserve it. Suggest to others that they find their way into next year's goals and your budget, over the scrutiny of public opinion. If there is truly some of the pie left, perhaps it should go to a cause such as reducing the membership fee for low-income groups who do not qualify for welfare medical assistance.

Public Relations and Marketing

Politics are at work everywhere, visibly and invisibly affecting membership outcomes. If legislation is required for public sector involvement, and sometimes even if it isn't, those seeking to begin service may find themselves at direct odds with private sector providers who are suspicious of the proposed program. Even if they have no intentions of providing it themselves, experience in two states has shown that they may vigorously oppose public sector membership. While it is helpful to have the support of various organizations, nothing stops private sector objections faster than public pressure on elected officials. Make sure the public knows the issues at stake before heading into a confrontation. Get whatever local political support is available—endorsements are preferred—even if there appears to be no opposition. Political support and endorsements add credibility to the program. Actively seek media support in the form of editorial endorsement and positive news coverage. And when the campaign is over, don't forget campaign thank-you's.

Expect some bureaucratic red tape and plan for extra time, energy, and money to accommodate it. There are reasons why government is best known for a conservative fiscal approach rather than entrepreneurial endeavors. If the plan of local government is to simply remove tax fund support from one part of your organization (i.e., from fire suppression) and replace it with membership revenue, this must be an open issue. As long as the action is taken for valid reasons (i.e., to eliminate a tax sub-

> Get whatever local political support is available—endorsements are preferred—even if there appears to be no opposition. Political support and endorsements add credibility to the program.

If providers are
doing their job,
consumers under-
stand more about
how to gain access
to ambulance
service and when
it's appropriate to
use or not use the
service.

sidy) and the public supports the concept, it should not inhibit member-ship. However, care should be taken that members are not asked to subsidize non-members. Therefore, if user fees to non-members can be raised to eliminate a tax subsidy, this is the preferred method.

Consider the effect of membership on nearby providers, then warn neighbors of the possible fallout. If local prices suddenly appear to be far more reasonable than neighbors, expect some unhappiness from neigh-boring consumers. Those in bordering areas may suddenly prefer service from the membership provider. At any rate, other providers may well feel the heat of public pressure for change, especially if electronic marketing efforts overlap into their area. This problem may be able to be solved with reciprocal membership agreements, which will be discussed later.

Probably the last place political adversity is expected is within the membership organization. Teamwork is a necessity of a smoothly func-tioning membership, so don't forget to nurture support on the inside. Don't even consider beginning with anything less than enthusiasm from the top and at least a conceptual check-off from field personnel. The "what's in it for me?" attitude is not necessarily bad, provided that those express-ing it intend to give the program full support. Set a goal that includes something for them, then stick to it.

Public opinion forms the backbone of support for membership programs. For this reason, every attempt must be made to help the con-sumer identify with the organization. Begin by eliminating the terms *sub-scription* and *subscriber.* Most subscribers do not develop a close sense of belonging to or identifying with a group. Usually, the subscriber pays and then receives something in return—and that's all there is to the re-lationship. On the other hand, give the public something to believe in, a program that saves lives and saves money, for example, and they are proud to belong to and identify with that program. The results are noth-ing short of amazing. Membership may become the hottest topic since Medicare for seniors—and they are the main consumer constituency and most frequent users. Those who may have hesitated to say nice things about service in the past because of the size of the bill will suddenly become number-one fans.

Now consider the effect of this change in consumer behavior. Uti-lization increases are the most obvious sign. Why? Public confidence and trust among members is at an all-time high. If providers are doing their job, consumers also understand more about how to gain access to ambu-lance service and when it's appropriate to use or not use the service. Finally, members don't fear the cost. As part of the deal, the public sector provider has become more responsive to consumer demand and is doing something positive to meet a community need. Not a bad package.

What's more, the same relationship can actually improve patient care and even save lives. It's no secret that if people suffering early warning signs of a heart attack would seek attention sooner, they would arrive in intensive care sooner and in better condition, having received early and proper prehospital care. In the same way, if equipment, training, or extra people are available specifically because of the membership, the beneficial effects are obvious.

The image of the membership provider should be one that is worth identifying with and one the provider can live up to. Just as a rose by any other name smells as sweet, the smell of something foul cannot be dressed up with a new name. Part of the image should be made using those heartwarming compliments now being received. If a member wants to know how to help, have a plan ready to use that help. Suggest a letter to the editor and provide the address. Use the member's story in testimonials for written materials or in news stories.

The image of membership as a form of "ambulance insurance" is a mixed blessing. Security is a powerful motivator for buying membership, but if the service comes away with only that image, those who may have contributed because of desire to support a worthy cause will be overlooked. Above all, the provider must calculate a personal, caring image. These consumers vote with their dollars in more ways than one. This may become the single most intimate relationship with any service of local government. A good feeling about that service may reflect in support of other programs.

Once the image that is desired has been given a name, the provider has made an investment. That investment should be protected from being tarnished by another program using the same name without putting the service behind it. Much like a business registers a name, public ambulance providers should consider protecting any special name that is part of an image that would be expensive to change. A check with the state agency responsible for such affairs would also prevent the unintentional use of a protected name, which could lead to similar expenses.

Marketing of healthcare services was discovered long ago but has only recently been made so visible by the advertising of hospitals, clinics, and other special care facilities. The type of visibility required for a true success in membership may require the use of billboards, television, radio, newspaper, direct mail, and public presentations. This sort of exposure is not customary for most governments, and the minds of many should be properly prepared. In a word, it's competition—competition for the attention of a public increasingly busy with all sorts of unrelated things. Yet membership is a service that must be sold, and advertising sells.

Negotiating a balance between paid public information spots and public service announcements and finding the best spots for advertising are not tasks for rank amateurs. Select a competent ad agency and give it the job. Its commissions come from discounts in the electronic media rates and therefore cost the provider nothing for TV and radio work. And don't consider handling direct mailing unless the number is fewer than a thousand. The special expertise and efficiency of a mail house can't be beat, and the frustration saved is well worth the price.

Marketing and enrollment periods should be kept short—not more

The type of visibility required for a true success in membership may require the use of billboards, television, radio, newspaper, direct mail, and public presentations.

Aggressive
management of
consumer misuse
of services is
necessary. Establish
a very firm policy
of action in case of
repeated misuse.

than 60 to 90 days—for several reasons. The cost of intensive advertising is expensive, and so is the overhead for year-round or full-time clerical help to answer phones, perform data input, etc. Given the chance to put off making a decision, many people will. That is, until they need help. If these people are allowed to buy on-the-spot, there is really no reason to buy any other way. Most people buying the service would also be using it. This would tip the cost-benefit scale over and result in financial failure for the membership system.

Other marketing considerations are best solved by prior planning. The marketing of an area served by multiple providers can best be solved with a reciprocal agreement. Each provider would agree to service the other's members and would be entitled to the insurance revenue. Monitoring of the results would be necessary to ensure mutually beneficial results. This same type of agreement can also be used to increase the area of any one membership by offering the same protection in neighboring jurisdictions, even when each area is served by only one provider.

In future years, when marketing efforts have reached near-saturation levels, the emphasis should change. Concentrate on taking good care of existing members and on finding out what sales obstacles may be overcome in non-member groups. This may involve a shift in dollars away from high-exposure media to direct presentation programs or other methods.

Field Operations

The primary effect on field operations is increased workload and equipment utilization related to increased demand. Some increase can be absorbed, but each system will have a point at which operational efficiency is reached, then surpassed. Workload increases may be handled in many ways, from a change in duties—i.e., personnel may no longer perform routine tasks that can easily be assigned to less-skilled labor—to adding additional production capacity during peak load hours. Simply ignoring production capacity overload will lead to a reduction in the level of service and most likely to a morale problem.

Aggressive management of consumer misuse of services is also necessary. Establish a very firm policy of action in case of repeated misuse. I have found that a "one, two, three, and you're out" policy works the best. On the first misuse, remind the customer politely that the service rendered is limited to the specific services included in the signed agreement and that other services are subject to regular fees. Some members are honestly not clear on what is included until this step has been taken. The first misuse is noted in a file. On the second misuse, the member is warned in writing that a third misuse will result in refund of the membership fee and revocation of the membership for violation of the agreement. A bill for services will be sent for the third such misuse. I have yet to reach the third step in two years of service. Training of hospital social services personnel and nursing home employees who often call for non-emergency services also reduces unnecessary calls.

The entrepreneurial voyage into a field that is typically so foreign to local government is not for the timid. Even when the trip is well planned, some risk is always present. In my case, the payoff has already been worth it. When Jim Page reported on the Eugene-Springfield area in the January 1986 issue of *JEMS*, he said, " . . . the administrative offices somewhat resembled an advertising agency these days." Jim was right. And the advertising worked. The FireMed program has lived up to the high ideals of what membership should stand for in every way. I have been fortunate to witness the addition of computerized defibrillators on every fire engine in this area, purchased solely because of FireMed. Within one month of initiating this service, the first life was saved. Other improvements have only just begun. I'm sold, and so are over 30,000 members.

Source

Reprinted with permission from JEMS, September 1987. Dennis Murphy is a fire chief with the Springfield, Ore., Department of Fire and Life Safety. He has over 25 years in the administration of both private and government services.

Fundraising for Volunteer EMS Organizations

Jay Fitch, PhD

Fundraising rates somewhere below scrubbing emesis basins on the priority lists of most EMS volunteers. In this article, the author tells how volunteer agencies can increase their net worth and member involvement by mastering this skill.

VOLUNTEER EMS ORGANIZATIONS find it increasingly difficult to locate willing givers in today's society. Yet without effective fundraising, many volunteer organizations would whither and die. Unfortunately, people have become hardened by the large number of appeals they receive—everything from their church or synagogue to the "save the snails" project. In part, this hardening is due to the "professionalization" of fundraising activities.

Over the past 30 years, an industry has developed around asking strangers for money. Professional fundraisers and "development" specialists offer their services and strategies for locating donors and extracting their full measure of generosity. The task of fundraising has become sophisticated, automated, and downright impersonal.

Let's face it: Most volunteers feel funny about asking for money. We don't like to think of ourselves as beggars. Pride and good manners trip us up. Successful fundraisers know a secret. People *like* to give. And, EMS organizations are ideally positioned to help fulfill that need to give. A volunteer EMS agency is visible, provides an essential "lifesaving" service, and has a positive, emotionally gripping story to tell.

People give to volunteer EMS organizations for a variety of reasons. Giving makes the givers feel good and enhances their self-image as generous people. Giving assuages guilt. Some give to get something—a free dinner or a write-off. And some support causes and organizations that they believe make a difference in others' lives. The most important reason people give, however, is that they are asked by the right person in the right way for the right amount at the right time.

There are several other advantages fundraising has for the volunteer EMS organization. Fundraising promotes membership, raises public profiles, provides opportunities to build social and political community awareness, and enhances the volunteer EMS organization's credibility.

Two primary types of campaigns are typically undertaken by volunteer services: the annual campaign used to fund the volunteer EMS agency's operating budget, and specific or specially targeted appeals. Targeted campaigns can range from building funds to a campaign to buy a particular piece of equipment. Special events can be used to support both annual giving programs and targeted campaigns.

Planning a Campaign

A five-step process should be followed in planning any fundraising campaign for an EMS organization.

Develop a clear and convincing case statement. A case statement tells people why they should support your activities. It should include a brief summary of the organizational mission, an overview of proposed and continuing programs that need financial support, statistics that support the EMS agency's service and effectiveness, an estimate of total program costs, and the squad's future plans.

Delve into the history and records. Look at the records of past campaigns. Which donation sources provided the highest yield—individuals, community groups, or corporations? Make sure that your budgets and financial records are in order if a major donor requests to see an audit. Look for previous letters of endorsement or clinical testimonials. Check the squad's general brochure to see how well it supports the fundraising effort.

Analyze the steps in each fundraising project. A healthy fundraising program uses a wide variety of tools. Over the years, the squad or volunteer corps can develop an entire battery of effective mechanisms. Determine the steps in each approach and select the approaches that match the overall objectives and the availability of volunteer members to staff the campaign.

Set your fundraising goals. Once you've selected the fundraising tools, delineated the various strategies, constructed timelines, and assigned tasks, it's time to specify just how much money is to be raised. At this point, the historical information is again helpful. Goals should inspire, not overwhelm. Analyze the rate of increase over the past three to five years. A goal of five to 10 percent above that number should be attainable. Unless there is an extraordinary commitment, setting goals beyond that may prove self-defeating.

Get started early. After constructing a solid working draft, submit it to key board members for their informal input. The more people who feel that they helped construct the plan, the more likely that those same individuals will be supportive. This strategy also works well with long-term donors. Some groups then use these long-term donors' contributions as an "advance gift" to jump-start the campaign.

Who Gives

A frequent error made by EMS organizations is trying to solicit everyone. It may be more effective to solicit specifically targeted donors. Primary categories of supporters for EMS organizations include individuals, foundations, associations, governments, and corporations. Each requires a customized approach that identifies the giver, determines the type of donation that particular person or group is likely to give, and ascertains both how and when the request is to be made.

Individuals. This group may represent the largest number of donors, and those hardest to reach. A volunteer squad can define its constituency by subgroups of individuals such as former patients, local officials, members of community groups, and those living within the service area. Utiliz-

> Primary categories of supporters for EMS organizations include individuals, foundations, associations, governments, and corporations.

The most essential lesson of fundraising is that in order to receive a donation, you must ask for it. The key is making the right approach to the right person at the right time.

ing commercially available mailing lists has become sophisticated. If using this method, the squad should select lists that mail to individual names rather than to all "occupants" in a particular zip code. Personally addressed mail receives a better response than "junk mail" addressed to "occupant."

Foundations. Large foundations rarely give to annual operating campaigns, but may provide support to specialized campaigns. For example, a number of years ago, the Ewing Kauffman Foundation, started by the late owner of the Kansas City Royals baseball team, provided a gift of $250,000 to initiate Kansas City's "CPR Now!" campaign. That program was responsible for training over 100,000 people in CPR in less than two years.

Associations. Clubs, fraternal organizations, community groups, neighborhood organizations, and professional societies are also prospects to support the annual campaign. Groups may provide human resources to assist one of the squad's fundraising events, or conduct their own event and make the squad the recipient. A number of ambulances have plaques saying "Donated through the generosity of the Lions Club" emblazoned on their sides.

Governments. State and local governments are also an excellent source of funds. For example, the State of Florida has a matching grant program to encourage volunteers. State agency directors can be helpful when trying to find out what funds are available from which programs. Local government agencies that would otherwise have to provide the service may also be willing donors of cash or in-kind gifts. In Richmond, Va., the city supports the volunteer squads by including their membership/donation requests in the municipal utilities mailings. Other in-kind gifts could be the use of buildings, radio systems, or gasoline.

Corporations. Begin with those firms located in the service area that have associations with the corps. From that point, develop potential donor lists by working closely with the local chamber of commerce. Corporate appeals should be addressed to specific persons; "Dear Sir or Madam" letters rarely work. Again, both cash and in-kind gifts should be welcomed. One successful corps receives discounted repairs from the local Ford dealer, tires from the Chevrolet dealer, and all routine oil changes from the Dodge dealer.

The most essential lesson of fundraising is that in order to receive a donation, you must ask for it. Funds are not, in fact, raised. They are solicited, requested, demanded, cajoled, enticed, and finagled. The key is making the right approach to the right person at the right time. Successful EMS fundraising may involve using a variety of strategies and techniques.

Direct Mail

Direct mail can be a cost-effective tool. Volunteer EMS services that have failed to obtain the desired result with direct mail indicate it was because their literature was poorly designed or because they addressed mail to "occupant." Some direct mail houses will help design effective mailers.

Some squads have had success getting brochures designed and printed in return for mentioning that those firms donated their services. Presorting labels by zip code can also save several cents mailing cost for each piece. Nonprofit permits can help reduce mailing costs where appropriate.

One of the most effective mail campaigns can be the "friends of friends" program. In this approach, high-profile community leaders write a letter on the squad's behalf asking their friends to join them in supporting the EMS agency. When a business person receives a letter from the owner of the primary industry in the area, who may also be a customer, you can bet the letter will be read and acted upon.

Special Event Ideas You Can Use

Whether planning an annual fundraising drive or a targeted or special campaign, a well-promoted special event may be helpful in focusing attention on the EMS organization and infusing excitement into the fundraising process. A special event is often held to help kick off the direct mail or general solicitation campaign.

Here are just a few ideas compiled from the files of volunteer agencies: anniversary celebrations; antique auto shows; art exhibits; award dinners; boot blocks; talent shows; bake sales; bazaars; book sales; raffles; luncheons/dinners/breakfasts (pancake, spaghetti, fish fry, pig roast, chili, etc.); carnivals; car washes; celebrity parties; charity balls; concerts; dinner dances; flower and plant sales; golf matches; house and garden tours; telethons; tennis/racquetball tournaments; walk-a-thons; jog-a-thons; and CPR contests.

The list of possible events is as endless as your creativity. There are 12 broad categories of special events—sales, games of chance, eating events, amusements, "a-thons," auctions, parties, tours, services (e.g., car washes), publications, radio and TV marathons, and tournaments. The choice of the category and the particular event should match both the character and personnel resources of your squad. Some events require significantly more effort than others. If a particular event not previously used is considered, try to locate another squad or volunteer agency to check their experience with that event.

The Donor Solicitation Process

When you are face-to-face with a prospective donor, a four-step process can enhance the chances for success. The steps are opening, involvement, presentation, and closing. Remembering these steps may be particularly helpful when soliciting corporate and municipal gifts. These same steps can also be used, in an abbreviated form, when making door-to-door solicitations.

Opening. In this step, warmth, rapport, and a relationship are created between the person requesting the gift and the donor. The opening explains the purpose of the visit and sets the tone. During this time, the

There are 12 broad categories of special events— sales, games of chance, eating events, amusements, "a-thons," auctions, parties, tours, services, publications, radio and TV marathons, and tournaments.

need for EMS in the community and how your volunteer agency is meeting that need is explained. At this point, you are discussing mission and organizational goals—not dollar needs—with the prospective donor.

Involvement. Explore the prospect's personal experience with the service. For example, "Has a member of your family or someone else you know used the EMS system in the past five years?" Ask questions that provide an understanding of the individual's perception of the need for high-quality EMS service.

Presentation. It is during this phase that you begin to zero in on your agency's needs. Keep it simple. Don't overwhelm the prospect with facts. Simply identify the benefits of having a high-quality volunteer EMS program. Identify the benefits to them personally. For example, you might say, "We would like you to support the volunteer EMS program now so we will be there when you or someone you love needs service." Identify benefits to the community; explain that the cost of providing service with municipal employees would be much higher than what it costs to provide the service with volunteers. And finally, explain the importance of volunteerism to the community. This could be done by saying something like, "We are an organization of neighbors helping neighbors. Our tradition of volunteerism dates back 100 years, and we need your help to continue that tradition." The presentation should be brief and to the point.

Closing. Restate the volunteer EMS agency's key features and why the service is best suited to meet the community's needs. Listen for the prospective donor's reaction. If there is agreement, ask for the donation. If there is no agreement, you have to restate the need. Discuss what might happen if the need is not met, e.g., longer response times, higher fees/taxes. Don't debate a prospect. Instead, quietly respond to any stated objections and, when you have the prospect agreeing with you, ask for the donation. Key phrases that may be helpful include

- Will you join others. . . ?
- Would you consider a donation of. . . ?
- Will you set the pace for others. . . ?
- Your donation is tax deductible. . . .

If the prospective donor says yes, then collect the donation or pledge card. If the prospect says maybe, then probe to find out what is keeping them from saying yes. If the prospect says no,

---

The 12 Truths of EMS Donor Solicitation

1. Attitude. Be positive, enthusiastic, and confident.
2. Do your homework. Know your service's case inside and out. Know the prospective donor.
3. Practice and "role play." This gives you an opportunity to prepare for the unexpected.
4. Listen. Hear the cues that will support you in reinforcing the prospective donor's willingness to give.
5. Be relaxed. Work in pairs so that conversation with the prospective donor flows naturally.
6. Be clear and direct. The prospective donor can always tell if you're timid and mealy mouthed about asking for money.
7. Know the answers. Make sure the answers to common questions are known to everyone involved in the campaign.
8. Ask for the donation. A wise fundraiser once told me, "Annual campaigns do not fail because people do not want to give; they fail because people are not *asked* to give."
9. Don't be embarrassed by a no! It will happen.
10. Be positive.
11. Effective solicitation is the right person soliciting the right prospective donor at the right time.
12. Say thank you.

determine why. Win, lose, or draw, make sure to thank the prospective donor for their time and/or donation when you leave.

Source
Original article.

Recognize the Donor's Generosity

Basic fundraising protocol requires the acknowledgment of each donation. But there is also a practical reason for doing so—to ensure that the donor continues to support the volunteer EMS agency. In fundraising terms, this is called "future cultivation." Here are some other ideas to encourage ongoing support of the squad:

- Publish an honor roll of donors.
- Place a plaque with the names of major and long-term donors in a prominent location.
- Prepare news stories about the campaign, listing major donors.
- Hold a donor recognition day, with festivities honoring contributors.
- Send regular updates or a newsletter to donors to keep them informed of the squad's accomplishments throughout the year.
- Invite donors to a special tour or reception in their honor.

You can add your own ideas to this list. The important thing is to acknowledge the support and build the case that your agency is worthy of the donor's ongoing support.

Conclusion

For a number of volunteer EMS agencies, the excitement of fundraising has to be first sold inside the organization. Sell the idea that the organization is worthy of the community's support, that campaigns require careful planning and execution to be effective, and that fundraising can be fun.

Fundraising is really selling ideas. You should sell the idea that lack of EMS is a major problem for the community, that your squad is the most effective mechanism to provide the service, and that the volunteer EMS organization is both deserving of the donation and will use it wisely. Finally, you are selling the idea that they enjoy donating as a way to do their part to help family, friends, and neighbors.

Case 3

Medicare Mistakes Can Be Costly

Almost everyone in EMS agrees that Medicare is complex. Remaining faithful to the regulations can be frustrating on good days and can drive staff to distraction when things do not go well. Here are two real-life examples of costly errors that were made, and how the government handled the cases.

Example 1

"You've got to be kidding," the EMS administrator exclaimed when told of allegations that the service fraudulently billed Medicare and Medicaid for medical transportation services. Apparently, the service had provided over 7,000 transports to nursing home residents between 1988 and 1991. The allegation was that the nursing home residents were provided (and billed for) ambulance transportation rather than wheelchair transportation, and that these transports were not medically necessary.

The charges came to light in 1991 when the insurance carrier conducted a routine audit of the provider's records, notifying both the agency and the government when the billing errors were discovered. Both federal and state officials began investigating. In the meantime, the company began its own investigation and discontinued the practice of billing ambulatory patients as ambulance patients. Medicare prohibits payments for transportation by ambulance when a lesser form of transportation would have been appropriate.

The government claimed that the organization violated the Federal False Claims Act, the state's Deceptive Fair Trade Practice Act, and the Consumer Fraud Act when it submitted and was paid for the ambulance claims. The company indicated that it simply provided the type of transportation requested by the nursing home. In a public statement about the incident, the company spokesperson said, "The Attorney General's Office stated that we should not have made errors in the billing process. And, with that we concur. But the Attorney General found no evidence of criminal intent. It was a mistake, an honest mistake, and we corrected it."

In a pre-litigation settlement, the organization agreed to provide $1.2 million in restitution and pay an additional $1.7 million in damages. The firm also had to provide over $100,000 in free transports to indigents, train employees involved in submitting claims, and implement a routine audit plan over the next three years. The organization admitted no liability in the settlement.

Example 2

The front page headlines screamed, "Medicare Ripoff Suspect Guilty." Following a four-day trial and six hours of jury deliberations,

Kevin O'Brien, the former owner of Beverly Ambulance Service in Beverly, Mass., showed no emotion as the jury foreman responded "guilty." He was convicted of 420 counts of submitting false ambulance reimbursement claims, according to newspaper reports.

The 35-year-old O'Brien was described by his attorney as an inexperienced young man who was thrust into the leadership role of his family business. He told the jury O'Brien was targeted as a scapegoat for "bureaucratic bungling."

Prosecutors, however, painted a different picture, describing O'Brien as a cash-strapped company president who directed a Medicare fraud scheme to exploit the government. Witnesses testified that they were not transported in ambulances, as O'Brien claimed, but in vans and station wagons. They also testified that they often traveled in groups of two to five people, rather than alone as O'Brien indicated on claim forms. Employees testified that records were knowingly altered to reflect inflated services and charges. They told of being directed to present bogus time sheets, assignment schedules, and phony transportation worksheets.

In August 1993, O'Brien was sentenced to federal prison.

Case Questions

1. Describe how these two cases are similar. How are they different?
2. Did the government handle the two cases differently? If so, why?
3. What specific Medicare regulations were violated?
4. What processes should your service routinely employ to ensure that violations are not being committed?
5. If notified of a pending investigation, what are the specific steps an EMS administrator should take?

Part Four

Managing the Changing Clinical Environment

Even if you are on the right track, you will get run over if you just sit there.

—Author Unknown

Many EMS leaders feel smugly comfortable, assuming that the future will be a linear extension of the past. But an accurate assessment of the changing clinical and technological environment reveals that this will not be the case. Too many EMS leaders and systems sit idly by, even though they are on the right track.

Medical direction and control, quality improvement processes, research issues, litigation, and new medical interventions are forcing EMS leaders to choose between the comfort of further inertia and the efforts of planned action. The articles compiled for Part Four challenge us to take action—to move down the track toward the future and avoid getting run over.

—Jay Fitch

Part Four Contents

Medical Control

Why EMS Needs Physicians

Joseph G. Ferko III

Paramedics and EMTs are not independent practitioners. Most state statutes require physician involvement in local EMS programs, but few provide meaningful guidelines for that involvement. While organizations such as the American College of Emergency Physicians and the National Association of EMS Physicians continue to define the physician's extended practice utilizing prehospital care personnel, the author of this article provides a non-physician perspective on the important role physicians play in EMS programs.

IN THE TWO DECADES that have followed the landmark publication of the White Paper in 1966, prehospital emergency medicine has undergone extensive changes. As the level of sophistication of prehospital personnel has increased, the need for increased physician involvement has become more apparent.

The Emergency Physician

The physician has been and will remain the "institution" of medicine. The complexity of the system associated with the art of healing the sick and injured requires much more than a strictly academic approach toward medicine. The physician must function as administrator, researcher, technical adviser, professor, and friend of the patients and professionals who compose his environment. This diverse environment may contribute to the various problems encountered by the physician. This factor, in conjunction with personal interests and a desire to improve the quality of patient care, has driven the physician, as well as the entire medical community, toward human system specialization.

The field of emergency medicine requires a physician who is a "generalized" specialist. The diversity of traumatic injuries further requires the emergency physician to possess the skills of a "generalized" surgical specialist. Although it is clear that all physicians must be versed in the basics of stabilizing the critically injured or ill, it was not until 1979 that emergency medicine was officially declared an area of physician specialization. Box 4.1 presents the definition that the American Medical Association (AMA) has attached to this area of specialization.

This definition further describes the scope of the practice of emergency medicine: "The emergency medicine specialist must be the definitive authority on all aspects of clinical management related to acutely ill or injured patients." Furthermore, the physician in this role is charged with identifying all of the patient's needs and referring the patient to the appropriate specialist or facility that may provide for these needs. This applies both in and out of the hospital. Clearly, this responsibility requires the emergency medicine specialist to acquire "an in-breadth base of knowledge as opposed to the in-depth interests required by traditional specialties," according to D. K. Wagner in "Emergency Medicine: An Important Specialty Today" (*Emergency Medicine*, 1980).

Physicians in Prehospital Care

Obviously, the field of emergency medicine requires a very special type of physician. While there is a tendency to focus solely on the emergency medical specialist, consideration must be given not only to the individuals specializing in emergency medicine, but also to the general practitioner or specialist in another area of medicine who either by choice or by demand is involved with emergency care. It is primarily these individuals who are involved with prehospital care, since the field of emergency medicine is still in its infancy.

Four reasons for physician involvement with prehospital emergency medicine can be identified. They are mandated involvement; a physician's "bad" personal experience, which leads to involvement; previous military experience, where a physician wishes to apply knowledge obtained; and personal enjoyment. Clearly, a correlation may be identified between the reason for physician involvement in prehospital emergency medicine and the role that the physician intentionally, or unintentionally, assumes. Four specific roles may be identified: precipitator, mediator, blocker, and neglecter.

Obviously, the roles most desirable are precipitator and mediator. These orientations provide for problem solving and coordinated advancement within the profession. Advancement in this case may be defined as the improvement of medical care available to the community. The third role, that of blocker, may be assumed by parties interested in precipitating advancement in the prehospital field and by those who prefer to conform to established standards. An example of a blocker with "good intentions" would be the physician whose extraordinary enthusiasm toward prehospital care interferes with his ability to rationalize other viewpoints, project his viewpoint, suppress the viewpoints of cohorts and subordinates, and/or overemphasize an issue and therefore create resentment toward that issue. A physician who reluctantly complies with changes in regionalized medical protocol simply to avoid the legalities of non-compliance may directly or indirectly function as a blocker. Finally, the physician who must by mandate or political pressure participate in prehospital emergency medicine may purposely neglect his responsibilities, complying only with those that are legally binding. An overtaxed physician may also neglect responsibilities simply due to a lack of time. Either case may result in the failure to maintain or advance the quality of care.

Identifiable qualities of individuals who most often assume roles that

Box 4.1

AMA Definition of Emergency Medicine

The House of Delegates of the American Medical Association defined the emergency physician as a physician trained to engage in

- The immediate initial recognition, evaluation, care, and disposition of patients in response to acute illness and injury

- The administration, research, and teaching of all aspects of emergency medical care

- The direction of the patient to sources of follow-up care, in or out of the hospital as may be required

- The provision when requested of emergency, but not continuing, care to in-hospital patients

- The management of the emergency medical system for the provision of prehospital care

American College of Emergency Physicians. "Standards for Residency Training Programs in Emergency Medicine," as approved by the American Medical Association House of Delegates on June 17, 1975.

produce a positive effect on prehospital medicine have been suggested by Margaret Gunter, PhD (Box 4.2). Most interesting is the fact that Gunter's list reflects the traits of a good administrator or manager and fails to address medical interests or competency. Gunter has examined the types of physicians and the roles that are most frequently assumed by these individuals. This knowledge should be applied to orienting the medical student toward the prehospital environment.

Orienting the Physician Toward Emergency Medicine

The American College of Emergency Physicians (ACEP) published *Guidelines for Undergraduate Education in Emergency Medicine* in 1980. The rationale behind this ACEP publication was that a "knowledge of emergency medical systems and services is appropriate for every physician, even if the physician is not involved in the delivery of such care."

This training should consist of a minimum of three elements that may be defined as EMT didactic course instruction, orientation to EMS systems didactic instruction, and EMS systems practicum, including direct interaction with a provider unit. In addition, it is suggested that the medical student be introduced to research methodologies and needs in emergency medicine. This orientation should begin with the first year of the medical program and may then be enhanced as the student progresses through the regular curriculum. Ironically, although this philosophy has been widely proclaimed by ACEP as a necessary change in educational practice, few teaching institutions have incorporated such programs in their curriculums. Instead, a trend in post-graduate education in emergency medicine has been observed. This training is, therefore, limited to individuals pursuing emergency medicine as a career.

Practitioners in specialties other than emergency medicine must acquire knowledge of the field either through firsthand encounters with prehospital emergency situations or through local physician training programs. The latter is usually not associated with any form of continuing education credit or formal certification and therefore requires the physician to put forth the effort to attend based solely on personal desire to obtain the information presented. One such program has been developed by Cooper and Ornato.

The Base Station Physician training course was designed to orient the general practitioner to prehospital emergency medicine. Cooper and Ornato have identified seven objectives of the course. They are awareness of EMT-P training content and skills; appropriate expectations of the EMT-P team faced with field situations; familiarization with radiotelemetry communications; knowledge of legal authority, responsibility, and limits; knowledge of content and proper use of medical protocols; familiarization with overall operation of the prehospital rescue team; and field experience for the physician.

The didactic course requires eight hours to complete and is aug-

---

Box 4.2

Typical Characteristics of Prehospital-Oriented MDs

- Dedicated
- Innovative
- Action-oriented
- Non-traditional
- Willing to take risks
- Personal charisma
- Taste for adventure
- Great energy
- Infectious enthusiasm for EMS
- "Maverick" (but well respected)
- Tactful
- Diplomatic
- Low-key
- Highly flexible

Gunter, M. J., et al. "Physician Involvement: A Critical Factor in the Development of Community Emergency Medical Services." *Emergency Medical Services* (May 1979): 48-61.

mented with field practice. Physicians are then encouraged to become involved with the local Paramedic Policy Procedures committee and the education program for the field providers. The participating physicians listed the following as benefits of the course: enhanced awareness and respect for the job paramedics do in the field; awareness of the difficulty and responsibility of acting as a base station physician; increased motivation to become familiar with the medical protocols; decreased "fear" of talking on the radio; and better understanding of the laws, rules, and regulations governing the paramedic program.

A comparison of the course objectives and the physician participants' comments clearly indicates that the course served its purpose. The problem of maintaining levels of attendance appears to be the primary concern at this time. Once the physician has been oriented to the prehospital environment, attention may be given to the numerous identifiable functions of the physician in that environment.

Identifiable Functions of the Prehospital-Oriented Physician

In a paper published in 1982, ACEP stated that "all aspects of the organization and provision of emergency medical services require the active involvement and participation of physicians." These aspects should "incorporate design of the EMS system prior to its implementation; continual revision of the system; and operation of the system from initial access to prehospital contact with the patient, through stabilization in the emergency department."

To optimize physician involvement, the American College of Physicians listed the items presented in Box 4.3 as both desirable characteristics of physicians involved in prehospital care and identifiable functions of such individuals. Gunter has also identified 11 areas of specific physician involvement in prehospital care. This information is presented in Box 4.4. Comparison of Boxes 4.3 and 4.4 reveals a very close similarity between the two. Education of field personnel, system design, research, and medical supervision are elements of both lists. As the medical expert of the prehospital team, the physician is also valuable as an educator of the public and the political community. In addition, when indicated, the physician as primary provider may offer additional levels of medical assistance in the field setting. Since the field provider is the physician extender in the prehospital system, it is the medical control and coordination that remains the primary function of the "prehospital-oriented physician."

The Medical Director's Role

Medical control may be defined as consisting of five elements: quality assurance; employee performance appraisal; prospective phase of field medical control; immediate phase of field medical control; and retrospective phase of prehospital medical control.

Box 4.3

Characteristics and Functions of Emergency Physicians

According to the American College of Emergency Physicians, the following characteristics reflect the role of the emergency physician:

- Familiarity with the design and operation of prehospital EMS systems
- Experience in prehospital emergency care of the acutely ill or injured patient
- Routine participation in base station radio control of prehospital emergency units
- Experience in emergency department management of the acutely ill or injured patient
- Routine active participation in emergency department management of the acutely ill or injured patient
- Active involvement in the training of basic and advanced life support prehospital personnel
- Active involvement in the medical audit review and critique of basic and advanced life support personnel
- Participation in the administrative and legislative process affecting the regional/state prehospital EMS system

American College of Emergency Physicians. "Medical Control of Prehospital Emergency Medical Services." *Annals of Emergency Medicine* 11, no. 7 (1982): 387.

Prospective control refers to the education and training of the EMS community. Immediate control is the on-scene medical supervision of field personnel via a two-way radio communication system, while retrospective control consists of a system of immediate and delayed evaluation by physicians of the performance of prehospital personnel. Among these, immediate medical control is the area of most debate. Specifically, the appropriateness of standing orders versus on-line command is under question.

In an article entitled "Standing Orders vs. Voice Control," R. C. Hunt found that there was no statistically significant (positive or negative) difference on patient outcome between the two types of command. However, it is suggested by the author that in regard to standing orders (algorithms) for certain patient populations, specifically cardiac arrest and traumatic hypovolemic patients, certain trends indicating improved patient outcome can be identified. In addition, paramedic attitudes were stated to reflect a positive position toward the operations effectiveness of standing orders.

In a similar study, the ACEP Algorithm Review Subcommittee found that standing orders were not effective in regard to patient care. In fact, the study was never fully completed because of resistance from the medical communities under investigation. Therefore, the use of standing orders should be confined to concurrent on-line medical command or reserved for settings that prohibit on-line medical direction. The physician clearly retains control of field medical practice via this method of immediate medical control.

Box 4.4

Physician Involvement Identifiable Functions

- Medical expertise for overall system function
- Promote legitimacy of EMS activities
- Recruitment of specialized teaching personnel
- Provide linkages to organized medicine
- Provide prehospital medical control
- Assist with public sector activities, i.e., writing and promoting local/state legislation
- Educate elected officials/assist with funding
- Assist with technical aspects of design (EMS)
- Participation in mechanisms of coordination and decision making (task forces/councils)
- Data collection and evaluation
- Education

Gunter, M. J., et al. "Physician Involvement: A Critical Factor in the Development of Community Emergency Medical Services." *Emergency Medical Services* (May 1979): 48-61.

References

American College of Emergency Physicians, Algorithm Review Subcommittee. "Evaluation of an EMS Algorithm System." *Annals of Emergency Medicine* 9, no. 10 (1980): 534-536.

American College of Emergency Physicians. "Guidelines for Undergraduate Education in Emergency Medicine." *Annals of Emergency Medicine* 9, no. 4 (1980): 222-228.

American College of Emergency Physicians. "Medical Control of Prehospital Emergency Medical Services." *Annals of Emergency Medicine* 11, no. 7 (1982): 387.

American College of Emergency Physicians. "Standards for Residency Training Programs in Emergency Medicine," as approved by the American Medical Association House of Delegates on June 17, 1975.

Ballinger, J. A. "Using Physicians On-Scene." *JEMS* (November 1982): 39-42.

Boyd, D. R., S. H. Micik, C. T. Hambrew, and T. L. Romano. "Medical Control and Accountability of Emergency Medical Services (EMS) Systems." *IEEE Transactions On Vehicular Technology* VT-28, no. 4 (1979).

Committee on Trauma of the American College of Surgeons, Subcommittee on Emergency Services—Prehospital. "Medical Control in Trauma Care." *American College of Surgeons Bulletin* (October 1985).

Cooper, M. A., and J. P. Ornato. "Involving and Educating Base Station Physicians in Paramedic Programs." *Annals of Emergency Medicine* 9, no. 10 (1980): 524-526.

Frank, M. "Medical Director vs. Fire Chief." *JEMS* (June 1984): 46-48, 55.

Gunter, M. J., et al. "Physician Involvement: A Critical Factor in the Development of Community Emergency Medical Services." *Emergency Medical Services* (May 1979): 48-61.

Hoff, J. "Emergency Medical Services and the Neurosurgeon." *Clinical Neurology* 27 (1980): 363-367.

Hunt, R. C. "Standing Orders vs. Voice Control." *JEMS* 7, no. 11 (1982): 26-31.

Jacobs, L. M. "The 23rd Specialty." *Emer. Health Ster. Quar.* 1, no. 1 (1980): 85-95.

Johnson, J. S. "A New Approach To Medical Control." *Emergency* 10, no. 3 (1978): 42-43.

Latessa, E. M. "Rx for Medical Control." *JEMS* (April 1984): 39-41.

Leroux, R. "Emergency Medicine: A New Reality." *L'Union Medicale du Canada* 102, no. 3 (1973).

McCann, J. "Medical Control of Trauma Systems Seem Necessary to Save More Lives." *Emergency Department News* 4, no. 1 (1984).

McSwain, N. J. "Medical Control of Prehospital Care." *Journal of Trauma* 2 (1984): 172.

McSwain, N. J. "Medical Control—What is It?" *Journal of the American College of Emergency Physicians* 7, no. 3 (1978): 114-116.

Moorman, R. C., and L. J. Tiscornia. "Doctor's Stethoscope Reaches Across Town." *Emergency Product News* 8, no. 3 (1972).

Newman, B. G. "EMS Medical Control—Doctor Shoppers Need Not Apply." *JEMS* 7, no. 11 (1982): 43-44, 46.

Open Forum. "The Role of EMS Medical Directors." *Emergency Medical Services* 15, no. 2 (1986): 38-49.

Page, J. O. "Medical Control." *Paramedics International* 2, no. 2 (1977): 26-29, 41.

Page, J. O. "Medical-Legal Considerations in Prehospital Care." *Topics in Emergency Medicine* 1, no. 1 (1980): 55-59.

Page, J. O. "The Physician and EMS." *Annals of Emergency Medicine* 10, no. 1 (1981): 64-65.

Pozen, M. W. "Effectiveness of a Prehospital Medical Control System: An Analysis of the Interaction between Emergency Room Physicians and Paramedic." *Circulation* 63, no. 2 (1981): 442-447.

Rafalik, D. "Emergency Medicine: Up From the Pit." *The New Physician* (December 1974).

Rosen, P., N. Dinerman, P. T. Pons, R. Marlin, et al. "Prehospital Care—Integrated Concept of Emergency Medicine." *Topics in Emergency Medicine* 1, no. 1 (1980): 19-26.

Shub, M. G. "Chain of Command." *The EMT Journal* 2, no. 3 (1978): 86-87.

Soderstrom, C. A., R. A. Cowley, and B. H. Kaplan. "Helicopter Transport of Trauma Victims: The Physician's Role." Maryland Institute for Emergency Medical Services (1986).

Stewart, R. D. "Prehospital Care—Education, Evaluation and Medical Control." *Topics in Emergency Medicine* 1, no. 1 (1980): 67-82.

Subcommittee on Medical Control, Committee on EMS, National Academy of Sciences. *Medical Control in Emergency Medical Services Systems*. Washington, D.C.: National Academy Press, 1981.

Sutnik, A. J., and D. K. Wagner. "Emergency Medicine as an Academic Discipline." *Journal of the American Medical Association* 238, no. 2 (1977): 147-148.

Thompson, C. T. "The Emergency Physician, The Trauma Surgeon, and the Trauma Center." *Annals of Emergency Medicine* 12, no. 4 (1983): 235-237.

Wagner, D. K. "Emergency Medicine: An Important Specialty Today." *Emergency Medicine* (1980): 383-390.

Editor's Note: Since the original publication of this article, important aspects of physician involvement direction have been discussed in the texts *Prehospital Systems and Medical Oversight* and *Principles of EMS Systems* published by The National Association of EMS Physicians and The American College of Emergency Physicians, respectively.

Source

Reprinted with permission from JEMS, *September 1987. At the time of original publication, Joseph G. Ferko III worked at the Maryland Shock Treatment unit and had been involved in EMS for nine years. He is the recipient of the congressional award of merit.*

Determining Domain: The Issue of Medical Control

Carol J. Shanaberger

"Who's in charge?" is a question with many answers, depending on the situation and who is asking. This article describes a legal case in which medical control authority was defined and upheld in the courts. It illustrates the need to clarify responsibilities for medical supervision.

ALL EMTS AND PARAMEDICS know that they function as an extension of a particular physician who provides medical supervision and support through both off-line and on-line medical control. The authority of that medical director should then logically include the right to curtail and withdraw that extension. However, exercising that right can place the medical director and EMS personnel at odds.

If the EMS provider is an employee of an ambulance service or is a civil servant, can he then be authorized by his employer to continue to work in the field against the desires of the medical director? Because of the unique tripartite (three-party) relationship among the medical director, EMS provider, and ambulance service employer, the answer is not likely to please all prehospital care providers.

Who's in Charge?

Logic would dictate that a medical director should not be compelled to supervise an EMS provider whom he believes cannot practice prehospital medicine safely. The legal system, however, has a way of distancing itself from the realities of the day-to-day operations of prehospital care. For example, in the case of *County of Hennepin v. Hennepin County Association of Paramedics and Emergency Medical Technicians*, the hearing officer failed to consider the importance of time and distance in making decisions regarding prehospital care or the value of a medical license.

Prior to a decision being reached in the Hennepin case, an arbitrator at a grievance hearing determined that a discharged paramedic could return to work in the field—even though he had a less-than-outstanding work history and even though the medical director believed that the paramedic could not practice prehospital medicine safely.

The Facts of the Case

The Hennepin case arose when a paramedic, employed by Hennepin County Medical Center, amassed five verbal warnings, two written warnings, and at least 11 counseling sessions concerning his work in less than two years. The incidents in question involved inadequate or incomplete documentation on run reports, "violations of various protocols," inappropriate use of pneumatic antishock garments (PASG), including one incident of PASG inflation without physician authorization, and various other "errors in judgment." This latter category included an incident in which the paramedic told a "patient's family and [the] fire department that another ambulance was closer but was not dispatched." The paramedic's date of hire was September 26, 1986; by the end of April 1988, his performance appraisal was rated as an "overall NI (needs improvement)."

In November 1988, the paramedic in this case was involved in another incident in which he advised the relative of a patient who was complaining of chest pain that the patient should have been transported to the hospital by car instead of enlisting 9-1-1 assistance for an ambulance. Of course, his behavior was contrary to protocol. Following this incident, the paramedic was dismissed by the county, which found that his conduct was "substantially inadequate" because he failed to take a good medical history and obtain information from the first responder on scene and, subsequently, did not correctly assess the patient's needs or condition.

The paramedic then filed a grievance to contest the county's decision. In December 1989, the paramedic received notification from the county that it intended to first suspend him and ultimately dismiss him from employment. Pursuant to a collective-bargaining agreement with the local union, the county is allowed to discipline employees "only for just cause." An administrative hearing upheld the county's dismissal of the paramedic, who then appealed the case to arbitration for resolution of the matter. (Many contracts, such as collective-bargaining agreements—contracts between an employer and a union—include a provision for arbitration in the event that the parties disagree on the final decision in a grievance process.)

The Issues

The following two issues were submitted to arbitration: Was the paramedic discharged for "just cause," and if not, what constituted the appropriate disciplinary action in this case?

A point of particular legal significance was the arbitrator's limited range of authority as specified in the collective-bargaining agreement. This agreement specifically provided that the arbitrator could only rule on the issues submitted to him and that the resulting decision had to be consistent with existing rules, regulations, or laws.

Medical Control on the Stand

The medical director for the service testified at the arbitration hearing. He stated what all professional EMS providers know and what all knowledgeable medical directors have been saying for years—that paramedics function under a medical director as "essentially physician extenders." Regarding the paramedic in this case, it was clear that the medical director believed that the medic should not be allowed to function in the field. The medical director stated that, based on his personal knowledge and a review of the records, this paramedic's conduct had been inconsistent and, further, "I think he represents a potential risk to myself and the service and his peers." He concluded that the paramedic "was not competent at the time of the discharge."

The medical director explained his responsibilities to the arbitrator

It is certainly arguable that the authority and respect afforded medical control in EMS is a matter of importance for a community as a whole and not simply the medical director, the paramedic, or an individual patient.

as follows: The medical director is "the only individual authorized to decide whether [the paramedic] could operate as a paramedic under [his] license or be placed on medical probation." Yet, despite the physician's unequivocal testimony, it was not accepted by the arbitrator. The arbitrator entered a decision that reinstated the paramedic, with back pay, placed him on "medical probation" for a minimum of one year, and required retraining in "clerical and medical procedure."

Needless to say, the medical director was disconcerted by the decision. The case was appealed to the district court, which vacated (or voided) the arbitrator's decision. This decision was then appealed by the paramedic's union to the district court.

The medical director submitted affidavits for the district court's consideration, one of which included the following statement:

> . . . I cannot, as medical director, trust . . . or ensure that [this paramedic], even if on medical probation, would recognize important symptoms, conduct necessary physical examinations, make the proper assessments, accurately report these back for physician diagnosis and treatment, and appropriately carry out physician instructions or necessary medical procedures. . . .

Medical Control and Public Policy

The fact that the district court overruled the arbitrator's decision is noteworthy in itself. It is also significant that the court did so on "public policy grounds." Unfortunately, the court of appeals did as most courts in the same circumstances would: It based its decision on the available statutes that adequately addressed the relevant issues, and it chose not to rule on the county's public policy argument (choosing instead the narrowest grounds on which to rule).

The concept of public policy has been noted in other editions of "The Legal File" (see May 1986 and June 1989 issues of *JEMS*). Public policy is a vague but valuable legal doctrine that is used as a basis for ruling, in which the court deems an interest as being expedient for the benefit of the community; it is also used in cases in which it is necessary to prevent an individual from doing something that is injurious to society or to another person or is otherwise "against the public good."

Although the value of relying on public policy for a legal decision is debatable, it is certainly arguable that the authority and respect afforded medical control in EMS is a matter of importance for a community as a whole and not simply the medical director, the paramedic, or an individual patient. The trial court's view in the Hennepin case that medical control was a matter of public interest may be an argument voiced more often in the future.

Recognition of Medical Control

In the Hennepin case, the state court of appeals analyzed the role of the medical director, giving unprecedented recognition to the uniqueness of delegated medical practice and the impact a paramedic can have on a medical director's license to practice medicine. The court of appeals agreed with the county's argument that the arbitrator had "exceeded the authority granted to him in the collective-bargaining agreement by ordering the medical director to employ [the paramedic] as a paramedic under the medical license of the medical director and against his best medical judgment."

The court of appeals further stated that local ambulance services are already "heavily regulated"—that there are existing standards regarding equipment and staffing that have been implemented for the protection of the health, safety, and welfare of the people of the county. Through the medical director, an integral component of the EMS system, "each paramedic practices pursuant to a physician's license." The court emphasized in its decision that an ambulance service must have a medical director who, by statute, "accepts responsibility for the quality of care provided by drivers and attendants of an advanced ambulance service." That medical director is required to be involved in setting standards for training and in authorizing recertification of paramedics based on their skills proficiency. All of these obligations, the court noted, "impose potential tort and disciplinary liability on a medical director for actions of unfit paramedics."

The court of appeals cited the testimony of the medical director at the original arbitration hearing when asked about complying with the arbitrator's ruling regarding probation: "I have to trust a paramedic in order to allow him to practice under my license." Consequently, the appellate court held that the arbitrator exceeded his authority by essentially forcing the medical director to permit a paramedic to work under his license "when [the medical director], in his best medical judgment, believes a person should not work as a paramedic. The arbitrator's remedy purports to dictate medical decisions legally delegated to the medical director."

Interestingly, the court added in a footnote (which is of no legal value) that the arbitrator could have ordered the paramedic to be reinstated subject to the approval of the medical director, and the court recommended that the paramedic be offered employment (e.g., a desk position) within the county system subject to the medical director's approval.

Sadly, it has taken until December 31, 1990 (the date the court of appeals' decision was rendered) for a state appellate court to recognize the role and responsibilities of medical control, which most medical directors have accepted as the standard of care, and to acknowledge the risks inherent in the supervision of paramedics. EMTs and paramedics should not overlook either of these points when engaging in patient care or when evaluating their own skills and knowledge in the practice of medicine in the field.

Source

Reprinted with permission from JEMS, *July 1991. Carol J. Shanaberger is an attorney and a paramedic. She lectures to EMS providers throughout the country and is a member of the legal committee for the National Association of EMS Physicians.*

References

County of Hennepin v. Hennepin County Association of Paramedics and Emergency Medical Technicians, 464 N.W.2d 578 (C. App. Minn. 1990).

Gilmer, W. *Cochran's Law Lexicon,* 5th ed. Cincinnati: The Anderson Co., 1973.

Minn. R. 4690.0100, subp. 2 (1989).

Overcoming Adversarial Administrative and Medical Relationships

Christine M. Zalar, RN, MA

A poor relationship with the medical director is like flying directly into the path of a tornado. If the administrator is lucky enough to survive, there is almost always widespread devastation after landing. EMS leaders need to develop and nurture positive, growing relationships. This article suggests methods for smoothing out "bumpy flights" and avoiding system devastation.

THE RELATIONSHIP BETWEEN EMS administrators and their medical directors has historically been quite turbulent. The adversarial relationship is an outgrowth of a lack of clarity about responsibilities, roles, and scope of authority. This article will identify factors that lead to adversarial relationships between EMS administrators and their medical directors; define areas in the service's operations that may be exposed to liability due to limited or no physician involvement; and develop strategies for prospectively improving the administrative/medical relationship in EMS organizations.

Clarify Roles and Develop Consensus

EMS administration has increasingly focused on the business side of the organization. This means budgets, bookkeeping, accounts receivable and payable, hiring and firing—all those things necessary to keep the organization running. This is true regardless of the type of EMS system in which the organization participates or who delivers the care. The administration of EMS organizations has evolved and matured significantly as financial and operational performance standards—coupled with sophisticated high-technology approaches—have become key benchmarks for effective EMS. Funding and reimbursement have become major factors in the success of EMS administrators as they strive to make their organizations more efficient.

Efficiency, at times, has been accomplished at the expense of other critical components that make the EMS system a *medical* system. The business of EMS has become somewhat of a distraction for EMS administrators, leaving the provision of care and medical control to stand on the laurels of previous performance. Fortunately, physicians have become increasingly sophisticated in their role in the EMS system, and have developed the "medical director" as an official position. The result has been a stronger role for the physician and for medical control.

Medical control and the scope of responsibility of the medical director are based on the traditional EMS system. Primary activities include developing and implementing standards that reflect the medical community's standard of care and monitoring compliance to those standards. Overall, the medical director's job is to develop a sound, competent, and accountable medical care system that is in the best interest of the patient. For medical control to be effective, it must be the official authority for clinical practice in the prehospital system. There are four clearly defined areas of medical control.

Prospective medical control. Traditionally called off line, prospective medical control creates the infrastructure for all medical control activities. It includes protocols, training standards, local certification requirements, education, and continuing education based on outcomes of quality improvement activities.

Interactive medical control. Interactive medical control, or on line, is the ability to talk with a physician or surrogate via radio or telephone to communicate field personnel findings and gain physician input. This leads to a concurrence in decisions regarding the patient's care and treatment, as well as collaboration for transport and destination assignments.

Retrospective medical control. Retrospective medical control includes the quality improvement activities of the organization. This typically involves reviewing the care and treatment delivered in all aspects of the EMS system through audits, morbidity and mortality conferences, and case presentations.

Influential medical control. Influential medical control is where leadership and the professional status of the physician medical control in the community can positively affect patient care for the public good.

EMS organizational failures have occurred because of the lack of— and the "fight" for—medical control in one or more of these four areas. Further, there has been an unfortunate impact on EMS systems when medical control has not been incorporated as one of the planning and operating components of the system. This problem is not unique to EMS organizations, but has occurred in the development of medical communications centers and first responder programs as well.

Historical Problem Areas

The need for a medical director and medical control has historically been associated with high-volume, advanced life support EMS systems. The criteria determining the need for medical control has been patient volume, as opposed to patient care. In rural EMS systems, closer physician monitoring should be more intense than in the urban setting, due to longer ambulance response times and distances to the appropriate facilities. Coupled with this is the issue of proficiency of the rural prehospital care providers who encounter a low number of patients and transports. From the patient's perspective, there should be an inverse relationship between the intensity of medical control and the number of patient transports.

Gray areas regarding the role of the EMS medical director have often evolved from the EMS environment itself. Often, the physician in this position has very little authority, and there are few funds available. Historically, this has meant that physicians have worked "on their own time," with no secretarial or clerical staff support, and have had no formal position in the organization's structure. The lack of authority the EMS medical director previously experienced obstructed his ability to impact change both internally and externally. It also led to conflict and "turf" issues with the EMS administrator.

EMS administrators must recognize the evolution of the medical director's operating environment, but must also prioritize the clinical performance aspects of their organizations.

As EMS organizations matured, so did the role of the medical director and the environment in which he functioned. Research data indicate that 69 percent of medical directors receive some degree of funding for their positions. The same research indicates that 62 percent are now provided with malpractice coverage, and 89 percent receive some form of clerical support. It is important to note that most of the statistics represent medical directors in larger EMS systems. These are the higher-volume patient care providers, but they represent the smallest number of EMS systems.

EMS administrators must recognize the evolution of the medical director's operating environment, but must also prioritize the clinical performance aspects of their organizations. The gray areas of confrontation between administrators and medical directors have not solely been based on the lack of medical director job descriptions, contracts, or salaries. Confrontation has also stemmed from a lack of clarity in regard to the scope of responsibility and authority, and equitable distribution of the organization's resources for the clinical management of the system.

This lack of clarity has resulted in an open arena for employees, government officials, and other external participants in the EMS system to create tension between the organization's administrative and clinical leadership by effectively polarizing one side against the other. EMS administrators must look to close the gap—and eliminate the gray areas—in order for a healthy EMS organization to progress, regardless of how big the organization is.

Discipline and Other Issues

The simple question, "Who is responsible for employee discipline, and under what circumstances?" creates controversy in every EMS system unless a formal structure for dealing with this issue is established. If someone shows up late, not in uniform, etc., these are clearly administrative areas that are solved by the disciplinary policies and procedures of the organization. However, the administrator's authority in the "discipline" for clinical practice deviations is not as clear.

Does the medical director have the right to fire somebody for consistent substandard care, persistent mistakes, or problems in their practices on the street? Medical directors have the right to decide who practices under their licenses, but administrators are usually empowered with hiring and terminating employees.

Most EMS organizations require that the medical director focus on clinical performance, discovering problem areas and determining remedial activities to resolve problems. Administrators must be involved to help determine if remedial activities have indeed resolved the problem. What happens to the paramedic under "administrative" reprimand? This is not necessarily the medical director's responsibility, yet clearly there is potential here for conflict between the medical director and the administrator. If you have a structure for limiting an employee's privilege to practice, you *must* have a strong, interactive base of administrative and medical support in setting the standards for what happens.

Medical directors and administrators must work collaboratively to ensure that the right people are hired from the beginning. Local, county, and state certification should be considered part of determining an individual's "fit" into the organization's values and culture. Without a thorough understanding of all these areas by the medical director and administrator, conflicts will occur.

The classic challenges of recruitment, education, and training are often found in rural systems. Administrators in rural areas have ongoing difficulties retaining volunteers because of increasing education and training requirements. Medical directors in these systems may require people with higher certification and education, but soon discover that these requirements have depleted the staff. Losing people because they can't keep up with continuing education demands (especially in rural areas) is an increasing concern for both administrators and physicians.

How many ambulances and what staffing configuration does the EMS system require? Medical directors and administrators will likely have two different answers, even if they are from the same area. Focusing on response times, and balancing this with the resources that are affordable, can reduce conflict areas between administrator and medical director perspectives.

Finally, there are destination policies. This gray area can be costly. Other than federal anti-dumping laws, there are few regulations that tell you where to take a patient. A lack of physician involvement in diversion policies has cost EMS organizations significant monetary damages. Juries do not take kindly to those who use EMS for reasons other than optimal patient care.

Consider the case of *Hospital Authority of Gwinnett County v. Jones.* In this case, a patient sustained burns over 75 percent of his body in a multiple-vehicle accident. Before even arriving on the scene, the EMT squad was told by a non-physician at the control center where to take the patient. The EMT arrived on scene and wanted to send the patient by helicopter (overhead and ready to land) to a burn center, but the EMS hospital control center insisted that the patient be ground transported to a "sister" hospital that was not nearby. When the ambulance arrived at this hospital, the emergency physician ordered the patient to the burn center by helicopter. The helicopter picked up the patient, had an accident en route, and the patient was again loaded into an ambulance for a 15-mile journey to the burn center. The original hospital transport to the burn center would have taken 20 minutes by ground.

It was proven in court that the hospital authority had a policy to transport within its own system ("sister" hospitals). Diversion instructions, however, came from a non-physician administrator. There was no medical justification for the transfer, and no medical protocols or destination policies supported the activities of the hospital authority. The nominal

Losing people because they can't keep up with continuing education demands (especially in rural areas) is an increasing concern for both administrators and physicians.

The use of medical advisory or administrative oversight committees helps create a balance in decision making.

damages were only one dollar, because the additional injuries to the patient were minor. However, the jury awarded $1.3 million in punitive damages because there was a clear presumption of conscience: Even though the hospital authority knew the consequences of its policies, it elected to ignore them.

Implications for administrators and their medical directors center on diversion or destination policies having medical input prospectively, and in this case, on line. Choosing the appropriate vehicle for the transport must be based on the patient's medical needs and the capabilities of the receiving resources within the EMS system. Obviously, the need for physician input and involvement in proactive policies, as well as in on-line enforcement and decision making, is well demonstrated in the Gwinnett County case.

Broaden the Support Base

A number of gray areas that can create adverse relationships have been touched on. It is important to deal in these overlapping areas with a goal toward a synergistic relationship and not a competitive one. Many systems have failed because they did not focus on the gray areas. Learn from them. You also need to learn from systems that have done the right things—administratively—in these gray areas. There are many examples of these.

Communities often bring in experts on both the administrative and medical sides to broaden perspective and involvement, and reduce conflict. Medical oversight committees, or physician advisory boards, need to be formalized to evaluate the EMS system clinically on behalf of the patient.

The size of your system is not related to the size of this committee. The qualifications should be that, as a group, the physicians have the interest, involvement, and clout to oversee clinical performance and outcomes. If the bottom line is true accountability to the patient, then both the medical director and administrator should be accountable to a respective oversight committee (e.g., medical and administrative committees).

The use of medical advisory or administrative oversight committees helps create a balance in decision making. In many systems, the administrator may be directly accountable to the administrative oversight committee and, similarly, the medical director to the medical committee. Each of the oversight boards is responsible, within its area of expertise, for making policy and creating systems for monitoring the organization's performance and evaluating the leaders it has appointed. Clearly, an oversight committee or board should not be involved in the system's daily operations or clinical management. The EMS administrator can be a leader in forming such independent boards or committees. The clear advantage of these types of governing structures is that they can eliminate a maverick administrator or medical director and provide an appropriate forum for resolving personality clashes and disagreements between administrative and clinical directives.

Remember the importance of performance and accountability, particularly regarding this bottom line: When you have adversarial relationships between medical directors and administrators, morale will go down. The staff will feel the tension, they will be confused about who their boss is, and ultimately patient care will suffer.

Successful systems balance the two powers of administrative and medical control. Regardless of the size of your system—one ambulance and one hospital, or 20 ambulances and 50 hospitals—you need that balance and broad involvement. A highly structured oversight committee will ensure that the balance of power ignores adversarial relationships and tilts toward the patient.

References

Hospital Authority of Gwinnett County v. Jones, 261 Ga. 613, 409 SE 2d 501 (1991); after remand 711 S.Ct. 1298; 259 Ga. 759, 386 SE 2d 120 (1989).

Swor, R. A., and R. L. Krome. "Administrative Support of Emergency Medical Services' Medical Directors: A Profile." *Prehospital and Disaster Medicine* 5, no. 1 (1990): 25-30.

Source

Original article. Christine M. Zalar is a partner at Fitch & Associates, Inc. She is widely recognized as one of the nation's leading experts on air medical and hospital-based EMS/medical transportation systems. She is also a principal author of the book EMS Management: Beyond the Street, *2nd ed.*

Quality Improvement

Total Quality Management: A Style for the Future

James N. Eastham, Jr, ScD

EMS systems take many circuitous paths in the journey toward quality. Dr. Jim Eastham offers a straightforward explanation of the process that includes quality planning, control, and improvement. In an accompanying article, Jerry Allison describes how quality can be used as a noun when defining objectives.

MORE THAN EVER BEFORE, all of healthcare, including emergency medical services, is under pressure to be fiscally, clinically, and morally accountable. Beyond our own ethical responsibility to provide the highest quality care possible, government agencies and the public are demanding justification that EMS is meeting their needs.

The principal reasons for this increased concern about quality in healthcare are the high costs of that care and the need for cost-containment. In this worldwide recession, taxpayers are less willing to provide money for healthcare without accountability.

Another major factor driving quality awareness is variation in clinical practice. Around the world—from country to country and from city to city—there are dramatic differences in the training levels of EMS personnel, in types of equipment and clinical practices, in response times to emergencies, and in the mortality and morbidity rates that result from trauma and medical emergencies. Finally, increased focus on healthcare quality is also being driven in some countries by the relatively high rate of litigation following poor outcomes from medical practice.

EMS and healthcare in general are having problems with their traditional methods for assessing quality. The authors of the book *Curing Health Care: New Strategies for Quality Improvement* discuss limitations of current methods of healthcare quality management and point out that the healthcare industry itself is rapidly realizing that it does not have a good set of tools with which to manage quality assessment and quality improvement (QI).

This is because the rather extensive quality assurance (QA) literature is decidedly academic, full of complicated jargon and complex methodology that speaks effectively to the scientist but not to most EMS system managers and field personnel. Also, the literature and methods currently available focus extensively on clinical issues and rarely on the administrative and organizational issues that are the foundation of clinical care. The existing quality management methods in EMS are elegant at the art of describing faults but weak when it comes to exploring causes and presenting methods for resolving problems.

Today's prevailing field-level EMS QA methodology usually involves having supervisors audit human performance. This system rarely involves investigating the system deficiencies that make operations inefficient or that make human performance failure inevitable. Instead, it focuses on human behavior as the primary target for change and promotes fear and resentment among personnel.

Fearful staff members may respond to the quality management system by trying to subvert it, either by not fully participating or by doctoring information to make themselves look better. All too often, QA programs are viewed by personnel as unfair, mistake-catching expeditions run by people who are too far removed from the process of field work to really understand how the EMS system operates.

It is apparent that we need to change our approach toward quality management. The theoretical model, commonly referred to as total quality management (TQM), is the result of the pioneering efforts of people such as W. Edwards Deming, Joseph Juran, and Kaoru Ishikawa and has been successfully guiding quality management in industry for more than 40 years, most notably in Japan. Recently, Donald Berwick and his colleagues at Harvard University conducted a successful demonstration project of TQM in hospitals in the United States.

Total Quality Management for EMS

TQM requires all people involved in EMS, from administrators to EMTs, to view the entire EMS system from a different perspective. EMS needs to change its emphasis from finding and correcting people's mistakes to producing a better EMS production system, a system whose basic operating objective is to develop internal (within the organization) and external (patient) customer satisfaction.

An EMS system can be described as a series of interrelated processes that produce information as well as administrative, technical, and clinical services. The creation of EMS system products involves the interaction of numerous people, including physicians, nurses, administrators, paramedics, EMTs, communications specialists, automotive mechanics, supply clerks, and secretaries.

All of these people relate to each other as internal suppliers and customers of internal EMS system products. The public is viewed as the external customer, who consumes the clinical care product of the EMS system (Table 4.1).

Each person in the EMS system should be encouraged to identify ways in which individuals or the system can do a better job of meeting internal and external customers' needs and increasing satisfaction with the products. By constantly striving to meet these needs and improve

TQM requires all people involved in EMS, from administrators to EMTs, to view the entire EMS system from a different perspective.

customer satisfaction levels, the EMS system will continually improve, as will the quality of patient care.

For example, in a typical EMS system, radio dispatchers use a process that produces an information product to guide their customers—the responding paramedics or EMTs—to the scene of an illness or injury. As customers, the responders depend on the dispatcher's information product to be high quality; if it isn't, the paramedics or EMTs may get lost, arrive late, or arrive at the patient without the proper equipment.

In a TQM system, every dispatcher continually works to maximize responder satisfaction with the information product. An organized effort is made to regularly assess and improve the entire process of how the information product is assembled and delivered to the responder/customer. The goal of this assessment is to ensure that the customer's information needs are being met and that the information production process is efficient. Under this system, dispatchers, supervisors, and field personnel meet periodically to review past activities and discuss potential ways to improve the dispatch product from both the supplier and customer viewpoints.

As indicated in Table 4.1, there are many other supplier/customer relationships within the EMS system, and each example points to the need for interdepartmental communication focused on enhancing both production efficiency and customer satisfaction. TQM also requires that EMS avoid the temptation to focus solely on clinical practice. Every aspect of the EMS system is important and supports the ultimate system goal: to keep patients satisfied and reduce morbidity and mortality.

The TQM Trilogy

Joseph Juran describes TQM using the Juran Trilogy model. The trilogy includes quality planning, quality control, and quality improvement. The rationale behind quality planning is that operations or processes should be designed and planned to meet and exceed customer needs. Too often, suppliers design production systems and products without asking customers what they need; the supplier simply assumes he knows the answer. Anyone who has ever been on the receiving end of sloppy work, vague instructions, or unexpected delays may be a victim of supplier ignorance about customer needs.

When planning an EMS production process, suppliers must determine their customers' needs, ensuring that they design products

Table 4.1

Examples of EMS System Production Process Relationships

Suppliers	Products	Customers
Dispatcher	Patient/scene information	Paramedic/EMT
Physician	Treatment protocols	Paramedic/EMT
Mechanic	Fleet maintenance	Paramedic/EMT
Secretary	Typed reports	Administrator
Administrator	Office policies	Secretary
Personnel officer	Personnel recruitment	Shift supervisor
Programmer	Dispatch software	Dispatcher
EMS instructor	Continuing education	Paramedic/EMT
Paramedic/EMT	Trip report data	Quality manager
Paramedic/EMT	Medical care	Patient

to include features the customer is looking for. Such features might include ease of use, rapid availability, clear instructions, safe working environment, adequate supplies, timely delivery of supplies, and compassionate and professional care. After designing such a product, the plan is put into production.

After execution of the quality plan, the manager is concerned with making sure that the production process remains as reliable and predictable as possible. This is called quality control. Any EMS production process will inevitably vary due to a variety of human, mechanical, and environmental factors. This variation in the production process will in turn cause the features of each product to vary. For example, changes in traffic patterns or overall call volume may cause ambulance response times to differ. The manager's role, then, is to ensure that this variation does not get out of control.

To do this, a quality control program must be put into operation to evaluate an operating system's performance. This program will include continual sampling and descriptive statistical analysis of the key variables of all major production processes within the EMS system. The findings from the statistical analysis are compared to the organization's goals and standards, and when statistically significant differences are found, personnel can act to bring the system back in control. An EMS system manager, for example, should be interested in the quality of the ambulance response—a key measure of which is response time. This measure should be carefully and continually analyzed on quality control charts.

To measure response time on a quality control chart, plot the proportion of calls that fall above and below an agreed-on quality control standard response time on a regular basis (e.g., every shift or every day). The variations in response times for a particular day or shift then should be analyzed against an average variation existing in the system over a longer time period (e.g., the previous six months or year). The trends in the chart should be reviewed (sometimes daily if necessary) for data points outside the norm or for problematic trends that need immediate correction or that indicate potential for long-term improvement projects.

Every EMS process that produces a product is subject to variation. But if quality is to be reliable, EMS organizations must continually strive to reduce this variation in their production systems. To do this, they must be aware of the components involved in making that product. If a company is to reduce variation in ambulance response time, for example, its personnel must have a firm understanding of the human, mechanical, and environmental factors that can cause response time to exceed quality control standards.

Ultimately, we must work to improve performance levels to new levels of achievement. This is known as quality improvement, which is the third—and most important—component of TQM.

As Juran states, "Quality improvement is the organized creation of beneficial change; the attainment of unprecedented levels of perfor-

"Quality improvement is the organized creation of beneficial change; the attainment of unprecedented levels of performance . . . a breakthrough!"

mance . . . a breakthrough!" QI is more than just putting out a fire. Rather, it relates to developing better methods of operation so the fire will not flare up again.

QI is accomplished by having in place a specific infrastructure that will encourage experimentation to improve clinical, administrative, and operations production systems. A QI program should be designed to regularly solicit QI projects from the entire EMS system workforce. These projects should then be worked on by teams of system employees who

So, Just What Is Quality?

Jerry A. Allison, NREMT-P

Many people think of the word "quality" as an adjective. But quality can be used as a noun; it is like rain, a car, or a pulse. It can be heavy or light, fast or slow, strong or weak. Just to say "quality" leaves the word's definition open to perception. And if we have no true definition of quality, how can we define a quality improvement (QI) program? We can do it by thinking of quality as a series of steps or a set of values on which to base our work or lives.

To define and develop a QI program, we must first know what we believe in. This means establishing a set of values on which to base all future actions. If we don't know what we believe in, we will find it difficult to reach our goals or to convince others to support our purpose.

In the January 1992 issue of *JEMS*, Publisher Jim Page stated that it has taken "square pegs" to bring EMS to where it is today and that only square pegs will keep EMS evolving as a profession that defines and delivers excellent prehospital care. These square pegs share some common values: No one has the right to deliver mediocre care; excellence can only be achieved through mutual understanding and seeking to meet the needs of both customers and EMS providers; and EMS caregivers are capable of understanding their responsibilities and should be held accountable for their actions.

Obviously, you don't need to share these exact values to set up a QI program, but you do need to have some foundation on which to set program goals. Once you understand your individual values, you can identify the purpose of your QI program and set objectives.

QI Objectives

The first objective of a QI program is to identify the system's principal strengths and develop mechanisms for reinforcing them. This is one of the most important functions of a QI program, since it prevents throwing out the good with the bad and creates a positive frame of mind. Certainly, it is easy to develop a negative perspective when identifying areas that need improvement. But often, when reinforcing the good in a system, some of the smaller problems work themselves out.

The second objective in a QI program is to identify weak areas in the system and develop, implement, and monitor programs—typically educational—to strengthen those areas. When identifying weaknesses, look for and identify strengths as well; people are more likely to work toward improvement if they know their strengths are also recognized. (Avoid such negative words as "problem," since they close doors to improvement.)

The third objective is to set goals. Both short- and long-term goals are an integral part of any program, but they must be attainable and measurable. To set goals, then, you must have standards. But how and by what do you establish these standards? The answer is simple: Look at where your system is right now, and establish standards according to current expectations. These standards may not be where you think they ought to be or where the system requires them to be, but you need to start somewhere.

Remember, standards are not only something to reach for—they are the foundation on which to measure progress. If you think your standards should be higher, make higher standards part of your goals. Take care, however, not to base your standards on what other systems are doing. Each system is unique, and you must consider your system's needs and capabilities when setting standards.

are given the appropriate resources to conduct proper experimentation.

QI requires the existence of "quality councils" designed to launch, coordinate, and "institutionalize" annual QI. These quality councils should be staffed by upper- and middle-level managers who represent all supplier and customer departments within an EMS system.

The quality council has six major responsibilities. First, it formulates overall quality policy for the EMS system. Second, it solicits QI project ideas from all members of the local EMS workforce. An ongoing quality

When you do reach your goals, acknowledge the fact by making some "hoopla." Since our society has created an expectation of quick gratification, make sure to set enough short-term goals to keep people from getting discouraged.

QI Techniques

In many systems, the largest quality problems identified are caused by lack of education. But those problems are also the most easily solved. Education is one of the most important components in any system, and that's particularly true of EMS. Both prehospital caregivers and administrators must stay abreast of current changes and trends if true quality is to be achieved.

If you are involved in QI, let everyone in the system help you—QI cannot be accomplished by one person or by a small group of people. This is where QI differs from traditional quality assurance (QA) programs. QA sets up figures of authority who focus on what went wrong and who did wrong. QI programs, on the other hand, rely on everyone in the system focusing on what goes right and who does well. By identifying weaknesses and improving them through education and placing less emphasis on punitive measures by a "governing" body, QI can elicit abundant support and enthusiasm.

You can encourage help by probing. Develop mechanisms to obtain data, suggestions, and comments from all participants in the system. Encourage participants to provide positive feedback before they offer suggestions for improvement.

A good QI program must provide communication and feedback to the people involved. Medical professionals should be treated as being capable of solving their own problems. They also want to be appreciated for their thoughts and ideas. The role of good management is to facilitate feedback by posting data analysis and providing written comments in answer to suggestions—regardless of whether they were used.

Many companies attribute much of the success of their QI programs to the use of "quality circles," or roundtable discussions, and to frequent interaction among system participants. Discussion is an important component of a QI program, as it stimulates thoughts and plans. But you must try to keep the discussions positive. Emphasize compliments before criticism and solutions before problems.

Conclusion

There is no uniform definition of quality. If you want to improve quality, you must develop values, goals, and standards and then strive to exceed them. To determine how much QI has been attained, measure the difference between the old standards and the new standards.

QI is not a patient care-only program; chart reviews are only a small portion of QI. Instead, QI is a way to raise standards in all departments—patient care, vehicle maintenance, communications, and marketing.

Finally, while it may be easy to identify "problems" in a system and to see many things that need improvement, we must remember that plenty is being done right as well. After all, people are being helped, and lives are being saved.

Reference
Page, J. "Publishers Page." *JEMS* (January 1992).

Source
Reprinted with permission from JEMS, *January 1993. At the time of original publication, Jerry Allison, NREMT-P, was the EMS coordinator in Saipan, Mariana Islands. Previously, he was the director of an EMS service in northern Ohio.*

Source

Reprinted with permission from JEMS, *January 1993. Dr. Eastham is an associate professor of emergency health services as well as the chair of the emergency health services department at the University of Maryland, Baltimore County. He received his doctor of science degree in health services research from the Johns Hopkins School of Hygiene and Public Health in Baltimore; he holds bachelor's and master's degrees in sociology.*

control database in each department is also an important source of information for defining potential QI projects.

Third, after careful review of each improvement project proposal, the council selects projects for implementation. Fourth, the quality council recruits interdepartmental teams to work on the QI projects, ensuring that the supplier and customer departments involved in the process to be improved are included on the team. Fifth, the council monitors the progress of the various QI teams and ensures that the teams have the resources to get the job done.

Finally, the council has the responsibility to ensure that appropriate rewards and recognition go to those members of the organization who participate on QI teams.

Organization Start-Up

When considering introducing TQM to an EMS organization, leaders must first ensure that they fully understand the program. Using outside consultants as coaches can be helpful, but cannot serve as a substitute for having internal leaders who understand the TQM process and are committed to its success. A TQM education program for top leaders is an essential first step. Including the physician/medical director in the initial TQM education process will work to destroy the myth that the physician alone is ultimately responsible for the quality of an EMS system.

Furthermore, the most important atmosphere to develop in an EMS system is one that breaks down communication and trust barriers between staff and supervisors and between functional departments. Without an atmosphere of open communication and cooperation, quality management as described here will not exist. Ultimately, all leaders and managers must work to eradicate fear among employees, and everyone should be encouraged to make recommendations for improvement without fear of reprisal or of being ignored.

Above all, every employee in an EMS system must be educated about how TQM works and about the concepts of EMS production systems and product quality variation. They must also learn that an EMS system must ration its improvement efforts to those projects that will provide the most good for the most people. Having this knowledge, the workforce and managers can work together in an atmosphere of cooperation.

All people working in an EMS system must be empowered to believe that their work matters. They should also know that through TQM they have a real opportunity to provide better products for the internal and external customers who depend on them.

References

Berwick, D. M., A. B. Godfrey, and J. Roessner. *Curing Health Care: New Strategies for Quality Improvement.* San Francisco: Jossey-Bass, 1990.
Deming, W. E. *Out of the Crisis.* Cambridge, Mass.: MIT-CAES, 1986.
Ishikawa, K. *What is Total Quality Control?* Englewood Cliffs, N.J.: Prentice-Hall, 1985.
Juran, J. M. *Juran on Leadership for Quality.* New York: Free Press, 1989.

Performance Standards: What Standards Are Good Enough?

Terry Abrams, MSC, EMT-P

"WE MET THE STATE STANDARD for practicing medics. Why do we have to meet higher department standards?" This lament, frequently heard by training personnel, will probably increase as the concept of quality improvement progresses through our industry. Just as the consumer movement shook up the North American manufacturing industries, the consumer movement is now shaking up the service industries, including emergency medical services. The demand for proficient, competent, compassionate service has never been higher.

Who sets the required "standard of care" for a service? As the primary benefactor of EMS, the patient does. Every medic working for a given agency must be able to handle the difficult calls as well as the more frequent "easy" calls. If a service operates a split crew system—a paramedic/EMT or an EMT/driver—the team must be competent. Patients do not "prebook" their emergencies, or make appointments through 9-1-1 for emergency ambulances. If they did, it would be reasonable that only the best, most competent employees would be allowed to handle those calls. But the real world just doesn't operate that way. The key is to prepare everyone to the level required and expected by the consumers.

Determining and Describing a Standard of Care

The standard of care can be determined by first reviewing the types and severity of calls most frequently encountered by a service. The local medical control authority is another good source of information. A review of the types of calls, the frequency of call types, and the status of the patients will help develop a patient profile and skills inventory. For example, a review of the rapid transport of an urban service, combined with short transport times, may produce a different list of required skills than a similar review of a rural service. Differences in staff qualifications and level of delivered service—advanced life support, basic life support, Rapid Zap, etc.—may result in different skill needs for staff members. An inter-hospital transfer service will have a different service profile than a pure emergency service. A rotary-wing air ambulance may be different from a fixed-wing air ambulance in terms of the types of patients transported and the skills required by the crew.

Representatives of the field staff should be encouraged to participate in setting "street-relevant" performance standards. Begin by listing all the skills performed in this field. The skills list should also include non-medical skills, such as map reading and radio communication. This list can then be sorted into major categories, i.e., airway maintenance, assessment skills, splinting skills, etc.

In this article, paramedic instructor Terry Abrams answers the question, "Who should set the standards of care?" He describes standards as dynamic expectations and explains how to develop and reinforce standards in any EMS organization.

Once the list is developed, each skill is examined to determine the agency-acceptable methods of performing the skill. Again, input from the practitioners is beneficial. The textbook method is not always the same as the street method. The opposite is also true. Sometimes the patient benefits when the street method is modified to more closely conform to the textbook method. Local medical control should be an integral part of the entire process. To ensure that the standard for a skill performance is objective, ask each member of the input group, "How do you know you have successfully completed this skill?"

Introducing the Standards

The next step, following the distribution of the skills list and the acceptable methods of skills performance, is an evaluation and feedback for each individual practitioner. Simulations and actual call experience are extremely beneficial. The issue of "examination versus assessment" is now at hand. Both procedures have a role to play. Regular testing is often incorporated into requalification or license renewal. Assessment and feedback are usually associated with the educational process. Ensuring that standards are met, while remaining objective and dispassionate, is a test of endurance, personal integrity, and commitment. The process of development, refinement, education, and evaluation of the standards is not a short-term project.

The issue of managerial/supervisory staff participation in these types of assessments is a thorny one. Every employee likely to aid a patient using company equipment must be capable of administering the "difficult call." Although patient care may be only a small part of the job description, everyone delivering patient care should meet the agency's standards. From an educator's point of view, having managers accountable to the same standards of care greatly assists in breaking down the rift that may exist between the street staff and the management staff. By evaluating field and management staff alike, the specter of a double standard can be removed. This step will help reduce the anxiety and fear of job loss associated with implementing performance standards. Further, everyone will identify with the experience. Buying into the process then becomes easier. Of course, the teacher is also a pupil. Teaching staff must be as fully capable of delivering the same level of care as a full-time provider, in addition to being able to teach.

Reinforcing the Standards

A difficult managerial problem is what to do when a medic fails to either attempt the standard or successfully meet the standard. Issues such as continuing responsibilities on the ambulance, ability to continue to provide advanced skills and techniques to the patient population, implications on wages or status, opportunities for additional attempts at the standard, reinstatement procedures, disciplinary actions, and the mechanisms by which performance standard competence will be evaluated all need to be discussed and formulated in an agency policy.

When the question, "What happens if someone fails?" is considered before a program is implemented, time is available to evaluate the legal, moral, ethical, and labor relations issues the question raises. In some services, three attempts to meet the performance standards are allowed. If the individual is unsuccessful on the third attempt, that person is no longer eligible to be "in charge" of a unit. When qualification exams are held again, the person can retake the exams to attain "in charge" status.

Hiring With Standards

When setting performance standards for a given agency, two types of employees must be considered: the new employee or applicant, and the person already employed in the system. It would be ideal to allow all new applicants to demonstrate their professional prowess on a truly life-threatening call. The next best method is to examine the candidates under simulated conditions using a standardized patient and evaluation form—the scenario. If possible, several scenarios reflect more reliable results. The testing scenarios should be based on calls done by the service. By using realistic scenario evaluations of new applicants, a reasonable picture of the candidate's performance potential can be gleaned at the least cost in terms of time, money, or liability. The candidate also gets a picture of what the service's expectations are. A reputation for hiring only the best people has never hurt an employer's status in any industry. In the event a candidate applies again for employment with the same agency, the additional training undertaken by the applicant to meet the entrance standard will benefit the employer, the employee, and the patient.

The Evolution of Standards

Performance standards are dynamic expectations. They may be initially set so that all members of the staff can meet them with only minimal additional work and training. As the staff becomes more proficient in managing the more common patient types, the standard should be raised to cover the next level of commonly encountered patients. As medical knowledge advances and regional treatment trends evolve, they should be reflected not only in staff training but also in performance standards. Strong medical control is a great asset in deciding what patient types, based on working diagnoses, are the greatest priority to the system's evolution.

Prehospital care is a service industry. Patients are consumers. Keep in mind that a patient's criteria of good service is different from what the technical experts define as good service. The patient is watching for compassion and "tender loving care" as well as technical competence. If a customer gets "lousy service," what is the likelihood of that service being used again? Performance standards help ensure that a service and its employees provide consistent, competent, and caring assistance to every patient who calls for it regardless of time, day, or responding ambulance crew. The agency's standards of care are an expression of commitment to the customer.

Source

Original article. Terry Abrams has worked as a standards and assessment officer in the Staff Development Division of the City of Calgary EMS Department for six years. He is involved in the design and implementation of competency-based training systems, including setting and evaluating performance standards.

Investing in Your People

Martha Libby, BS, EMT-P, and Scott Vahradian, BA, EMT-P

If the statement, "A leader can't motivate—he can only provide an environment for self-motivation to occur," is true, then the same holds true for quality. In this important article, the authors describe how staff members become empowered to improve quality.

WHAT MAKES PEOPLE STRIVE to do their very best work? The answer to this question is really quite simple: People strive to succeed—and excel—when they feel invested in the work they do.

One system that helps people feel invested in their work is peer-driven quality improvement (PDQI). PDQI in prehospital care means that the people responsible for improving the quality of care delivered in the field are the same people who deliver that care. PDQI works. It is based on fundamental assumptions about what makes people care about the work they do and what motivates them to strive for excellence. It gives them ownership and control.

Traditional QA Programs

Traditional prehospital quality assurance (QA) programs are structured to parallel the established medical hierarchy. Physicians, of course, are at the top of this hierarchy, followed by nurses and other medical professionals, including EMS personnel.

The problem with this type of "quality" program is the assumption that field providers are not competent or clinically sophisticated enough to devise performance standards and programs to monitor compliance with these standards; the people at the top of the hierarchy do it for them. In addition, there is the issue of the fox minding the chicken coop: Having field providers monitor other field providers, so the theory goes, could compromise the entire QA process. Therefore, the monitoring part of EMS field provider QA programs has been left to doctors and nurses.

Programs that use a hierarchical approach to QA tend to focus on the outcomes of EMS provider practice and measure competencies based on these outcomes. These programs, therefore, enforce minimum standards by "error trapping" (solving mistakes as they arise) rather than by adopting a proactive, educational approach to ensuring continual quality field care.

For these and other reasons, traditional QA programs have often lacked credibility among field staff. EMS field personnel are constantly required to make decisions influenced by constraints that rarely exist in clinical settings, such as hazardous scenes or a lack of adequate working space and lighting. It's understandable, then, that field providers have a certain amount of anxiety about being evaluated and monitored by people who potentially don't understand these constraints.

At the same time, a growing number of field providers see themselves as medical professionals. Many are now EMS managers and educators who design EMS systems, formulate EMS policies, and train future EMS colleagues. This professionalization has led many EMS providers to ask why someone else judges their daily field performance when they themselves possess the critical balance of clinical sophistication, system know-how, and street sense that arguably makes them best suited for the job.

Recognizing that field providers are medical professionals and that they know their own jobs better than anybody else possibly could, American Medical Response (AMR) West, located in central California's Santa Clara County, has abandoned the traditional QA program in favor of the PDQI process. AMR West's paramedic division is creating a dynamic process in which field providers create their own standards for field practice. They monitor each other's field work and provide feedback to educate their co-workers. This way, the providers themselves can affirm that the best practice models are actually being realized in the field.

PDQI Overview

AMR West's field personnel are empowered to make judgments that could have serious consequences for their patients. Yet with empowerment comes accountability, which is best managed through a peer process. The point of PDQI is to facilitate this process by involving field providers in all elements of the program.

Herein lies the greatest benefit of PDQI. Field staff set performance standards, monitor performance, and train their peers. These duties make them responsible for their own system—and this responsibility has a host of ripple effects: It reduces the burnout associated with powerlessness; it actively engages field providers in improving the overall quality of care their service delivers; and, most importantly, ownership of the system by all field staff brings new voices and fresh ideas to the QI process.

As with all such programs, there is a system of checks and balances. For instance, all aspects of the program are subject to medical director approval and audit. Yet the medical director's confidence in field personnel, which has been generated by the PDQI program, has enabled him to expand the providers' scope of practice and increase their autonomy from direct base station control.

PDQI Doesn't Spank

Traditional QA programs often adopt a "no news is good news—spank 'em if they screw up" attitude. If customers don't complain, it is assumed that quality has been ensured. If they do complain, the offending providers are sought out and reprimanded. While these reprimands might be cloaked in the guise of "re-education," they tend to have a punitive feel. In fact, personnel who make it through re-education are said to have been "QA'd," an adult form of spanking.

To avoid this punitive function, the QI department is not part of AMR West operations. Instead, QI personnel report directly to the vice president of ALS operations as a completely independent department. The QI division has no disciplinary power whatsoever and makes no person-

> The greatest benefit of PDQI: Field staff set performance standards, monitor performance, and train their peers.

Creating clear
standards for field
care practice
provides employees
with a benchmark
for gauging their
performance.

nel decisions regarding hiring and firing. To complete the metaphor, it doesn't have the ability to "spank" personnel.

These departmental divisions are drawn quite clearly since the entire focus of the QI department is educational, not punitive. The purpose is to eliminate fear-motivated changes in behavior, which occur only to avoid painful consequences rather than through a person's desire to improve.

The philosophy of AMR West's QI department is that performance issues are training issues until proven otherwise. The department believes that people want to excel at their work. The department's goal is to use several strategies—meetings, independent research, and clinical and field remediation—to help paramedics do just that.

It All Starts With Standards

One of the most prevalent problems associated with monitoring field performance is the lack of clear expectations. Employees cannot be held accountable for performance expectations that are vague or nonexistent.

Creating clear standards for field care practice provides employees with a benchmark for gauging their performance. Medical protocols outline the medical treatment algorithms for specific medical and traumatic emergencies, while field performance standards define generic performance expectations in areas such as call management, patient assessment, and patient treatment.

Working within the peer theory, a group of experienced paramedics called field training officers (FTOs) drafted the AMR West performance standards for field paramedics and paramedic interns, which were based on the medical protocols the medical director drafted. The resulting standards are quite rigorous, but because they were written by paramedics, the field staff feels invested in seeing that they are met. The paramedics are held accountable for maintaining their standards.

These standards are flexible, however, to account for the situational constraints that affect most calls. They also focus on processes rather than outcomes. For example, the performance standard for IV starts specifies that the paramedic identify when it is or is not appropriate to start an IV depending on patient acuity, ETA to the emergency department, patient compliance, etc. If the paramedic determines that an IV is indeed appropriate, he must choose the correct vein and catheter and IV set size, ensure sterile conditions, and use the correct cannulation technique. Although important, successful placement of the catheter on any particular attempt is a secondary issue.

An Evolutionary Process

The people who write and implement the programs and standards also must live by them. Indeed, a poor fit between QI-derived standards and actual field staff needs becomes readily apparent, and when performance standards or programs don't fulfill their purpose, they are changed.

For example, AMR West's FTO position has changed significantly during the past four and a half years. Initially, a core group of FTOs set performance standards and developed core programs, such as the chart audit, in which paramedics review charts to see that documentation meets prescribed standards. They also developed new employee field orientation programs.

With these goals accomplished, there was no need for such a centralized group of core FTOs. In addition, the FTO workload became too great, and AMR West wanted to open various training and auditing positions to other field staff. The resulting model now consists of a small group of QI specialists who design and oversee programs and a larger group of training officers who implement the programs and conduct training in both the classroom and field.

Taking a Look Ahead

Prospective QI at AMR West prepares people to work in the field with such programs as field internships, employee hiring, and new employee orientation. For example, having paramedics on the employee hiring panel ensures that candidates have the experience necessary to work in the field before they are hired.

Field paramedics interview all job applicants and then ask themselves questions: Would I want to work with this person? Is this provider safe and competent? The pragmatic self-interest the field staff brings to the hiring process is a powerful way to ensure quality at the front end.

AMR West's internship program is guided by intern performance standards drafted by paramedic preceptors and directed by an experienced paramedic who serves as education coordinator. (All preceptors complete a preceptor training course designed by a co-worker.) Field preceptors manage the internships, select interns, and make recommendations regarding internship completion, extensions, and failures. With such peer involvement, internship failures have decreased by more than 35 percent. It seems ownership of the program has also empowered paramedics to substantially affect the future quality of their EMS system.

New employee orientation also uses a peer-driven approach. Subjects such as patient care report documentation, spinal immobilization, and driver safety are taught by paramedics. In fact, training programs throughout the ALS division are conducted almost exclusively by paramedics. During the past two years, paramedics have trained the entire paramedic field staff in PALS, PHTLS, spinal immobilization methods, and medical protocols and procedures. These courses are designed to elevate the standard of care throughout the system.

The benefits of peer-driven training are numerous. Training concerns are couched in language that other paramedics understand. Courses that may not have strict prehospital application, such as PALS, can be tailored to deal specifically with the constraints of field practice. And instructors can monitor the effectiveness of their courses as they work daily with their trainees.

Praise Where It's Due

Newly hired paramedics are placed in the field with an experienced training officer. The training officer serves as a guide through an extensive field orientation program that includes check-off sheets covering everything from correct use of the LifePak 10 to cleanup of the crew's quarters. Additionally, the paramedic trainer evaluates the new paramedics' field performance for several months.

AMR West's field coaching program makes up a large part of its PDQI process. Within this program, the field care coordinator—a certified paramedic—completes several ride-alongs with field paramedics in the county. The strategy of the program is to coach rather than grade. Using the paramedic field performance standards, the field care coordinator gives paramedics immediate feedback about their performance on calls. Strengths are acknowledged, while problems with field practice are articulated and worked through using the standard in question.

The field care coordinator also enters individual call evaluations into a database. While the subjective component—comparing witnessed field performance to the standards—is never entirely lost, this database shows individual and system-wide performance trends by numerically comparing both to the performance standards. This information is used to verify competency and identify individual and system-wide training needs.

A run of 1,200 call evaluations has shown that, overall, system performance is meeting performance standards at AMR West. A sample of new paramedics scored below standard in 12 percent of the performance categories. Consequently, the program has been modified to provide intensive coaching for new paramedics.

A Look Back at Performance

In addition to the database element of the field coaching program, the Paramedics Advancing Care Excellence (PACE) program at AMR West provides a glance back at field performance. It calls for field paramedics to rotate into the office to review all patient care reports (PCRs) according to charting standards developed by paramedics and approved by AMR West's medical director. After auditing the PCRs using these standards, the PACE auditor offers paramedics positive feedback and suggestions for improving their charting.

During the past three years, AMR West's paramedics have improved from filling in 70 percent of all the blanks on a PCR to filling in more than 96 percent. This indicates that clear standards have led to more organized and complete PCRs. The PACE program is now focusing on protocol compliance, the quality of report narratives, and overall patient care standards.

Additional components of retrospective PDQI are call and incident reviews. Conducted by the director of the QI department, this program seeks to resolve complaints and concerns voiced by patients, base hospitals, first responders, regulatory agencies, and other field providers. Again, the focus here is an educational one; an analysis of complaints from October 1989 to November 1992 shows that more than 97 percent of all complaints required customer or provider education rather than disciplinary action.

PDQI Challenges

Committing to a peer-driven approach to ensure competent field practice is not without its difficulties. At first, field staff expressed reticence about taking constructive feedback from peers, saying, "What right do you have to tell me how to run a call or fill out a run form or resolve conflicts with a local fire department crew?" Yet once people realized their co-workers were giving them feedback to improve their field practice rather than to establish a hierarchy or gain power, they accepted it more freely.

Another difficulty for some providers was believing that the information being gathered about their performance would not be used against them. This thinking reflects past experiences with more hierarchical, punitive approaches to ensuring quality field care. While this will probably always be a concern, paramedics have learned to trust that the programs are designed to help improve field practice, not punish people.

PDQI is also time intensive. Like the democratization of any hierarchical organization, it can be inefficient and slow in the beginning as people learn their jobs. This can be exacerbated by management, which has a tendency to hold onto decision making for the sake of efficiency and centralization of control.

Finally, PDQI must contend with those people in the medical community who believe field providers do not have the competency to monitor performance. The irony here is that the medical community has long depended on peer review as a method of ensuring quality medical care delivery.

Conclusion

PDQI works. It is a viable alternative to traditional top-down QA programs. By involving field providers in the monitoring of their own performance, PDQI fosters pride, commitment, and empowerment among field staff. Personnel are encouraged to see the performances of their peers as their responsibility.

PDQI programs have credibility because they are designed and implemented by the people doing the job. They diminish the always deadly "us versus them" perspective fostered by a workforce consisting of two camps: those who do the job and those who sit behind desks and "armchair" their performance.

Once people realized their co-workers were giving them feedback to improve their field practice rather than to establish a hierarchy or gain power, they accepted it more freely.

Source

Reprinted with permission from JEMS, *June 1994. Martha Libby, BS, EMT-P, is the director of quality improvement and education for American Medical Response (AMR) West in California's Santa Cruz and Santa Clara counties. Scott Vahradian, BA, EMT-P, is the field care coordinator for AMR West in those same counties.*

PDQI programs empower field staff by teaching them skills to further their professional growth long after they have decided to stop working the streets. Giving feedback, maintaining objectivity, and performing in front of and teaching one's peer group can test one's subject knowledge and classroom management skills. PDQI programs also encourage organizational skills, computer and writing skills, and statistical and research skills.

PDQI creates a "win-win-win" situation for all involved in EMS. Field providers win because they experience empowerment, better self-esteem, and professional recognition and growth. The agency wins because its providers are happier and more motivated to do good work. And finally, patients win because they receive care that is competent and caring.

What EMS Research Can Mean to an Organization

Research Lessons from the Past: A Guide for the Future

Elizabeth A. Criss

In recent years, the importance of clinical and operational research in EMS has become quite clear. New methods and techniques must be adapted to meet the challenges of the future. In this thought-provoking article, the author outlines how to develop an EMS research project and how to share your findings.

THE TWENTIETH ANNIVERSARY of the landmark Emergency Medical Services Systems Act of 1973 has come and gone. Although we have grown in size, we still lack meaningful data that demonstrate the effects of EMS on out-of-hospital illness and injury. In the mid-1970s, cardiac care moved from the hospital to the street and demonstrated an impact on sudden cardiac arrest. But it was not until 1991 that a standardized data set related to cardiac arrest was established so that out-of-hospital cardiac care could be uniformly evaluated and the outcomes could be compared. Analogous information exists for no other type of injury or illness, making system comparison difficult, if not impossible.

Dr. Ron Stewart, one of the first and foremost researchers in EMS, stated in 1983 that the time had come for our "initiative and innovative spirit" to solve the problems of EMS. "If our methods and techniques are not changed to conform to what is medically needed, EMS as we know it will fast fade from the medical scene." More than 10 years have passed since Dr. Stewart made this statement, and we are still no closer to answering the important questions related to system design, the effectiveness of trauma care, or the impact of advanced life support in urban, suburban, or rural environments.

To answer these and other important questions about EMS, we need more than our personal experiences; we need to develop factual data. Therefore, we must become active participants in the research process. We have learned a great deal during the past 20 years, but we have a great deal more to learn.

This article provides an introduction to the steps in the research process. The intent is to develop an understanding of the importance of research and the need to incorporate it into all aspects of EMS, including the evaluation of protocols, medications, procedures, and equipment. To assist in understanding the research process, examples from current lit-

Research should be thought of as an organized method of examining or evaluating a topic. It is a set of systematic steps, designed to lead to a well-defined outcome.

erature will be included. We will conclude with a look at the future of EMS and EMS research, examining the changes that will be required in the coming decade.

Idea Formation

Research should be thought of as an organized method of examining or evaluating a topic. It is a set of systematic steps, designed to lead to a well-defined outcome. A standardized format is used to provide meaningful information at the conclusion of the evaluation. A worthwhile project need not be complicated or involve a complex design. Often the most interesting and unique ideas for research come from field personnel asking that ever-present question: "Why?"

The first step in the process is to identify a topic or question for evaluation. The idea should be something that will provide important information for use in decision making or provide program justification. Ideas can be generated from any aspect of EMS. They need not be strictly related to patient care issues. For example, in 1989, Valenzuela, et al., published research on the thermal stability of ALS medications in the desert heat. The idea for this topic was generated by numerous questions from paramedics regarding the apparent ineffectiveness of certain medications. The study results demonstrated that most ALS medications could tolerate the extreme temperatures of the Arizona summer. This topic does relate to patient care, but it also answers an important system issue related to medication storage.

Once a possible topic has been determined, discuss the idea with a variety of people, including your medical director or another established researcher. Their input may prove valuable in refining or focusing the idea into a more manageable project. Sharing an idea is a very important step in the development of a research project. Without obtaining some outside input, the idea may not be clearly focused or stated, resulting in little or no usable data. Idea sharing may also assist in determining the general interest of others in participating in the potential project.

The next step is to formulate a hypothesis. The hypothesis is a statement or estimate, based on your knowledge of the expected outcome of the research. Spaite, et al., in "A Prospective Evaluation of the Impact of Initial Glasgow Coma Score on Prehospital Treatment and Transport of Seizure Patients" defined the hypothesis clearly in the abstract. They stated, "The initial Glasgow Coma Score (GCS) obtained by prehospital personnel on seizure victims is associated with the likelihood of treatment and transport." This hypothesis is based solely on the clinical judgment of the researcher and serves to focus and direct the remainder of the study.

For the project to be successful, the resources for evaluating the topic and subsequent hypothesis must be available within your system or agency. In the preceding example, Dr. Spaite knew that the local EMS system evaluated approximately 1,200 seizure patients per year and recorded a GCS on each patient. Therefore, the resources to evaluate the hypothesis did exist. If the types of patients needed for the study are limited, you might re-evaluate the idea or consider joining forces with another agency or system that is similar. This will provide you with additional patients and additional assistance with data collection.

It is important to discuss the hypothesis with the medical director or other experienced researchers. Their continued input, especially early in the research phase, can prove valuable in developing a well-focused research project.

Literature Review

Once the idea has been formulated and a hypothesis established, it is important to evaluate the current literature related to the selected topic. This can be accomplished in several ways. The most common method is the computerized literature search. Library services found at a university, medical school, or public library can be very helpful in the development of this computerized search. The librarians at these facilities can assist you in determining the appropriate subject headings for the search and the best type of search to be done. These searches may cost a few dollars unless the libraries have personal computer-based systems that allow individual access free of charge.

Reference sections from review articles in the subject area can be another method for obtaining articles pertinent to the research. This is a little more time-consuming than a computerized literature search but can provide valuable resources if access to a large library is limited. Articles cited in these review papers can also be helpful in setting up the computerized literature search. Having specific citations will assist you and the librarian in determining search parameters.

It is important that an attempt be made to obtain and read all the articles pertinent to the subject area before moving on in the design of the project. This will provide a strong foundation for project design and implementation.

Information from the literature review can also assist in refining and focusing the question and hypothesis. Examples from similar projects can provide useful guidelines for new researchers. Research is not always original; it's often a process of validating another individual's work. It is acceptable to use aspects of other research projects that have proved useful. If the science of emergency medicine is to advance, learning must result from mistakes and progress from successes. Re-evaluation of a similar topic does not make it an unacceptable project. The uniqueness of each EMS system provides the variation that can offer valuable new information. Validating research on a specific topic contributes to the growth and understanding of EMS.

Research Design

Begin the design phase of the project once the literature review is

> Research is not always original; it's often a process of validating another individual's work.

completed. If a research mentor has not already been located, it is recommended that one be identified and utilized for the remainder of the research process. Since very few projects can be developed with only a single variable to evaluate, inclusion of a statistician or experienced researcher increases the likelihood of a worthwhile project.

There are several components to the research design phase. They include defining the type and format of the project, developing inclusion and exclusion criteria for the population, determining sample size, and obtaining appropriate approvals. This phase is the essence of the project, and careful attention should be paid to each component. This careful scrutiny will result in a more organized research project.

Project Type and Format

There are basically four types of research projects. Each has a different application to EMS research, and each has its own unique characteristics. The topic selected for evaluation will assist in determining which type of study is most appropriate.

Epidemiological. These studies identify trends found within a particular environment. This type of project lends itself well to topics related to system utilization and determining educational needs. In "A Prospective Analysis of Injury Severity Among Helmeted and Non-Helmeted Bicyclists Involved in Collisions with Motor Vehicles," Spaite, et al., identified characteristics that were specific to each patient population and the resulting injury patterns. Information from this project is used to assist in citizen education programs.

Historical. Historical studies relate patient presentation and treatment to outcome. These studies lend themselves to quality improvement issues. To determine if standing orders could decrease scene time, Gratton, et al., reviewed 197 trauma cases. Findings did not support the original hypothesis but did outline areas for further study.

Feasibility. Typically, these are short-term studies with a purpose of gathering preliminary information on new treatment possibilities or equipment. Information from a feasibility study is often used to prepare a grant or develop a proposal for continuing study on the area of interest. New helicopters are added to EMS systems often without complete understanding of their potential impact. In "A New Model for Evaluating the Impact of Major System Changes on Emergency Air Medical Scene Responses in a Regional EMS System," Spaite, et al., posed a model, based on retrospective data, that could assist in determining impact. This is termed a feasibility study because it proposes a model but requires further studies for validation.

Clinical. These projects introduce a new aspect or alter an existing aspect of care and evaluate the effects related to patient outcome. This type of study is important in the evaluation of protocols and new medications. Most of the changes in EMS in recent years are the result of clinical studies. McCabe, et al., in "Intravenous Adenosine in the Prehospital Treatment of

Paroxysmal Supraventricular Tachycardia," evaluated adenosine in the out-of-hospital environment. Although limited in size, the project was important to the expansion of hospital medications to the prehospital environment.

In addition to the four types of research projects, there are also two formats that must be considered: retrospective or prospective. Three of the four project types can be done in either format, while clinical studies are almost exclusively prospective.

Retrospective. Retrospective formats use data that have already been collected, usually medical records or prehospital run sheets. These projects are inexpensive and quick to complete, as the information is readily retrievable from existing sources. Research done in this format is, however, weak, and the conclusions are not transferable to other studies. Valenzuela, et al., used a historical type and a retrospective format to evaluate the effect of air transportation on critically ill patients. The project reviewed records on 118 patients transported by air and 50 similar patients transported by ground in an effort to support the hypothesis.

Prospective. Prospective studies involve the pre-establishment of inclusion criteria and the ongoing entry of patients into the project. Patients entered into the study are followed to a predetermined end point, usually discharge from the hospital. This format is more difficult, but the conclusions are more reliable and comparable to similar projects. The Spaite, et al., evaluation of helmeted versus non-helmeted bicyclists is an excellent example of the various aspects of a prospective evaluation. The patient population is clearly identified and followed through to discharge or death.

Criteria and Sample Size

When research projects are going to involve selecting a specific group of patients or people for evaluation, it is essential to develop inclusion and exclusion criteria. Inclusion criteria outline the specific characteristics that are required before a patient can be entered into the study. Conversely, exclusion criteria specify those patients who are not to be included in the project. For example, a study evaluating the effect of albuterol versus isoetharine in asthmatics might specify adults, history of asthma, decreased breath sounds with wheezing, and no sensitivity to either product. The exclusion criteria might include children, history of COPD, and hypertension. It is important to clearly define both types of criteria, especially if others will be involved in the data gathering. When developing these criteria, refer back to the literature for possible suggestions. Using similar patient populations will make the results of your research more comparable to existing research.

At this point, it is important to discuss sample size with the statistician or research mentor. Discuss the type and format for the study and the potential patient population. If possible, estimate the frequency of this type of patient over a one-year period of time. This will help determine the approximate length of the project.

There are several things to consider regarding the sample size. A

Any research project that involves human subjects must be reviewed by an Institutional Review Board (IRB).

sample size that is too small may not yield results that prove or disprove the hypothesis. Without an adequate number of patients, it may not be possible to determine if the event or intervention in question is random or truly a result of the study. A large sample will result in powerful conclusions; however, the more data needed for a project, the longer the project will continue. Continuing the project past a necessary limit exposes more patients to the study protocol, which may be an unnecessary risk. Utilizing the statistician will ensure that an adequate sample size is obtained and appropriate conclusions can be reached.

Project Approvals

Any research project that involves human subjects must be reviewed by an Institutional Review Board (IRB). These committees are established by hospitals and universities to review the validity of the research design as well as the ethics of a project. Even something as simple as chart review for a retrospective study should have the "stamp of approval" of the IRB. Your research mentor should be familiar with the submission process and can help obtain the appropriate approvals.

Some project designs necessitate the use of animals. Animals have been used in research for centuries, and the information gained from these experiments has been invaluable. Despite the possible gains for humankind, some individuals find animal use intolerable. Due to this persuasive faction, animal research is very controlled and carefully reviewed. If you are considering the use of an animal model, review your institution's policy for specific guidelines. These research projects are subject to a similar IRB review process.

Another source for project approval may be within the agency itself. Most agencies are aware of the need to participate in the research process but appreciate being included in the review of the project design. If the project involves alteration in patient treatment protocols, the agency may request that its risk management department review and approve the research proposal.

Data Collection

Collecting data for the project may prove to be the most difficult part of the process. Without it, there is no research process, and if done poorly, the study will fail to reach any reliable conclusions. This phase contains several components that require special attention. These include identification of the data to be collected, developing a data collection tool, and educating field personnel.

Data Identification

Begin the process of identifying what data to collect by reviewing the hypothesis and research design. After this review, generate a list of possible items that need to be collected for the data analysis. Review this list with the research mentor or statistician. Make sure that the list contains all pertinent information related to the topic, because once data collection begins, additional data points cannot be easily added.

Once the list is established, determine if a source is available for each item. For example, is information on incident location already recorded on the run sheet, or will an additional sheet be required? Another example may be use of restraint systems—is the information routinely recorded, or will separate documentation be needed? Once this process is complete, review the list again. For each of the data items that does not have a readily available source, determine what will be necessary to obtain the data. For example, if autopsy data is necessary to complete the project, it must be determined if that information is accessible. Another example may be outcome data from another hospital. These details must be anticipated in advance, otherwise the project could run into some significant problems.

Data Collection Tools

With the data items established and appropriately reviewed, it is time to develop the data collection tools. If field personnel are to be used in the data collection process, the tools must be "user friendly" and not interfere with patient care tasks. Developing tools that can be incorporated into normal routine will increase compliance with the project protocol. If additional information is required, be sure it is information that field personnel are likely to encounter while on the scene or completing tasks at the hospital. Keep in mind that missing or invalid data will prolong and possibly weaken the project.

During the development of the actual data collection form, request input from field personnel. Incorporate their ideas into the format. This will make them feel like a valuable part of the team and ensure that the form will conform to their needs. If possible, limit the information to be gathered by the field personnel to one page. This will assist in overall compliance.

Training

Education of the data collectors is vital to the successful completion of the research project. It may be helpful to develop a project protocol to assist in the education and training of the potential data collectors. This guideline should be designed to be used as both a training tool and a resource document during the data collection phase. The format of the protocol can be either a simple list or a flow chart outlining each step in the process. This type of resource document can be easily posted for future reference.

During the training phase, attempt to meet with each person who will be collecting data for the project. This individual attention will allow the collectors to gain insight into the development of the project. It will ensure that each person receives the same information regarding patient inclusion/exclusion criteria and use of the data collection form.

It is important that the results be examined only in the context of the system in which they were gathered.

Results

The results evaluation begins after the appropriate number of patients have been documented and all the data have been entered into a database for analysis. It is time to return to the research mentor and statistician for guidance. Begin by reviewing the hypothesis again, this time in the context of the available data. Ideally, all the data points that were requested have been completed on all patients. In reality, this may not be the case. It is not uncommon that data points may be missing or not available for some project patients. If the amount of missing data for a certain question is significant, that data point may have to be discarded. This is why it is important to consult with a statistician before and after data collection.

Once the data have been reviewed, it is time to begin extracting results that prove or disprove the hypothesis. The type of tests that will be required will be determined by the statistician. Some general information, demographic or descriptive results about the population, can be done without the assistance of the statistician. These demographic or descriptive results can include the total number of participants, age ranges for the patients, frequency of each sex, or frequency of each type of injury or illness, if applicable. In Spaite's article comparing the injury severity scores between helmeted and non-helmeted bicyclists, the results section begins with demographic information related to the patient population. It states, "A total of 98 patients met study criteria. Sixty-six (67.3 percent) were male, and 32 (32.7 percent) were female. Mean age was 34 years with a range of four to 87 years." The next paragraph in this section reviews the mechanism of injury frequencies and ISS score distribution. All of these frequency distributions are very important to the discussion of the project. They require simple addition and calculation of percentages, yet they provide a strong base for discussing the impact of the project.

This type of analysis, in most cases, will not replace statistical testing; it is meant only as a supplement to describe the population. In most research projects, there are other types of data analyses that are required to determine the significance of the findings. These may include "t" tests, one-way analysis of variance, chi-square analysis, or Fisher's exact test. Because it is important to the validity of the findings, a statistician must be consulted to determine the correct tests. Statisticians can also be helpful in interpreting the results.

After all the data have been evaluated and the results of the demographic and statistical analyses have been assembled, the process of evaluating how it relates to the hypothesis begins. It is important that the results be examined only in the context of the system in which they were gathered. It is easy to want to extrapolate results to all other EMS systems, however, differences in protocols and field conditions make that type of assumption difficult. Extrapolation can be effective only if all the conditions between systems are matched very closely.

Information Sharing

Once the project has reached this point, the difficult part is over and congratulations are in order. Developing and implementing a research project is a rewarding experience. At this point, consideration should be given to how to prepare a written report on the project or a manuscript for possible publication. It is also important to be able to effectively read published research projects. Therefore, in this section, we will discuss aspects involved in communicating or extrapolating relevant information about a research project.

Research manuscripts usually follow an organized format, whether the findings are being reported to the company CEO or the National Association of EMS Physicians. To assist both the reader and the writer, manuscripts utilize the following headings: introduction, methods, results, and discussion. Each heading contains separate and useful information.

Introduction. This section will contain information relevant to the problem and hypothesis used in the project. Some general background information is usually in this section as a means of introducing the problem area.

Methods. The methods section discusses the type and format of the project. It should include inclusion and exclusion criteria, sample size, specific data collection tools, and statistical methodology. The purpose of this section is to relay the specific aspects of how the project was designed and implemented.

Results. This section often begins with demographic data on the patient population, followed by the statistical findings. It is important that this section include only results and leave the conclusions to the discussion section. Readers will often find graphs and charts helpful resources for this section. Reading a lot of numbers can be confusing.

Discussion. The reader should find a brief restatement of the hypothesis at the beginning of this section. The hypothesis is often followed by more background information as it applies to the hypothesis or findings. At this point, the reader should find an individual review of the results and their impact on the agency or system. Some writers find it helpful to include a discussion of limitations of the study, i.e., format, data collection, compliance with protocol, etc. This can provide useful information for other researchers.

Whether you are writing or reading, it is important to understand what information is contained in each section. Keep in mind that research manuscripts are not novels. Each section should be clear, concise, and contain only relevant material. Readers should be able to move quickly through each organized section.

The Future

EMS, as Dr. Stewart pointed out 10 years ago, must undergo some changes if it is to stay current and flexible. The future of EMS research will focus on the entire system, incorporating both clinical and operational aspects into the research process. This type of systems-based research will develop more fiscally responsible organizations with state-of-the-art patient care capabilities.

Continued emphasis will be placed on outcome studies that will determine the impact of EMS on patient care. Outcome-based research to date has been limited. The best example is the trauma literature and the concern over scene time in trauma patients. The literature is replete with discussions debating "stay and play" versus "scoop and run" in the trauma patient. The debate centers on the use of ALS procedures at the scene and the resulting increase in on-scene times. In outcome-based systems research, the focus is broadened to determine where the delays occur and how the delays relate to the final patient outcome. Currently, there are a limited number of systems-based research projects, but the results of the projects are interesting and enlightening.

During the past 20 years, the scope of practice has broadened far beyond care of the cardiac patient. Today, the scope of paramedic practice ranges from cardiac to trauma to pediatric to neonatal—but where does it make the most difference? What types of patients and care will the future paramedic provide? These questions have yet to be asked and the research design for answering them has yet to be validated. Nevertheless, these are the exciting issues facing EMS and the EMS researcher of the future.

Conclusion

Dr. Stewart summed up the point of research best when he said, "We can never hope to be respected by peers or others in other specialties if we do not base what we do on sound scientific findings." This is why research is necessary and why involvement at all organizational levels is critical to establishing a sound basis for why EMS exists and should continue to exist in the future.

None of us will ever win the Nobel prize for our research, but patient care and the operations of our systems will be strengthened and the future of EMS will be well served by our efforts. For some, this process will come easily and for others it may take longer—but don't get discouraged. Enjoy it.

References

Aprahamian, C., B. Thomson, J. Taune, et al. "The Effect of a Paramedic System on Mortality of Major Open Intra-Abdominal Vascular Trauma." *Journal of Trauma* 23 (1983): 68.

Brill, J., and J. Greiderman. "A Rationale for Scoop and Run: Identifying a Subset of Time-Critical Patients." *Topics in Emergency Medicine* 3 (1981): 37.

Cummins, R. O., D. A. Chamberlain, N. S. Abramson, M. Allen, et al. "Recommended Guidelines for Uniform Reporting of Data from Out-of-Hospital Cardiac Arrest: The Utstein Style." *Annals of Emergency Medicine* 20 (August 1991): 861-874.

Emergency Medical Services System Act of 1973. P.L. 93-154.

Gratton, M. C., R. A. Bethke, W. A. Watson, and G. M. Gaddis. "Effect of Standing Orders on Paramedic Scene Time for Trauma Patients." *Annals of Emergency Medicine* 20 (December 1991): 1306-1309.

Jacobs, L., A. Sinclair, A. Beiser, et al. "Prehospital Advanced Life Support Benefits in Trauma." *Journal of Trauma* 24 (1984): 8.

McCabe, J. L., G. C. Adhar, J. J. Menegazzi, and P. M. Paris. "Intravenous Adenosine in the Prehospital Treatment of Paroxysmal Supraventricular Tachycardia." *Annals of Emergency Medicine* 21 (1992): 358-363.

Smith, J. P., B. I. Bodai, and A. S. Hill. "Prehospital Stabilization of Critically Injured Patients: A Failed Concept." *Journal of Trauma* 23 (1983): 317.

Spaite, D. W., M. Murphy, E. A. Criss, T. D. Valenzuela, and H. W. Meislin. "A Prospective Analysis of Injury Severity Among Helmeted and Non-Helmeted Bicyclists Involved in Collisions with Motor Vehicles." *Journal of Trauma* 31 (1991): 1510-1516.

Spaite, D. W., T. Brophy, T. D. Valenzuela, H. W. Meislin, et al. "A New Model for Evaluating the Impact of Major System Changes on Emergency Air Medical Scene Responses in a Regional EMS System." *Prehospital and Disaster Medicine* 7 (1992): 19-23.

Spaite, D. W., T. D. Valenzuela, H. W. Meislin, E. A. Criss, and J. Ross. "A Prospective Evaluation of the Impact of Initial Glasgow Coma Score on Prehospital Treatment and Transport of Seizure Patients." *Prehospital and Disaster Medicine* 7 (April-June 1992): 127-132.

Stapczynski, J. S., and P. M. Paris. "Conducting Prehospital Research." In *Principles of EMS Systems: A Comprehensive Text for Physicians,* ed. W. R. Roush, 201-211. Dallas: ACEP, 1990.

Stewart, R. D. "Is the Honeymoon Over?" *JEMS* (1983): 32-34.

Stewart, R. D., J. Dernocoeur, and E. A. Criss. "The Nuts and Bolts of Prehospital Care Research: Designing for Success." Paper presented at the Ninth Annual EMS Today Conference, 1991.

Valenzuela, R. D., E. A. Criss, M. K. Copass, G. K. Luna, and C. L. Rice. "Critical Care Air Transportation of the Severely Injured: Does Long Distance Transport Adversely Affect Survival?" *Annals of Emergency Medicine* 19 (1990): 169-172.

Valenzuela, T. D., E. A. Criss, W. M. Hammargren, K. H. Schram, et al. "Thermal Stability of Prehospital Medications." *Annals of Emergency Medicine* 18 (February 1989): 173-176.

Source

Reprinted with permission from the Research Evaluation, February 1993. Elizabeth A. Criss is an EMS consultant and senior researcher at the University of Arizona in Tucson.

Cardiac Arrest and Resuscitation: A Tale of 29 Cities

Mickey S. Eisenberg, MD, PhD; Bruce T. Horwood, MD; Richard O. Cummins, MD, MPH, MSc; Robin Reynolds-Haertle, MS; and Thomas R. Hearne, PhD

This landmark article is considered an EMS research classic. EMS researcher Dr. Mickey Eisenberg and his team review clinical studies published between 1967 and 1988, comparing the types of EMS systems and the factors that improve cardiac arrest outcomes.

MORE THAN TWO DECADES have passed since Pantridge introduced the mobile intensive care unit (MICU) in Belfast, Ireland. Since then, prehospital emergency care programs have spread rapidly throughout the world. But published survival rates for out-of-hospital cardiac arrest vary widely.

Ten years ago, we reviewed the scientific literature for articles that described the success of paramedic systems in resuscitating patients with cardiac arrest. In the past 10 years, additional types of emergency systems have developed. The published experiences of 29 communities with out-of-hospital cardiac arrest are described in this article. From this review, five types of EMS systems are defined and their success rates compared. The way characteristics of a particular system may explain differences in survival rates is also indicated.

Methods

Peer-reviewed articles published between January 1967 and December 1988 that reported survival rates for patients with out-of-hospital cardiac arrest were selected for review. Thirty-four articles selected for evaluation met two criteria. First, they reported outcome data on a minimum of 100 cases. Second, they provided enough information to characterize the prehospital system.

All published studies could be classified into one of five types of EMS systems:

- Basic EMT—ambulance or response unit staffed with personnel trained in basic cardiac life support (BCLS)
- EMT-defibrillation (EMT-D)—basic EMTs also trained in the use of defibrillators
- Paramedic—personnel trained in advanced cardiac life support (ACLS) and able to provide definitive care (defibrillation, medication, endotracheal intubation)
- Basic EMT/paramedic—a double-response system with the first responder unit being a basic EMT unit and the second responder unit being a paramedic unit
- EMT-D/paramedic—a double-response system with the first responder unit being an EMT-D unit and the second responder unit being a paramedic unit

Units primarily staffed with paramedics but assisted by a physician or nurse were placed under the paramedic classification. Systems with prehospital emergency care units staffed by only physicians or nurses were excluded.

Often several reports provided information about the same EMS system. To have a single set of information and to prevent double counting, the study that reported the largest number of cases was, in general, chosen. There were several exceptions to this criterion. Data from one community were updated with unpublished data (personal communications used with permission, A. J. Gray and A. D. Redmond, Stockport, England) that represented a more fully implemented system. In one instance, two articles that reported data over different times were combined to give a more accurate representation of that type of system. For King County, Wash., unpublished data describing experiences with EMT-D/ paramedic services for the years 1982 through 1987 were added to previously published data for the years 1979 through 1982. Some community reports were of more than one type of system.

In addition to information about the type of system and survival rates, data were also recorded, when available, on average age, percent male, percent cardiac arrest witnessed, average EMT response time, average paramedic response time, percent bystander CPR, and percentage of patients found in ventricular fibrillation (VF). Summary discharge rates were calculated for each of the five systems.

Results

Thirty-four articles on 39 EMS programs in 29 communities met the study criteria. Seven communities reported experiences with two or more systems. The 29 locations were dispersed throughout eight countries: Australia, Canada, England, Iceland, Israel, New Zealand, Sweden, and the United States. The settings varied from rural to urban.

Information gathered on the 39 programs is summarized in Table 4.2. There were eight basic EMT programs, five EMT-D programs, 14 paramedic programs, 10 basic EMT/paramedic programs, and two EMT-D/ paramedic programs.

Variations occurred in case definitions and other variables. Fourteen EMS programs used cardiac arrest due to cardiac etiology as the case definition, eight reported all etiologies, three reported only ischemic heart disease cases, four excluded trauma cases, and two excluded cases with trauma and previous treatment by physicians before EMS personnel arrival. The remaining eight programs did not provide a definition.

In 13 programs, emergency personnel were allowed to withhold treatment where resuscitation was considered impossible, but the criteria for "impossible resuscitation" were not defined. In the remaining programs, either the emergency personnel were required to treat all patients in cardiac arrest or information on this issue was not provided.

Twenty-one locations reported the percentage of cases receiving bystander CPR before the arrival of an EMT or paramedic unit. The range for the percentage of patients receiving bystander CPR was eight to 55 percent. When reporting bystander CPR, the majority of programs reported

Table 4.2

Patient Characteristics and Survival from Out-of-Hospital Cardiac Arrest

Type of EMS System and Location	No. of Attempted Resuscitations	Average Age (yr)	Percent Male Patients	Percent Witnessed	Average EMT Response Time in Minutes	Average Paramedic Response Time in Minutes	Percent With Bystander CPR	No. in All Rhythms Discharged (%)	No. in VF (%)	No. in VF Discharged (%)
Basic EMT*										
Durham	126			47†	6.5		35†	11 (9)	61 (48)†‡	7 (11)†
Goteborg	189			100				3 (2)†	23 (12)	
Iowa	52	64	69	73	7		31	1 (2)	31 (60)	1 (3)
King County	323	64†	68†	51†	4.3†		19†	19 (6)†	147 (57)†	18 (12)†
Minnesota	118		79†	100			37†	3 (3)		
Reykjavik	222	63	75†		7.3			21 (9)	90 (41)†	18 (20)
Vancouver	110						16†	6 (6)†		
Winnipeg	849							33 (4)	226 (27)‡	24 (11)
EMT-D*										
Iowa	110	68	75	70	5.7		20	12 (11)	64 (58)	12 (19)
King County	54	62	89	79	4.3		22	10 (19)	38 (70)	10 (26)
Minnesota	100	70	73†	70	10 (84%)		50†	6 (6)	51 (51)	6 (12)
Stockholm	307							11 (4)†	144 (47)†‡	9 (6)†
Stockport	103							15 (15)	70 (68)	15 (21)
Paramedic										
Auckland	405		75				55	72 (18)†		
Brighton	356							39 (11)		
Charleston	100	56	72†			7	19	7 (7)		
Cincinnati	147		74†					22 (15)		
Israel	2,995	68	71	82	6		8	210 (7)	839 (28)	126 (15)
Los Angeles	300	65	68	41	5		35†	30 (10)	135 (45)	19 (14)
Lucas/Kent	2,171					4.7		169 (8)		
Miami	301	63	75			4 (80%)			301 (100)	42 (14)†
Minnesota	46		80†	100			48†	5 (11)	26 (57)	5 (19)
N. Westminster	227							21 (9)†	116 (51)†	15 (13)†
Oregon	210							38 (18)†		
Pittsburgh	187	68†				6	19†	18 (10)†	98 (52)†‡	15 (15)
Tampa	296	58				5 (87%)			296 (100)	68 (23)
Torrance	120		82†			4 (70%)		16 (13)	50 (42)†	15 (30)†
EMT/Paramedic										
Columbus	129				3	5		32 (25)		
Durham	168				6.5§	8.7		7 (4)		
Goteborg	176					5		19 (11)	87 (49)†	
King County	1,297	65†	78†	100	4.4	9.1†	45†	344 (26)†	947 (73)†	312 (33)
Milwaukee	1,905			100	2	5	31†	303 (16)	779 (52)◊†	183 (23)
Minneapolis	514							83 (16)		
New S. Wales	434			55†			30	91 (21)	369 (85)	81 (22)
Seattle	725			67	3	6.5§	40		725 (100)	181 (25)
Vancouver	244						12†	28 (11)†		. . . (24)
York Adams	1,066	67	69	79				68 (6)†	454 (43)†	51 (11)†
EMT-D/ Paramedic										
Seattle	687	65	81	79	3.6	8.8	36	98 (14)†	276 (40)	83 (30)
King County	4,068	66	75	55	4.2	10	54	741 (18)	2,117 (52)	615 (29)

* EMT, emergency medical technician; EMT-D, emergency medical technician-defibrillation
† Calculated from available data
‡ Includes VF and ventricular tachycardia
§ Estimated from available data
◊ Includes coarse VF only

CPR by non-professionals; however, in several locations, both professional and laypersons were included.

Eighteen locations reported the percentage of cardiac arrests that were witnessed. Five recorded witnessed events only, and 13 others reported witnessed and non-witnessed events. The percentage of patients with a witnessed arrest ranged from 41 to 82 percent.

The average EMT response time reported for 14 communities ranged from two to 7.3 minutes. The response time was defined in three communities as the interval from receipt of the call by the emergency dispatcher to the arrival of the emergency unit near the scene. Time of actual arrival of the personnel at the patient's side was not recorded. The average paramedic response time was reported in 16 programs and ranged from a minimum response time of four minutes (or less in 70 percent of the cases) to a maximum response time of 9.1 minutes.

Twenty-seven locations had information on the percentage of patients who initially were found to be in VF. In three instances, only patients in VF were reported. In 24 programs, the percentage of patients found in VF ranged from 12 to 85 percent. In reporting VF cases, four programs included ventricular tachycardia in the VF group and one reported coarse VF.

The percentage of patients resuscitated from cardiac arrest in all rhythms and discharged from the hospital alive is shown in Table 4.2. The eight basic EMT programs had a discharge rate varying from two to nine percent. Discharge ranged from four to 19 percent for the five EMT-D programs. In the 14 paramedic programs, the discharge percentage ranged from seven to 18 percent. The 10 basic EMT/paramedic programs recorded a range from four to 26 percent. The two EMT-D/paramedic programs reported discharge rates of 13 and 18 percent. The range of discharge rates for each type of system is shown in Figure 4.1.

Also included is a summary discharge rate calculated by weighting each system in proportion to the square root of the number of cases. The square root of the number of cases was selected as an adjustment factor to take into account the widely varying number of cases in each program as well as to reduce the effect of programs that reported large numbers on the

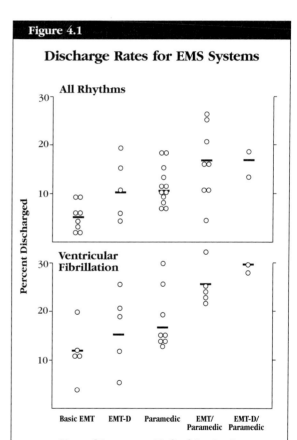

Figure 4.1

Discharge Rates for EMS Systems

Percentage discharged from out-of-hospital cardiac arrest in all rhythms (top panel) and ventricular fibrillation (bottom panel) from five EMS systems. Circles represent the percentage discharged from individual communities, and horizontal lines represent the weighted mean discharge rate.

summary rate. The summary discharge rates for the EMT, EMT-D, paramedic, EMT/paramedic, and EMT-D/paramedic systems for all cardiac arrests are five percent (95 percent confidence intervals, three to seven percent), 10 percent (six to 16 percent), 10 percent (nine to 13 percent), 16 percent (10 to 19 percent), and 17 percent (13 to 19 percent), respectively. Confining the analysis to the 26 U.S. locations reveals summary discharge rates of five percent, 11 percent, 16 percent, and 18 percent, respectively.

The percentage of patients discharged from the hospital alive who were initially found in VF is summarized in Table 4.2. In the five basic EMT programs that reported survival from VF, the percentage discharged ranged from three to 20 percent. In five EMT-D programs, the survival rates ranged from six to 26 percent. Of the eight paramedic programs reporting survival from VF, the range varied from 13 to 30 percent. The range for the six EMT/paramedic programs was 11 to 33 percent. In the two EMT-D/paramedic programs, the discharge rates were 29 and 30 percent.

The range of discharge rates for patients in VF in each system is also shown in Table 4.2. Adjusted discharge rates for VF for the five types of systems were calculated weighting each discharge rate based on the square root of the number of cases. The adjusted discharge rates for VF for the five systems were 12 percent (95 percent confidence intervals, six to 16 percent), 16 percent (10 to 23 percent), 17 percent (14 to 21 percent), 24 percent (17 to 27 percent), and 29 percent (29 to 30 percent). For U.S. locations, the discharge rates were 10 percent, 18 percent, 24 percent, and 29 percent, respectively.

Discussion

The survival rates for the 29 communities and 39 programs varied widely. Not only were there large differences among the five EMS systems, but there also were large variations within each system.

Previous Research

Previous research has demonstrated that shorter times from collapse to the start of CPR and from collapse to definitive care are associated with improved survival from cardiac arrest. To be effective, CPR must be initiated within four to six minutes of the time of collapse. We have suggested previously that early initiation of CPR prolongs the duration of VF and prevents the deterioration of coarse VF to fine VF. This increases the likelihood that VF will last longer and that the response to defibrillation will be positive. When CPR is delayed or the time to defibrillation is more than 10 to 12 minutes after the start of CPR, it is more likely the patient will be in fine VF and will convert to asystole.

Time to definitive care is also recognized as a major factor associated with survival from cardiac arrest. Most studies use the term definitive care to encapsulate all ACLS interventions, including defibrillation, IV medications, or intubation. In large part, such studies are impossible because it has become the standard of care for these advanced procedures to be used. Intubation allows better oxygenation, and administration of medications stabilizes electrical conduction and inhibits recurrence of VF. An awareness of the therapeutic interventions provides a basis for understanding differences in survival rates among systems.

Differences in Survival Among Systems

The variability in survival among the five EMS systems conceivably could be explained solely by differences in methodologies and inconsistencies in terminology and case definitions. These differences and their effects on survival rates are difficult to quantify but must be acknowledged as a partial explanation for the variance in survival rates. However, the upward trend in survival among the five EMS systems suggests that the type of system correlates with survival. As seen in Figure 4.1, a general improvement in survival occurs as the type of EMS system increases in sophistication with the largest increase occurring between single- and double-response systems.

Although such improvement was expected, what is the explanation? To answer this question, the specific therapies brought to a resuscitation must be considered: CPR, defibrillation, IV medications, and endotracheal intubation. The most obvious differences among the systems are the times required to provide these therapies because each system delivers different elements from this menu of interventions at different times. Conceptually, these therapeutic interventions can be considered to alter the survival curve after cardiac arrest. Most survival curves are defined in months or years; however, the survival curve for cardiac arrest is defined in minutes. It can be argued that the natural history of cardiac arrest without any intervention is biologic death within 10 minutes.

The cardiac arrest survival curves of the five EMS systems (Figure 4.2) are hypothetical models that display the effect of various therapeutic interventions on survival. They are a means to explain intersystem survival differences. The discharge rates of the models are

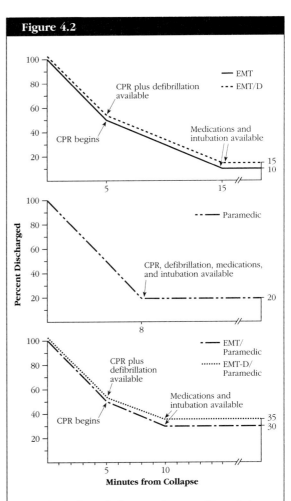

Figure 4.2

Hypothetical survival curves for out-of-hospital cardiac arrest treated by five types of EMS systems. Basic EMT and EMT-D services are depicted in the top panel, paramedic services in the middle panel, and EMT/paramedic and EMT-D/paramedic services in the bottom panel.

based on the adjusted observed discharge rates for the five systems.

The survival curves, while hypothetical, propose that the ability to resuscitate is a function of time, type, and sequence of therapy. The curves display a sequence of interventions occurring at different times: CPR, defibrillation, intubation, and medication. It is not self-evident, however, whether other sequences could result in higher survival rates. For example, would intubation performed by basic EMTs improve survival compared with an EMT/paramedic or an EMT-D/paramedic system? In a tiered-response system, is early intubation preferable to early defibrillation? The curves, while unable to provide an answer to these questions, suggest a theoretical framework to understand resuscitations in which sequentially applied interventions occur.

The Five Systems

Several assumptions are made in portraying survival curves for the five EMS systems. The probability of survival after cardiac arrest falls linearly with time and varies depending on the therapeutic intervention. The slope of the survival curve is steepest without any intervention; the probability of survival is zero after 10 minutes without CPR. In all systems, the survival curve starts at 100 percent, because, at the moment of collapse, there is a theoretical 100-percent chance of resuscitation. The slope of the survival curve improves after CPR and defibrillation and stabilizes after medication and intubation are provided (medication and intubation are considered simultaneous interventions).

The average interval from collapse to CPR is five minutes in systems with EMTs and EMT-Ds. The average interval to paramedic care is eight minutes in a single-response paramedic system and 10 minutes in a double-response system.

EMT System

The hypothetical survival curves and sequence of events during resuscitation in the five types of EMS systems are portrayed graphically in Figure 4.2. With each passing minute without CPR, the probability of survival falls steeply toward zero probability at 10 minutes. When CPR is initiated by the EMTs (at an average interval of five minutes), the survival curve improves. Survival probability continues to fall but at a slower rate. The ultimate result, however, is still poor because of the long time to reach the hospital, which is where definitive care can begin. The few lives that are saved are those in situations with rapid response times and short drives to the hospital.

EMT-D System

The EMT-D system demonstrates the benefit of early CPR combined with early defibrillation. The probability of survival initially falls, as in the EMT system (Figure 4.2). In an EMT-D system, however, CPR and defibrillation are brought to the patient simultaneously. The survival curve is shifted with a flatter slope than exists with CPR alone. The slope still continues downward because medications are not available at the scene and cannot be given until arrival at the hospital. Results from King County demonstrated the opportunity to save almost 20 percent of all patients with out-of-hospital cardiac arrest with an EMT-D system.

Paramedic System

Generally, paramedic systems have slower average response times than EMT systems. In EMT systems, vehicles are staffed with EMTs who often respond from local stations. A given geographic area will be covered by a relatively large number of stations. In King County, for example, EMT-Ds already trained as firefighters are located in 96 different fire stations. Such a system, layered on an existing fire suppression service, does not incur significant extra personnel costs. Paramedic systems use specially trained individuals who generally are not able to serve in a dual capacity. Because of these extra costs, the number of paramedic vehicles is less than the number found in an EMT system. Thus, a given geographic area will be covered by much fewer units. In King County, for example, eight paramedic stations cover the same area as the 96 fire stations.

In single-response paramedic systems, the interval from collapse to care is eight minutes on the average. CPR is administered later and defibrillation is delayed compared with EMT-D systems. While this should theoretically decrease the survival rates, they are, in fact, often equal to or better than those of EMT-D systems. This is most likely a result of the early medications and intubation that paramedics provide. The probability of survival in a paramedic system is depicted in Figure 4.2. Compared with basic EMT and EMT-D systems, the probability of survival initially falls more sharply (owing to the longer response time). However, once the paramedics arrive, all therapies (CPR, defibrillation, medication, and intubation) are available at the scene. Then, survival is stabilized.

It should be pointed out that these graphic representations are slightly deceptive. If a victim had no CPR for eight minutes, there would be little chance of survival. Average response times are displayed; individual times will be less than eight minutes 50 percent of the time. The low discharge rate of seven percent in Charleston, S.C., with a response time of seven minutes, emphasizes the importance of early CPR. On the other hand, Torrance, Calif., with a VF survival rate of 30 percent, demonstrates the potential for success when CPR and definitive care are provided early; 70 percent of the victims were reached within four minutes after the call for help.

EMT/Paramedic System

The basic EMT/paramedic system uses EMT units to provide early CPR, which helps delay rhythm deterioration until the paramedic unit can arrive to administer defibrillation and medications. In a basic EMT/paramedic system, initiation of CPR by the EMT unit increases the chance of survival compared with a system without EMT care. The probability of survival is twice that of a paramedic system (Figure 4.2). The probability of survival is stabilized when the paramedic unit arrives to deliver defibrillation, medication, and intubation. Survival from VF in EMT/paramedic systems consistently approaches 25 percent (one system reported a 33-percent survival rate).

EMT-D/Paramedic System

The best therapeutic situation is provided by an EMT-D/paramedic system. On arrival, a unit staffed with EMT-Ds can provide both CPR and defibrillation. When paramedics arrive several minutes later, medications, intubation, and additional defibrillation can be provided. The probability of survival initially is similar to that of an EMT-D system (Figure 4.2). However, because paramedics can provide the same therapy as a hospital, survival is stabilized at the arrival of paramedics. To date, very few studies have been done on this type of system. Information available from Seattle and King County demonstrates the potential benefit of this system. The discharge rates for VF patients were 29 percent for King County and 30 percent for Seattle.

Differences in Survival Within Systems

The above models may explain differences in survival among the five systems, but they do not explain the wide variation in discharge rates within each system. For example, survival within the basic EMT system for VF ranges from three to 20 percent.

There are several possible explanations for the wide intrasystem variations in discharge rates. One explanation may lie in physiologic variations among populations. It is conceivable that a patient with a cardiac arrest in Reykjavik, Iceland, is physiologically different and more easily resuscitated than a cardiac arrest patient in Los Angeles. While intriguing, this possibility cannot be measured easily.

A second explanation may lie in the quality of the program. A resuscitation is a complex, dynamic process with many interventions. Systematic problems or deficiencies in performing CPR, paddle placement in defibrillation, rhythm recognition, or sequence of medications could affect overall survival rates. It is possible that some communities have better EMS programs because of these quality factors. Quality, while undoubtedly important, is difficult to measure. Local pride may stimulate some locations to claim high-quality EMTs or paramedics. It is just as likely that all communities have some extremely competent and some less-than-competent personnel, suggesting that the quality factor may neutralize itself.

A third explanation may lie in the demographic and program characteristics of each community. Predictive scores relating the probability of discharge to characteristics such as age, witnessed collapse, percentage of patients in VF, and response time of emergency personnel demonstrate the importance of a variety of factors. Much intrasystem variation can be explained by variations in these factors. For example, a low resuscitation rate in Durham, N.C., may be explained by older patients, fewer witnessed arrests, less bystander CPR, and longer response times. Other explanations for variations in survival rates may be improved in-hospital care during the past decade or system differences in thresholds for initiation of CPR. There often is no clear demarcation between someone "dead on arrival" (DOA) and someone who potentially can be resuscitated. A system selecting a disproportionate number of DOAs will have a lower survival rate.

It is difficult to quantify the role of these demographic and program factors because few programs report such variables and variation exists in terminology. The term *response time*, for example, may involve all or some of the following: recognition time, decision-to-call time, calling time, dispatch interview time, dispatching time, time from station to arrival at scene, and time from scene to arrival at patient's side.

In addition, variations in definitions exist for such basic terms as cardiac arrest, bystander CPR, witnessed arrest, VF, and admission. Rather than this Babel of resuscitation terminology, there should be common definitions and a common format for reporting outcomes from out-of-hospital cardiac arrest. If most systems used a common reporting format, observed differences in survival rates would have more meaning. In addition, it would be possible to address issues such as quality assurance and optimal therapeutic interventions.

Quality assurance means that objective goals are set for an EMS system. The average success recorded for various system configurations is shown in Figure 4.1. By using such data, both national and international organizations can compare their program's cardiac arrest survival rate with that recorded for similarly configured programs. Major discrepancies can serve as a stimulus for refinement and reorganization.

Additional Determinants of Survival

The survival rates for the five types of EMS systems appear to reflect how rapidly and effectively the system can provide CPR, defibrillation, medication, and intubation. There are additional factors that affect the performance of an EMS system. One major determinant is bystander CPR before EMT or paramedic arrival. High rates of bystander CPR permit earlier initiation of CPR. Frequent bystander CPR can occur as a result of widespread CPR training or as a result of dispatcher-assisted telephone CPR programs.

A second factor is for defibrillation to occur before EMT or paramedic arrival. The use of automatic defibrillation by laypersons has the potential to bring defibrillation even quicker to the individual in cardiac arrest. Although these devices are not widespread at the moment, pilot projects have occurred for high-risk patients and in community locations such as airplanes, community centers, office buildings, senior centers, and fairgrounds.

Are Higher Survival Rates Possible?

Our presentation and discussion of each type of system have focused on the range of survival rates. It appears, however, that as one moves from the basic EMT system to the more advanced double-response systems, the survival rates plateau at approximately 25 to 30 percent for witnessed arrests in VF. Can higher survival rates be obtained, or is this the maximum percentage of victims who can be saved? Have the systems of today reached a theoretical ceiling for survival rates, or can fine-tuning of the systems produce greater survival? Can new techniques and treatment be developed that will increase survival from out-of-hospital cardiac arrest? A community survival rate of 30 percent for witnessed cardiac arrests in VF should be the standard of excellence given current technology and unchangeable variables, such as the percentage of witnessed cases, percentage of cases in VF, and realistic response times.

The success of the five EMS systems, as measured by discharge rates, appears directly related to the ability of each to rapidly provide CPR, defibrillation, medications, and intubation. An awareness of these factors and the strengths and weaknesses of each system can allow other communities to rationally build EMS systems and allocate resources.

Conclusion

Prehospital programs for out-of-hospital cardiac arrest can be grouped into five systems based on the personnel who deliver CPR, defibrillation, medications, and endotracheal intubation. Reported discharge rates ranged from two to 25 percent for all cardiac rhythms and from three to 33 percent for VF. Although there was considerable variation within each type of system, survival appeared to be highest in the systems that combined EMT or EMT-D with paramedic services. The combined response allows CPR to be started early, which permits definitive procedures, including defibrillation, medications, and intubation, to be more effective.

Acknowledgments

The authors wish to thank Alfred Hallstrom, who provided suggestions for analysis of data, Mary Pat Larsen, who assisted in data analysis, and Judy Prentice and Janet Weideman, who assisted in manuscript preparation.

References

Amey, B. D., E. E. Harrison, and J. E. Straub. "Sudden Cardiac Death: A Retrospective and Prospective Study." *Journal of the American College of Emergency Physicians* 5 (1976): 429-433.

Bachman, J. W., G. S. McDonald, and P. C. O'Brien. "A Study of Out-of-Hospital Cardiac Arrests in Northeastern Minnesota." *Journal of the American Medical Association* 256 (1986): 477-483.

Carter, W. B., M. S. Eisenberg, A. P. Hallstrom, et al. "Development and Implementation of Emergency CPR Instructions Via Telephone." *Annals of Emergency Medicine* 13 (1984): 695-700.

Chadda, K. D., and R. Kammerer. "Early Experiences with the Portable Automatic External Defibrillator in the Home and Public Places." *American Journal of Cardiology* 60 (1987): 732-733.

Chadda, K., R. Kammerer, J. Kuphal, et al. "Successful Defibrillation in the Industrial,

Recreational and Corporate Settings by Laypersons." *Circulation* 76 (suppl IV) (1987): IV-12.

Cobb, L. A., and A. P. Hallstrom. "Community Based Cardiopulmonary Resuscitation: What Have We Learned?" *Annals of New York Academic Sciences* 382 (1982): 330-341.

Copley, D. P., J. A. Mantle, W. J. Roger, et al. "Improved Outcome for Prehospital Cardiopulmonary Collapse with Resuscitation by Bystanders." *Circulation* 56 (1977): 902-905.

Crawford, C. G., M. Denton, C. A. Fisher, et al. "Resuscitation Outside Hospital in Auckland." *New Zealand Medical Journal* 99 (1986): 452-455.

Cummins, R. O., and M. S. Eisenberg. "Prehospital Cardiopulmonary Resuscitation: Is it Effective?" *Journal of the American Medical Association* 253 (1985): 2408-2412.

Cummins, R. O., M. S. Eisenberg, A. P. Hallstrom, et al. "Survival of Out-of-Hospital Cardiac Arrest with Early Initiation of Cardiopulmonary Resuscitation." *American Journal of Emergency Medicine* 3 (1985): 114-118.

Cummins, R. O., M. S. Eisenberg, J. E. Moore, et al. "Automatic External Defibrillators: Clinical, Training, Psychological and Public Health Issues." *Annals of Emergency Medicine* 14 (1985): 755-760.

Cummins, R. O., M. S. Eisenberg, L. Bergner, et al. "Automatic External Defibrillation: Evaluations of Effectiveness in the Home and in Emergency Medical Systems." *Annals of Emergency Medicine* 13 (1984): 798-801.

Diamond, N. J., J. Schofferman, and J. W. Elliot. "Factors in Successful Resuscitation by Paramedics." *Journal of the American College of Emergency Physicians* 6 (1977): 42-46.

Eisenberg, M., A. Hallstrom, and L. Bergner. "The ACLS Score: Predicting Survival from Out-of-Hospital Cardiac Arrest." *Journal of the American Medical Association* 246 (1981): 50-52.

Eisenberg, M., L. Berner, and A. Hallstrom. "Paramedic Programs and Out-of-Hospital Cardiac Arrest: I. Factors Associated with Successful Resuscitation." *American Journal of Public Health* 69 (1979): 30-38.

Eisenberg, M. S., A. P. Hallstrom, M. K. Copass, et al. "Treatment of Ventricular Fibrillation with Emergency Medical Technician Defibrillation and Paramedic Services." *Journal of the American Medical Association* 251 (1984): 1723-1726.

Eisenberg, M. S., E. Hadas, I. Nuri, et al. "Sudden Cardiac Arrest in Israel: Factors Associated with Successful Resuscitation." *American Journal of Emergency Medicine* 6 (1988): 319-323.

Eisenberg, M. S., J. Moore, R. O. Cummins, et al. "Use of the Automatic External Defibrillator in Homes of Survivors of Out-of-Hospital Ventricular Fibrillation." *American Journal of Cardiology* 63 (1989): 443-446.

Eisenberg, M. S., L. Bergner, and A. Hallstrom. "Out-of-Hospital Cardiac Arrest: Improved Survival with Paramedics Services." *Lancet* 1 (1980): 812-815.

Eisenberg, M. S., L. Bergner, and T. Hearne. "Out-of-Hospital Cardiac Arrest: A Review of Major Studies and a Proposed Uniform Reporting System." *American Journal of Public Health* 70 (1980): 236-239.

Eisenberg, M. S., M. K. Copass, A. P. Hallstrom, et al. "Treatment of Out-of-Hospital Cardiac Arrests with Rapid Defibrillation by Emergency Medical Technicians." *New England Journal of Medicine* 302 (1980): 1379-1383.

Eitel, D. R., S. L. Walton, A. D. Guerci, et al. "Out-of-Hospital Cardiac Arrest: A Six-Year Experience in a Suburban-Rural System." *Annals of Emergency Medicine* 17 (1988): 808-812.

Goldstein, S., J. R. Landis, R. Leighton, et al. "Characteristics of the Resuscitated Out-of-Hospital Cardiac Arrest Victim with Coronary Heart Disease." *Circulation* 64 (1981): 977-984.

Gray, A. J., A. D. Redmond, and M. Martin. "Use of the Automatic External Defibrillator-Pacemaker by Ambulance Personnel: The Stockport Experience." *British Medical Journal* 294 (1987): 1133-1135.

Gudjonsson, H., E. Baldvinsson, G Oddsson, et al. "Results of Attempted Cardiopulmonary Resuscitation of Patients Dying Suddenly Outside the Hospital in Reykjavik and the Surrounding Area." *Acta Med Scand* 212 (1982): 247-251.

Guzy, P. M., L. M. Pearce, and S. Greenfield. "The Survival Benefit of Bystander Cardiopulmonary Resuscitation in a Paramedic Served Metropolitan Area." *American Journal of Public Health* 73 (1983): 766-769.

Holmberg, S., and B. Wennerblom. "Out-of-Hospital Cardiac Arrest." *American Journal of Emergency Medicine* 2 (1984): 222-224.

Jakobsson, J., N. Nyquist, N. Rehnquist, et al. "Prognosis and Follow-Up of Patients Resuscitated from Out-of-Hospital Cardiac Arrest." *Acta Med Scand* 222 (1987): 123-132.

Lauterbach, S. A., M. Spadafora, and R. Levy. "Evaluation of Cardiac Arrest Managed by Paramedics." *Journal of the American College of Emergency Physicians* 7 (1978): 355-357.

Lewis, R. P., J. M. Stang, and J. V. Warren. "The Role of Paramedics in Resuscitation of Patients with Prehospital Cardiac Arrest from Coronary Artery Disease." *American Journal of Emergency Medicine* 2 (1984): 200-203.

Liberthson, R. R., E. L. Nagel, J. C. Hirschman, et al. "Prehospital Ventricular Defibrillation: Prognosis and Follow-Up Course." *New England Journal of Medicine* 291 (1974): 317-321.

Lund, I., and A. Skulberg. "Cardiopulmonary Resuscitation by Lay People." *Lancet* 2 (1976): 702-704.

Lund, I., and A. Skulberg. "Resuscitation of Cardiac Arrest Outside Hospitals: Experiences with a Mobile Intensive Care Unit in Oslo." *Acta Anas Scand* 53 (suppl) (1973): 13-16.

Mackintosh, A. F., M. E. Crabb, R. Grainger, et al. "The Brighton Resuscitation Ambulances: Review of 40 Consecutive Survivors of Out-of-Hospital Cardiac Arrest." *British Medical Journal* 1 (1978): 1115-1118.

Martin, T. G., N. S. Hawkins, J. A. Weigel, et al. "Initial Treatment of Ventricular Fibrillation: Defibrillation or Drug Therapy." *American Journal of Emergency Medicine* 6 (1988): 113-119.

McSwain, G. R., W. B. Garrison, and C. P. Artz. "Evaluation of Resuscitation from Cardiopulmonary Arrest by Paramedics." *Annals of Emergency Medicine* 9 (1980): 341-345.

Moore, J. E., M. S. Eisenberg, E. Andresen, et al. "Home Placement of Automatic External Defibrillators Among Survivors of Ventricular Fibrillation." *Annals of Emergency Medicine* 15 (1986): 811-812.

Moore, J. E., M. S. Eisenberg, R. O. Cummins, et al. "Lay Person Use of Automatic External Defibrillation." *Annals of Emergency Medicine* 16 (1987): 669-672.

Pantridge, J. F., and A. A. J. Adgey. "Prehospital Coronary Care: The Mobile Coronary Care Unit." *American Journal of Cardiology* 24 (1969): 666-672.

Pantridge, J. F., and J. S. Geddes. "A Mobile Intensive Care Unit in the Management of Myocardial Infarction." *Lancet* 2 (1967): 271-273.

Pressley, J. C., M. P. Raney, B. H. Wilson, et al. "Assessment of Out-of-Hospital Resuscitation." *American Journal of Emergency Medicine* 2 (1984): 215-216.

Rockswold, G., B. Sharma, E. Ruiz, et al. "Follow-Up of 514 Consecutive Patients with Cardiopulmonary Arrest Outside of the Hospital." *Journal of the American College of Emergency Physicians* 8 (1979): 216-220.

Rose, L. B. "The Oregon Coronary Ambulance Project: An Experiment." *Heart Lung* 3 (1974): 753-755.

Roth, R., R. D. Stewart, K. Rogers, et al. "Out-of-Hospital Cardiac Arrest: Factors Associated with Survival." *Annals of Emergency Medicine* 13 (1984): 237-243.

Sammel, N. L., K. Taylor, M. Selig, et al. "New South Wales Intensive Care Ambulance System: Outcome of Patients with Ventricular Fibrillation." *Medical Journal of Australia* 2 (1981): 246-550.

Stueven, H., P. Troiano, B. Thompson, et al. "Bystander/First Responder CPR: Ten Years Experience in a Paramedic System." *Annals of Emergency Medicine* 15 (1986): 707-710.

Stults, K. R., D. D. Brown, and R. E. Kerber. "Efficacy of an Automated External Defibrillator in the Management of Out-of-Hospital Cardiac Arrest: Validation of the Diagnostic Algorithm and Initial Clinical Experience in a Rural Environment." *Circulation* 73 (1986): 701-709.

Stults, K. R., D. D. Brown, V. L. Schug, et al. "Prehospital Defibrillation Performed by Emergency Medical Technicians in Rural Communities." *New England Journal of Medicine* 301 (1984): 219-223.

Swenson, R. D., D. L. Hill, J. S. Martin, et al. "Automatic External Defibrillators Used by Family Members to Treat Cardiac Arrest." *Circulation* 76 (suppl IV) (1987): IV-463.

Thomas, J. W., and C. G. Cayten. "EMS System Planning and Control." In *Principles and Practices of Emergency Medicine,* 2nd ed., eds. G. R. Schwartz, P. Safar, J. H. Stone, et al., 566-576. Philadelphia: WB Saunders, 1986.

Tweed, W. A., G. Bristow, and N. Donen. "Resuscitation from Cardiac Arrest: Assessment of a System Providing Only Basic Life Support Outside of Hospital." *Canadian Medical Association Journal* 122 (1980): 297-300.

Vertesi, L. "The Paramedic Ambulance: A Canadian Experience." *Canadian Medical Association Journal* 119 (1978): 25-29.

Vertesi, L., L. Wilson, and N. Glick. "Cardiac Arrest: Comparison of Paramedic and Conventional Ambulance Services." *Canadian Medical Association Journal* 128 (1983): 809-813.

Vukov, L. F., R. D. White, J. W. Bachman, et al. "New Perspectives on Rural EMT Defibrillation." *Annals of Emergency Medicine* 17 (1988): 318-321.

Weaver, W. D., L. A. Cobb, A. P. Hallstrom, et al. "Considerations for Improving Survival from Out-of-Hospital Cardiac Arrest." *Annals of Emergency Medicine* 15 (1986): 1181-1186.

Weaver, W. D., L. A. Cobb, C. E. Fahrenbruch, et al. "Use of the Automatic External Defibrillator in the Management of Out-of-Hospital Cardiac Arrest." *New England Journal of Medicine* 319 (1988): 661-666.

Weaver, W. D., M. K. Copass, D. Bufi, et al. "Improved Neurologic Recovery and Survival after Early Defibrillation." *Circulation* 69 (1984): 943-948.

Wilson, B. H., H. W. Severance, Jr., M. P. Raney, et al. "Out-of-Hospital Management of Cardiac Arrest by Basic Emergency Medical Technicians." *American Journal of Cardiology* 53 (1984): 68-70.

Source

Reprinted with permission from Annals of Emergency Medicine, *February 1990. The authors include Mickey S. Eisenberg, MD, PhD; Bruce T. Horwood, MD; Richard O. Cummins, MD, MPH, MSc; Robin Reynolds-Haertle, MS; and Thomas R. Hearne, PhD, from the Center for Evaluation of Emergency Medical Services, King County, Wash., Health Department, EMS Division, and the departments of Medicine and Biostatistics, University of Washington, Seattle.*

Controlled Studies in the Prehospital Setting: A Viable, Important Venue for Clinical Research

Paul E. Pepe, MD, FACEP

In this short editorial, Houston Fire Department's medical director, Dr. Paul Pepe, explains the importance of controlled studies in the prehospital environment. Dr. Pepe, a member of the faculty at Baylor College of Medicine and past president of the National Association of EMS Physicians, recognizes the long-term value of scientific research in the field.

Since almost all life-threatening injuries and the great majority of cardiac arrests occur outside of the hospital, there would seem to be no better place to test early lifesaving interventions than in the prehospital setting. Not only does the earliest intervention make a difference, but the prognosis for out-of-hospital arrest is far better than in-hospital arrest. However, the question arises as to whether scientific research actually can be accomplished successfully and reliably in the prehospital setting. The question relates to the fact that, in the United States, the actual prehospital emergency medical care is not provided by physician-scientists, but by persons who are physician surrogates (EMTs, paramedics). Some doubt that these EMS personnel can conduct reliable research using scientific methods. The issue is complicated further by the question of patient consent in the prehospital setting.

Nevertheless, the capacity to conduct well-designed, prospective, controlled clinical studies in the prehospital setting has been demonstrated for cardiac arrest patients and for certain trauma interventions. For example, results of studies with the pneumatic anti-shock garment (PASG) and with infusions of 7.5-percent (hypertonic) saline/dextran 70 have demonstrated the ability to evaluate the efficacy of these interventions with well-matched populations in the prehospital setting. Prospectively collected demographic and study/control group comparison data have validated the investigational designs. Thus, in these studies, the only difference between the study and control groups was the single intervention being examined.

Caveats for Success in Prehospital Research

In accepting the fact that successful execution of well-controlled, prospective clinical studies using large patient populations is feasible in the prehospital setting, certain caveats must be acknowledged. The first qualification is that in those prehospital emergency medical care systems that have demonstrated the successful conduct of such research, the physician-director of the EMS system essentially has controlled the entire system. Furthermore, these respective medical directors share a common philosophy in which they regard the prehospital emergency care system to be part of their personal practice of medicine. Therefore, a key element in the systems that have effected sound clinical research is that the EMS medical director has the attitude that the standard of care given to patients by EMS personnel must be the best that the medical director personally could offer. In turn, this provides reasonable assurance that the paramedics under the medical director's supervision are competent and reliable, and that their performance will be predictable. The results of such commitment are reflected in the remarkable survival statistics for critically ill and injured patients.

The second caveat for success in prehospital EMS research is that all of the EMS *system* personnel involved (and the care delivered by them) are rigidly controlled; that is, the control of patient care extends into the hospital. This control is enhanced in certain locales where the EMS medical directors also are supervising faculty in the receiving facilities. By extending the control over protocol to include the care being delivered in the hospital, better scientific control extends through the emergency department, operating suites, and the intensive care units. In turn, this further ensures rigorous compliance with the research protocols.

A third caveat for success in prehospital research is the inclusion of the EMS personnel (who will be executing the protocol) in the early discussions regarding rationale, study design, and methodology. In retrospect, this key element may be the feature missing in EMS systems that have experienced difficulties in protocol execution.

A highly active, responsible EMS medical director actually creates a more controlled situation than is possible in most other clinical research settings. With a single, responsible physician in control of all medical procedures, the same standardized care is delivered by each of the paramedics under his direction, particularly if a strict protocol is effected. On the other hand, in a hospital environment, one is more apt to find many physicians with an equal number of approaches, styles, and philosophies. As a result, protocols often are modified by such independent spirits. In contrast, in a paramilitary EMS organization (under intensive, singular medical direction), there exist better guarantees of rigid, standardized, systematic implementation of study protocols. Again, this rigid standardization helps to ensure that the intervention under investigation is the only factor separating a study group from a control group.

There are other factors that make the prehospital setting an excellent venue for the performance of clinical investigations. Beyond the exceptional occupational enthusiasm of EMS personnel, one usually finds in the urban North American paramedic a specialized expertise for dealing quickly and effectively with cardiac and trauma resuscitation. This expertise is reinforced by the high volume of cases that EMS personnel encounter. Compared to the average emergency department physician, they more regularly see patients requiring resuscitation and their skills are honed further by regularly scheduled performance reviews and retraining, as well as by the constant feedback of a streetwise, intensely involved medical director. In essence, paramedics can follow resuscitation protocols closely because they specifically do that for a living. And when they do it every day, they do it well in supervised systems.

One more factor that enhances the feasibility of scientific research in the prehospital setting is the large number of patients that can be studied.

With a single, responsible physician in control of all medical procedures, the same standardized care is delivered by each of the paramedics under his direction, particularly if a strict protocol is effected.

A major proviso in the willingness of paramedics to carry out studies is the reliability and quality of on-scene physician involvement in the event of an unanticipated problem.

Large study populations are possible because the entire catchment of the whole EMS system potentially is available. It is less likely that a statistically desirable number of resuscitation patients can be entered into a study from a single hospital emergency department. The longer the period over which a study is conducted, the more likely it is to be affected by other factors.

Special Considerations

Since investigational studies classically have originated as an in-hospital phenomenon, there are some philosophical and logistical problems that have to be considered for prehospital studies. These hurdles include

- Seeking permission to bring study patients to and continue the protocol at various receiving hospitals
- Developing deferred consent procedures
- Assuring the paramedics that they will be protected from liability

In highly complex or highly experimental interventions (e.g., the prehospital use of thrombolytic therapy by paramedics), some of these problems can be addressed by limiting the number of EMS personnel that actually carry out the protocol, at least initially. For example, in the Houston system, the three senior supervisors, who oversee each of the three different 24-hour shifts of paramedics, often are used initially in resuscitation research using investigational drugs. They drive their own response vehicles and usually are available to respond to all cardiac arrests that occur in the prehospital setting, usually an average of 25 cardiac arrests per senior supervisor per month.

Prior to the project, detailed instructions and training are given to these three senior supervisor paramedics whose job it may be to initiate administration of the experimental therapy in the field. These instructions usually involve study entry and exclusion criteria as well as the background information relevant to the study. However, for the most part, because they usually help in study design, instruction is relatively easy. In addition, better care and stricter protocol adherence have been rendered during any protocol because paramedic supervisors arrive at practically every arrest in the city (three to four per day). Furthermore, because they are under extremely close scrutiny by physicians who specialize in prehospital care and cardiac arrest management, these paramedics' skills, judgment, and performance in such cases generally exceed that of most physicians.

A major proviso in the willingness of paramedics to carry out studies is the reliability and quality of on-scene physician involvement in the event of an unanticipated problem. Physicians who regularly provide supervision to the paramedics, and are the usual resource for the paramedics in case of complications, best suit this purpose.

In terms of deferred consent and receiving hospital approval, the case can be presented to institutional review boards that the overwhelming majority of patients who have major injury or who arrest from primary cardiac disease, are dependent on care rendered in the prehospital setting. If some time-dependent therapies are initiated only after the patient arrives at the hospital, fewer study patients would benefit from them (let alone survive). Paramedics can be very capable in cardiac resuscitation, and there is no better time to administer a new interventional drug than "immediately." And what is the alternative? A proposed complication seems to be inconsequential in someone who has no other option but death. As long as the study is carefully designed, carefully executed, and carefully monitored and scrutinized for safety, any complications that occur can be addressed accordingly.

Conclusion

The prehospital setting provides an excellent venue for conducting prospective, controlled clinical trials. This venue offers a potential for the implementation of excellent, standardized research protocols and a large patient base from which to enroll study participants. Moreover, it provides an arena in which early therapeutic care has the best potential to significantly improve the outcome for many people. With thousands and thousands of injuries that may be amenable to some new therapy, and nearly 250,000 potentially treatable cases of sudden death in the United States occurring each year, the obvious magnitude of impact of even a small improvement in care will be profound.

The prehospital setting offers a potential for the implementation of excellent, standardized research protocols and a large patient base from which to enroll study participants.

References

Beatrice, Colonel Edwin S., Commander, U.S. Army Institute of Research, Division of Military Trauma Research, personal correspondence, San Francisco, 15 December 1986.

Bickell, W. H., P. E. Pepe, C. H. Wyatt, et al. "The Effect of Antishock Garments on Patients with Penetrating Abdominal Injuries." *Annals of Emergency Medicine* 16 (1987): 653-658.

Bonnin, M. J., P. E. Pepe, and P. S. Clark. "Key Role of Prehospital Resuscitation in Survival from Out-of-Hospital Cardiac Arrest." *Annals of Emergency Medicine* 19 (1990): 466.

Bonnin, M. J., P. E. Pepe, and P. S. Clark. "Survival Prognosis for the Elderly Following Out-of-Hospital Cardiac Arrest." *Annals of Emergency Medicine* 18 (1989).

Copass, M. K., M. R. Oreskovich, M. R. Bladergreen, and C. J. Carrico. "Prehospital Cardiopulmonary Resuscitation of the Critically Injured Patient." *American Journal of Surgery* 148 (1984): 20-26.

Emergency Medical Services in the City of Houston. Houston: City of Houston Fire Department, 1989.

Haynes, R. E., T. L. Chinn, M. K. Copass, and L. A. Cobb. "Comparison of Bretylium Tosylate and Lidocaine in Management of Out-of-Hospital Ventricular Fibrillation: A Randomized Clinical Trial." *American Journal of Cardiology* 48 (1981): 353-356.

Heller, M. B., J. B. Melton, R. M. Kaplan, et al. "Data Collection by Paramedics for Prehospital Research." *Annals of Emergency Medicine* 17 (1988): 414-415.

Mattox, K. L., P. A. Maningas, P. E. Pepe, et al. "Hypertonic Saline/Dextran 70 in Prehospital Management of Post-Traumatic Hypotension: Preliminary Observations." *American Journal of Surgery* 157 (1989): 528-534.

Mattox, K. L., W. H. Bickell, P. E. Pepe, and A. D. Mangelsdorff. "Prospective

Source

Reprinted with permission from Prehospital and Disaster Medicine, *July-September 1990. Paul Pepe, MD, FACEP, is the medical director for the Houston Fire Department and a faculty member at the Baylor College of Medicine.*

Randomized Evaluation of Antishock MAST in Post-Traumatic Hypotension." *Journal of Trauma* 26 (1986): 779-784.

Pepe, P. E., and M. J. Bonnin. "Limitations and Liabilities." *Emergency* (1989): 2140-2143.

Pepe, P. E., and M. K. Copass. "Prehospital Care." In *Early Care of the Injured.* 4th ed., American College of Surgeons Committee on Trauma. Ed. E. E. Moore, 37-55. Philadelphia: B. C. Decker, Inc., 1990.

Pepe, P. E., and R. D. Stewart. "Role of the Physician in the Prehospital Setting." *Annals of Emergency Medicine* 15 (1986): 1480-1483.

Pepe, P. E., K. L. Mattox, and F. D. Prentice. "Impact of Full-Time Physician Supervision on an Urban EMS System." *Prehospital and Disaster Medicine* 5 (1989): 7.

Pepe, P. E., R. D. Stewart, and M. K. Copass. "Prehospital Management of Trauma: A Tale of Three Cities." *Annals of Emergency Medicine* 15 (1986): 1484-1489.

Pepe, P. E., R. R. Bass, and K. L. Mattox. "Clinical Trials of the Pneumatic Antishock Garment in the Urban Prehospital Setting." *Annals of Emergency Medicine* 15 (1986): 1407–1410.

Pepe, P. E., W. H. Bickell, and K. L. Mattox. "The Effect of Anti-Shock Garments on Prehospital Survival: The Need for Controlled Clinical Studies." *Prehospital and Disaster Medicine* 3 (1987): 40-45.

Taffet, G. E., T. A. Teasdale, and R. J. Luchi. "In-Hospital Cardiopulmonary Resuscitation." *Journal of the American Medical Association* 260 (1981): 2069-2072.

Weaver, W. D., L. A. Cobb, M. K. Copass, and A. P. Hallstrom. "Ventricular Fibrillation: A Comparative Trial Using 175-J and 320-J Shocks." *New England Journal of Medicine* 307 (1982): 1101-1106.

For more than two decades, EMS systems have proliferated primarily due to governmental impetus and funding at the federal, state, and local levels. Although many of the foundations of patient care rendered in these systems have been based on intuitive logic, the understanding of the impact on patient outcome is poor, at best. The reasons for the current status are varied, but five issues are pre-eminent:

- The authority for the development of these medical systems has been based primarily in political and bureaucratic institutions that have little or no medical expertise.
- Little attention has been paid to system evaluation, particularly in the area of cost effectiveness.
- Few academic medical institutions have become involved in EMS research.
- Traditional approaches to medical research primarily are disease-specific and are not multidisciplinary. Thus, these are not useful for evaluating and understanding the highly complex and uncontrolled environmental interactions that typify EMS systems.
- The process of efficiently and reliably collecting accurate data in the prehospital setting is extremely difficult.

The foundation of all EMS research is based on the assumption that important information about prehospital patients and systems can be obtained reliably. Unfortunately, it has become clear that this assumption is not necessarily true. There are enormous barriers that make prehospital data collection difficult in the best of settings. Perhaps the best evidence that supports the concept that EMS research remains in its infancy is the fact that researchers are just beginning to scratch the surface of understanding the *problems* involved in data collection. The recent emphasis on identifying these problems has unearthed many distressing realities. However, it is fortunate that attention now is given to these issues.

Obtaining answers to the pressing questions about the efficacy and cost effectiveness of prehospital care begins with identification of the problems that exist with accessing EMS system data. The following is a discussion of the major problems involved in EMS data collection. This list certainly is not exhaustive, and numerous important issues will not be discussed. The purpose is to focus specifically on problems intrinsic to the prehospital data collection process itself.

Barriers to Clinical Evaluations of EMS Systems: Problems Associated With Field Data Collection

Daniel W. Spaite, MD, FACEP; Terence D. Valenzuela, MD, FACEP; and Harvey W. Meislin, MD, FACEP

Why has scientific research in EMS been lacking until all but the last few years? The authors describe common problems associated with EMS research and a dozen helpful ideas to break down barriers to valid research.

Methods for ensuring a high degree of confidence in the data collected must be developed and should be a priority in future EMS research.

Problem One: Assumptions About What Data Are Available May Be Wrong

Most, if not all, EMS systems have at least a simple form of data collection for purposes that vary from evaluating patient care to billing for patient transport. Although there is enormous variability in the structure, format, and information collected, most of these data collection tools contain at least basic medical information. Because of this, there is a general sense among most EMS administrators, medical directors, and researchers that simple questions about prehospital care can easily be answered. An example of such a question might be "What prehospital interventions are carried out on hypertensive patients?" The basic assumption would be that vital signs are measured in the field, and hence, hypertensive patients can be identified. Unfortunately, in some systems, even this simple assumption is not true.

We evaluated the prehospital care of 229 patients from 20 ALS agencies throughout the state of Arizona. An in-field observer timed and recorded each event as it occurred during EMS runs. This investigation revealed that no blood pressure was measured in 27 percent of the patients. Unfortunately, these results showed that, in Arizona as a whole, it would have been impossible to reliably answer the above research question, despite its simplicity.

Of course, many involved in EMS hope to be able to answer much more complex and pertinent questions. An example is the attempt to develop low-yield criteria that potentially could identify seizure patients that can be left safely at the scene after evaluation by prehospital personnel. The assumption involved in such an endeavor is that an accurate and appropriate physical assessment is obtained on all prehospital seizure patients. The attempts to answer such complex questions must be based on reliable information.

Therefore, future research must be directed specifically at Problem One or there will be no hope of answering many of the most important EMS system questions. Methods for ensuring a high degree of confidence in the data collected must be developed and should be a priority in future EMS research.

Problem Two: Providing a Good Data Collection System Does Not Guarantee Good Data Collection

Currently, many EMS systems are spending significant amounts of money in an attempt to provide a good data collection system. This is the foundation for any system evaluation. In 1986, the Tucson, Ariz., Fire Department desired to improve its ability to develop, direct, and evaluate its system. One priority was to develop a data collection tool that would be reliable and useful for answering administrative as well as research questions. Numerous possibilities were considered, and a decision was made to revise the system that was in place.

Part of the impetus to improve data collection was to evaluate prehospital cardiac arrest in the Tucson system. However, prior to using the data collection system for this purpose, data entry compliance with the newly implemented tool was evaluated. During the first month of the study, nearly 25 percent of cases were missing all medical data items. During months three and four, data entry compliance improved markedly and achieved an acceptable rate for patient and system evaluation (96-percent compliance). Subsequently, entry compliance from months seven and eight was evaluated to identify long-term compliance and was found to have remained at an excellent level.

The implication from this study was obvious. Attempts to evaluate essentially any aspect of the prehospital care of cardiac arrest victims using the data from the first few months after implementation would have been problematic. Decisions for system alterations that might have affected patient care significantly could have been based on flawed information. However, evaluating the data collection tool allowed us to ensure the completeness of the data. Subsequently, useful information was obtained using this tool, and those data have had profound implications for this system.

It is important to remember that the best data collection system, no matter how sophisticated or expensive, does not guarantee good data collection, but must be evaluated for data entry compliance and data validity prior to its use for system analysis.

Problem Three: Human Factors Might Be More Important Than Structural Factors

A significant body of EMS research deals with computer systems, data collection tools, information storage, interactive databases, and other structural factors. However, the human factors that may be important have received essentially no attention in the literature. Issues such as interest, motivation, stress, sleep deprivation, volunteer versus paid status, private versus public status, perceived importance of the data, educational level, perceived consequences of non-compliance, tendencies to underplay or delete "bad" information, and others essentially remain unstudied.

In traditional medical research, data tend to be collected by a small number of personnel in controlled environments. On the other hand, EMS data are collected in a large number of uncontrolled and highly unusual circumstances by personnel who are under stress, conceivably in danger, and maybe near exhaustion. Clearly, the assumption that the data collected in such a setting can be assumed to be reliable is suspect. Investigations regarding human factors and how to alter and control them are needed desperately. If the impact of such issues is not evaluated in the future, the usefulness of even the most impressive and sophisticated data collection systems will be greatly handicapped.

> It is important to remember that the best data collection system, no matter how sophisticated or expensive, does not guarantee good data collection, but must be evaluated for data entry compliance and data validity prior to its use for system analysis.

A major thrust of future EMS research must be directed toward the provision of careful attention to identify those data items that reflect outcome alterations and those that do not.

Problem Four: Researchers May Be Collecting the Wrong Data

One of the major problems associated with our attempt to collect data in the field has been the fact that the actual data items collected have been chosen arbitrarily. In fact, until 1991, more than two decades of cardiac arrest research were done without a unified model or even a consistent definition of terms. Data collection for essentially all other clinical entities remains even more suspect, since the minimum data sets and definitions of terms that have been suggested have not been widely accepted.

One example to expose the collection of convenient but "wrong" data occurred in the evaluation of the association between on-scene interval and survival from out-of-hospital cardiac arrest in Tucson. One primary impetus of this investigation was the belief that an association would exist, and that this association most likely was due to two factors.

First, on-scene intervals were defined as the time elapsed between the unit reporting arrival at the scene and the personnel reporting departure from the scene. Thus, in situations in which getting to the patient's side took a long time, the on-scene interval would be expected to be increased. It was surmised that this might even be significant enough to be associated with poor survival.

Second, the patients most likely to survive also were expected to have early successful resuscitation with little likelihood of remaining on scene for a prolonged time. Indeed, significantly higher survival was found in patients with on-scene intervals less than 12 minutes (13.9 percent versus 6.5 percent, $p < 0.05$). Several investigations indicate that the key issues in improving survival from out-of-hospital cardiac arrest are the time from collapse to CPR and from collapse to defibrillation. As in many systems, the data collection at that time was limited only to the time of initial call and the time of paramedic arrival at the scene. It could not be identified when defibrillation occurred. In response, a system was subsequently developed that allowed precise recording of the actual times that were pertinent to survival by real-time, simultaneous audio and ECG recordings. A program of follow-up interviews of bystanders also was instituted to most accurately identify the time of collapse. Institution of these programs indicated that the actual mean interval in this system from paramedic arrival at the scene until delivery of the initial defibrillatory shock was 3.1 minutes. It is possible that differences in this "patient access interval" explain these findings of improved survival in patients with shorter on-scene intervals in the previous investigation. In any case, this revealed the problem of assuming that the response interval for a system is equivalent to the call-to-defibrillation interval.

A major thrust of future EMS research must be directed toward the provision of careful attention to identify those data items that reflect outcome alterations and those that do not. Mere associations no longer will do—we must begin to collect the right data.

Problem Five: Methods of Data Collection Are Suboptimal

A long-established paradigm in science is that the foundations of all knowledge start with simple observations. Amazingly, after more than two decades of EMS system development, we still have very little information about what actually transpires in the field. To our knowledge, only four investigations have involved systematic in-field observation. Any major improvement in the understanding of EMS systems will require specific, accurate, timed observations. One of the concerns for this type of investigation is the impact of the Hawthorne effect. That is, in some settings, merely studying a clinical entity can lead to alterations in the care. Despite this limitation, the failure to observe what actually goes on in the field in EMS systems leaves an enormous hole in understanding EMS.

Another arena of suboptimal data collection methodology is the failure to utilize many technologies that already are available. As discussed in Problem Four, one good example of this is the event documentation unit available for monitor-defibrillator equipment. This allows a record, in real time, of cardiac rhythm and surrounding audio information during patient encounters. The awareness of the limitations in the initial data collection system for cardiac arrest research in Tucson (see Problem Four) led to the decision to utilize such a tool. Whenever the unit is turned on, simultaneous real-time recording begins. Thus, when a reference point is set (i.e., the unit reports leaving the scene), precise times for all other recorded events automatically are established from this reference point. The EMS personnel are trained to speak out loud as they carry out each intervention and task, allowing precise timing of events. Thus, time intervals that actually impact survival, such as time to defibrillatory shock, are automatically established independent of any estimates by the personnel involved in the resuscitation.

Problem Six: Much of the Data Relies on Perceptions and Estimates

An investigation by Jurkovich and associates indicated that the perceptions of elapsed time by EMS personnel intrinsically are unreliable. This investigation evaluated the ability of EMS personnel to estimate the total prehospital interval involved in EMS patient encounters. If an accuracy within one minute of actual total prehospital interval was required, the error rate was 60 percent in very short runs and approached 100 percent at 30 minutes. Even if an accuracy interval of five minutes in either direction was allowed, significant error rates were present (30 percent). Unfortunately, many systems treat information that is based on perceptions and estimates as "hard" data.

An excellent example of a frequently used estimation that is extremely important but highly suspect is "downtime" in cardiac arrest. Estimations made by EMS personnel in such a stressful setting are likely

The failure to observe what actually goes on in the field in EMS systems leaves an enormous hole in understanding EMS.

Box 4.5

Five Potential Sources of Prehospital Data

- Estimates and perceptions
- Informal recording
- Routine notification of an independent recorder (i.e., dispatcher)
- Real-time event recording
  - ECG
  - Audio
  - Video
- Direct in-field observation

From *Prehospital and Disaster Medicine* © 1993, Spaite et al.

to be inaccurate at best and blatantly misleading at worst. This awareness has led several systems to use research personnel to establish the time of events based on retrospective interviews with bystanders (Seattle, Tucson). Although such a structured interview process still is based on estimates, data acquired using this process are likely to be significantly more accurate than are data collected at the time of arrest. The combination of this methodology and real-time event documentation technology in this system has allowed the evaluation of important intervals such as collapse-to-CPR and collapse-to-defibrillation intervals.

The five potential sources of prehospital information are listed in Box 4.5 in order of increasing reliability. Unfortunately, the vast majority of systems use the top three sources. As discussed above, a few systems currently use real-time ECG and audio recording on an ongoing basis for evaluation of the cardiac arrest process. However, currently no systems are using audio recordings of all patient encounters.

Problem Seven: In Different Systems, the Problems May Not Be the Same

In the statewide system in Arizona, blood pressure measurement omissions occurred more frequently among non-urban personnel (34 percent) than among urban personnel (20 percent) ($p < 0.027$). This investigation revealed that regional variations impacting data collection may significantly alter information reliability. Once again, this information highlights the fact that human factors such as motivation, training, volunteer versus paid status, and other issues may profoundly impact data validity. In a broad sense, the problem of "skills retention" in the rural setting may not be limited solely to medical procedures, but may also impact data collection and reliability.

Unfortunately, the variations that occur in different systems are limitless. An enormous number of issues impact every aspect of each system and each patient. Thus, the barriers to proper data collection may be so variable in different systems that problems that may be well defined in one system essentially may be irrelevant to others. This problem underlies the quagmire in which researchers find themselves when trying to compare outcomes from cardiac arrest in various systems.

Potential Answers to EMS Data Collection Problems

The preceding discussion highlights the enormity of the problems that face those who collect EMS data with the intent of evaluating systems. Although these problems are large ones, there are potential answers to some of these problems that may help to break down many of the barriers.

Develop professional relationships. Medical directors of EMS systems must develop close professional relationships with key personnel in the system. The type of personnel that are relevant to this issue may vary widely from one system to another. Fire chiefs, paramedic supervisors, law enforcement personnel, communications system personnel, ambulance company owners, or others may play an important role in a given system.

Evaluate data collection methods. It is key that the system medical director find someone who really cares about system evaluation and improvement. Unfortunately, the personnel involved in many systems never take the time to concern themselves with these issues. The relationships developed with key personnel discussed above may fulfill this need; however, interested persons in the system need not be administrative personnel. Once the relationships are developed, this small group must take the time to meet specifically regarding data collection issues. A plan should be developed to evaluate the current data collection system, if one exists, and potentially alter it or develop a new one. Necessary preparation for this process requires that the medical director be aware of pertinent scientific publications.

Unfortunately, many data collection "improvements" instituted with good intentions are done in a vacuum and recapitulate errors that have been identified and solved in other systems and reported in EMS literature. This problem is not unique to EMS and has been identified to exist within medicine in general.

Involve an expert consultant. The EMS system leaders should consider involving an expert consultant with significant experience in data collection, reliability evaluation, data analysis, and research.

Minimize worthless data items. When developing an EMS data collection tool, it is important to minimize worthless data items. There is a strong tendency to desire to capture every conceivable piece of information when developing a new data collection system. This tendency must be avoided since the importance of non-targeted information will be ambiguous to EMS personnel and the process may collapse due to lack of interest or disillusionment.

Be realistic about data collection. It is very important to be realistic about how ambitious the data collection system needs to be. Some systems that collaborate closely with research-based institutions may develop sophisticated data collection tools. However, unless personnel with the expertise to manage such complex information systems are available for development, utilization, and analysis, simplicity should be a priority.

Minimize estimating. It is very important to minimize the number of data items that require estimates in the "heat of battle." As previously discussed, "downtime" during cardiac arrest is a good example of such an estimate that is very inaccurate.

Involve system users in the development. During the development and institution of a new data collection system, the users of the data collection tool should be involved. An "ivory tower" syndrome must be avoided to help prevent data entry non-compliance by field personnel.

Develop a plan for supervisory data review. When feasible, this

The problems of data collection are enormous. However, the need to better understand EMS systems in the future mandates that we must overcome these barriers.

plan should include EMS agency supervisors as well as the medical director. It is important that incomplete forms or those that are filled out improperly are returned to the personnel for completion or correction. If EMS personnel know there is a process in the system that identifies incomplete or obviously incorrect information, they will be far more likely to enter data properly the first time.

Make the EMS system a "laboratory." Since the problems associated with various EMS systems vary widely, it is important that the leaders of essentially all systems perceive themselves as being in the business of evaluation. The scope and sophistication of this system evaluation obviously will vary with the resources and expertise of the personnel but will remain extremely important, even for small systems.

Empower the agency to receive recognition. The EMS personnel collaborating in the study should be co-authors on publications, and the agency's name should be included. This was found to be important because it empowers the EMS agency to receive national recognition that they otherwise would not obtain. In Tucson, this does wonders for consolidating the commitment by EMS administrators, supervisors, and personnel to be attentive to data collection. Developing such a collaborative relationship can significantly increase the likelihood that the system will support research projects.

Consider new technology. Consider implementing new technology that does not rely on personnel for data collection. Programs such as real-time cardiac event recording or audio recording of all patient encounters in the system could be implemented. If EMS personnel are trained to verbalize each task and procedure, enormous amounts of information potentially could be obtained by simple audio recording of patient encounters. Such innovations would lead to a marked improvement in understanding EMS systems.

Involve an observer. Consider placing an independent observer in the system. As previously discussed, there has been a near absence of carefully designed, specific, timed system observation. In the future, an observer should be considered as essential to EMS systems as having a radio or a defibrillator. In the scope of things, at least in large systems, this is a relatively inexpensive way to allow continuous system evaluation.

Conclusion

The problems of data collection are enormous. However, the need to better understand EMS systems in the future mandates that we must overcome these barriers. Indeed, solving the problems associated with field data collection is absolutely essential if we hope to compete successfully for the societal resources that are needed to continue EMS system development.

References

Becker, L. B., M. P. Ostrander, J. Battett, et al. "Outcome of CPR in a Large Metropolitan Area—Where are the Survivors?" *Annals of Emergency Medicine* 20 (1991): 355-361.

Bell, J. M., M. Moody, C. E. Wiles, et al. "Computer Management of Prehospital Information." *JEMS* 7 (1982): 33-38.

Bowman, W. D. "The Development and Current Status of Wilderness Prehospital Emergency Care in the United States." *Journal of Wilderness Medicine* 1 (1990): 93-102.

Braun, O., J. Turns, R. McCallion, et al. "Necessity for Objective Evaluation of EMS System Performance." *Annals of Emergency Medicine* 17 (1988): 415. Abstract.

Braun, O., R. McCallion, and J. Fazackerley. "Characteristics of Mid-Sized Urban EMS Systems." *Annals of Emergency Medicine* 19 (1990): 536-546.

Campbell, J. C., M. C. Gratton, and W. A. Robinson. "Meaningful Response Time Interval: Is it an Elusive Dream?" *Annals of Emergency Medicine* 20 (1991): 433.

Campbell, J. C., M. C. Gratton, J. A. Salomone, et al. "Time-to-Patient Interval: The Hidden Component of Response Time." *Annals of Emergency Medicine* 21 (1992): 643. Abstract.

Cohen, H. C. "Assessment of EMT-P Medications Used by Baltimore County Fire Department Supervisors/EMT-Ps." *Prehospital and Disaster Medicine* 5 (1990): 19-24.

Cummins, R. O., D. A. Chamberlain, N. S. Abramson, et al. "Recommended Guidelines for Uniform Reporting of Data from Out-of-Hospital Cardiac Arrest: The Utstein Style." *Annals of Emergency Medicine* 20 (1991): 861-874.

Dean, N. C., P. J. Haug, and P. J. Hawker. "Effect of Mobile Paramedic Units on Outcome in Patients with Myocardial Infarction." *Annals of Emergency Medicine* 17 (1988): 1034-1041.

Donovan, P. J., D. M. Cline, T. W. Witley, et al. "Prehospital Care by EMTs and EMT-Is in a Rural Setting: Is the Advancement of Service Justified?" *Annals of Emergency Medicine* 17 (1988): 415. Abstract.

Eisenberg, M., A. Hallstrom, and L. Bergner. "The ACLS Score: Predicting Survival from Out-of-Hospital Cardiac Arrest." *Journal of the American Medical Association* 246 (1981): 50-52.

Eisenberg, M., L. Bergner, and A. Hallstrom. "Paramedic Programs and Out-of-Hospital Cardiac Arrest: I. Factors Associated with Successful Resuscitation." *American Journal of Public Health* 69 (1979): 30-38.

Eisenberg, M. S., L. Bergner, and T. Hearne. "Out-of-Hospital Cardiac Arrest: A Review of Major Studies and a Proposed Uniform Reporting System." *American Journal of Public Health* 70 (1980): 236-240.

Eisenberg, M. S., R. O. Cummins, S. Damon, et al. "Survival Rates from Out-of-Hospital Cardiac Arrest: Recommendations for Uniform Definitions and Data to Report." *Annals of Emergency Medicine* 19 (1990): 1249-1259.

Eitel, D. R., S. L. Walton, A. D. Guerci, et al. "Out-of-Hospital Cardiac Arrest: A Six-Year Experience in a Suburban-Rural System." *Annals of Emergency Medicine* 17 (1988): 808-812.

Hedges, J. R., and S. M. Joyce. "Minimum Data Set for EMS Report Form: Historical Development and Future Implications." *Prehospital and Disaster Medicine* 5 (1990): 383-388.

Heller, M. B., J. B. Melton, R. M. Kaplan, et al. "Data Collection by Paramedics for Prehospital Research." *Annals of Emergency Medicine* 17 (1988): 414-415. Abstract.

Herrman, N., C. G. Cayten, J. Senior, et al. "Interobserver and Intraobserver Reliability in the Collection of Emergency Medical Services Data." *Health Services Research* 15 (1980): 127-143.

Jones, S. E., T. P. Nesper, and E. Alcouloumre. "Prehospital Intravenous Line Placement: A Prospective Study." *Annals of Emergency Medicine* 18 (1989): 244-246.

Joyce, S. M., and D. E. Brown. "An Optically Scanned EMS Reporting Form and Analysis System for Statewide Use: Development and Five Years Experience." *Annals of Emergency Medicine* 20 (1991): 1325-1330.

Joyce, S. M., and E. Criss. "Guidelines for Development of EMS Reporting Forms: Nationwide Survey." *Annals of Emergency Medicine* 16 (1987): 508. Abstract.

Jurkovich, G. J., L. D. Campbell, J. Padrta, et al. "Paramedic Perception of Elapsed Field Time." *Journal of Trauma* 27 (1987): 892-897.

Maio, R. F., and R. E. Burney. "Improving Reliability of Abstracted Prehospital Care

Data: Use of Decision Rules." *Prehospital and Disaster Medicine* 6 (1991): 15-20.

Mueller, B. A., F. P. Rivara, and A. B. Bergman. "Urban-Rural Location and the Risk of Dying in a Pedestrian-Vehicle Collision." *Journal of Trauma* 18 (1988): 91-94.

Pointer, J. E., M. Osur, C. Campbell, et al. "The Impact of Standing Orders on Medication and Skill Selection, Paramedic Assessment and Hospital Outcome: A Follow-Up Report." *Prehospital and Disaster Medicine* 6 (1991): 303-308.

Polsky, S. S. "Medical Record Keeping." In *Principles of EMS Systems,* ed. R. R. Roush. Dallas: American College of Emergency Physicians, 1989.

Pons, P. T., E. E. Moore, J. M. Cusick, et al. "Prehospital Venous Access in an Urban Paramedic System—A Prospective On-Scene Analysis." *Journal of Trauma* 28 (1988): 1460-1463.

Pressley, J. C., H. W. Severance, M. P. Raney, et al. "A Comparison of Paramedic Versus Basic Emergency Medical Care of Patients at High and Low Risk During Acute Myocardial Infarction." *Journal of the American College of Cardiologists* 12 (1988): 1555-1561.

Roth, R., R. D. Stewart, K. Rogers, et al. "Out-of-Hospital Cardiac Arrest: Factors Associated with Survival." *Annals of Emergency Medicine* 13 (1984): 237-243.

Saunders, C. E. "A Computer Simulation Study of the Effects of Priority Dispatch and Lights and Sirens Operation on Ambulance Response Time." *Prehospital and Disaster Medicine* 7 (1992): S22. Abstract.

Saunders, C. E., P. Amick, and J. Applegarth. "Analysis of Ambulance 'Response Time' and Component Intervals: Suggestions for Standard Definitions." *Prehospital and Disaster Medicine* 6 (1991): 382. Abstract.

Shuster, M., and J. Chong. "Pharmacologic Intervention in Prehospital Care: A Critical Appraisal." *Annals of Emergency Medicine* 18 (1989): 192-196.

Spaite, D. W., and M. Joseph. "Prehospital Cricothyrotomy: An Investigation of Indications, Technique, Complications, and Patient Outcome." *Annals of Emergency Medicine* 19 (1990): 279-285.

Spaite, D. W., E. A. Criss, T. D. Valenzuela, et al. "A Prospective Evaluation of Prehospital Patient Assessment by Direct In-Field Observation: Failure of ALS Personnel to Measure Vital Signs." *Prehospital and Disaster Medicine* 5 (1990): 325-334.

Spaite, D. W., E. A. Criss, T. D. Valenzuela, et al. "Analysis of Prehospital Scene Time and Survival from Out-of-Hospital, Non-Traumatic Cardiac Arrest." *Prehospital and Disaster Medicine* 6 (1991): 21-28.

Spaite, D. W., T. D. Valenzuela, H. W. Meislin, E. A. Criss, and J. Ross. "A Prospective Evaluation of the Impact of Initial Glasgow Coma Scale on Prehospital Treatment and Transport of Seizure Patients." *Prehospital and Disaster Medicine* 7 (1992): 19-24.

Spaite, D. W., T. D. Valenzuela, H. W. Meislin, et al. "Prospective Validation of a New Model for Evaluating EMS Systems by In-Field Observation of Specific Time Intervals in Prehospital Care." *Annals of Emergency Medicine* 21 (1992): 643. Abstract.

Spaite, D. W., T. Hanlon, E. A. Criss, et al. "Prehospital Cardiac Arrest: The Impact of Witnessed Collapse and Bystander CPR in a Metropolitan EMS System with Short Response Times." *Annals of Emergency Medicine* 19 (1990): 1264-1269.

Spaite, D. W., T. Hanlon, E. A. Criss, et al. "Prehospital Data Entry Compliance by Paramedics after Institution of a Comprehensive EMS Data Collection Tool." *Annals of Emergency Medicine* 19 (1990): 1270-1273.

Steele, R. *Development of a Minimum Data Set for Emergency Medical Services Patient Record Keeping.* National Technical Information Service, PB243822, July 1974.

Stewart, R. D., J. Burgman, G. M. Cannon, et al. "A Computer-Assisted Quality Assurance System for an Emergency Medical Service." *Annals of Emergency Medicine* 14 (1985): 25-29.

Thompson, B. M., H. A. Stueven, R. J. Mateer, et al. "Comparison of Clinical CPR Studies in Milwaukee and Elsewhere in the United States." *Annals of Emergency Medicine* 14 (1985): 750-754.

U.S. Congress, Office of Technology Assessment. Rural Emergency Medical Services. *Special Report, OTA-H-445.* Washington, D.C.: U.S. Government Printing Office, November 1989.

Valenzuela, T. D., A. L. Wright, E. S. Venkatraman, et al. "Collapse of CPR and Defibrillation Intervals in Out-of-Hospital Sudden Cardiac Death: Ethical Thresholds for Prospective, Randomized Trials." *Prehospital and Disaster Medicine* 7 (1992): S15. Abstract.

Valenzuela, T. D., and E. A. Criss. "Data Collection and Ambulance Call Report Design." In *EMS Medical Directors' Handbook*, ed. A. E. Kuehl. St. Louis: CV Mosby, 1989.

Valenzuela, T. D., D. W. Spaite, H. W. Meislin, et al. "Case and Survival Definitions in Out-of-Hospital Cardiac Arrest." *Journal of the American Medical Association* 267 (1992): 272-274.

Valenzuela, T. D., D. W. Spaite, H. W. Meislin, et al. "Emergency Response Intervals Versus Collapse to CPR and Defibrillation Intervals: Monitoring EMS System Performance in Sudden Cardiac Death." *Annals of Emergency Medicine* 21 (1992): 648. Abstract.

Valenzuela, T. D., E. A. Criss, D. W. Spaite, et al. "Cost-Effectiveness Analysis of Paramedic Emergency Medical Services in the Treatment of Prehospital Cardiopulmonary Arrest." *Annals of Emergency Medicine* 19 (1990): 1407-1411.

Valenzuela, T. D., E. A. Criss, et al. "Computer Modeling of EMS System Performance." *Annals of Emergency Medicine* 19 (1990): 898-901.

Valenzuela, T. D., K. T. Keeley, E. A. Criss, et al. "Implementation of a Computerized Prehospital Management Information System in an Urban Fire Department." *Annals of Emergency Medicine* 18 (1989): 573-578.

Valenzuela, T., E. A. Criss EA, K. Facter, et al. "Medical Versus Regulatory Necessity: Regulation of Ambulance Service in Arizona." *Journal of Emergency Medicine* 7 (1989): 253-256.

Warnke, W. J., and M. J. Bonnin. "Direction and Motivation of Prehospital Personnel to Do Research: How to Do it Better." *Prehospital and Disaster Medicine* 7 (1992): 79-83.

Weaver, W. D., D. Hill, C. E. Fahrenbruch, et al. "Use of the Automatic External Defibrillator in the Management of Out-of-Hospital Cardiac Arrest." *New England Journal of Medicine* 319 (1988): 661-666.

Weaver, W. D., L. A. Cobb, A. P. Hallstrom, et al. "Considerations for Improving Survival from Out-of-Hospital Cardiac Arrest." *Annals of Emergency Medicine* 15 (1986): 1181-1186.

Wiederhold, R. "Integrated Information Management System." *Prehospital and Disaster Medicine* 7 (1992): 161-166.

Witte, M. H., A. Kerwin, C. L. Witte, et al. "A Curriculum on Medical Ignorance." *Medical Education* 23 (1989): 24-29.

Source

Reprinted with permission from Prehospital and Disaster Medicine, *January–March, 1993. The authors include Daniel W. Spaite, MD, FACEP; Terence D. Valenzuela, MD, FACEP; and Harvey W. Meislin, MD, FACEP. At the time of original publication, the authors were associated with the Arizona Emergency Medicine Research Center, College of Medicine, at the University of Arizona, Tucson.*

Why and How the Law Is Driving Patient Care Issues

Respecting a Patient's Right to Refuse Treatment

Spencer A. Hall, MD, JD

Dying with dignity is an increasingly accepted concept. Unfortunately, the legal framework governing EMS personnel's interaction with terminal patients has been slow to change. This article outlines the underlying legal doctrines and implications for medical transportation services.

ONE AREA OF MEDICINE HAS BEEN largely ignored when issues of patient refusal of treatment are discussed—EMS. EMS personnel are a diverse group, running the gamut from basic EMTs (with approximately 120 hours of training), who render care that is largely first aid, to highly trained paramedics (with more than 1,000 hours of training), who may establish airways, defibrillate, and administer drugs. These individuals may be volunteers who leave their routine jobs or households when paged or paid providers who make their living delivering EMS care.

What links these groups is the fact that they are usually the first individuals to encounter seriously ill patients entering the healthcare system. Thus, it is the EMS personnel who in many cases must decide, with input from medical control, whether to begin aggressive resuscitative efforts—efforts that are currently difficult for the patient or family to refuse. Given the lack of EMS training in this area, EMS personnel are probably also the least prepared to make this decision.

There is no need to recount the long history of court decisions and changes in public attitudes that have increasingly recognized an individual's right to refuse unwanted medical treatment as an integral part of personal autonomy. This personal autonomy is commonly defined by the phrase made famous by Judge (later U.S. Supreme Court Justice) Benjamin Cardozo, who said, "Every human being of adult years and sound mind has a right to determine what shall be done with his own body." This may also be stated in the negative as recognizing that "it is wrong to subject the actions (including choices) of others to controlling influences."

Advance Directives

This recognition of the importance of the right to refuse treatment has evolved to the point where by law—the Patient Self-Determination

Act (PSDA)—most institutional healthcare providers, such as hospitals and nursing homes, must inform individuals of their right to use advance directives to refuse treatment. This creates a problem, however. Although EMS personnel will encounter advance directives more often than before patients were informed of these rights, there is still no clear policy on how they may—or must—deal with them. Perhaps more troubling is how often EMS providers are taking the responsibility of withholding resuscitation into their own hands regardless of their legal ability to do so.

In the healthcare arena, advance directives usually involve either a living will or a durable power of attorney for healthcare. Living wills typically state that if a person has a terminal (i.e., fatal) condition that is confirmed by more than one physician, the stipulations of the document will be carried out. But the standard requirement for physician certification—usually not something available in the field—largely limits the living will to institutional use. Additionally, the common requirement that this document be a valid will under state law requires expertise that is not part of an EMS provider's routine training.

Durable powers of attorney for healthcare also have their shortcomings. These are documents that appoint someone other than the patient (called the surrogate) to make healthcare decisions for the patient. Again, the healthcare provider on the scene must determine whether the document is valid and whether it applies. Often, these factors are based on a determination of the surrogate's competency, which is legally beyond the scope of EMS providers. It also may be impossible to contact the designated surrogate decision maker before a decision must be made.

There are other reasons why advance directives may be ineffective in the prehospital setting. Both types are written documents and may be difficult to locate when urgently needed. Also, the decision whether to begin resuscitation must be made rapidly; the setting is a field situation, such as the patient's house or a ditch on the side of the road in the rain; the atmosphere is tense; and the personnel who must make the decision possess only minimal training and experience with respect to advance directives.

Attempts to remedy some of these shortcomings have been made in a number of states and are pending in others. And, while the National Association of State EMS Directors has now approved a consensus document that outlines suggested guidelines for recognizing prehospital refusals, each state has largely instituted its own plan, by statute or regulations, to deal with identifying individuals who do not want to receive prehospital resuscitation attempts. These advance directive systems allow a rapid, positive, and relatively precise identification, commonly by means of a bracelet, of those individuals who do not wish resuscitation by EMS personnel. The bracelets are not removable without destruction of their integrity. Removal or tampering constitutes voiding their effect.

The ethical shortfall lies in how—and which—individuals may obtain this bracelet in the first place. Usually a bracelet may be obtained only on a physician's authorization and often only on that physician's

Advance directives usually involve either a living will or a durable power of attorney for healthcare.

certification that the patient has a terminal medical condition. In some states, such as Virginia, the physician signing this document does not even have to be licensed to practice in that state or have any experience in dealing with EMTs.

Unfortunately, while these plans may aim to further patient autonomy, in practice they largely do not do this because of the number of stipulations imposed. Additionally, they raise some legal questions concerning the reciprocal honoring of the regulations of one state by the EMS personnel of another. EMTs are only licensed to practice in a certain state, usually under the medical control of a physician licensed to practice medicine in that state. It is potentially problematic for an EMT from one state to function under a physician licensed in another, as could occur when someone with a prehospital refusal valid in one state travels to another.

What seems to be happening in current prehospital right-to-refuse treatment practices is that individuals' rights to choose what happens to them are limited in several ways. For example, only the terminally ill are able to take advantage of the right to refuse EMS interventions. Furthermore, their refusal may only be applicable for a limited amount of time (e.g., monthly in New York, yearly in Virginia). Finally, implementation of this right is not the individual's sole personal decision; a physician must validate the person's wishes.

Restrictions on Refusal of Lifesaving Treatment

Several arguments support putting restrictions on refusal or limitation of potentially life-prolonging or lifesaving medical treatments. Many of these are similar to those made in the context of do-not-resuscitate (DNR) orders. (DNR orders are somewhat different than the issues being discussed here, although many of the ethical questions are similar. DNR orders are usually restricted to an institutional setting and are valid only for the length of the patient's stay in that institution.) The arguments seem to try to protect the medical profession's integrity by justifying providers' nonaction as someone dies.

The first argument concerns the traditional idea that consent for EMS is a given. Anyone calling for an ambulance is presumed to consent to whatever EMS personnel—and, later, physicians—do to them. There may be a problem, however, in applying this generalization to all people coming into contact with prehospital providers. Often, the person who calls EMS has no real relationship with the individual for whom he calls. For example, EMS may be called by a bystander or police officer who has neither knowledge of the individual's wishes in regard to life-prolonging treatment nor any actual authority to make medical decisions on the patient's behalf.

The second argument calls for withholding emergency treatment only for reasons of futility; it is considered acceptable to allow someone to refuse treatment if that person will not benefit from the treatment. Thus, if a patient is going to die anyway, there is no problem with allowing terminal patients to decline EMS treatment. For example, given the actual results of CPR without defibrillation, futility is often a given.

"Proper" Physician Involvement

The issue of "proper" physician involvement in refusal of prehospital care is somewhat ambiguous. Clearly, physicians are the only individuals who can provide the information necessary to allow someone to make an informed decision about refusing medical care. In fact, U.S. law allows lawsuits based on uninformed refusals.

The problem with prehospital right-to-refuse-treatment strategies is that the physician allowing the refusal often has nothing to do with the patient's later interaction with EMS. The physician signing the document is neither required to be knowledgeable about EMS nor, in some cases, to even be licensed in the state for which he is signing off. On the other hand, it is clearly impossible to foresee which physician will come into contact with a given EMS patient. Thus, what we think of as proper informed refusal may never be able to take place in this context. Yet this is no reason to preclude potential EMS patients—or anyone, for that matter—from their right to refuse treatment.

Currently, physician involvement in prehospital refusal of treatment seems to serve two purposes. The first is to determine if individuals wishing to invoke this right are competent and able to understand what their decision may mean to them in the future. The second is to ensure—at least in some states—that only terminally ill patients are able to make these types of decisions.

Challenges for EMS

By presuming consent to treatment and limiting treatment refusals to terminal patients, EMS does a disservice to those it serves; there is no reason to use people's illnesses or misfortunes to strip them of their right to personal autonomy. All individuals have a right to determine what happens to them. This includes refusing life-prolonging or lifesaving treatment.

Properly administered, EMS provides a valuable service by delivering what may well be lifesaving medical care to those who need it. Unwanted resuscitation attempts, on the other hand, often provide tragedy for families and friends. They also may violate personal autonomy.

Refusal of prehospital resuscitation does not require recognition of the problematic "right to die." It merely recognizes a person's basic right to refuse unwanted medical treatment.

Besides healthcare reform, the U.S. medical system is now struggling with an increased awareness of personal autonomy and the implementation of the PSDA requirements, and new awareness that CPR does not save as many lives as advertised. Surely, then, this is the appropriate time to extend recognition of personal autonomy to the prehospital sphere by implementing national standards for refusal of prehospital resuscita-

U.S. law allows lawsuits based on uninformed refusals.

Source

Reprinted with permission from JEMS, *May 1994. Spencer A. Hall is an emergency department physician in New Mexico. He is currently working to develop and write state regulations giving prehospital providers the right to recognize patient refusals.*

tion. It is also the time to allow individuals who do not want to receive aggressive prehospital resuscitation attempts to identify themselves in a manner less radical than that of the Arizona physician who had a DNR order tattooed on his chest.

There may be a way to do this. A national organization, the National Conference of Commissioners on Uniform State Laws, writes laws on important topics such as banking and business and tries to get the same laws passed in all states. The organization recently drafted the Uniform Health-Care Decisions Act, which simplifies the process anyone has to go through to create an advance directive and widens the scope of healthcare providers who may honor these without the necessity of further regulations. If enacted into law, this act would respect personal autonomy and make it easier for EMS to honor these autonomous decisions. As several states have done, EMS may want to look at this law closely and think about supporting it.

Whatever happens in healthcare during the next few years, EMS personnel are going to be making increasingly difficult decisions regarding patient care. It is important that the EMS industry take a united stand to ensure providers are legally protected and trained to make these decisions.

References

Areen, J. "Advance Directives Under State Law and Judicial Decisions." *Law, Medicine and Health Care* 19, no. 1-2 (1991): 91-200.

Bonnin, M. J., et al. "Distinct Criteria for Termination of Resuscitation in Out-of-Hospital Setting." *Journal of the American Medical Association* 270, no. 12 (1993): 1457-1462.

Childress, J. F. "The Place of Autonomy in Bioethics." *Hastings Center Report* 20, no. 1 (1990): 13.

Cohen, E. H. "Refusing and Forgoing Treatment." In *Treatise on Health Care Law*, eds. M. G. MacDonald, et al. New York: Matthew Bender, 1992.

"Giving Life to Patient Self-Determination." *Hastings Center Report* 23, no. 1 (1993): 12-24.

Gray, W. A. "Prehospital Resuscitation: The Good, the Bad and the Futile." *Journal of the American Medical Association* 270, no. 12 (1993): 1471-1472.

Hall, S. A. "New Act Compels EMS to Define New Roles." *JEMS* 17, no. 1 (1992): 19-20.

Iserson, K. V., and R. F. Rouse. "Case Studies: Prehospital DNR Orders." *Hastings Center Report* 19, no. 6 (1989): 17-19.

Iserson, K. V. "The No-Code Tattoo: An Ethical Dilemma." *West I Med* 156 (1992): 309-312.

Johnson, D. R., and W. A. Maggiore. "Resuscitation Decision Making by New Mexico Emergency Medical Technicians." *American Journal of Emergency Medicine* 11, no. 2 (1993): 139-141.

Kass, L. R. "Is There a Right to Die?" *Hastings Center Report* 23, no. 1 (1993): 34-43.

Kellerman, A. L., et al. "Predicting the Outcome of Unsuccessful Prehospital Advanced Cardiac Life Support." *Journal of the American Medical Association* 270, no 12 (1993): 1433-1436.

Neighmond, P. "Health Care in the United States" on National Public Radio's Morning Edition, 11-15 January 1993.

Rosoff, A. J. "Consent to Medical Treatment." In *Treatise on Health Care Law*, eds. M. G. MacDonald, et al. New York: Matthew Bender, 1992.

Sachs, G. S., et al. "Limiting Resuscitation: Emergency Policy in the Emergency Medical System." *Annals of Internal Medicine* (1991): 114-151-154.

Schloendorff v. Society of New York Hospital, 211 N.Y. at 129-130, 105 N.E. at 93.

The Patient Self-Determination Act (PSDA). In the *Omnibus Budget Reconciliation Act (OBRA) of 1990*, 42 USC §1395cc.

Truman v. Thomas, 611 P.2d 902 (1980).

Withholding Resuscitation: The Medical, Legal, and Ethical Concerns

W. Ann Maggiore, NREMT-P

THE ISSUE OF WITHHOLDING and withdrawing resuscitation in the prehospital emergency setting is fraught with controversy. Because EMTs and paramedics enter the field with limited training in medicine, law, or ethics, they are often unequipped to make defensible decisions regarding the merits of resuscitative measures in a given situation.

While a great deal has been written on the subject of withholding resuscitation in the hospital setting, little information exists regarding the prehospital provider's role when faced with the decision to initiate resuscitation when the patient is unlikely to benefit from such efforts or has expressly refused these measures via a living will. The medical community has long understood that resuscitative efforts may not be in the best interest of some patients. A New Jersey Supreme Court first granted the legal right to die to Karen Ann Quinlan in 1975. In the years since then, more than 40 states have enacted some type of right-to-die legislation. Yet the withholding and withdrawal of medical procedures continues to be a volatile medical, legal, and ethical issue. The following three case studies are indicative of the types of scenarios EMS providers are encountering in the field today.

Case Study One

EMTs responded to a call for a 30-year-old male who had suffered a grand mal seizure and gone into cardiac arrest. The patient had a history of chronic alcoholism. Family members initiated CPR and, shortly after, contacted 9-1-1. A BLS crew arrived about 35 minutes later, due to the remoteness of the residence. The patient presented with fixed and dilated pupils and had no pulse or spontaneous breathing. The EMTs elected not to continue resuscitation and did not contact their medical director from the scene.

Case Study Two

Urban paramedics were called to the home of an unresponsive patient. On arrival, they found an 88-year-old woman who was pulseless and apneic. There were no signs of rigor mortis or dependent lividity. Family members said the death was expected, as the patient was a terminal cancer victim, and they did not want resuscitation initiated. The paramedics applied a cardiac monitor and documented the presence of asystole. They did not initiate resuscitation, nor did they contact their medical director from the scene.

Author Winnie Maggiore explores the medical, legal, and ethical issues related to withholding resuscitation in the field. The complexity of these issues is highlighted through three common scenarios encountered by paramedics. The author reviews position statements of several national organizations and how "do not resuscitate" protocols have been successfully implemented by EMS agencies.

An oral refusal of CPR by a competent patient prior to illness and physician orders have also been recently recognized as constituting valid, legal reasons for withholding resuscitation.

Case Study Three

EMTs arrived at the scene of a motor vehicle accident that had occurred approximately 15 minutes earlier. A 60-year-old male was found inside the cab of an overturned pickup truck. The first EMT to arrive was told by a police officer at the scene that the patient was dead; no resuscitative efforts had been initiated by police or bystanders. When the EMT began to evaluate the patient, however, he found a weak pulse. The patient's airway was opened, and ventilation was initiated. Twenty minutes later, after he was extricated from the vehicle, the pulse was lost, and definitive airway management and CPR were begun. Upon arrival of an ALS crew, the patient was noted to be in asystole, and an order to discontinue resuscitation was elicited from a medical control physician over the radio.

EMS Training

The current U.S. Department of Transportation national standard curriculum for EMTs affords only one to two hours of discussion to the topic of medical-legal roles and responsibilities in the prehospital arena. During these lectures, terms such as ethics, do-not-resuscitate (DNR) orders, and standard of care are barely defined, and no substantive suggestions are offered for dealing with cases in which CPR might not benefit the patient.

Most paramedics receive specialized training in advanced cardiac life support (ACLS), an American Heart Association (AHA) certification that must be renewed either annually or biannually. An algorithm of treatment for each type of cardiac arrest rhythm is provided as a guideline. It is important to note that the AHA guidelines are simply that—guidelines to be used with other factors that define a legal standard of care. Because EMS training incorporates AHA guidelines for CPR, certain scenarios are adequately covered: CPR is to be initiated on all patients found pulseless and not breathing when there is a possibility that the brain is viable and when there is no legally or medically legitimate reason to withhold it. These reasons are defined as the presence of rigor mortis or dependent lividity, decapitation or transection of the body, and injuries in which brain matter is severely extruded. AHA standards allow for withdrawal of CPR only when the rescuer is exhausted or if the patient regains a pulse.

However, there are clearly other situations in which the administration of CPR may not benefit the patient. The duration of CPR efforts has been cited as being a possible criterion for deciding to withhold or terminate CPR, as it has been conclusively shown that failed prehospital resuscitative efforts continue to prove futile in the hospital.

With the advent of DNR orders and living wills, the medical system has also begun to recognize the rights of the patient in such matters. An oral refusal of CPR by a competent patient prior to illness and physician orders have also been recently recognized as constituting valid, legal reasons for withholding resuscitation. Such criteria raise particular concerns for EMS providers, who have only seconds in which to decide whether to begin resuscitation. In most cases, the provider has no prior relationship with the patient, no way to determine the patient's medical status prior to cardiac arrest and no way to know of his personal wishes about resuscitative efforts. In addition, attempts to discover how long a patient has been in cardiopulmonary arrest prior to the arrival of EMS units are usually futile, making it difficult to quantify the length of time the brain has been without oxygen. This lack of history puts the EMS provider at a great disadvantage when faced with the decision to begin resuscitative efforts.

EMS Practice

In addition to limited formal training on the issue of patient resuscitation, the medical-legal framework that governs local policies and protocols differs from state to state. A recent study showed that, out of 70 responding medical control physicians, 47 had no formal written policy or protocol regarding DNR orders. Without the benefit of such protocols, providers have no way of knowing what is allowed or expected in practice.

Developing training programs that address situations in which resuscitative efforts may not benefit a patient would ultimately help protect EMS providers from potential litigation. In addition, developing protocols that allow providers to make decisions based on patient survival statistics, such as the impact of time frames and distances from the hospital, would go a long way toward establishing legal protection in such instances.

For example, the EMTs in the first case study were well aware that their patient had little or no chance of survival. However, withholding resuscitation in this case was a deviation from AHA guidelines. Although the decision to withhold CPR probably had no effect on this patient's outcome, the EMTs' actions would probably be indefensible in the courts of many states. Proper training for this type of scenario could preclude assuming liability in such cases.

In the second case study, the paramedics ignored their existing protocols for patients in asystole, which specify that CPR, advanced airway management, and drug therapy should be initiated in such patients. These providers assumed serious legal risks in not doing so without physician consent. Additionally, the withholding of resuscitation in this case did not meet AHA guidelines, since there was no rigor or livor mortis. These paramedics might thus be subject to wrongful death litigation (from family members who were not present) for not acting in accordance with the standard of care. In many EMS systems, quality assurance reviews would target this behavior as a protocol violation. Once again, the existence of training and protocols for making such decisions would have helped to protect the paramedics in this case.

Furthermore, even in cases in which medical and ethical justification for such decisions exists, legal backing often does not. Studies have conclusively shown that patients who do not survive initial ACLS-level

Developing training programs that address situations in which resuscitative efforts may not benefit a patient would ultimately help protect EMS providers from potential litigation.

Because EMS providers are often not the first responders at the scene, they typically have to rely on determinations made prior to their arrival.

resuscitation in the field have extremely poor chances for neurologically intact survival when they reach the hospital. Yet, despite the fact that medical literature supports the decision to discontinue resuscitation after initial attempts, the legal backing for a provider's decision to discontinue resuscitation is often not articulated in protocols.

Another problem encountered in the field is that existing DNR orders or living wills are often not presented to EMS providers. And many EMTs and paramedics are trained to ignore this type of documentation when supplied by family members or nursing home staff due to liability concerns and lack of communication between private physicians and field providers. Even in situations in which a terminally ill patient is taken home to die, families often change their minds and summon EMS when the patient stops breathing. Especially trying are situations in which family members are divided, with one group insisting on immediate resuscitation, while the other camp threatens litigation if CPR is initiated. Confusion and high emotional drama are common at these scenes, and the EMS providers are under a great deal of pressure to make a quick decision.

Another frequent dilemma arises when prehospital providers are called to transport a patient from a nursing home to a hospital. While patients may have enacted a valid living will or be covered by a DNR order, providers may be restrained from recognizing that patient's wishes. Many areas require full resuscitative efforts for all patients, prompted by a fear of subsequent litigation.

Because EMS providers are often not the first responders at the scene, they typically have to rely on determinations made prior to their arrival. For example, in the third case study, the decision to withhold resuscitation was made 15 minutes prior to the arrival of EMS. Police officer training in patient assessment varies across the nation, from police who are cross-trained as paramedics to those who have never received any CPR training. The local police in this case study had no training whatsoever and therefore were in no position to perform patient assessment or make treatment decisions.

The second problem in this scenario involved the order to discontinue resuscitation. A radio order of this nature may have legal ramifications in a state such as New Mexico, which has no provisions for physicians transferring such responsibilities to field providers, a concept known as delegated practice. Yet while a New Mexico physician may not legally delegate practices that fall outside of the scope of EMT licensure, he can place limitations on situations in which resuscitation is initiated. The legal concern is that delegated practice has its limitations—the physician may be delegating a practice that is not within the scope of the EMT licensure.

Again, while the standard of withholding resuscitation in the trauma setting may be medically and ethically correct, it may not be legally defensible in the absence of training and protocols allowing this practice. The region covered in the third case study had no protocols or training to address situations in which withdrawal of CPR was appropriate. Still, the providers in the third case study had valid medical reasons to request permission to discontinue resuscitative measures.

Studies show that fewer than one percent of blunt-trauma victims who present without vital signs survive. However, many protocols either do not specifically allow EMS providers to withhold resuscitation from these patients or do not address the issue.

Solving the Problem

Several EMS systems have attempted to solve these dilemmas by devising systems in which those who may be involved in decisions to withhold resuscitation coordinate their efforts. Hennepin County, Minn., adopted DNR guidelines for long-term care facilities in 1985 and for hospice facilities in 1986. To date, there have been no legal challenges to Hennepin's system, and the local medical community has expressed considerable appreciation for the system. The system uses a standardized form, updated regularly with validation stamps, which the EMS providers recognize as a valid order to withhold resuscitative efforts.

Dallas County EMS in Texas has established a DNR protocol that identifies patients via a bracelet system. Patients who have completed the appropriate steps for DNR status constantly wear distinctive plastic bracelets that indicate their status; this eliminates the need to examine paperwork and the problems that can arise if the arrest does not occur at home. Providers are instructed to resuscitate these patients if the bracelets are altered or damaged in any way, which affords patients the opportunity to change their minds.

In 1980, the Los Angeles County EMS Agency instituted a policy that defines situations in which CPR may be withheld. The policy was revised in April 1988, after an individual who was pronounced dead in the field was later found to be exhibiting signs of life.

The American College of Emergency Physicians (ACEP) has also released a set of guidelines for withholding resuscitation in the prehospital setting. ACEP supports the notion that, in the absence of a valid DNR document and/or physician involvement, prehospital personnel should follow standard AHA guidelines. ACEP's position is that, although overtreatment may be the result, resuscitative efforts can be withdrawn in a controlled setting (i.e., hospital) when a more informed medical, legal, and ethical decision can be made by physicians. ACEP may not, however, have considered rural and wilderness situations, in which hours may elapse before the patient arrives at a hospital. ACEP guidelines specifically require that the decision not to resuscitate a patient in the prehospital setting be made by the on-line medical control physician (the one giving orders on the radio at the time of the incident).

The answer to the medical, legal, and ethical dilemmas of withholding or withdrawing resuscitation lies in the thorough integration of EMS providers with the medical and legal components of the decision-

> The answer to the medical, legal, and ethical dilemmas of withholding or withdrawing resuscitation lies in the thorough integration of EMS providers with the medical and legal components of the decision-making process.

making process. EMS providers and physicians must work with agencies such as the AHA and the Department of Transportation to revise the national curriculum and standards for prehospital resuscitation. The standard of care needs to be changed to ensure that the wishes of patients are recognized and that treatment that is not beneficial is no longer automatically rendered.

The answer also lies in the training and preparation of providers for the decisions that lie ahead in practice. Training is both part of the problem and part of the solution: EMS training needs to be updated to include current legal frameworks, modern ethical values, and the findings of recent medical studies.

When developing local protocols, EMS providers and medical control directors should first examine the legal relationship set forth by their state. Within that framework, protocols and training programs should be developed that reflect how a patient's wishes will be incorporated in prehospital care, as well as how providers will handle situations in which resuscitative efforts may not benefit the patient.

Prehospital providers should request that their medical directors write clear protocols that have been reviewed by legal counsel. Additionally, medical directors should ensure that the emergency responders follow them through quality assurance programs. Any time that doubt exists as to the validity of a DNR order or a living will, resuscitation should be initiated, and voice contact should be made with on-line medical control.

Right-to-die legislation will also play a role in how EMS handles resuscitation issues. Situations in which CPR may be withheld need to be clearly outlined by law in a cooperative effort by all participants. Methods for EMTs and paramedics to recognize living wills and DNR orders should be devised. In states in which legislation does not address these issues, efforts must be undertaken toward that end. Legislation may be needed to support the medical community, help avoid malpractice litigation, and provide care in accordance with medical standards and the patient's wishes.

While common EMS practices may be medically defensible, they often raise serious legal and ethical concerns. EMS providers should not make on-scene decisions to withhold or withdraw resuscitative efforts without enlisting physician involvement. The legal relationship between field providers and physicians in a given state should guide the type of physician involvement necessary. Criteria for decision making should be thoroughly discussed in both training and protocol development.

References

American College of Emergency Physicians. "Guidelines for Do Not Resuscitate Orders in the Prehospital Setting." *Annals of Emergency Medicine* (October 1988).

American Heart Association. *Textbook of Advanced Cardiac Life Support*. Dallas: American Heart Association, 1987.

American Medical Association. "Standards and Guidelines for Cardiopulmonary Resuscitation and Emergency Care." *Journal of the American Medical Association* 227 (June 1986).

Ayres, J. "Current Controversies in the Prehospital Resuscitation of the Terminally Ill Patient." *Prehospital and Disaster Medicine* (January–March 1990).

Ayres, J. "Do Not Resuscitate Orders." *Emergency Department Law* (28 September 1989).

Baruch, B. "Resuscitating a Patient with No Vital Signs." *Ethics in Emergency Medicine.* Williams & Wilkins Publishing, 1986.

Bonnin, M. "Outcomes in Unsuccessful Field Resuscitation Attempts." *Annals of Emergency Medicine* (May 1989).

"Calling 911 Preempts Power of Living Wills." *Arkansas Democrat,* 1 October 1990.

Crimmins, T. "The Need for a Prehospital DNR System." *Prehospital and Disaster Medicine* (January–March 1990).

Department of Health Services, County of Los Angeles. *Withholding or Discontinuing Resuscitation* (prehospital care policy manual). Los Angeles: Los Angeles Department of Health Services, 1989.

Haynes, et al. "Letting Go: DNR Orders in Prehospital Care." *Journal of the American Medical Association* 254 (26 July 1985).

In the Matter of Karen Quinlan. 70 N.J. 10, 355 A2d 647 (1976).

Kellerman, A. L. "In-Hospital Resuscitation Following Unsuccessful Prehospital Advanced Cardiac Life Support: Heroic Efforts or an Exercise in Futility?" *Annals of Emergency Medicine* (June 1988).

Miles, S., and T. Crimmins. "Orders to Limit Emergency Treatment for an Ambulance Service in a Large Metropolitan Area." *Journal of the American Medical Association* 254 (26 July 1985).

Shanaberger, C. J. "Medical Control Physicians and DNR Protocols." *Annals of Emergency Medicine* (July 1988). Abstract.

Stratton, S. "Withholding CPR in the Prehospital Setting." *Prehospital and Disaster Medicine* (January–March 1990).

U.S. Department of Transportation, National Highway Safety Administration. *Emergency Medical Technician-Paramedic: National Standard Curriculum.* Washington, D.C.: U.S. Department of Transportation, 1985.

Source

Reprinted with permission from JEMS, *July 1991. W. Ann (Winnie) Maggiore, NREMT-P, has over 10 years of rural and urban paramedic experience. Her firm, New Mexico MedLegal Consultants, provides EMS training and paralegal consulting.*

A Review of Prehospital Care Litigation in a Large Metropolitan EMS System

Richard J. Goldberg, MD; John L. Zautcke, MD, FACEP; Max D. Koenigsberg, MD, FACEP; Ron W. Lee, MD, FACEP; Frank W. Nagorka, JD, EMT-P; Mark King, MD; and Sharon A. Ward, RN

Dr. Goldberg and his associates conducted a 12-year study of patient care-related lawsuits filed against the Chicago Fire Department's EMS program. The results indicated, among other things, that incidents of litigation were increasing. This analysis provides insight on "common acts of omission" that could subject an EMS system to litigation.

DURING THE PAST DECADE, the practice of medicine has changed radically. A significant factor in this change has been an increase in malpractice claims. As a clearly recognized component of the healthcare system, emergency medical services personnel are likely to be affected by this trend. The impact of the legal system on the delivery of prehospital care may be significant and long-lasting.

National and state trends in hospital- and physician-targeted litigation have been well documented. In Illinois, a steady increase in malpractice claims has been noted during the past decade. While reviews of malpractice trends and litigation involving physicians and hospitals have been widely addressed and discussed, there are limited data on the incidence of malpractice in the prehospital setting. Soler, et al., published a retrospective review of prehospital litigation incidence in Dade County, Fla., from 1972 through 1982. Their data indicated an incidence of approximately one lawsuit for every 24,000 paramedic-patient encounters. A trend of increasing litigation during the study period was noted. However, the number of cases was too small to determine any statistical significance.

This study involved a retrospective review of all prehospital care-related litigation filed against the city of Chicago and city paramedics during the 12-year period from 1976 through 1987. In addition to quantifying the incidence of lawsuit claims within our system, we sought to determine whether the number of claims was increasing. Our hypothesis was that litigation incidence in the prehospital setting would parallel the increasing trend seen elsewhere in our healthcare system. In addition, we sought to identify various descriptive aspects of EMS-related litigation to better understand the high-risk liability areas in prehospital care. The economic and legal outcomes of the litigation were also reviewed.

Methods

The Chicago municipal ambulance service serves a population of more than three million. The fire department ambulances furnish initial response for emergencies when the call for assistance comes through the 9-1-1 system. All municipal ambulances are equipped with advanced life support (ALS) capabilities. Two paramedics staff each ambulance, with the paramedics working 24-hour shifts (8 a.m. to 8 a.m.). Overall, fire department ambulances respond to approximately 170,000 calls per year and transport more than 100,000 patients per year.

The 9-1-1 system is organized to provide police intervention first. If a medical problem is identified, emergency calls are subsequently forwarded to the fire ambulance dispatch. The system design provides for medical control jurisdiction only after the paramedics are contacted.

Criteria for patient transport in this system are very liberal. Patients who are competent to refuse treatment or transport and decide that they do not want to be taken to the hospital will not be transported.

We conducted a retrospective review of lawsuits brought against the Chicago Fire Department EMS Bureau. Cases that involved a paramedic as a city employee and not as a healthcare provider were excluded. Cases involving solely dispatch irregularities before paramedic contact were also excluded. Because the 9-1-1 dispatch system is not formally incorporated within the EMS system, there is no medical control accountability until the paramedics are notified.

Data collection involved an in-depth review of prehospital run forms, resource hospital telemetry forms, pretrial depositions, pretrial motions, trial proceedings, and receiving hospital records. Each case underwent a primary review by one of the authors to extract the initial data and a secondary team review to establish the completeness and validity of the original findings. The second team consisted of one or more base station physicians, an off-line prehospital medical control director, a base station mobile intensive care nurse, and a paramedic lawyer.

While the general descriptive data included cases through 1987, the incidence data were derived for cases from 1976 through 1985 only. (The statute of limitations had not yet expired for 1986 and 1987, and new claims continued to be filed.) Consequently, any analysis of the incidence of lawsuit claims includes a sample size of 60, whereas the descriptive data include six additional cases from 1986 and 1987. Because cases often named more than one defendant and more than one alleged cause of action, analysis of the data involved a larger number of sample items (Figures 4.3 and 4.4). Where appropriate, x^2 goodness-of-fit statistical analyses were used.

Results

The total number of lawsuit claims during the incidence study period (1976 through 1985) was 60. The overall incidence during this

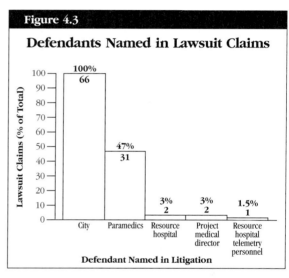

Figure 4.3

Defendants Named in Lawsuit Claims

Lawsuit Claims (% of Total) vs. Defendant Named in Litigation

- City: 100%, 66
- Paramedics: 47%, 31
- Resource hospital: 3%, 2
- Project medical director: 3%, 2
- Resource hospital telemetry personnel: 1.5%, 1

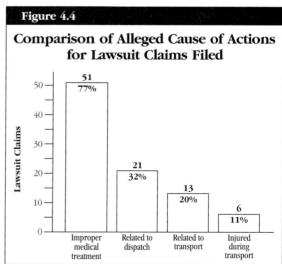

Figure 4.4

Comparison of Alleged Cause of Actions for Lawsuit Claims Filed

Lawsuit Claims

- Improper medical treatment: 51, 77%
- Related to dispatch: 21, 32%
- Related to transport: 13, 20%
- Injured during transport: 6, 11%

10-year period was one lawsuit per 27,371 paramedic-patient encounters and one lawsuit per 17,995 patient transports. Paramedic-patient encounters included all patients evaluated by paramedics in the field regardless of whether they subsequently were transported to the hospital.

As expected, the city, perceived as the "deep pocket," was named in all cases. The paramedics were specifically named in 47 percent of the cases (Figure 4.3). The resource hospital, project medical director, and telemetry personnel were rarely named as defendants.

The majority of cases (65 percent) involved adults ages 21 to 60 years (Figure 4.5). Male patients were involved in a slightly larger number of cases (55 percent versus 45 percent). An equally large number of cases involved African-Americans and Caucasians (46 percent each), whereas fewer cases involved Hispanics (six percent) or other ethnic groups (two percent). Except for the low number of cases involving Hispanic patients, these findings appear consistent with overall city demographics. A determination of whether certain demographic variables increase the relative likelihood of litigation could not be made because the fire department does not keep statistics on the demographic characteristics of patients served.

The percentages of claims based on the patient's problem (medical versus traumatic) and outcome are shown in Figure 4.6. All non-traumatic conditions such as obstetric, pediatric, and medical are grouped together as "medical" in our classification. Nearly one-third of the cases involved cardiac arrest. Claims involving traumatic death were the second largest group (22 percent). Patients with non-lethal traumatic injuries accounted for 15 percent of lawsuit claims, whereas those with primary respiratory arrest were the next largest group, accounting for 12 percent of the claims. However, trauma was not associated with increased litigation disproportional to its share of paramedic runs. Trauma-related cases accounted for approximately 33 percent of all system runs during the study period and trauma cases accounted for 37 percent of all litigation during this same period ($p > 0.05$). On the other hand, patient death, regardless of the cause, did increase the likelihood of litigation ($p < 0.01$).

A relatively larger number of lawsuit

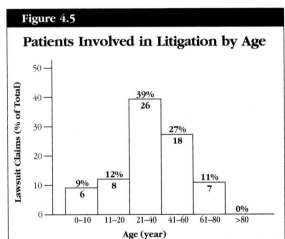

Figure 4.5

Patients Involved in Litigation by Age

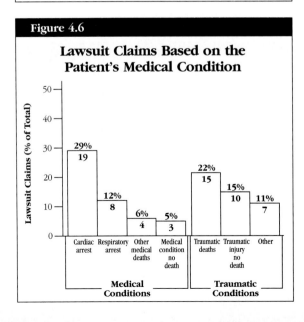

Figure 4.6

Lawsuit Claims Based on the Patient's Medical Condition

claims were generated from events that occurred toward the end of the paramedics' 24-hour shift (Figure 4.7). However, this was not statistically significant ($p = 0.13$).

In the beginning of the study period, only one or two lawsuits per 100,000 ambulance runs were noted, whereas toward the end of the decade, four to seven lawsuits per 100,000 ambulance runs were noted (Figure 4.8). When total ambulance volume was nearly constant, the number of lawsuit claims increased (Figure 4.9). A comparison of lawsuit claims from the first five years of the study period and the second five years showed that three times as many suits were filed during the period from 1981 through 1985 (45 cases) than during the period from 1976 through 1980 (15 cases) ($p < 0.0001$). The total number of ambulance runs was nearly identical during each of the five-year periods.

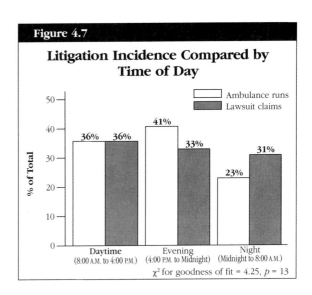

Figure 4.7

Litigation Incidence Compared by Time of Day

Cause of action was classified into four groups: those related to improper medical treatment, those related to dispatch (after paramedic notification), those related to transport, and those related to injuries occurring during transport. Improper medical treatment involved such allegations as improper technique, omission of treatment, missed diagnosis, and inappropriate care for the specific condition of the patient. Cases related to dispatch involved delays in ambulance arrival at the scene. Cases related to transport included situations with alleged transport delays once at the scene, transport to an inappropriate medical facility, or patients not being transported who later developed a deterioration of their condition.

Lawsuit claims often listed more than one alleged cause of action. More than three-fourths of lawsuit claims alleged improper medical treatment, whereas just less than one-third of the cases involved alleged delays in ambulance arrival (Figure 4.4). A smaller percentage of cases involved problems related to transport or injury during transport.

Litigation outcome data revealed that, to date, 25 cases (38 percent) have been closed (i.e., dropped by the plaintiff or settled, either in or out of court). Of the closed cases, seven (28 percent) were dropped by the plaintiff without money changing hands. More than two-thirds of these cases involved out-of-court settlements in which an agreed-upon sum of money was given to the plaintiff (without judgment)

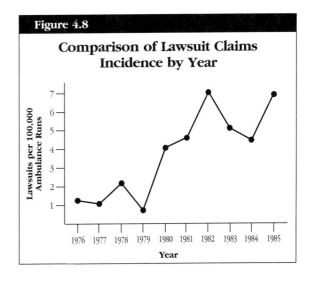

Figure 4.8

Comparison of Lawsuit Claims Incidence by Year

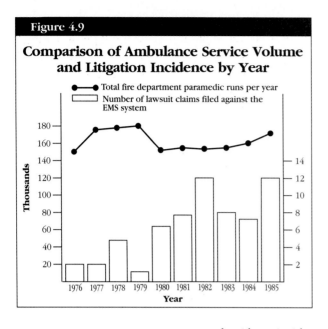

Figure 4.9

Comparison of Ambulance Service Volume and Litigation Incidence by Year

in exchange for having the plaintiff drop the case. Less than one-third of all closed cases involved awards of more than $5,000. The majority of cases involved small awards or no money awarded at all; 17 awards (68 percent) were $5,000 or less. The mean award was $13,664 (range, $0 to $150,000). Total monies awarded for all closed cases was $341,600. Only two of the 25 closed cases went to trial. Of these, one case was dropped by the plaintiff before the verdict, while the other case was ruled in favor of the defendant without any monetary award.

Discussion

The incidence of lawsuit claims involving the Chicago city paramedics was relatively low and comparable to previous rates reported, with an incidence of approximately one per 27,000 paramedic-patient encounters. However, there was a definite trend of increasing litigation during the study period. While many factors, including recent medical malpractice law reforms, make it difficult to anticipate future prehospital litigation incidence, these data suggest that increases in prehospital medical litigation may continue.

These data also show that resource hospitals, project medical directors, and base station telemetry personnel are rarely named in prehospital litigation. Whether personal injury lawyers in the future will view medical control personnel and institutions as another "deep pocket" remains to be seen.

Although trauma patients accounted for one-third of litigation, traumatic conditions are not associated with increased litigation relative to other medical conditions. However, poor patient outcome (i.e., death), whether from trauma or serious medical conditions, greatly increases the likelihood of litigation.

Our review indicated that the most common cause of legal action involved acts of omission. Examples of omitted actions included not arriving in a timely fashion, not providing ALS care, not transporting in a timely fashion, and not transporting a patient who refused care. We conclude from this that prehospital providers should be encouraged to provide aggressive management when any doubt exists. Periodic continuing education sessions on these medicolegal aspects of prehospital care might be useful in accomplishing this.

The study had certain limitations. We cannot be certain that all appropriate EMS-related litigation during the study period was located and included, although every effort was made through manual and computer searches to find all appropriate cases. In addition, because our analysis did not include cases of dispatch irregularities that involved problems with police forwarding of calls, potentially significant cases may have been omitted. These types of cases do not directly impact medical control liability, but they cannot be treated lightly in the context of overall system liability exposure. Further, there may be incidence data inaccuracy involving pediatric cases due to the extended statute of limitations. The statute allows for delayed filing until the age of 18 years. However, our data have shown no cases being filed any more than two years from the time of the alleged incident.

Although our incidence data appear comparable to data in the literature, the descriptive aspects of our data may not apply to other EMS systems. Factors such as system organization, structure, and size; types of communities served; and level of prehospital care service are likely to influence the incidence and types of prehospital litigation in a given system. Furthermore, our study does not address the question of prehospital litigation involving private ambulance providers. Private providers in the study system did respond to a very small number of emergency cases (not through the 9-1-1 system). A study of liability and the legal and economic impact on private providers might reveal a different set of incidence and descriptive data. This is particularly true as a large percentage of private provider transports involve nursing home patient transfers, which is clearly a different patient population.

The economic impact of litigation in the Chicago EMS system has been relatively small ($341,600 for the entire 12-year period). However, this figure does not include the cost of Chicago's large in-house governmental legal department and so may greatly underestimate the actual economic impact of prehospital litigation in other systems.

Because approximately two-thirds of claims are still open cases, the outcome data may be unrepresentative of the full data set. This large group of open cases may be attributable to the county's backlog of legal cases; for example, the Cook County court backlog for personal injury cases is nearly 70,000 cases.

Conclusion

Prehospital litigation in the Chicago EMS system shows an overall lawsuit claims incidence of one lawsuit for every 27,371 paramedic-patient encounters, comparable to rates reported in the literature. During the 10-year period from 1976 through 1985, a significant trend of increasing litigation was noted. Resource hospitals, project medical directors, and telemetry personnel were rarely named as defendants. While patient death increases the likelihood of litigation, traumatic conditions are not associated with increased litigation.

While the majority of prehospital litigation cases are still open and unresolved, an analysis of the closed cases indicates that many cases are

Source

Reprinted with permission from Annals of Emergency Medicine, *May 1990. At the time of original publication, authors Richard J. Goldberg, MD; John L. Zautcke, MD, FACEP; Max D. Koenigsberg, MD, FACEP; and Mark King, MD, were with the University of Illinois Affiliated Hospitals Emergency Medicine Residency. Ron W. Lee, MD, FACEP, and Frank W. Nagorka, JD, EMT-P, were with the Department of Internal Medicine, Loyola University of Chicago. Sharon A. Ward, RN, was with the Chicago North EMS System, Illinois Masonic Medical Center, Chicago.*

settled without money changing hands. Of the 25 closed cases, only two actually went to court. The total monies awarded for all closed cases to date is only $341,600, exclusive of government legal expenses. However, with the majority of cases still open, interpretation of the litigation outcome data must be made with caution.

Acknowledgments

The authors extend special thanks to Mary Slattery for manuscript preparation as well as to Quin Heath and Mylowe Wooley for graph and figure preparations.

References

Illinois State Medical Inter-Insurance Exchange. *Annual Report.* Chicago: ISMIIE, 1986.

Rapp, J. A., M. T. Rapp, R. E. Rapp, et al. *Illinois Medical Malpractice: A Guide for the Health Sciences.* St. Louis: CV Mosby Co., 1988.

Soler, J. M., M. F. Montes, A. B. Egol, et al. "The Ten-Year Malpractice Experience of a Large Urban EMS System." *Annals of Emergency Medicine* 14 (1985): 982-985.

U.S. Department of Commerce. *1980 Census of Population. General Population Characteristics, Pt 15: Illinois.* Washington, D.C.: U.S. Department of Commerce, August 1982, 15-76.

The Most Effective Intervention: Electricity in the Field

AN INCREASING NUMBER of EMS agencies and first responder organizations nationwide are developing early defibrillation programs, in which automatic or semi-automatic external defibrillators (AEDs) are used by basic EMTs and first responder/public safety personnel. As more of these programs are implemented, there is an increasing need for good systems by which to report, collect, and manage outcome data. A recent article in the *Journal of the American Medical Association*, for instance, outlines a comprehensive framework for early defibrillation developed by the state of California that includes statewide requirements for reporting outcomes. Such efforts are likely to be initiated by other states as well.

The collection and management of outcome data from early defibrillation programs is useful for a number of reasons, but primarily for assisting EMS personnel in improving survival rates. Because rapid delivery of defibrillation by first responders increases the chance of survival in cardiac arrest patients, it is crucial that EMS providers document and analyze how defibrillation and other components of the EMS system affect patient outcome. It is only through documentation that new programs can be justified and old programs improved.

Currently, there is no standardized method for collecting and managing early defibrillation data. As a result, EMS agencies and first responder organizations have taken it upon themselves to create systems that best suit their individual needs. Only by understanding the value of defibrillation data and becoming familiar with the various data collection and management systems available can services be at the forefront of implementing successful early defibrillation programs.

Why Collect Data?

"The bottom line for any EMS system is to save lives," said Vicki

The Data Game: Making the Most of Early Defibrillation

Cynthia L. Pollock, MSJ

If early defibrillation is to become more widely accepted as an integral component of EMS, then additional data must be collected at the local level to demonstrate its effectiveness. This article outlines minimum data elements that must be collected and suggests options for creating a collection system that works.

Data from early defibrillation programs have multiple uses, from assessing an individual crew member's performance to justifying program and personnel expenditures to tracking statewide or national trends.

Ginger, RN, clinical nurse specialist with the Houston Fire Department. "Statistical information can help us show how many lives actually are saved by early defibrillation. This type of data can prove why the first responder role is so critical."

Data from early defibrillation programs have multiple uses, from assessing an individual crew member's performance to justifying program and personnel expenditures to tracking statewide or national trends. Probably the most important reason for EMS and first responder agencies to collect and manage these data, however, is to ensure a high level of patient care. "One of our primary goals is to make sure that deviations don't happen and our patients are treated correctly," commented John Strock, division instructor with the San Diego Fire Department (SDFD).

Early defibrillation data also can reveal how an EMS system performs regarding cardiac arrest patients. Data derived from these patients are often more complete than the information that is gathered from trauma victims and thus can serve as one of the prime indicators of the EMS system's performance, according to Paul Anderson, director of the Idaho EMS system.

Finally, hard data that quantify the success of early defibrillation can help EMS agencies obtain the support and funding necessary to create or expand an early defibrillation program. "A lot of information is needed to find out if you're doing the right thing for the right people—to see if there is something [you] can do to change the death rate from cardiac arrest," remarked Sheldon Glazer, MD, a medical consultant to the British Columbia Ambulance Service in Canada.

The type of defibrillation data collected and reported by EMS agencies and first responder organizations to local and state authorities varies widely throughout the nation. In California, for example, an outcome-reporting requirement mandates that all defibrillation programs involving basic EMTs, first responders, or other public safety personnel collect and report annually to the state's Emergency Medical Services Authority the following information:

- The number of patients defibrillated
- The number of these patients who suffered a witnessed cardiac arrest and were initially in ventricular fibrillation
- The number of the patients initially in ventricular fibrillation who were discharged from the hospital

Other types of defibrillation data typically collected include

- Age and sex of patient
- Arrest location
- Length of time a patient was unattended after cardiac arrest
- Whether bystander CPR was initiated and by whom
- Response times
- Initial monitored rhythm
- Identification of crew members
- Whether protocol was properly followed

- Whether defibrillator equipment had been checked daily
- Equipment failures
- Shockable calls versus non-shockable calls
- Outcome

Because time is so crucial to ensuring the success of early defibrillation, most EMS agencies and fire departments with early defibrillation programs routinely check that response time standards are being met. "If you want to know if your system and field personnel are working properly, you need to know response time," Glazer explained. "How long did it take from the time of the call for the first responders to get to the scene?" he asked. "How long did it take from the time they got to the scene until they delivered the first shock? What were the times between shocks?"

At some point in the near future, there likely will be more standardization in the type of information gathered during prehospital cardiac resuscitation. Standardization will become increasingly important as more data are captured and analyzed on an international basis. However, emergency medical systems around the world still use different definitions of such common terms as "CPR," "basic life support," "admission," and "survivor."

To help standardize nomenclature for reporting outcome data from cardiac arrest, members of the international medical community met at a conference in December 1990 and created a set of data reporting recommendations called the "Utstein style." These recommendations include a template approach to gathering cardiac arrest data and reporting outcomes that allows EMS systems to compare their results with each other and to improve their internal method of quality assurance. The Utstein style and future recommendations of this sort should help ensure that every EMS system is collecting data in the same manner and using the same definitions.

Consolidation and review of defibrillation data in a city, county, state, or national database can help public safety agencies (police, fire, and EMS) track trends—both from an internal standpoint and in comparison to departments elsewhere. "When data are consolidated in a database at a central office somewhere, you're able to see trends that you wouldn't necessarily see looking at individual communities," Idaho's Anderson explained.

Defibrillation data also allow for feedback to EMS personnel regarding performance and patient outcome. Many early defibrillation programs track the outcome of all cardiac arrest patients. This information is then relayed to specific crew members—usually in the form of a letter generated by the medical director of the defibrillation program—to provide feedback on their performance.

The San Francisco Fire Department, which has collected cardiac arrest information for more than six years, has fostered a good working relationship with hospitals in that city. This allows the department to easily obtain information about patients within one week, according to Odie Braun, MD, the department's medical director.

> Consolidation and review of defibrillation data in a city, county, state, or national database can help public safety agencies (police, fire, and EMS) track trends—both from an internal standpoint and in comparison to departments elsewhere.

"When delivering early defibrillation, the EMS crew must receive clear feedback to help them learn what they're doing right and wrong," Braun explained. "If we notice that one crew member is having specific problems, we address that in a letter. If the problems continue, we retrain the person. If we notice that all defibrillator operators are making the same kinds of mistakes, we change our training process."

Reviews of defibrillation data allow problems—with either the operator or the equipment—to be spotted and resolved immediately. Periodic critique sessions using data from actual defibrillation run recordings also improve training, ultimately enhancing patient care.

Facilitating Data Management

Having the right kind of equipment for data collection and management improves an EMS system's ability to monitor the performance and training of the providers as well as its overall system performance.

During operation, most AEDs or semi-AEDs automatically collect critical patient and device information for later review and analysis. Thus, complete documentation of the defibrillation is available immediately after use of the defibrillator.

AEDs currently on the market use either a memory module or tape recorder-based system to gather information on cardiac arrest runs. Both systems capture and store EKG information as well as device data, such as time, date, serial number, messages, and shock information. AEDs that rely on memory modules also come with two-channel tape recorders to record operators' voices and any backup EKGs. The information stored in memory modules can be downloaded into a computer or printed out through a memory-module reader. The data stored with the tape-based defibrillators can be played back using special players and can be loaded into a computer or printed out on a strip-chart recorder.

Once defibrillation information is collected by EMS personnel during a run, it can be transferred to a central location for review. EMS agencies and first responder organizations transfer data from memory modules and tapes in different ways—via car, mail, modem, or facsimile—depending largely on the department's size and geographic location and on the degree of its computer and communication capabilities.

The process of data entry varies by department, and some systems use a variety of techniques. For many departments, memory-module readers and tape recorders are used to download information directly into computers, while tape players are used to review the recordings of the defibrillator runs. Supplementary documentation is entered manually on a keyboard.

Sophisticated computer hardware and software programs promote efficient and quick analysis and storage of information on line. Such programs save data from the memory modules and tapes in the computer to be viewed on screen, copied, or distributed to other locations.

The latest communications capabilities allow EMS systems—particularly larger ones that often need to move data to a central location for collection, processing, and analysis, such as the largely rural Idaho EMS—to connect a central computer with any number of remote computers through standard telephone lines and modems. This type of system allows incident information to be entered remotely, thereby reducing the amount of data entry by a system clerk. It also enables states to consolidate their information to create a statewide network and database. Such a system will also prove useful as more EMS data are collected on a nationwide basis.

Other features of advanced software packages include

- Creation of individual defibrillation run records
- Ability to review and edit data
- Analysis of data
- Creation of customized reports
- Tracking and evaluation of EMS
- Performance

Creating a System that Works

The following case studies reveal the diversity of data collection/management systems currently used by EMS agencies and first responder organizations.

The first case study presents an in-depth look at the San Diego Fire Department (SDFD), outlining the specific tasks involved in defibrillation data collection and management. The second case study, of the Idaho EMS system, describes an approach that a rural area has taken to improve efficiency. The third case details a new method of data handling implemented by several first responder organizations in San Diego County.

SDFD—Straightforward and Thorough

Every fire engine and truck company in the city of San Diego has a defibrillator under the review of the SDFD. In a typical cardiac arrest run, engine companies in the city are usually the first on the scene with semi-AEDs. San Diego uses a simple, straightforward system of collecting and managing data from its defibrillation program—a system that works well but relies heavily on manual data input.

Once a cardiac patient has been transported, the company captain receives the time of the incident via pager and then completes a generic EMT-D cardiac arrest report form. When the crew members return to the station, they restock their defibrillator with a new microcassette tape and a fresh memory module. The used memory module, tape, and EMT-D/cardiac arrest report are placed in a special EMT-D mailer and are sent via interoffice mail to the EMS coordinator. A crew member also calls the coordinator about the run and reports any problems, deviations from protocols, or equipment failures.

Once the coordinator receives the EMT-D mailer containing all of the run data, an EMT-D control number is assigned to the incident. These assigned numbers are divided into two categories—shockable and non-shockable—and are recorded in an EMT-D incident log. The EMS coordinator then reviews the cardiac arrest report for completeness and accuracy, transfers information from the memory module to the EMT-D database, and stores it on disk (the module is then returned to the crew for reuse in the field). He next prints the event log and EKG, evaluates event logs and tapes, and determines patient outcome. The incident is then logged in the EMT-D quality assurance tracking file.

After auditing the tape and reviewing the cardiac arrest report, event log and EKG, the coordinator identifies any issues of note about the run and documents these on the QA form. Any actions that may be needed are listed along with any follow-up that has been completed.

The coordinator then compiles a package for the base hospital consisting of the incident tape, cardiac arrest report, event log, EKG, and QA form. The medical director or designee at the base hospital reviews all of the paperwork and tapes, identifies any other issues, and makes any additional actions or recommendations. One copy of the event log and QA form is kept with the medical director, and two copies are returned with the remaining paperwork and tape to the coordinator for further review.

The crew then receives feedback about the run and takes any necessary action as indicated on the QA form, recording its compliance in the follow-up section. This form is then returned to the coordinator for filing and future audits.

Any deviation—defined by the SDFD as an act, procedure, or departure from established policies and protocols—that appears to have occurred is documented in the EMT-D deviation log, after which the coordinator contacts the base hospital to discuss the possible deviation. The medical director or designee and the coordinator then collectively determine what actions should be taken.

Idaho EMS System—Linking Rural Areas

This statewide program has 200 ambulance and quick response units (QRUs), all of which will one day be equipped with semi-AEDs. Four field offices oversee the provider units in specific geographic areas of the state; these offices are interconnected via software and modem, creating a statewide network. This enables defibrillation data to flow easily and quickly from each field office into a central office in Boise, consolidating information on all automated defibrillator arrest runs into one statewide database.

After a typical cardiac arrest run, the EMS crew or unit delivers or mails the memory module, the tape, and a copy of the run sheet or report to the field office, where the information is transferred into a computer.

A training specialist and medical director review a copy of the run report as well as information from the memory module and tape. Information from each incident is stored at the field office in an individual file. A hard-copy printout of the memory-module information and the memory module itself are returned to the appropriate EMS personnel or unit for review. At a designated time, the field office computer autodials the modem at the main office in Boise and transmits the new data, which are then reviewed by a state training coordinator and added to the statewide database.

San Diego County—Modems Speed Data Delivery

A number of fire departments in San Diego County are now on the cutting edge of collecting and managing defibrillation data. When four fire departments—San Miguel, Bostonia, Alpine, and Lakeside—began developing early defibrillation programs in 1989, they ran into a major hurdle: They did not like the idea of transporting the defibrillators' memory modules by car to the base station after each run or sending them via the mail. They solved the problem by contracting with an information processing company that helped them create a system to send information over the phone lines.

The system's simple design allows information from the memory module to be downloaded into a computer directly at the fire station using a memory-module reader and special software. The data are transferred to the base station over a phone line by modem.

The goal eventually is to link all of the departments in the area by modem to improve the overall defibrillation information system by saving time and money.

Conclusion

Defibrillation data can reveal much about the efficiency and effectiveness of personnel, equipment, and specific procedures throughout an EMS system. While many EMS agencies and first responder organizations still have to overcome the fear of managing such an immense quantity of information, the challenge is worth it. "Don't be afraid to keep track of lots of information," said Criss Brainard, a captain with the SDFD. "The data will prove worthwhile immediately and down the line."

New technologies are making the handling and management of data easier and more practical. They help improve efficiency, safeguard information, and facilitate communication between various locations. Computer data management systems are no longer beyond the reach of the average EMS agency—in fact, they have become a necessity.

EMS agencies and other organizations with early defibrillation programs need to devote the time, personnel, and money necessary to set up an efficient and thorough method for data collection and management. Improved quality of care, system-wide, will be the outcome.

Source

Reprinted with permission from JEMS, *July 1992. Cynthia L. Pollock, MSJ, has been a professional medical writer for over 12 years. She has published articles in numerous national magazines, including* OMNI, The Physician and Sports Medicine, Emergency Medicine, *and* Physician's Weekly.

References

Beeler, J. "Heartland Departments First to Use Modems with Defibrillators." *The California Fire Service* (May 1990).

Haynes, B., et al. "A Statewide Early Defibrillation Initiative Including Layperson Outcome Reporting." *Journal of the American Medical Association* 266, no. 4 (1991): 545–547.

Ensuring the Effectiveness of Community-Wide Emergency Cardiac Care

Lance B. Becker, MD, and Paul E. Pepe, MD, FACEP

Drs. Becker and Pepe outline recent developments that have influenced the treatment of cardiac arrests. They also walk the reader through each of the "links" in the chain of survival and describe specific steps for improving the survival rate in local communities.

To IMPROVE EMERGENCY CARDIAC CARE (ECC) on the national or international level, we must translate to the rest of our communities the successes found in cities with high survival rates. In recent years, important developments have evolved in our understanding of the treatment and evaluation of cardiac arrest. Some of the most important of these developments include

- Recognition of the chain of survival, which is necessary to achieve high survival rates
- Widespread acceptance that survival rates must be assessed routinely to ensure continuous quality improvements in the emergency medical services system
- Development of improved methods for performing survival rate studies that will maximize the effectiveness of information gathering and analysis

While each community should determine how to optimize its own ECC services, some general guidelines are useful. Successful treatment of cardiac arrest starts in the community with prevention and education, including early recognition of the signs and symptoms of cardiovascular ischemia. Obtaining 9-1-1 service (and preferably enhanced 9-1-1) should be a top priority for all communities. EMS dispatchers should dispatch the unit to the scene in less than one minute, provide critical information to the responders regarding the type of emergency, and offer the caller telephone-assisted CPR instructions. The EMS first responders should strive to arrive at the patient's side in less than four minutes, be able to immediately defibrillate if necessary, and begin basic CPR. An excellent strategy for accomplishing this is to equip and train all firefighting units in the operation of automatic external defibrillators and dispatch them as a first responder team.

To manage the cardiac arrest patient, a minimum of two rescuers trained in advanced cardiac life support plus two or more rescuers trained in basic life support are needed. Furthermore, an EMS system is not complete without ongoing evaluation. Therefore, the 1992 National Conference on CPR and ECC strongly endorses the position that all ECC systems assess their survival rates through an ongoing quality improvement process and that all members of the chain of providers should be represented in the outcome assessment team.

We still have much to discover regarding optimal techniques of CPR, optimal methods for data collection, and optimal structure of an EMS system. Research in these areas will provide the foundation for future changes in EMS systems development.

Overview of Issues

The purpose of basic life support (BLS) and advanced cardiac life support (ACLS) training is to increase the number of patients who survive a cardiac arrest. Unfortunately, though some communities enjoy survival rates greater than 15 percent, the overall survival rate from out-of-hospital cardiac arrest in the rest of the country has been estimated to be much lower, almost certainly less than five percent. While informal surveys support this assertion, no comprehensive data confirm this statistic. The very fact that no reliable national data currently exist is an additional argument favoring more widespread evaluation of community survival rates. Understanding the causes of the low overall survival rate and improving care for the majority of our citizens are major challenges facing emergency cardiac care today.

How do we improve ECC in our communities? How do we translate the critical components for success found in communities that have high survival rates to the rest of the country and the international community? In recent years, important developments have evolved in our understanding of the treatment of cardiac arrest. Some of the most important of these changes involve the following:

- The understanding that a strong chain of survival is necessary to achieve high survival rates
- The realization that survival rates must be assessed to ensure continued improvements in the emergency medical services system
- The development of improved methods for performing survival rate studies that will maximize the usefulness of the information gathered and the proper interpretation of subsequent data analysis

This article considers the structural components of a chain of survival that are generally necessary to save victims of out-of-hospital cardiac arrest, the rationale for community-wide evaluation of the ECC system, and contemporary methods to perform such an evaluation. Note that for many of the recommendations presented here, there are dissenting views (e.g., "the use of automatic external defibrillators [AEDs] on every fire apparatus should *not* be mandatory"). These dissenting views usually are based on political and cost considerations. Because so little research is available regarding the cost-benefit of certain EMS services, these concerns should be faced and addressed in future investigations.

The central issue is whether a community's ECC system provides optimal chances for patient survival. Again, achieving the optimal survival rate for out-of-hospital cardiac arrest in every community will be our main challenge as ECC enters the next century. However, what is optimal in one community may not be possible in all communities. The early reports of high survival in mid-size cities provided the prototype for EMS models subsequently adopted by most communities. However, the obstacles to providing care in rural and large metropolitan areas can create different challenges for EMS systems. It is unlikely that a single, specific EMS structure will provide optimal care in all communities. Therefore, each community will need to examine and devise its own standards and mechanisms to achieve the goal of optimal patient survival. Ensuring effectiveness in the management of cardiac arrest should be expanded to examine the whole ECC system from beginning to end. This is based on the concept that there is a chain of survival necessary for optimal outcome.

The Chain of Survival

Survival following cardiac arrest depends on a series of critical interventions that occur in a rapid and sequential manner. If one of these critical actions is neglected or delayed, chances of survival are severely compromised. This sequence of critical interventions has been termed the "chain of survival" (Box 4.6). This chain has four major interdependent links: early access, early basic CPR, early defibrillation, and early ACLS. While intrinsically rational, these remain arbitrary divisions. One can imagine many different chains of survival with dozens of links, one for each event that occurs during a cardiac arrest. Regardless of how one defines the links, the chain-of-survival concept underscores several important principles:

- If any one link in the chain is inadequate, the result will be less-than-optimal survival rates.
- While all links must have strength, rapid defibrillation is generally the most important single factor in determining survival. It is not completely understood to what degree and under what circumstances the other links contribute to optimal survival. While their positive effect is clear, we have not yet clearly delineated the *relative* importance and exact time dependency of factors such as bystander CPR, IV medications, and airway management.
- Because the chain of survival has many links, one cannot test the effectiveness of a system by examining an individual link. Rather, one must test the whole system. Because the survival rate has emerged as the gold standard for the effectiveness of the treatment of cardiac arrest, some general guidelines may assist communities in strengthening their own chain of survival.

Early Access

The first link in the chain is early access. Early access encompasses all of the events initiated immediately after the patient's collapse until the arrival of EMS personnel at the patient's side prepared to deliver care. It should include widespread recognition of early warning signs, such as chest pain and shortness of breath, as well as a community education program that encourages patients or bystanders to call 9-1-1 even prior to a patient's collapse. The major "access" events that must occur rapidly include

---

Box 4.6

The Chain of Survival

Early Access

Early CPR

Early Defibrillation

Early Advanced Care

Reproduced with permission. From *Textbook of Advanced Cardiac Life Support,* © American Heart Association, 1987, 1990.

- Early identification of patient collapse (or impending collapse) by a person or persons who can activate the system
- Rapid notification (usually by telephone) of the EMS dispatchers that a cardiac arrest is occurring or imminent
- Rapid recognition by dispatchers of a probable or potential cardiac arrest
- Rapid deployment instructions to the closest available EMS responders (first/second/third-tier EMS personnel) to guide them to the patient
- Rapid arrival of EMS responders at the address
- EMS responder arrival at the patient's side with all necessary equipment
- Identification of the cardiac arrest and rhythm

All of these events must take place before defibrillation or advanced care can occur. Each event is therefore a vital part of the early access link. In most communities, responsibility for these events falls under the 9-1-1 telephone system, the EMS dispatch system, or the EMS responder system.

The 9-1-1 telephone system. In the United States, widespread use of 9-1-1 has simplified and expedited emergency assistance. Many other countries also have established universal telephone numbers within their borders (for example, 03 in Russia, 120 in China, 119 in Japan). Currently, the European community is planning to establish a universal number for all member nations. Unfortunately, many U.S. communities are still without 9-1-1 service.

A more recent development is the implementation of "enhanced 9-1-1" in many communities. This option provides dispatchers with automatic electronic displays of information regarding the caller's address and phone number, which may not only save valuable time but may avoid catastrophic errors due to misinformation. The only real disadvantage to enhanced 9-1-1 is that it is more expensive. Although it is intuitively advantageous, many communities may be unwilling to spend additional dollars for a technology that has not yet been proven scientifically to save lives.

The EMS dispatch system. Rapid dispatching of EMS responders (including first responders and ambulance units) is a vital part of the early access link that has been neglected in past discussions of the chain of survival. The organization, structure, and protocols of EMS dispatchers vary worldwide. Nevertheless, EMS dispatchers must perform several vital steps.

The dispatcher must answer the call rapidly. Periods of unanswered ringing and busy signals are unacceptable.

The dispatcher must quickly identify that a cardiopulmonary arrest (or at least a high-priority medical emergency) has occurred while determining the exact location. This is often difficult. Obstacles include confused, anxious callers, language barriers, inability to identify the exact location, and perception among some dispatchers that the majority of calls will be for trivial medical problems.

Early access encompasses all of the events initiated immediately after the patient's collapse until the arrival of EMS personnel at the patient's side prepared to deliver care.

The dispatcher must identify not only the most available but also the most appropriate EMS response unit(s). How this is accomplished varies by location and community needs. Criteria-based dispatch procedures appear to be an excellent method for not only accomplishing rapid dispatch but also increasing the availability of appropriate units.

The dispatcher must rapidly contact the EMS responders, alert them to a possible cardiac arrest, and give exact details for the location. It is not acceptable for EMS responders to arrive at the scene of a cardiac arrest without having been informed of the nature of the medical emergency (when it is known). This should be considered a communication failure on the part of the dispatcher.

The critical measure of effective dispatch is a short interval from the initiation of the 9-1-1 call until the time that the ambulance is dispatched to the scene. This "call-to-ambulance-dispatch" interval should be no more than one minute (preferably less). For larger systems, this can best be accomplished by automatic prioritization of cardiac arrest calls in dispatch queues.

While the EMS responders are being dispatched, the caller should be asked to remain on the line. Dispatchers then may collect additional information or, whenever possible, give pre-arrival instruction to the caller on how to perform bystander CPR until the EMS responders arrive. Dispatcher-assisted bystander CPR has been shown to be feasible and effective. It may also be helpful as an "instant refresher" to CPR-trained individuals. Many of the people who call 9-1-1 for a cardiac arrest are extremely motivated to perform CPR. Controlled studies have demonstrated that emergency dispatchers following a standardized protocol can provide safe and effective CPR instruction to a bystander at the time of need. A dispatcher-directed CPR program can supplement community CPR training efforts. Therefore, telephone CPR is a logical extension of dispatcher responsibility. The training of dispatchers for this specific function usually requires only two to four hours.

Emergency medical dispatch has emerged as a vital ingredient in EMS systems. Dispatchers must have formal training in rapid interrogation and determination of the nature and severity of medical situations. Several nationally recognized programs have been established that provide specific guidelines regarding training, continuing medical education, quality improvement monitoring, and medical control.

The EMS responder system. The EMS responder system usually is composed of both BLS- and ACLS-trained responders. The system may be structured for either a single- or multi-tiered level of response. Most single-tier systems use ACLS-trained (paramedic) responders; however, others may provide only BLS care. Two-tiered systems generally provide first responder units that are staffed with EMTs or firefighters who are in close proximity to the scene. This first responder tier, capable of providing basic CPR and often defibrillation, is followed by the second tier of ACLS responders. It is generally held that two-tier systems, in which the first responders are trained in early defibrillation, are the most effective deployment systems for delivering rapid cardiac care.

Once dispatched, EMS responders must arrive quickly at the address of the patient in cardiac arrest. They then must locate and arrive at the patient's side with all of the necessary equipment.

The EMS transit interval, or the time elapsing while an EMS responder drives to the scene, is critical for cardiac arrest survival. Communities have learned to shorten this interval by strategic placement and deployment of response vehicles, adding supplementary response/transport crews, and improving traffic paths for ambulances. Multi-tiered systems appear to have the fastest response intervals due to increased numbers and availability of first responder units. Many communities report an EMS transit interval of approximately five minutes (or less) for first responders. Unfortunately, this is still too long when considering the goal of providing basic CPR and defibrillation within the initial four minutes following collapse.

Few studies have actually measured the time interval from when the EMS responders arrive at the address until they arrive at the patient's side. This interval, often assumed to be negligible, is difficult to document, because most systems do not have a means to accurately record the time spent locating the patient. However, recent studies have attempted to examine this interval more closely, and their results suggest that time spent locating the patient may be a significant factor, particularly in large urban areas.

The first EMS responders dispatched to a cardiac arrest must carry a defibrillator, oxygen, and airway management equipment. It is irrational for the EMS responders to leave these necessary pieces of equipment in the vehicle when survival is dependent on the earliest possible treatment. Today's defibrillators are lighter, easier to operate, and should be carried to each patient. Some EMS responders only carry the defibrillator to the patient when they are expecting the situation to be a cardiac arrest; this should be considered substandard care. Rationalizations for not carrying the defibrillator to the patient (such as cumbersome equipment, lack of personnel to carry the equipment, lack of training in the use of automated defibrillation, and inadequate dispatch information) indicate serious system deficiencies and require immediate correction.

Early Bystander CPR

The second link in the survival chain, bystander CPR, is most effective when started at the time of patient collapse. In most clinical studies, bystander CPR has been reported to have a significant positive effect on survival. The one possible exception to this occurs in situations in which the call to defibrillation interval is extremely short. Bystander CPR rarely causes significant injury to people, even when started inappropriately on people not in cardiac arrest.

Training in basic CPR also teaches citizens how to access the EMS system more efficiently, thus shortening the time to defibrillation. The 1992 National Conference on CPR and ECC recommended that community-

> Bystander CPR has been reported to have a significant positive effect on survival.

Increased utilization
of AEDs by larger
numbers of people
appropriately
trained in their use
may be the key
intervention that will
increase the survival
of out-of-hospital
cardiac arrest
patients.

wide citizen CPR training programs should be developed and augmented wherever possible (including at schools, military bases, housing complexes, workplaces, and public buildings). Communities need to remove any barriers that may discourage citizens from learning and performing basic CPR. CPR training has benefits beyond the provision of respiratory and circulatory support for cardiac arrest victims. Training programs inform the public about the dangers of heart disease and cardiac risk factors. Training increases the recognition of cardiac arrest and highlights the need for rapid activation of the EMS system. In addition, training people to provide the medical priorities of airway, breathing, and circulation can be lifesaving in many other medical emergencies (such as respiratory arrest, drug overdose, seizure, obstructed airway, near-drowning, etc.). CPR training should be inexpensive and widely available (e.g., free videotapes, public service announcements, mass training, etc.). Some have suggested or implemented the completion of CPR training as a requirement for high school graduation. Communities could reinforce training with an easy-to-remember phone number for CPR information (e.g., "225-4CPR").

Although bystander CPR is clearly of value in adult cardiac arrest, it is only temporary and loses its value if the subsequent links (early defibrillation and ACLS) do not follow rapidly. Therefore, if alone, the bystander first should call 9-1-1 for help, then initiate CPR. In the case of children, where respiratory problems are the usual ideology of arrest, a minute of basic rescue efforts is still advised. When notifying dispatchers or telling others to call 9-1-1, witnesses should not just state "we need an ambulance" but instead instruct the caller to state specifically that the person is not breathing or that CPR is in progress. This will quickly alert the dispatchers to the gravity of the situation and guarantee an appropriate level of response.

Early Defibrillation

The third and most important link in the chain of survival is early defibrillation. Increased utilization of AEDs by larger numbers of people appropriately trained in their use may be the key intervention that will increase the survival of out-of-hospital cardiac arrest patients. The American Heart Association (AHA) has strongly endorsed the position that every emergency vehicle that may respond to and transport potential cardiac arrest patients should be equipped with a defibrillator, and furthermore, that the emergency personnel should be trained in the use of the device and permitted to operate it. Toward this goal, the International Association of Fire Chiefs has proposed that every fire suppression unit in the United States be equipped with an AED and that all personnel be trained to operate the device.

Currently, there are several options for rapid defibrillation. Defibrillation can be performed using either manual, automatic, or semi-automatic external defibrillators. Manual defibrillation requiring interpretation of a monitor or rhythm strip is usually performed by ACLS-trained responders. However, manual defibrillation by emergency medical technicians (EMTs) who have been trained in the recognition of ventricular fibrillation has been shown to significantly improve survival in systems without ACLS (paramedic) service or when the response time for paramedics is relatively long.

Automated external defibrillation using automatic, automatic advisory, or semi-automatic external defibrillators has been shown to be safe and effective in increasing the survival from out-of-hospital cardiac arrest. These devices analyze the rhythm, charge themselves in appropriate cases, and then either automatically provide the countershock or advise the operator to press the defibrillator button. The widespread effectiveness and demonstrated safety of AEDs have now made it acceptable for "non-professionals" to effectively operate the devices as well. Such individuals still must be trained in basic CPR and in the proper application and use of the device under accountable physician supervision to ensure appropriate use.

Shortening the interval from cardiac arrest until defibrillation can be achieved through community education, enhanced 9-1-1, improved dispatch, additional EMS personnel with defibrillators (including AEDs), and faster response strategies, such as those in systems with multiple tiers of responders and those that emphasize a rapid first responder. In the current atmosphere of tight EMS budgets, defibrillators should be prioritized for purchase over other expensive medical devices (such as automatic transport ventilators or 12-lead ECGs). Using current technology, the cost of defibrillators could be reduced from the current levels of $5,000 to $7,000 to nearly $2,000. Ultimately, inexpensive defibrillators would increase the availability of these devices.

While strategies for earlier defibrillation first should be directed at speeding the initial links in the chain of survival, more creative use of AEDs in the near future by non-professionals (e.g., police officers, security guards, health club personnel, sports coaches) may result in improved survival. Because of their ease of operation and the need to integrate their use with basic CPR, AEDs can now be considered a "basic" life support intervention.

Early ACLS

The fourth link, early ACLS, usually is provided by paramedics (or physicians in some situations). In some systems, paramedics call a designated EMS base station for orders. In many systems, paramedics operate under the standing orders of the medical director. The ACLS link involves advanced judgment skills, cardiovascular monitoring, and invasive procedures.

In the management of cardiac arrest, EMS systems should have sufficient staffing to provide a minimum of two rescuers trained to an ACLS level throughout the emergency. Obviously, additional responders should be present. In systems that have attained survival rates higher than 20 percent for patients presenting with ventricular fibrillation, the attending response teams had a minimum of two ACLS providers plus a minimum of

> **The ACLS link involves advanced judgment skills, cardiovascular monitoring, and invasive procedures.**

two (usually four) BLS personnel present at the scene. Most experts feel that four responders (at least two ACLS trained and two BLS trained) are the absolute minimum required to properly treat a patient with cardiac arrest. In reality, not every EMS system can currently attain this level of response. However, all systems should strive to eventually achieve this goal.

Both basic and advanced responders need locally applicable training regarding field operations, communications, telemetry equipment, defensive driving, and local geography. Also, these persons must know how to interact with other agencies, especially those responsible for establishing security, traffic, and crowd control.

Medical Supervision

Medical supervision is defined as the authority exercised by a designated physician (medical director) to supervise and direct the medical care provided by any and all personnel involved in the EMS system. In most states, this function and authority is mandated by law. EMS personnel are not independently licensed and therefore may not function as independent practitioners. Medical authority and control is necessary in all EMS systems because EMS personnel are performing medical acts on behalf of the responsible physicians. Whether they are providing BLS or ACLS procedures, these are still medical acts. Medical supervision need not necessarily include administrative or fiscal control, but the medical director must have significant influence on administrative or fiscal decisions when they affect medical care.

Putting It All Together

One of the best methods for evaluating both the individual links and the overall strength of the chain of survival is to assess the survival rates achieved by the entire EMS system. However, to gain the most information, it is necessary to make relative comparisons between EMS systems. For example, community leaders may be interested in the fact that bystander CPR was performed in 30 percent of cardiac arrests, but it is more useful to compare this figure with that achieved in similar communities.

If useful comparisons are to be made, however, standardized definitions and terms of reference are needed. Until recently, uniform terminology has not been available, producing a cardiac arrest "Tower of Babel." With reported survival rates in the literature ranging from two to 44 percent, we need to delineate whether these profound variations are due to differences in population, treatment protocol, system organization, rescuer skills, or simply definitions and reporting practices.

Considerable efforts recently have been directed at creating clear, unambiguous terminology and at establishing a uniform method of reporting data (Box 4.7). These efforts have improved methodology for cardiac arrest research. There is now international consensus on the importance of using standard terminology and methods when evaluating the chain of survival (Box 4.8).

The motivation for these efforts is the underlying concern that thousands of deaths each year could be prevented if the ECC system in every community was optimized. Improving the ECC system, however, first requires an accurate measurement of the current survival rate for each community. The AHA strongly endorses the position that all ECC systems assess their survival rates through an ongoing quality improvement process.

Consensus Terminology

To address the recommendations stated above, the terms and definitions listed in Box 4.8 have been developed by a combined task force of the AHA, the European Resuscitation Council, the Heart and Stroke Foundation of Canada, and the Australian Resuscitation Council. This consensus has been referred to as the "Utstein style." These terms are intended to be a starting point for achieving uniform terminology. While all terms may not be ideal, they collectively represent a significant improvement over previous practice. The emphasis has been placed on developing terms that will not only assist in comparisons between communities and have a degree of universal applicability but also will replace imprecise terms previously used in cardiac arrest literature.

In-Hospital Data

In our enthusiasm for evaluating cardiac arrest in the out-of-hospital setting, we should not neglect the opportunities for cardiac arrest research within the hospital. The outcome of patients with in-hospital cardiac arrest has received some attention in the literature, yet these data have not been analyzed extensively. Researchers have expressed concerns regarding a number of methodological problems encountered during study of the in-hospital arrest population. The analysis is extremely complicated due to confounding co-morbid variables, such as terminal diseases and serious underlying illnesses, which may lead to a disproportionate number of deaths. The claim has also been made that out-of-hos-

---

Box 4.7

Minimal Recommended Data to Be Collected for Cases of Cardiac Arrest With Attempted Resuscitation

- Location and time of the cardiac arrest
- Any precipitating event/obvious non-cardiac etiology
- Time of receipt of call for help
- Time of dispatch of the emergency vehicle
- Time first-response vehicle departs for and stops at scene
- Confirmed cardiac arrest (witnessed or unwitnessed)
- Bystander CPR performed and time initiated
- Delineation of arrests occurring after the arrival of EMS personnel
- Time of first CPR efforts
- Initial presenting ECG rhythm found on monitor
- Treatment provided and corresponding times
- Time of first defibrillation
- Return of spontaneous circulation and the time
- Final patient status at scene
- Patient status on arrival in emergency department
- Status after emergency department treatment
- Status at hospital admission
- Status at hospital discharge (with neurological assessment, if possible)
- Discharged alive or dead (time of death)
- Alive at one year (with neurological assessment, if possible)
- Demographics (age, sex, race, co-morbidity, and other risk factors, if possible)

Describe the method by which the data are obtained (estimated or measured)

Cummins, R., D. Chamberlain, N. Abramson, et al. "Recommended Guidelines for Uniform Reporting of Data from Out-of-Hospital Cardiac Arrest: The Utstein Style." *Circulation* 84 (1991): 960-975.

Box 4.8

Glossary of Definitions and Terminology Used in ECC

Cardiac arrest. Cardiac arrest is the cessation of cardiac mechanical activity. It is a clinical diagnosis, confirmed by unresponsiveness, the absence of detectable pulse, and apnea (or agonal respirations).

Cardiopulmonary resuscitation (CPR). CPR refers to attempting any of the broad range of maneuvers and techniques used to restore spontaneous circulation. CPR can be further classified as advanced, basic, successful, unsuccessful, bystander, or other depending on the setting and techniques.

Basic CPR. Basic CPR is the attempt to restore circulation using the techniques of chest-wall compression and pulmonary ventilation.

Bystander CPR, layperson CPR, or citizen CPR. These terms are synonymous; however, bystander CPR is preferred. Bystander CPR is an attempt at basic CPR provided by a person who happened to be near the scene of a cardiac arrest and is not (at that moment) part of the organized emergency response system.

Basic cardiac life support (BLS). This refers to the education program that provides medical information including basic CPR, as access to the EMS system, and recognition of cardiac arrest.

Advanced CPR or advanced cardiac life support (ACLS). These terms refer to attempts at restoration of spontaneous circulation using basic CPR plus advanced airway management, endotracheal intubation, defibrillation, and IV medications. ACLS also may refer to the educational program that provides the standards and guidelines for these techniques and their implementation.

Emergency medical services (EMS) or emergency personnel. Persons who respond to medical emergencies in an official capacity are emergency (or EMS) personnel responsible for receiving, interpreting, and prioritizing the call for help as well as dispatching EMS responders to the scene of medical emergencies. They also provide telephone instructions to bystanders at the scene while professionals are en route.

pital cardiac arrests represent a more homogeneous population and therefore should not be compared to in-hospital cardiac arrests.

However, the facts do not support all these concerns. First, not all in-hospital cardiac arrest patients die. Conversely, many out-of-hospital patients also have terminal diseases or underlying illnesses. Jastremski reported that the cumulative survival rate of seven recent in-hospital studies was 11 percent (199 hospital discharges out of 1,804 arrests), a survival rate better than those achieved in some recent out-of-hospital studies. While there may be important differences in the pathophysiology of some in-hospital cardiac arrests (e.g., a higher percentage of pulmonary emboli, hyper-kalemia, etc.), the majority of in-hospital cardiac arrests appear to have many similarities to out-of-hospital arrests.

In fact, there are many advantages to studying in-hospital patients. Documentation is often more accurate, and "arrest-to-defibrillation" intervals are often shorter. Research protocols and data collection techniques that require advanced or invasive monitoring procedures are usually more feasible and can be implemented rapidly in the in-hospital setting. Most hospitals have a code team that responds to all cardiac arrests. If trained and structured appropriately, such teams can be used to facilitate uniform treatment protocols and monitoring. In addition, the past medical history and conditions leading to the arrest often are documented in the patient's chart. Those patients who have do-not-resuscitate (DNR) status will be clearly identified as such, thus eliminating the situations encountered in the prehospital setting in which emergency response personnel are called to a patient who should not receive resuscitation efforts. Also, the complete cardiac arrest record is in the hospital chart, eliminating the need for the merging of multiple data sources. A single clock (the hospital clock) runs during the arrest, reducing the likelihood of a lack of synchronization between time points.

The Chain of Providers

If we accept a chain of survival for cardiac arrest treatment, another important dynamic should be considered when performing quality improvement studies of early access, early CPR, early defibrillation, early ACLS, and eventual outcome from cardiac arrest within a community. The chain of survival implies that a chain of providers is required for the successful treatment of cardiac arrest. It is this chain of providers who should perform the outcome assessment. Because the long-term goal is not merely to collect data but to improve the ECC system, all members of the chain of providers should be represented in the outcome assessment team. It is logical that all providers have a chance to be involved in the ECC assessment process, because the assessment will naturally produce actions that they must take to improve the system and enhance survival odds.

The outcome assessment team may benefit from participation by representatives of the various local and state health departments, first responders, and ambulance personnel, as well as members of the police department, hospitals, universities, industry, and organizations active in BLS and ACLS training. Often, a nonpartisan organization like the AHA can facilitate the genesis of this diverse team and function as an umbrella for the evaluation process.

Design of Cardiac Arrest Studies

The field of study design in cardiac arrest research is complex and beyond the scope of this text. Several excellent resources are available. Box 4.9 is provided as a generic outline for the data collection process. When developing a chain of survival assessment, one should remember that the process of this team working together may be as important as any scientific results.

For example, EMS personnel often feel threatened by the review process. It is common for paramedics to question why administrators wish to collect information regarding how long it takes to defibrillate. Likewise, not being part of the process, dispatchers may feel that they are being singled out for scrutiny. Hospitals that provide much of the outcome data are also reluctant to expose themselves to more outside scrutiny. In reality, local politics will always be difficult to separate from the assessment project. Some system modifications will always be necessary, even in the best of systems. If the assessment team is well represented by the various providers, most concerns can be addressed adequately for the improvement process to move forward.

Commentary

The following suggestions will ensure a better chain of survival in one's community.

Box 4.8 (cont.)

EMS responders. The EMS personnel who respond to medical emergencies by going to the scene in an emergency vehicle. They may be first responders, second responders, or third responders, depending on the EMS system. They may be ACLS or BLS trained, but they all should be capable of defibrillation. Emergency medical technician (EMT) usually denotes BLS training. Paramedic (or EMT-P) usually denotes ACLS training.

Emergency cardiac care (ECC) system. The ECC system includes all aspects of cardiac care, including that rendered by emergency personnel. The extended ECC system also includes bystander CPR, rapid activation of the EMS system, emergency departments, intensive care units, cardiac rehabilitation, cardiac prevention programs, BLS/ACLS training programs, and even citizen defibrillation.

Chain of survival. The chain of survival is a metaphor for describing the interdependence of survival chances following cardiac arrest upon each of the various sequential emergency responses in the community. This response is composed of four major links: early access, early CPR, early defibrillation, and early ACLS. A single weak or missing link will result in markedly diminished chances of survival, despite excellence in the rest of the ECC system.

Presumed cardiac etiology. Cardiac arrest due to presumed cardiac etiology is the major focus of ECC. Studies of cardiac arrest should attempt to exclude arrests due to obvious non-cardiac causes when reporting cardiac outcome data. Arrests from other etiologies will have different treatments and survival characteristics. Granted, this is a diagnosis of exclusion; however, due to practical considerations (lack of autopsy information, cost) all arrests are considered to be of presumed cardiac etiology unless an obvious non-cardiac etiology can be identified. Common non-cardiac diagnoses that should be separated during analysis of cardiac arrest outcome include sudden infant death syndrome, airway obstruction, drug overdose, suicide, drowning, trauma, exsanguination, and terminal states of illness.

Return of spontaneous circulation. Some researchers would define return of spontaneous circulation (ROSC) as the

Box 4.8 (cont.)

initial return of a spontaneous perceivable pulse lasting more than a minute without the need for providing chest compressions. Others use this term to refer to a more sustained ROSC (i.e., five minutes, 10 minutes, or no further recurrence of cardiac arrest). Specify the duration when reporting ROSC.

Time intervals. The Utstein recommendations have provided a more rational nomenclature for important time intervals. Time intervals should be reported as the A-to-B interval, which represents the period that begins at time point A and ends at time point B. These are more informative than imprecise terms such as *downtime* or *response time*. For example, the following terms are suggested:

9-1-1-call-to-dispatch interval. The interval from the time the call for help is first received by the 9-1-1 office until the time that the emergency vehicle begins to leave for the scene.

Vehicle-dispatch-to-scene interval. The interval from when the emergency vehicle departs for the scene until the EMS responders indicate the vehicle is stopping at the scene or address. This does not include the time interval until emergency personnel arrive at the patient's side or the interval until defibrillation occurs.

Vehicle-at-scene-to-patient-access interval. The interval from when the emergency response vehicle stops moving at the scene or address until the EMS responders are at the side of the patient.

Call-to-patient-access interval. The interval from the time the call is first received by the 9-1-1 center until the first responders are at the side of the patient.

Call-to-defibrillation interval. The interval from the call receipt at the 9-1-1 center until the patient receives the first countershock.

Cummins, R., D. Chamberlain, N. Abramson, et al. "Recommended Guidelines for Uniform Reporting of Data from Out-of-Hospital Cardiac Arrest: The Utstein Style." *Circulation* 84 (1991): 960-975.

Early Access

Obtaining 9-1-1 service should be a priority for all communities. The availability of funding for an enhanced 9-1-1 service may determine the feasibility of its implementation. Although there are not studies yet available to suggest that enhanced 9-1-1 results in improvements in survival, this system has clear advantages.

EMS Dispatch

System managers should ensure the ability of the EMS dispatch system to do the following:

- Immediately answer all emergency medical calls
- Rapidly determine the nature of the call
- Identify the closest and most appropriate EMS response unit(s)
- In the case of potential or confirmed cardiac arrest, dispatch the unit(s) to the scene in less than one minute
- Provide critical information to the EMS responders (while en route) regarding the type of emergency
- During the time until responders are present on the scene, offer telephone-assisted bystander CPR as needed

Although some believe that a one-minute standard time interval to achieve dispatch of responders is not feasible, this is a reasonable goal in mid-size and large cities. Rural areas may have difficulty getting volunteer units to respond in one minute. Also, some systems may be unable to afford the infrastructure and training that would allow dispatchers to perform at this level. Nevertheless, it should be recognized that this key link in the chain of survival eventually must be addressed.

EMS Responders

System managers should set a goal of first responders arriving at the patient's side in less than four minutes following the first call to 9-1-1. Also, first responders should be required to arrive with all of the necessary equipment to immediately defibrillate and begin CPR. It is recognized that this four-minute goal is quite difficult to achieve. Funding systems for a four-minute response is not always feasible, and fiscally, this goal may be quite burdensome. Most communities have begun to realize this goal or at least come close to it through use of neighborhood fire apparatus or police units.

Early CPR

ECC community leaders should develop widespread basic CPR training programs especially targeting subpopulations that are most likely to witness a cardiac arrest or have the opportunity to perform bystander CPR. During these training programs, priority should be placed on activating the EMS system and telling the dispatcher that CPR is in progress to ensure the appropriate deployment in priority dispatch systems. A single unassisted rescuer with an adult victim should activate the EMS system after establishing unresponsiveness. In pediatric arrest, the EMS system should be activated after rescue breathing is initiated. Usually in such cases, the child can be brought to the phone.

A few studies have questioned the need for bystander CPR in systems with very fast response times for first responders. They question whether funds spent on training citizens in bystander CPR might be better used elsewhere in the EMS system. However, the cost of such CPR training is minimal, and required training of high school students seems to be the most cost-effective approach. No study has yet demonstrated that "good" (perfectly performed) CPR is better than "bad" (poorly performed) CPR. Some have suggested that a simplified version of CPR, as effective as the current method, might be developed that would be easier to teach, learn, retain, and perform.

Early Defibrillation

It is now feasible to provide widespread placement of AEDs in the hands of a larger group of appropriately trained people. It makes medical and economic sense to equip and train all neighborhood firefighting units in the operation of AEDs. It also would be wise to facilitate the placement and use of defibrillators in gathering places that have greater than 10,000 people.

Box 4.9

Developing a Community Outcome Assessment

Step 1. Designate one to three project directors to lead the project. These may be the EMS system medical director, a resuscitation researcher, or someone recruited from the various teams of emergency care personnel.

Step 2. Create an outcome assessment team (which functions like a steering committee) by enlisting the assistance of representatives from applicable organizations such as the AHA (or, if applicable, the European Resuscitation Council, Australian Resuscitation Council, Heart and Stroke Foundation of Canada, or similar agency), EMS personnel, fire department, emergency medicine, cardiology, anesthesiology, nursing, police, public health, unions, and hospitals. If possible, include a statistician or epidemiologist and at least one senior scientist. Try to include as part of the team all individuals who provide access to necessary patient data and charts.

Step 3. Develop a data form to provide information on the current performance of the chain of survival, including outcomes. Determine the desirable goals for each performance category (i.e., call-to-first-responder-at-scene interval of less that five minutes in 90 percent of cases). These performance goals should include the recommended core data (see Utstein recommendations) as well as any other specific data developed by the team to benefit the community ECC system. Determine the degree of data necessary to evaluate whether or not actual performance meets the recommended goals.

Step 4. Attempt to establish funding for the project, including (at a minimum) data collection, coding, data entry, and data analysis.

Step 5. Perform pilot studies and obtain data acquisition agreements with hospitals (including confidentiality agreements) as well as data collection agreements with EMS providers. Hire personnel and resolve any difficulties in the data collection process. Develop a final data form and outline quality control measures and testing procedures. Make necessary modifications.

Step 6. Start the data collection period. Transpose the specified data from patient records to data collection forms and (when possible) to a computer database.

Step 7. Begin data analyses to answer questions regarding outcome variables and test whether the measured performance met the goals for each link in the chain of survival. Enter data onto the reporting template and compare results to those of other communities. Scrutinize data for areas of improvement and poor survival subgroups. The data should create more questions!

Step 8. Wherever feasible, improve the EC system at each step through modification of the weak links in the system. Use data to justify (and fund) solutions to these weaknesses. Re-examine the results after modifications to the ECC system to determine if the new system factors help to meet the goals. Report the results.

> System managers should develop a comprehensive evaluation process for each community. This analysis should include an accurate assessment of survival rates using standardized nomenclature and reporting methods.

If necessary, community leaders should enact legislation to enable EMS personnel and other trained rescuers to perform early defibrillation. Still, these recommendations may be too strong or premature; in some communities, placing an AED on every firefighting unit is perhaps unnecessary. Not every study has shown an improvement in survival with the use of AEDs. Funding remains a key factor for implementation.

Early ACLS

If possible, a minimum of two ACLS-trained rescuers plus two or more BLS-trained rescuers should be provided to manage the cardiac arrest patient. With the possibility of early defibrillation with the first responder team, the optimal interval from 9-1-1 call to ACLS arrival is not yet established. The more successful EMS systems have an average interval of eight minutes or less from 9-1-1 call to ACLS arrival.

Unfortunately, not every system currently can afford this level of prehospital ACLS care. In communities with few resources, it makes sense to first maximize the currently existing resources before establishing a more expensive and elaborate system. Citizens should first be trained to rapidly access the ECC system and to provide basic CPR. This can be followed with the purchase of AEDs for existing rescue apparatus or police units. When fiscal limitations create obstacles, creative means of providing care within the budget must be found. Expert medical control and supervision throughout the EMS system should be the rule, with active involvement in important aspects of dispatch, fire responders, early defibrillation, and ACLS care.

Evaluation of the Community ECC System

System managers should develop a comprehensive evaluation process for each community. This analysis should include an accurate assessment of survival rates using standardized nomenclature and reporting methods. This focus on quality improvement should identify practical goals (given the structure and demographics of the local system) and current performance, including the survival rate. It should then identify gaps between goals and current performance, evaluate strategies to improve system performance, and document whether performance indeed improves with these modifications. All providers at each link in the chain should be represented and should participate in this process. The funding for evaluation should be considered an integral part of the system.

Research Initiatives

Research will play an important role in the development of cardiac arrest treatment. Many areas will benefit from future studies. Three broad areas for future study include technique and training for bystander CPR, data collection methods that are accurate and provide the most information, and the optimal structure of the EMS system to maximize survival.

Many questions still exist regarding the physiology, critical timing, and optimal techniques of bystander CPR. For example, how does the quality of bystander CPR affect patient survival? What percent of the community should be targeted for training in CPR to obtain optimal survival rates? Who are the best subgroups within the community to target for CPR training (medical professionals, middle-aged couples, Boy Scouts, security guards, ushers, golf caddies, etc.)? What is the most effective method of CPR training? Can the current method of ventilation and compressions be modified (interposed abdominal compressions or compression/active decompression CPR) and still produce favorable or even improved results?

Accurate data collection is the second important area for future research. Few systems have been capable of accurately documenting those points in time when emergency personnel arrive at the patient's side, establish an airway, defibrillate the patient, establish an IV line, and detect return of spontaneous circulation. Fortunately, defibrillators and monitors with audio or event recorders, computer notebooks, bar codes, and other technology are becoming available that can help EMS responders better document each of these events. Such technology, when synchronized with the 9-1-1 clock, will establish a better system of analysis. However, new methods must be developed that are reliable, inexpensive, and do not interfere with duties at the scene. If such devices can be developed, they will help answer many questions posed by researchers and ECC system managers in future analyses of resuscitation efforts.

There are even more questions regarding optimal structure for community-wide ECC. How can we shorten the time interval until defibrillation? Can we use additional members of the community to deliver effective defibrillation (police or coaches)? What EMS structures or deployment strategies will work best in rural or urban areas? How many AEDs are needed for adequate survival rates? What is an appropriate survival rate for a community to achieve? We need further analysis to answer the question, "Is all of this cost and effort worth it?" For communities with extremely limited funding, where along the chain of survival should the dollars be spent in order to save the most lives?

Evaluation of neurological effects, overall performance categories, and even financial status (i.e., return to previous state of employment, cost of hospitalization) may be important outcome factors to examine. In addition to these easily measurable, objective factors, the subjective opinion of family as to the ultimate value of the resuscitation efforts is difficult to quantify yet may become the final and determining criterion for success of EMS systems. Therefore, future research should take these issues into account.

References

Agency for Health Care Policy and Research. "Medical Treatment Effectiveness Research." *U.S. Department of Health Care Policy,* March 1990.
American Heart Association. "Putting It All Together: Resuscitation of the Patient." In

Textbook of Advanced Cardiac Life Support, ed. A. Jaffe, 235-248. Dallas: American Heart Association, 1987.

American Heart Association. "Standards and Guidelines for Cardiopulmonary Resuscitation for Emergency Cardiac Care: Part VII: Emergency Cardiac Care Units (in EMS Systems)." *Journal of the American Medical Association* 255 (1986): 2974-2979.

Bachman, J., G. McDonald, and P. O'Brien. "A Study of Out-of-Hospital Cardiac Arrests in Northeastern Minnesota." *Journal of the American Medical Association* 256 (1986): 477-483.

Baskett, P., G. Carss, and D. Withers. "Resuscitation Guidance by Telephone." *The Journal of the British Association of Immediate Care* 7 (1984): 46-48.

Becker, L. B., ed. "Proceedings of the Chicago Symposium on Methodology in Cardiac Arrest Research." *Annals of Emergency Medicine* 22 (1993).

Becker, L., M. Ostrander, J. Barrett, et al. "Outcome of CPR in a Large Metropolitan Area: Where Are the Survivors?" *Annals of Emergency Medicine* 20 (1991): 355-361.

Bossaert, L., and R. Van Hoeyweghen. "Bystander Cardiopulmonary Resuscitation (CPR) in Out-of-Hospital Cardiac Arrest: The Cerebral Resuscitation Study Group." *Resuscitation* 17 (1989): S55-S69.

Campbell, J., M. Gratton, and W. Robinson. "Meaningful Response Time Interval: Is It an Elusive Dream?" *Annals of Emergency Medicine* 20 (1991): 433. Abstract.

Clawson, J. J. "Emergency Medical Dispatch." In *National Association of EMS Physicians: EMS Medical Directors' Handbook,* ed. A. E. Kuehl, 59-90. St. Louis: CV Mosby Co. 1989.

Clawson, J. J. "Emergency Medical Dispatching." In *Principles of EMS Systems: A Comprehensive Text for Physicians,* ed. W. R. Roush, R. D. Aranosian, T. M. H. Blair, et al. Dallas: American College of Emergency Physicians, 1989.

Cobb, L. A., and A. P. Hallstrom. "Community-Based Cardiopulmonary Resuscitation: What Have We Learned?" *Annals of New York Academic Sciences* 382 (1982): 330-342.

Cobb, L. A., H. Alvarez, and M. K. Copass. "A Rapid Response System for Out-of-Hospital Cardiac Emergencies." *Med Clin North Am* 60 (1976): 283-290.

Cummins, R., and M. Eisenberg. "Prehospital Cardiopulmonary Resuscitation: Is It Effective?" *Journal of the American Medical Association* 253 (1985): 2408-2412.

Cummins, R., D. Chamberlain, N. Abramson, et al. "Recommended Guidelines for Uniform Reporting of Data from Out-of-Hospital Cardiac Arrest: The Utstein Style." *Circulation* 84 (1991): 960-975.

Cummins, R., J. Ornato, W. Thies, et al. "The 'Chain of Survival' Concept." *Circulation* 83 (1991): 1832-1847.

Cummins, R. O., and J. R. Graves. "Clinical Results of Standard CPR: Prehospital and In-Hospital." In *Cardiopulmonary Resuscitation: Clinics in Critical Care Medicine,* eds. W. Kaye and N. Birchner. New York: Churchill-Livingstone, 1989.

Cummins, R. O., and W. Thies. "Encouraging Early Defibrillation: The American Heart Association and Automated External Defibrillators." *Annals of Emergency Medicine* 19 (1990): 1245-1248.

Cummins, R. O. "From Concept to Standard-of-Care? Review of the Clinical Experience with Automated External Defibrillators." *Annals of Emergency Medicine* 18 (1989): 1269-1275.

Cummins, R. O., M. S. Eisenberg, A. P. Hallstrom, et al. "Survival of Out-of-Hospital Cardiac Arrest with Early Initiation of Cardiopulmonary Resuscitation." *American Journal of Emergency Medicine* 3 (1985): 114-119.

Curka, P. A., P. E. Pepe, V. F. Ginger, et al. "Computer-Aided EMS Priority Dispatch: Ability of a Computerized Triage System to Safely Spare Paramedics from Responses Not Requiring Advanced Life Support." *Annals of Emergency Medicine* 20 (1991): 446. Abstract.

Dearmin, D. "California Develops Guidelines for Emergency Medical Dispatching." *Associated Public Safety Communications Officers Bulletin* (14-15 February 1986).

Eisenberg, M., B. Horwood, R. Cummins, et al. "Cardiac Arrest and Resuscitation: A Tale of 29 Cities." *Annals of Emergency Medicine* 19 (1990): 179-186.

Eisenberg, M., L. Bergner, and T. Hearne. "Out-of-Hospital Cardiac Arrest: A Review of Major Studies and a Proposed Uniform Reporting System." *American Journal of Public Health* 70 (1980): 236-240.

Eisenberg, M., R. Cummins, S. Damon, et al. "Survival Rates from Out-of-Hospital Cardiac Arrest: Recommendations for Uniform Definitions and Data to Report." *Annals of Emergency Medicine* 19 (1990): 1249-1259.

Eisenberg, M. S., A. P. Hallstrom, W. B. Carter, et al. "Emergency CPR Instruction Via Telephone." *American Journal of Public Health* 75 (1985): 47-50.

Eisenberg, M. S., L. Bergner, and A. Hallstom. "Out-of-Hospital Cardiac Arrest: Improved Survival with Paramedic Services." *Lancet* 1 (1980): 812-815.

Eisenberg, M. S., M. K. Copass, A. P. Hallstrom, et al. "Treatment of Out-of-Hospital Cardiac Arrest with Rapid Defibrillation by Emergency Medical Technicians." *New England Journal of Medicine* 302 (1980): 1379-1383.

Hoekstra, J. W., J. Banks, D. Martin, et al. "The Effect of First-Responder Automated Defibrillation On Time to Therapeutic Intervention During Out-of-Hospital Cardiac Arrest." *Annals of Emergency Medicine* 22 (1993).

IAFC on Scene (newsletter). Washington, D.C.: International Association of Fire Chiefs, 1987, 1.

Jaggarao, N. S., M. Herber, R. Grainger, et al. "Use of an Automated External Defibrillator-Pacemaker by Ambulance Staff." *Lancet* 2 (1982): 73-75.

Kellerman, A. L., B. B. Hackman, and G. Somes. "Dispatcher-Assisted Cardiopulmonary Resuscitation: Validation of Efficacy." *Circulation* 80 (1989): 1231-1239.

Kerber, R. E. "Early Defibrillation: Position Statement of the American Heart Association Emergency Cardiac Care Committee." *Circulation* 83 (1991): 2233.

McManus, W. F., D. D. Tresch, and J. C. Darin. "An Effective Prehospital Emergency System." *Journal of Trauma* 17 (1977): 304-310.

Murphy, D. M. "Rapid Defibrillation: Fire Service to Lead the Way." *JEMS* 12 (1987): 67-71.

Pack, W. "Program to Spur CPR Training in City Schools." *Houston Post,* 25 March 1992.

Paris, P. M. "EMT-Defibrillation: A Recipe for Saving Lives." *American Journal of Emergency Medicine* 6 (1988): 282-287.

Pepe, P. "Advanced Cardiac Life Support: State of the Art." In *Emergency and Intensive Care,* ed. J. L. Vincent, 565-585. Berlin: Springer-Verlag, 1990.

Pepe, P. E., and D. R. Almaguer. "Emergency Medical Services Personnel and Ground Transport Vehicles." *Problems in Critical Care* 4 (1990): 470-476.

Pepe, P. E. "Demonstrating the Efficacy of Basic and Advanced Life Support: A Cooperative Effort of Key Community Leaders." *Houston Heart Bulletin* 9, no. 1 (1991): 1-7.

Pepe, P. E., J. E. Kelly, M. V. Ivy, et al. "Resource Utilization and Impact of Using Fire Apparatus for a Fully Integrated EMS First-Responder Program." *Annals of Emergency Medicine* 20 (1991): 488. Abstract.

Pepe, P. E., K. L. Mattox, F. D. Prentice, et al. "The Impact of Intense Physician Supervision on the Success of Emergency Medical Services Systems." *Critical Care Medicine* (1993).

Pepe, P. E., M. J. Bonnin, and K. L. Mattox. "Regulating the Scope of EMS." *Prehospital and Disaster Medicine* 5 (1990): 59-63.

Pepe, P. E., M. J. Bonnin, D. R. Almaguer, et al. "The Effect of Tiered System Implementation on Sudden Death Survival Rates." *Prehospital and Disaster Medicine* 4 (1989): 71. Abstract.

Ritter, G., R. A. Wolfe, S. Goldstein, et al. "The Effect of Bystander CPR on Survival of Out-of-Hospital Cardiac Arrest Victims." *American Heart Journal* 110 (1985): 932-937.

Sammel, N. L., K. Taylor, M. Selig, et al. "New South Wales Intensive Care Ambulance System: Outcome of Patients with Ventricular Fibrillation." *Medical Journal of Australia* 2 (1981): 546-550.

Stewart, R. D. "Medical Direction in Emergency Medical Services: The Role of the Physician." *Emerg Med Clin North Am* 5 (1987): 119.

Stults, K. R., D. D. Brown, and R. E. Kerber. "Efficacy of an Automated External Defibrillator in the Management of Out-of-Hospital Cardiac Arrest: Validations of the Diagnostic Algorithm and Initial Clinical Experience in a Rural Environment." *Circulation* 73 (1986): 701-709.

Troiano, P., J. Masaryk, and H. Stueven. "The Effect of Bystander CPR on Neurological Outcome in Survivors of Prehospital Cardiac Arrests." *Resuscitation* 17 (1989): 91-98.

Weaver, W. D., D. Hill, C. E. Fahrenbruch, et al. "Use of the Automatic External Defibrillator in the Management of Out-of-Hospital Cardiac Arrest." *New England Journal of Medicine* 319 (1988): 661-666.

Wright, D., C. James, A. K. Marsden, et al. "Defibrillation by Ambulance Staff Who Have Had Extended Training." *British Medical Journal* 299 (1989): 96-97.

Source

Reprinted with permission from Annals of Emergency Medicine, *February 1993. At the time of original publication, Lance B. Becker, MD, was with the Section of Emergency Medicine, Department of Medicine, University of Chicago. Paul E. Pepe, MD, FACEP, is the medical director for the Houston Fire Department and a faculty member at the Baylor College of Medicine.*

Predicting Survival from Out-of-Hospital Cardiac Arrest: A Graphic Model

Mary P. Larsen, MS; Mickey S. Eisenberg, MD, PhD; Richard O. Cummins, MD, MPH, MSc; and Alfred P. Hallstrom, PhD

This article illustrates survival from cardiac arrest by tracking four elements: no treatment given; if and when CPR was started and by whom; when defibrillation was given and by whom; and when advanced cardiac life support measures were administered. Some of the results are predictable, while others may be surprising.

SURVIVAL TO HOSPITAL DISCHARGE from out-of-hospital sudden cardiac arrest depends in part on the timing of three critical prehospital interventions: CPR, defibrillation, and advanced care (e.g., intubation, medication). The shorter the time interval between collapse and these three interventions, the higher the probability of survival.

From the moment of collapse, the likelihood of survival decreases rapidly with each minute that elapses without initiation of lifesaving procedures. Prehospital interventions typically occur in a sequence: CPR is started by bystanders or EMS personnel followed by defibrillatory shocks administered by EMTs authorized to defibrillate or by paramedics and then followed by advanced care administered by paramedics. The average time to performance of these critical interventions determines a community's overall survival rate from sudden cardiac arrest.

We developed a model that describes the relationship between a community's average time intervals to these three critical interventions and its overall survival rate. The model is easy to apply, and its lessons are readily interpretable.

Materials and Methods

Since 1976, we have collected information on all patients with out-of-hospital cardiac arrests in King County, Wash., for whom emergency personnel attempted resuscitation (9,245). Data were obtained from multiple sources, including EMS run reports, hospital records, death certificates, and interviews with bystanders.

For all cases, we determined retrospectively the etiology of the cardiac arrest, whether the collapse was witnessed, and the cardiac rhythm associated with the arrest. For all witnessed cardiac arrests, we determined the time intervals to the three critical interventions: from collapse to CPR, from collapse to first defibrillatory shock, and from collapse to advanced care. Time of collapse may be biased by inaccurate recall of exact times surrounding such a stressful event. In our data, however, time of collapse is gathered consistently from dispatcher recordings and paramedic on-scene reports. We expect neither the nature of this potential bias nor the method of estimating time of collapse to change in the future. Thus, the timing guidelines proposed by the model should be no different for future cases than they would be for the cases on which the model is based.

We estimated time intervals to actual treatment as follows: the time interval to bystander-initiated CPR was taken from interviews with the bystander or from the incident report prepared by EMS personnel; the time interval to EMS-initiated CPR was estimated from the EMS response time plus one minute (the time needed for EMTs or paramedics to arrive at the scene, reach the patient's side, and position the patient); and the time interval needed for EMTs or paramedics to attach the defibrillator and clear the patient for defibrillation once CPR was in progress was estimated to be two minutes past EMT arrival or one minute past time of initiation of CPR by EMTs. In our data, the time interval from arrival of paramedics to the initiation of advanced care was estimated to be two minutes past paramedic arrival if defibrillation had taken place before paramedic arrival, three minutes past paramedic arrival if defibrillation had not yet taken place, and four minutes past paramedic arrival if the paramedics were the only EMS providers on the scene. These intervals to interventions are the best estimates of EMTs, paramedics, and EMS medical directors.

We recognize that "advanced care" by paramedics includes multiple interventions delivered over time (intubation, initiation of IV access, administration of multiple medications, rhythm assessment, hyperventilation). For simplicity of analysis, however, we focused on a single time interval, from collapse to the moment when paramedics were ready to perform advanced interventions.

To determine the effect of these three time intervals on survival, we selected a somewhat uniform group with a higher likelihood of survival: patients who had a witnessed cardiac arrest due to underlying heart disease, who were in ventricular fibrillation, and whose arrest occurred before arrival of EMS personnel (1,667). Survival was defined as discharge alive from the hospital.

We estimated the relative strength of influence of each time interval on survival using a multiple linear regression model with survival (discharge from the hospital) as the outcome and time interval from collapse to CPR (I_{CPR}), time interval from collapse to first shock (I_{DEFIB}), and time interval from collapse to advanced care (I_{ACLS}) as predictors. Age, sex, underlying morbidity, and time to various hospital procedures, although certainly relevant to the survival rate, were not included in the model because they were not considered to be under EMS control. The model is expressed as the following equation:

$$\text{Survival rate} =$$
$$C_{COLLAPSE} + C_{CPR}I_{CPR} + C_{DEFIB}I_{DEFIB} + C_{ACLS}I_{ACLS}$$

where C_{CPR}, C_{DEFIB}, and C_{ACLS} are the regression coefficients (relative strength of the effect) for the designated time intervals (I) and $C_{COLLAPSE}$ is the regression constant, which represents the survival rate expected when treatment is available immediately on collapse, i.e., the hypothetical situation in which a patient went into cardiac arrest at the exact moment that an endotracheal tube was inserted, an IV catheter entered a vein, and defibrillator paddles were placed on the chest. Although a term to account for random measurement error generally is included in regression models, we have omitted it for simplicity.

To test for the effects of interactions between terms or squared effects of any one term (a term multiplied by itself, such as $I_{DEFIB} \times I_{DEFIB}$), we also performed a stepwise linear regression using all possible products and squares of terms using a significance level of $p = 0.1$. None of these factors contributed significantly to the model, indicating that a simple, additive model was the most efficient.

All three time intervals, I_{CPR}, I_{DEFIB}, and I_{ACLS}, were limited to 20 minutes; cases with EMS arrival times in excess of 20 minutes were not included in the model. The survival rate is between 0 and 100 percent by definition. Within these limits, the model consists of a curve, the slope of which becomes more shallow with each intervention. Because the individual outcome measurement is discharge alive from the hospital and we are assessing the effect of prehospital treatments only, the decline in survival is considered to be zero after the delivery of advanced care.

The final step in the development of the model was the elimination of outliers, atypical observations that have undue influence on the fit of the model. We eliminated all observations with residuals (difference between the observed survival rate and the rate predicted by the model) that exceeded the ninety-eighth percentile (i.e., observations with residuals in the top two percent). After elimination of the outliers, the model was fit again, and the resulting coefficients were used to predict the rate of survival.

To assess the performance of our model, predicted survival rates obtained from the model were compared with rates reported for communities representative of different types of EMS systems: basic EMT, EMT-D (EMTs trained and authorized to defibrillate), paramedic, basic EMT/paramedic, and EMT-D/paramedic. For this comparison, we used data that contained EMS response times and survival rates for cardiac arrest cases in ventricular fibrillation. From the EMS response times available from these studies, time intervals to CPR, defibrillation, and ACLS were estimated as described above.

For EMT and EMT-D systems, we assumed that both defibrillation and advanced care occurred on arrival at the hospital 20 minutes after collapse. Although 20 minutes is an estimate, we know this is close to the reported times for systems with EMT-level care.

Results

Plotting the rate of survival as the resuscitation process unfolds demonstrates changes in the survival rate with each procedure (Figures 4.10 through 4.17). If nothing is done, the survival rate declines to zero rapidly. Any single point on this curve represents the predicted survival for the hypothetical situation in which CPR, defibrillation, intubation, IV medications, and so on, occur simultaneously; that is, nothing is done until a particular point in time, and then all interventions occur simultaneously. With the earlier performance of each critical procedure (CPR, defibrillation, ACLS), this decline becomes slower. The regression model gives the following coefficients (standard errors in parentheses) for the three time intervals: time to CPR, -2.3 percent per minute (0.7 percent, $p = 0.001$); time to first shock (DEFIB), -1.1 percent per minute (0.7 percent $p = 0.09$); time to paramedic arrival (ACLS), -2.1 percent per minute (0.3 percent, $p < 0.001$); and a regression constant of 67 percent (3 percent, $p < 0.001$). The F test for the regression model, 45.8 (3,1663 degrees of freedom), was significant at $p < 0.001$. Substituting these coefficients into the equation gives the following:

Survival rate =
67% - 2.3% x I_{CPR} - 1.1% x I_{DEFIB} - 2.1% x I_{ACLS}

which can be read as the following:

Survival rate =
67% at collapse - 2.3% per minute to CPR - 1.1% per minute to defibrillation - 2.1% per minute to ACLS

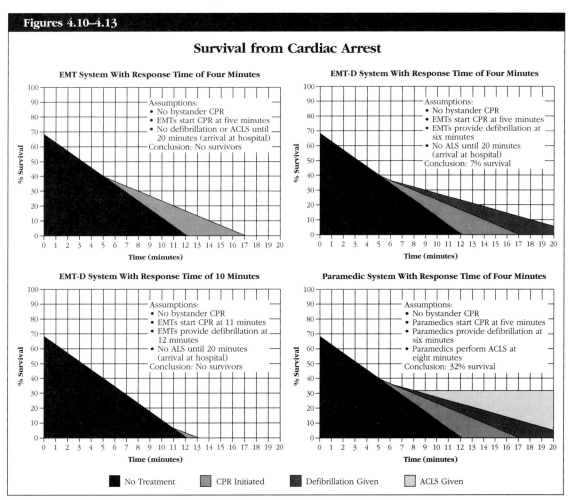

Figures 4.10–4.13

Survival from Cardiac Arrest

The regression constant, 67 percent, represents the probability of survival in the hypothetical situation in which all treatments are delivered to patients with prehospital cardiac arrest immediately on collapse. This probability is hypothetical because there are no actual patients in our database for whom time intervals to all three treatments is zero. The shortest time interval to CPR and defibrillation in our model is one minute, and the shortest time interval to ACLS is two minutes. Among 26 patients with prehospital arrest and CPR, defibrillation, and ACLS delivered within three minutes, however, the average survival rate was 50 percent. With delays in CPR, defibrillatory shock, and definitive care, the magnitude of the decline in survival rate per minute is the sum of the three coefficients (-2.3 percent, -1.1 percent, -2.1 percent), or -5.5 percent. For each minute to first shock after the start of CPR, survival declines by 3.2 percent (-5.5 percent + 2.3 percent); and for each minute to advanced care once CPR

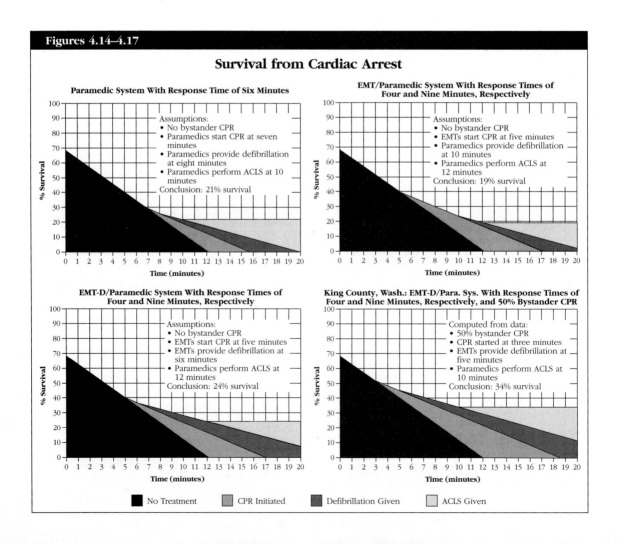

Figures 4.14–4.17

Survival from Cardiac Arrest

Paramedic System With Response Time of Six Minutes

Assumptions:
• No bystander CPR
• Paramedics start CPR at seven minutes
• Paramedics provide defibrillation at eight minutes
• Paramedics perform ACLS at 10 minutes
Conclusion: 21% survival

EMT/Paramedic System With Response Times of Four and Nine Minutes, Respectively

Assumptions:
• No bystander CPR
• EMTs start CPR at five minutes
• Paramedics provide defibrillation at 10 minutes
• Paramedics perform ACLS at 12 minutes
Conclusion: 19% survival

EMT-D/Paramedic System With Response Times of Four and Nine Minutes, Respectively

Assumptions:
• No bystander CPR
• EMTs start CPR at five minutes
• EMTs provide defibrillation at six minutes
• Paramedics perform ACLS at 12 minutes
Conclusion: 24% survival

King County, Wash.: EMT-D/Para. Sys. With Response Times of Four and Nine Minutes, Respectively, and 50% Bystander CPR

Computed from data:
• 50% bystander CPR
• CPR started at three minutes
• EMTs provide defibrillation at five minutes
• Paramedics perform ACLS at 10 minutes
Conclusion: 34% survival

■ No Treatment   ▨ CPR Initiated   ■ Defibrillation Given   ▢ ACLS Given has been started and the first shock has been given, survival declines by 2.1 percent (-5.5 percent + 2.3 percent + 1.1 percent).

Figures 4.10 to 4.17 show model representations of five types of community EMS services: EMT, EMT-D, paramedic only, EMT/paramedic, and EMT-D/paramedic. These plots demonstrate the change in survival rate as EMS arrival times vary for each system. When comparing survival rates predicted by the model and those observed in the literature (Table 4.3), the largest differences between the observed survival rates and those predicted by the model occurred at the lower end of the survival scale. The model predicted no patient survival to 20 minutes when EMTs provide CPR only, whereas observed survival rates for EMT-only systems in three different communities varied from three to 12 percent. For EMT-D systems with an arrival time of four minutes, a seven-percent survival rate was predicted, and a 26-percent survival rate was observed. Observed and predicted survival rates agreed more closely for paramedics, EMT/paramedics, and EMT-D/paramedics—systems in which all of these critical procedures were performed before hospital arrival.

To verify the stability of the model, we split the sample, using patient identification numbers ending in 0 through 4 as the first sample and those ending in 5 through 9 as the second sample. The coefficients of both split models were within two standard deviations of each other. Also, predicted values of both models were within seven percent of each other and within seven percent of the predicted value for the entire model.

Discussion

The model demonstrates the critical role that time plays in the success of resuscitation from sudden cardiac arrest. The shorter the time to critical interventions, the higher the survival rate. Although this is intuitive, the model demonstrates the quantitative contribution of each intervention to the survival rate. Each intervention used alone slows the rate of dying, and

Table 4.3

Reported and Predicted Survival Rates for Different Types of EMS Systems

EMS Agency Type	EMT Response Time (min.)	Paramedic Response Time (min.)	Estimated Time to (min.): CPR	Estimated Time to (min.): Defibrillation	Estimated Time to (min.): ACLS	Reported Survival Rate (%)	Predicted Survival Rate from Model (%)
EMT only	4		5	20	20	12	0
	7		8	20	20	3-20	0
EMT-D	4		5	6	20	26	7
	10		11	12	20	12	0
Paramedic	4		5	6	8	14-30	30
	6		7	8	10	15	21
EMT/Paramedic	3	7	4	8	10	25	28
	4	9	5	10	12	33	19
EMT-D/Paramedic	4	9	5	6	12	34	24
King County, Wash. (EMT-D/Paramedic)	4	9	3	5	10	34	34

the model clearly shows how placing each treatment earlier in the protocol improves the likelihood of survival. For instance, when an EMT-D/paramedic system is in place with average arrival times of four and nine minutes, respectively, a community bystander CPR program could decrease the average time to CPR by two minutes. Notice in comparing Figure 4.16 with Figure 4.17 that the effect of beginning CPR two minutes earlier enhances the contributions of the other procedures, making the total contribution to survival 10 percent, which is much more than the 2.1 percent per minute, or 4.2 percent, for the two minutes' earlier CPR. Putting defibrillators in the hands of EMTs makes a difference of five percent in the survival rate given EMT and paramedic arrival times of four and nine minutes, respectively.

Even though the EMS systems of different communities vary in their ability to provide CPR, defibrillatory shocks, and advanced care rapidly, the model can predict expected changes in survival rates for any of these systems given a hypothetical change in protocol. The model does not distinguish effects on survival rate due to factors not under EMS control, such as age, sex, underlying morbidity, and quality of hospital care. Customization of the model by computing coefficients from a community's data may be necessary when demographics, rate of bystander CPR, and hospital care standards differ from those in King County.

Of particular interest is a direct comparison between an EMT/paramedic system and an EMT-D/paramedic system, showing the effect of shifting the responsibility for defibrillation from paramedics to EMTs. Fortunately, observed times were available for both systems where the EMTs arrived in four minutes and the paramedics arrived in nine minutes. An EMT/paramedic system that gave an expected survival rate of 19 percent had an observed rate of 33 percent. An EMT-D/paramedic system with the same arrival times gave a predicted survival rate of 24 percent and an observed rate of 34 percent, showing a strong improvement in predicted survival rates when both CPR and defibrillation are provided early by EMTs. The current survival rate for King County, which has an EMT-D/paramedic system with an average EMT arrival time of four minutes, an average paramedic arrival time of nine minutes, and a bystander CPR rate of 50 percent is 34 percent, representing the payoff of the aggressive public education campaign on bystander CPR and the policy of training and authorizing EMTs to defibrillate.

In addition, recent research shows that an EMT-D program can improve the probability of survival in ways other than simply providing earlier defibrillation. Because it transfers the task of defibrillation out of the hands of paramedics, it allows paramedics to move more quickly to intubation and IV medication. This means that the specific elements of advanced care occur earlier in such systems. Furthermore, moving defibrillation earlier in an EMT-D system means that personnel will treat a greater number of persons in ventricular fibrillation because they arrive before the ventricular fibrillation has deteriorated to asystole.

Several assumptions weaken the model. First, we did not have exact times to CPR and defibrillation for all cases. We were forced to estimate these time intervals by adding constants to the EMS response times. These estimates, while consistently applied, are less accurate than measuring exact time intervals. Second, the model assumes that the start of delivery of ACLS is the last procedure that defines the survival rate. We know that this is not true but is merely a representation of the fact that no further information on treatment and response is provided until hospital discharge. Of course, additional interventions occur in the hospital, but the major prehospital interventions end with the performance of ACLS. Third, because the three time intervals are not independent (the same agency often provides at least two procedures), the model best describes situations where CPR, first defibrillatory shock, and advanced care follow each other in the order listed.

As Table 4.3 shows, the model does not agree with published data for EMT-only and EMT-D communities. One of the following factors may explain this. The published data were from many different sources, making it difficult to assess consistency of reporting among them. Average time intervals to first shock and advanced care were not available to EMT and EMT-D systems. The 20 minutes assumed to be the time interval for advanced care reflect the average hospital arrival time for these systems. The greater-than-expected number of survivors for the actual systems may reflect intervals of less than 20 minutes. Data for these systems tended to be much older and were obtained for communities with smaller populations, which would have allowed faster transport of patients to the hospital. The more advanced lifesaving procedures were not provided, saving time for transport (as the model shows, however, this option does not result in more lives saved). Sample sizes for these studies were smaller, making the effect of random noise greater. A high bystander CPR rate (rates as high as 35 percent were given) could account for positive survival times seen for these communities.

Conclusion

Knowledge of the relationship between EMS time intervals and survival rates can guide an EMS system to improvements that should increase its survival rate. The model is useful for planning EMS in any community and for comparing the different types of EMS systems. In addition, this model can reflect the variation in survival rates when response times differ within a single system. The model can be customized easily to describe any community. However, a linear least-squares regression on a binary outcome variable may not be valid on small sample sizes. Also, because the predictors (time intervals to CPR, first defibrillatory shock, and advanced care) are highly correlated, the model performs best when applied to systems where all three treatments are given before hospital arrival and the average times to treatment can be computed from the data rather than assumed.

An individual case of cardiac arrest has two possible outcomes—the individual lives or dies. However, this model shows each individual's probability of survival based on a community's ability to deliver CPR, defibrillation, and advanced care.

The model is a graphic representation of the "chain of survival" concept describing the linkage among access, CPR, defibrillation, and ACLS. Between survival and the time intervals by which these interventions are provided, life ebbs rapidly and the slope of death is steep, but the downward fall need not be an inevitable plummet into the jaws of death.

References

Cummins, R. O., D. A. Chamberlain, N. S. Abramson, et al. "Recommended Guidelines for Uniform Reporting of Data from Out-of-Hospital Cardiac Arrest: The Utstein Style" (AHA Medical/Scientific Statement Special Report). *Circulation* 84 (1991): 966-981.

Cummins, R. O., J. P. Ornato, W. H. Theis, et al. "Improving Survival from Sudden Cardiac Arrest: The 'Chain of Survival.'" *Circulation* 83 (1991): 1832-1847.

Cummins, R. O., M. S. Eisenberg, A. P. Hallstrom, et al. "Survival of Out-of-Hospital Cardiac Arrest with Early Initiation of Cardiopulmonary Resuscitation." *American Journal of Emergency Medicine* 3 (1985): 114-118.

Diamond, N. J., J. Schofferman, and J. W. Elliot. "Factors in Successful Resuscitation by Paramedics." *Journal of the American College of Emergency Physicians* 6 (1977): 42-46.

Eisenberg, M. S., E. Hadas, I. Nuri, et al. "Sudden Cardiac Arrest in Israel: Factors Associated with Successful Resuscitation." *American Journal of Emergency Medicine* 6 (1988): 319-323.

Eisenberg, M. S., L. Bergner, and A. Hallstrom. "Out-of-Hospital Cardiac Arrest: Improved Survival with Paramedic Services." *Lancet* 1 (1980): 812-815.

Eisenberg, M. S., L. Bergner, and A. P. Hallstrom. *Sudden Cardiac Death in the Community.* New York: Praeger Publishers, 1984, 74-100.

Eisenberg, M. S., L. Bergner, and T. Hearne. "Out-of-Hospital Cardiac Arrest: A Review of Major Studies and a Proposed Uniform Reporting System." *American Journal of Public Health* 70 (1980): 236-239.

Eisenberg, M. S., M. D. Copass, A. P. Hallstrom, et al. "Management of Out-of-Hospital Cardiac Arrest." *Journal of the American Medical Association* 243 (1980): 1049-1051.

Eisenberg, M. S., M. K. Copass, A. P. Hallstrom, et al. "Treatment of Out-of-Hospital Cardiac Arrests with Rapid Defibrillation by Emergency Medical Technicians." *New England Journal of Medicine* 302 (1980): 1379-1383.

Gudjonsson, H., E. Baldvinsson, G. Oddsson, et al. "Results of Attempted Cardiopulmonary Resuscitation of Patients Dying Suddenly Outside the Hospital in Reykjavik and the Surrounding Area." *Acta Med Scand* 212 (1982): 247-251.

Hoekstra, J. W., J. R. Banks, D. R. Martin, et al. "The Effect of First-Responder Automated Defibrillation on Time to Therapeutic Interventions During Out-of-Hospital Cardiac Arrest." *Annals of Emergency Medicine* 22 (1993): 1247-1253.

Kleinbaum, D. G., and L. L. Kupper. *Applied Regression Analysis and other Multivariable Methods.* North Scituate, Mass.: Duxbury Press, 1978, 131-147.

Liberthson, R. R., E. L. Nagel, J. C. Hirschman, et al. "Prehospital Ventricular Defibrillation: Prognosis and Follow-Up Course." *New England Journal of Medicine* 291 (1974): 317-321.

Pepe, P. E., and D. Mann. "The Effects of Early Defibrillation Programs on the Percent of People Found in VF." *Prehospital Disaster Medicine* 8 (1993).

Roth, R., R. D. Stewart, K. Rogers, et al. "Out-of-Hospital Cardiac Arrest: Factors Associated with Survival." *Annals of Emergency Medicine* 13 (1984): 237-243.

Stults, K. R., D. D. Brown, V. L. Schug, et al. "Prehospital Defibrillation Performed by Emergency Medical Technicians in Rural Communities." *New England Journal of Medicine* 301 (1984): 219-223.

Vukov, L. F., R. D. White, J. W. Bachman, et al. "New Perspectives on Rural EMT Defibrillation." *Annals of Emergency Medicine* 17 (1988): 318-321.

Weaver, W. D., L. A. Cobb, A. P. Hallstrom, et al. "Considerations for Improving Survival from Out-of-Hospital Cardiac Arrest." *Annals of Emergency Medicine* 15 (1986): 1181-1186.

Weaver, W. D., L. A. Cobb, C. E. Fahrenbruch, et al. "Use of the Automatic External Defibrillator in the Management of Out-of-Hospital Cardiac Arrest." *New England Journal of Medicine* 53 (1988): 68-70.

Wilson, B. H., H. W. Severance, Jr., M. P. Raney, et al. "Out-of-Hospital Management of Cardiac Arrest by Basic Emergency Medical Technicians." *American Journal of Cardiology* 53 (1984): 68-70.

Source

Reprinted with permission from Annals of Emergency Medicine, *November 1993. The authors include Mary P. Larsen, MS; Mickey S. Eisenberg, MD, PhD; Richard O. Cummins, MD, MPH, MSc; and Alfred P. Hallstrom, PhD, from the center for Evaluation of Emergency Medical Services, EMS Division, King County Department of Public Health and the Department of Medicine and Biostatistics, University of Washington, Seattle.*

Case 4

How Much Is a Life Worth, Anyway?

Example 1

The incident involved an 18-year-old victim whose car slid on ice and collided with a pickup truck. The service claimed the death was due to head injuries suffered in the accident. The family claimed that the death occurred because the young woman was chewing gum that became lodged in her throat, blocked her airway, and deprived her brain of oxygen. Both sides presented pathologists as expert witnesses to support their respective theories. The plaintiffs asked for $2.5 million in damages.

The EMS agency asked that the suit be dismissed due to a state law protecting EMS agencies and their personnel from lawsuits. The judge indicated that the law indeed protected the organization for its actions during the run, including its treatment of the patient. It could, however, be held responsible for negligence before responding to the accident, including neglecting to properly maintain equipment, the judge ruled.

The jury heard testimony that the light on the laryngoscope didn't work, preventing the medic from seeing the gum in the patient's airway. There were no replacement bulbs or devices on the unit. The family argued that the service should have been certain the light worked or carried a backup unit. Backup bulbs for this device are not required by state regulations.

The jury awarded the family $1.8 million.

The father said, "We feel that there's justice in the verdict, but, you know, nothing can bring her back.

Example 2

"OSHA to fine EMS agency $34,000," the headline proclaimed. The charge was "willful and serious" violations of federal health regulations that OSHA claimed jeopardized the safety of employees. The written statement went on to say, "The critical items cited here concern the inadequate protection for those employees, especially emergency medical technicians and paramedics, whose work duties may bring them into contact with blood, body fluids, or other potentially infectious materials, and therefore bloodborne pathogens." OSHA defines willful violations as those committed with "an intentional disregard of, or plain indifference to" the health and safety codes.

The four willful violations cited were

- Failure to write an exposure control program governing employee exposure to bloodborne pathogens
- Failure to clean laundry contaminated by blood and body fluids
- Failure to properly provide the hepatitis B vaccine to employees
- Failure to develop a hazardous communications program for employees

OSHA also cited the agency for serious

violations including locked and blocked exit doors, unguarded grinding machinery, some hazardous chemicals that weren't labeled, and lack of employee training on bloodborne pathogens.

The agency involved was in the midst of lobbying the city council to provide expanded service. The OSHA story dominated local headlines for several days.

Example 1 Questions

1. Who was internally responsible for the outcome of this incident—the paramedics and EMTs, the supply officer, the medical director, or top management? Why?

2. What actions could the EMS administrator have proactively taken to ensure that equipment failure was minimized?

3. As medical director, what actions would you take retrospectively to reduce future potential liability?

Example 2 Questions

1. As the administrator, what actions would you take to ensure that employee safety questions and concerns were internally reported and acted upon?

2. Describe a strategy to "limit the political damage" of this incident with the city council.

Part Five

System Design Issues and Options

The future is like heaven—everyone exalts it but no one wants to go there now.

—James Baldwin

In EMS, we are moving from what was to what will be. True to Baldwin's quote, a number of EMS leaders exalt the process of getting to the future, but few want to radically depart from their status quo to go there now.

Healthcare and EMS paradigms are shifting—and many EMS managers are resisting. Ready or not, changes are afoot in our world and in our profession that will have a profound effect on EMS systems in the decades ahead.

Some observers outside of our profession have accused us of lacking insight. The authors of the articles in Part Five are full of it (insight, that is). While they may espouse views that are different from your own, each has been selected because of his or her unique perspective.

The articles are organized in five sections. They include debates on EMS system design and politics, evolving systems and standards, discussions of different ways to accomplish the EMS mission, and finally, a peek into what the future may hold for public, private, and hospital-based systems.

—Jay Fitch

Part Five Contents

EMS System Design and Politics

Expecting the Best from Today's EMS Systems

Jay Fitch, PhD

Twenty-five years ago, the federal government identified 15 components that were considered necessary for any EMS system. As systems have evolved, the focus has moved from rigid components to understanding what makes a system effective. This article describes the eight essential elements or values that an EMS system and its leadership must embrace to become effective.

WHAT SHOULD WE EXPECT from our EMS system? This question is frequently asked by state and local community leaders. Despite consulting for over 10 years, in almost all 50 states and several foreign countries, I have found that there is no easy answer to that question.

In the 1970s, the federal government outlined 15 components to describe an EMS system. They were manpower, training, communications, transportation, facilities, critical care units, public safety agencies, consumer participation, accessibility, transfer of patients, standard medical record-keeping, public information, evaluation, disaster linkage, and mutual aid agreements. While these components are important, most now agree that simply having them in place does not ensure a well-functioning system. If this is the case, then what criteria can be used to analyze and improve an EMS system?

Community leaders should consider eight guiding principles or values in determining what to expect from their EMS program. They are speed of response, sophistication, competence, soundness and accountability, reliability, integration, ensuring value for money, and satisfaction. Let's take a look at each element and describe in detail what makes these elements essential to an effective EMS system.

Speed of Response

The principal aim of an EMS system is to minimize the time to definitive care for victims of certain types of illness and injury. To speed the response to those in need, EMS systems must consider how to minimize discovery and reporting times, improve dispatch and crew alert functions, effectively utilize first responders, reduce scene times, and transport to the appropriate facilities.

Discovering and reporting an incident is the first step in the response cycle. While EMS providers cannot be held accountable for discovery time, reducing the time that it takes for people to recognize the problem and enter the system is a meaningful mechanism for improving effectiveness.

Although media awareness and community education efforts continue to improve recognition, educational efforts need to be expanded. For example, statistics indicate that patients often delay reporting early symptoms of a heart attack for up to five hours. There are also significant delays in accessing care in rural areas. Reducing discovery and access delays can provide substantial reductions in morbidity and mortality.

Emergency 9-1-1 service has been one of the most important tools for improving access. However, it is still not universally available. According to Bill Stanton, executive director of the National Emergency Number Association (NENA), the statistics are telling. "It depends on how you look at the figures," he said. "For example, 90 percent of the 195 most populous cities in the United States are covered by E-9-1-1 (expanded 9-1-1, which includes automatic number identification and automatic location identification). Yet, geographically, only 26 percent of the country is covered by 9-1-1 service."

Call reception is another focus point that can speed the response. How is the call received and dispatched, and how is the crew alerted? How many telephone transfers are necessary before the caller reaches the right dispatcher? Is that person properly trained in medical dispatch procedures? Training in both telephone and radio skills are paramount. Communications personnel should also be medically trained, since they may need to relay medical instructions to the caller. Strong communications skills are a must, since this is the first contact between the patient and the system.

First responders are an effective intervention for those in life-threatening situations. The promptness and ability of the first responders impact their effectiveness. First responder programs today range from the highly sophisticated and fully integrated total response systems to a patchwork quilt of public safety agencies, often without any systemic direction or quality assurance mechanisms.

Rapid defibrillation by first responders has repeatedly demonstrated the ability to reduce morbidity and mortality. It has been shown to be a simple and cost-effective method of improving survival rates in cardiac patients.

Scene times and identification of high-risk patients for transfer are also major factors influencing the speed of the total system response. Effective EMS systems strive to reduce scene times and to transport patients by ground and air to the most appropriate facility. The phrase "the golden hour" was coined to define the maximum time from discovery to definite trauma care. As practitioners began studying outcomes, rapid intervention and transport have clearly been shown to increase patient survivability. Sophisticated systems routinely monitor scene times by type of call and work to reduce those times.

Rapid medical transport can be accomplished without traveling at reckless speeds using lights and sirens. Choosing when to transport by air can also be a key factor in survival. Systems should closely monitor scene times, improve on-scene procedures, and monitor the decision-making process used to determine both the method of transportation and the appropriate destination for the patient.

Systems must also monitor emergency department referral times for high-risk patients. Referral/transfer times impact the patient's outcome, particularly in trauma cases. Sophisticated systems monitor these decisions and time frames, making adjustments that reduce the time required to reach definitive care.

Improving the speed of the total system response as a guiding value involves incident reporting, dispatch, first responders, identification of high-risk patients, and quick delivery of the patient to the appropriate care facility.

Sophistication

The second guiding principle describes the level of care each system provides its patients. An EMS system is generally considered to be more sophisticated if it delivers "more powerful" treatment options to patients. That is, the higher the level of care provided, the more sophisticated the system. Using that definition, a BLS system with first responder defibrillation is more sophisticated than a BLS system with no first response. An ALS system would be considered more sophisticated than a BLS system.

Factors that impact the sophistication of a system's response include providing the highest level of care available, upgrading medical knowledge, making modern treatment modalities available, and promoting citizen EMS education.

Effective EMS systems strive to maximize the number of patients served by the highest level of prehospital care. While some believe it is impractical to serve all patients at the highest level of care, others think it is both more efficient and effective to do so. (See "ALS in Urban and Suburban EMS Systems," by Joseph Ornato, MD, et al., also in Part Five.) Forward-thinking systems work to maximize the proportion of patients served at the highest level of care. A number of factors influence the sophistication of the response.

Provider training is a key factor. States require minimum standards for certification. Many systems have accepted the minimum standard as the appropriate standard. Unfortunately, minimal standards are often substandard. A number of states still permit advanced first aid trained personnel or even non-medically trained personnel to participate in care as first responders or ambulance drivers.

A minimal standard for first responders should be completion of an approved first responder training program. Rescue and ambulance personnel should be trained to the EMT-basic level at the very least. Advanced care capabilities are always preferred, but must be weighed against the cost and potential good generated, plus the inability to retain skills that are seldom used.

The medical knowledge of each provider must be continually upgraded. Continuing medical education (CME) should be a requirement at all levels of prehospital care. This is particularly important for providers in rural areas, who do not have enough clinical and critical care exposure to maintain proper skills. The field of EMS continues to change at a rapid pace, and treatment modalities today may be contraindicated tomorrow. CMEs are available through journals, hospital-based and in-house programs, and regional and national conferences. They should be pursued at any opportunity.

A system is generally considered more sophisticated if it has a broad range of treatment capabilities available. This includes both equipment and procedures for providing definitive care. While effective systems ensure that their personnel have up-to-date equipment and fully understand how to use the equipment to the patient's benefit, more sophisticated systems keep abreast of the changing medical knowledge base. They work closely with medical advisors and are involved in clinical research. Their goal is to continually improve the outcome for the patient.

The final factor relating to sophistication involves citizen EMS education. Services should promote the education of their citizens, because the citizen's ability to perform some EMS functions can make a difference in the final outcome of certain types of illnesses. Numerous cities have adopted citizen CPR programs with positive results. Japan began implementing a program to train its citizens in EMS matters as a prerequisite for receiving a vehicle license. In the United States, organized statewide efforts should be implemented to promote citizen EMS education.

Sophistication involves providing the highest level of care available, upgrading medical knowledge, making modern treatment modalities available, and promoting citizen EMS education.

Competence

Regardless of the level of sophisticated care that a system is designed to deliver, to be effective it must deliver that care in a competent manner. Improving the competence of the response can be accomplished in a variety of ways. Factors that influence a system's competence include setting and enforcing standards, monitoring those standards, improving management skills, and providing both a quality education and an adequate certification process.

Service standards should be set, monitored, and enforced for licensed ambulance and first responder services. They should be monitored on a regular, but not predictable, basis. The range varies from states with no enforcement regulations to states that are stringent in their enforcement policies. Regulations that are standardized, preferably by the state, are needed to ensure proper medical care.

A system is generally considered more sophisticated if it has a broad range of treatment capabilities available. This includes both equipment and procedures for providing definitive care.

Standards for EMS personnel are also a factor impacting a system's competence. EMS personnel face a maddening process of certification regulations. A true national standard needs to be set and adopted by all states to facilitate competence. The National Registry attempted to accomplish this goal, but its standard has never been fully accepted. The fragmented nature of local regulations and certifications has made improving personnel competency difficult. Despite federal guidelines, there is no clear agreement between states on first responder, EMT, EMT-I, and EMT-P requirements. EMS personnel find it difficult to relocate and often get "stuck" in a single system rather than have a variety of experience. The ability to smoothly move from one system to another for career development is a factor that affects the competence and satisfaction of many providers.

Leadership is a major factor impacting the competence of many state and local EMS systems. The backbone of the EMS system lies in local services, and many of these are poorly managed. Increasing the competence of the total EMS system begins with increasing the competence of local EMS service management and with helping them understand that they are part of a larger system.

Developing local service leadership skills should be a high priority. There is no standardized core curriculum required for EMS supervisors and managers. The U.S. Fire Academy and the American Ambulance Association's Management Training Institute have developed programs to address this issue. Neither program has universal acceptance, however.

The availability and quality of EMS training varies greatly throughout the United States. Typically, overseeing initial and refresher training has been a state function. Well-developed systems and services recognize that the training required by various states represents a minimum standard. Sophisticated systems strive to intellectually challenge their staff members to a higher level of achievement. This can be accomplished in a variety of ways. For example, the decreasing cost of technology has made it possible to present information to providers via satellite, video, and computer-based training in an extremely cost-effective manner.

The final factor that affects the competence of the response is certification. While certification may be a dirty word to those EMS professionals who believe that they should be licensed like nurses and physicians, it is a necessary evil. Effective systems recognize that a regular competency-based certification process is necessary to ensure high-quality care. In fact, regular competency-based certification processes should be required for all medical disciplines.

The process should encompass more than just certification; it should include basic clinical education, continuing education, in-service training, quality improvement training, and training devoted to performance enhancement.

Ensuring that an EMS system is competent involves setting and enforcing standards, monitoring those standards, improving management skills, and providing both a quality education and an adequate certification process.

Soundness and Accountability

Soundness refers to active medical guidance that ensures current, proper treatment protocols based on thorough and continuing research. It involves developing mechanisms for accountability, including systems to collect data, objectively evaluate performance, and improve the system.

The first step in developing a sound EMS system is having defined standards of care at the state level. These should complement the national standards of care published by the American College of Emergency Physicians (ACEP) and the National Association of EMS Physicians (NAEMSP). Still, standards of care today are overwhelmingly defined by the local medical director or regional authority. The state EMS office should be encouraged to prescribe sound and appropriate patient care through the Board of Medical Examiners or a related agency.

Written protocols and medical control for uniform care delivery should be established. Patient care protocols will vary, depending on geography, transportation parameters, and designated medical facilities. However, a uniform set of regional protocols will facilitate consistent patient care among providers when care is transferred or mutual aid is required.

Services should review and conduct valid research on EMS tools, operational and clinical methods, and patient outcomes on a continual basis. Efforts directed toward doing original research should be coordinated and encouraged through the state health department, preferably in conjunction with a recognized teaching hospital.

Data systems must be developed, enhanced, and integrated. Data transmission and retrieval systems should be easy to use. Their interface capabilities should be varied in order to meet the needs of a variety of agencies. This will make valid research much easier to perform, and the analysis of past and future actions easier to accomplish. Justification of current practices can only be validated by analyzing accurate records of past performances. EMS has been traditionally slow to incorporate computerized systems into daily routines, including patient data and analysis programs.

The final item in considering soundness involves constantly striving to improve the system. It entails regularly reviewing the successes and failures in various components of the EMS system. Often referred to as QA or QI, a program must be free from fear of legal retribution in order to be effective. Positive components of the system must be reinforced and negative components modified on both a micro and a macro level. Quality improvement activities constantly reassess and update an organization's standards. The old management question of "who" has been replaced by "why" when defining quality and establishing standards for measuring the various EMS components.

To summarize, soundness—or ensuring appropriate medical guid-

Soundness—or ensuring appropriate medical guidance—includes striving for regionally accepted standards of care, establishing written medical protocols, continuously reviewing and conducting medical research, developing data systems to collect pertinent information, and regularly reviewing the successes and failures of the system.

Cooperation among agencies increases the combined resources and effectiveness of the entire system.

ance—includes striving for regionally accepted standards of care, establishing written medical protocols, continuously reviewing and conducting medical research, developing data systems to collect pertinent information, and regularly reviewing the successes and failures of the system.

Reliability

EMS systems rarely function *exactly* as they were designed. However, a system delivering a specific level of care to 95 percent of its patients is significantly better than one that delivers the same level of care to 75 percent. A reliable system can deliver quality care in stressful situations, including mass casualties and major disasters, as well as during day-to-day emergencies.

Factors that influence the reliability of the response include staffing, communications capabilities, cooperative agencies sharing resources, and vehicles properly equipped and maintained at optimal levels.

Adequate staffing at the highest technical level is one of the most difficult goals for many systems to achieve. Medics and EMTs are often in short supply. There are simply very few career tracks for EMS field providers. Working conditions and access to improved medical training may determine how long an EMT will volunteer or remain in a position offering a less-than-competitive salary. Developing and offering career paths as instructors, managers, field supervisors, physician assistants, and even product specialists will help challenge and retain a well-trained staff.

A comprehensive, reliable communications system is crucial to any EMS operation. Hospitals will continue to close for a variety of economic reasons, putting an added burden on medical transportation services. The healthcare team—from first responders to the staff at a designated hospital—needs to be in contact through pagers, telephones, computer terminals, and/or radios. This is particularly true for rural services that often transport longer distances to regional tertiary care facilities. Rapidly evolving communication technology can only help the EMS organization that stays abreast of these changes.

Cooperation among agencies increases the combined resources and effectiveness of the entire system. This has been accomplished even between for-profit providers who frequently compete for service areas and patients. It is another reason for sharing universal medical protocols, policies, training, and purchasing on a regional basis. Otherwise, services may spend funds needlessly and waste precious time and energy.

Emergency vehicles should be provided that are appropriately equipped and maintained. A statewide standard should exist that clearly spells out the minimum vehicle and equipment capabilities. Federal KKK ambulance standards offer a good beginning. Ambulances should not be allowed to operate if they do not meet minimal standards. Optimum vehicles and equipment should be determined in consultation with local medical authorities. Vehicles should receive preventive maintenance to ensure that no mechanical breakdown interferes with quality patient care. A service that owns a tow truck is spending funds foolishly.

Reliability means providing the highest level of training to staff, implementing a modern communications system, sharing resources with cooperative agencies, and properly equipping and maintaining vehicles.

Integration

Development of an integrated system of care, which is preplanned from roadside to rehabilitation, has been a guiding principle since the initiation of modern EMS systems. This concept is important because the various agencies involved in a patient's care are capable of acting independently. It has been generally recognized that a more coordinated network of facilities and specialty centers offers the greatest opportunity to optimize care for the patient. Sophisticated trauma systems, available in some states, are an excellent example of a highly refined, integrated approach that ensures optimum care for a particular patient type.

Factors that impact the integration of care include planning at the state, regional, and local levels, coordination by the state health department or other agency, and cooperation by local facilities and agencies.

Planning is the first and most essential ingredient in any successful EMS system. The most successful statewide systems use a regional approach that promotes quality care for all citizens. A regional system developed in conjunction with state health officials will facilitate a fully integrated statewide delivery system.

Medical facilities and their personnel must be involved in the state and regional planning process. Involvement by all parties translates into increased teamwork, compliance, cooperative ongoing system evaluation, and an improved response at all levels.

The relationships between the various divisions of the state health department must be used to facilitate coordination. The EMS division is traditionally a small part of the state health department. It is vital that EMS organizations use other health department resources to improve the efficiency and reduce the cost of state EMS system development.

Relationships outside the state EMS office, and even the state health department, may have regulatory responsibilities for EMS systems. It is essential that the state EMS division and the local and regional EMS systems develop and improve relationships with other agencies that hold EMS-related responsibilities.

Public, private, and government agencies frequently have overlapping areas of interest, responsibility, and scope. This overlap contributes to duplication, unnecessary expense, and poor utilization of human resources. Creating interagency ventures results in maximized resources, increased awareness, and a reduced overall financial impact.

Integration at the highest levels means planning with the state EMS division; incorporating medical facilities and their personnel in the plan-

Development of an integrated system of care, which is preplanned from roadside to rehabilitation, has been a guiding principle since the initiation of modern EMS systems.

Good value for dollars should always be pursued. This can be accomplished by understanding current costs, considering alternative methods of providing service, linking grant monies to local plans and objectives, and using state resources to assist in upgrading local provider efficiency.

ning process; getting all divisions in the state health department involved in EMS issues; reaching outside the state health department to involve other agencies that have EMS responsibilities; and encouraging public, private, and government agencies into cooperative ventures to reduce duplication of efforts and improve overall financial impact.

Ensuring Value for Money

Simply put, every EMS system should be cost effective. A number of factors positively contribute to gaining value from the dollars invested. They include encouraging local services to evaluate alternative system designs, developing deeper understandings of service costs, linking federal grant programs to local or regional EMS plans, and upgrading local programs.

Systems need to regularly evaluate and compare their current operations to alternative service delivery methods. To meaningfully accomplish this task, services must objectively determine their fixed and variable costs of operations.

Even more basic, many systems are not able to determine their actual cost of transporting a patient. They must consider a complex series of factors that may include subsidies; patient mix; sharing of overhead for items like communications, supplies, and exchanges with hospitals; a combination of delivery system types, including tiered, dual response, and emergency and non-emergency providers; and a host of other considerations. Alternative delivery methods can only be compared when the actual costs of delivery are known and understood.

Another area of potential funding for system planning can be found in state and federal grant programs. Linking grant programs to local or regional EMS plans can reduce the cost of implementing these plans. Most plans are structured around goals and objectives for a five-year period.

In many cases, state resources may be available to assist in upgrading local or regional systems. Monies for communication systems, leadership training, specialty equipment, disaster planning, or other items could be available to improve the clinical and operational aspects of local systems. Efforts should be regularly taken to improve the efficiency of local services. Many local EMS providers may not be operating at peak efficiency. Better efficiency and cost effectiveness equates to better value for dollars spent.

Good value for dollars should always be pursued. This can be accomplished by understanding current costs, considering alternative methods of providing service, linking grant monies to local plans and objectives, and using state resources to assist in upgrading local provider efficiency.

Customer and Worker Satisfaction

Quality, dignity, and respect are all reasonable expectations for every participant in the EMS system, from consumers to healthcare employees. Factors that contribute to the satisfaction of consumers and those working in the system include increasing awareness of the system, continually demonstrating best value for the dollars spent, focusing on worker health and safety, monitoring and enhancing worker satisfaction, and disseminating information about the system to all constituents.

One factor that needs regular work is improving system awareness. The exciting field of emergency services offers high-profile "sound bites" for local government officials and legislators in a host of one-time appearances. But the issues that are vital to the provision of EMS need exposure on a regular basis. Citizens, legislators, and providers alike need to be kept current on the issues affecting EMS systems.

The value of dollars spent must be demonstrated and reported to all concerned. Simply providing the best possible care in the most cost-effective manner is not enough. The mechanisms for monitoring and reporting care versus dollars must be well established and improvements promoted both within and outside the system.

Worker safety and health must also be ensured. Risk management has become a specialized field, primarily due to the potential adverse impact of liability and health-related issues. Services must provide health and safety protocols and environments that exceed federally mandated standards. Funds are currently being used for legal fees and lawsuit awards that would be better spent on resources and improved services.

The consequences of ignoring the priorities of worker safety and health are unnecessary death, injury, and employee turnover. It is in the best interest of the EMS system to control expenses, eliminate adverse situations, improve the overall operations, and better manage precious resources in this area.

Objectively monitoring worker satisfaction at regular intervals and developing positive mechanisms to deal with employee issues are important first steps. In addition, providing an opportunity for involvement in decisions that affect workers, whenever possible, is central to improving the internal organizational health of the system.

Finally, the level of satisfaction is directly related to the quality and quantity of information provided about the system. Information should be offered in a variety of media on a regular basis about the many efforts the system makes on the public's behalf.

Satisfaction with an EMS system is derived from increasing awareness, demonstrating best value for the dollars spent, worker health and safety, improving worker involvement and satisfaction, and disseminating information about the system to all constituents.

Conclusion

These eight system values embrace the view that a modern EMS system is dynamic, ever-changing, and striving to constantly improve. The values suppress the parochial view of EMS services as individual components. Use these principles as building blocks for improving the effectiveness of EMS systems.

Source

Original article.

The Whole is ALL of the Parts, Together

Marvin L. Birnbaum, MD, PhD

Have EMS systems become fractionalized and self-serving? EMS sage and editor of the journal Prehospital and Disaster Management, *Dr. Marvin Birnbaum presents his view in this brief and hard-hitting editorial.*

I AM INCREASINGLY CONCERNED that prehospital emergency medical services are becoming fractionated. Many providers have formed or are in the process of forming new organizations to meet needs that are perceived as not being met by the organizations currently in place in the EMS community. The issue is not whether the current organizations are able to meet these needs, but the perception that the needs are not being met. The inherent danger in the factionalization of prehospital EMS is that the discipline may be sucked into the parochialism that plagues the rest of the medical world. If we look to the other subspecialized disciplines of medicine as a model and mimic their failures, we too shall fail.

Prehospital EMS is distinct from other branches of medical care in that it truly is interdisciplinary. No other area of healthcare comprises persons of such different backgrounds and training. These special people provide the best care possible at a remarkably low cost with a profound commitment to helping their neighbors, friends, and community.

Each EMS system comprises many parts, like the fibers composing a rope. All in all, the predominant reason that EMS systems work is that each of the parts is mutually dependent. The system coordinates all of its component parts. It is sustained by close ties and mutual respect between and among the components. Common purpose and communications not present in any other branches of medicine link each of the components. The system forms the foundation of prehospital EMS. It is the system that distinguishes EMS in the medical community.

Independent Components

To understand the current problem, it is important to view each component strand from the perspective of how it came into existence: Each arose in answer to a perceived need, independent from stimulation or leadership by any of the other parts. Ambulance providers arose without the stimulation or leadership from the physician community. Initially, training of personnel was minimal, but later became mandatory, often at the state level—without significant physician involvement. Education was provided by instructors often selected by default. Each part fended for itself. Each struggled for its own survival and for recognition. Each formed with little regard to the system in which it had to function. Complete, functional systems were conceived and implemented only in exceptional circumstances. The EMS forest was planted, germination had occurred, and growth was under way. Similar patterns arose all over the world.

Centralized offices were a reaction to the many helter-skelter services—an effort to splice existing pieces into a rudimentary system. Functional systems came later. Since there was a general lack of medical input and commitment, government found itself in the position of having to mandate standards by regulation. Thus, intense rigidity became the rule. The EMTs, paramedics, nurses, physicians, pilots, educators, administrators, firefighters, and others came to meet most of their respective needs independently from the others.

Since each struggled long and hard for identity, each component continues to try to function independently to remain true to its original ideals. Therefore, each has come to view all of EMS parochially, often with little regard for the other components with which it has been forced through regulations to function within the "system." Only recently were there attempts to integrate all of the component parts into comprehensive EMS systems, and these attempts were often a series of heroic struggles. But, systems evolved and persons with common interests bonded together. In the United States, EMS systems developed at all governmental levels.

New Organizations—The Second Generation

But, when a segment of one of these groups felt that its needs were not being heard, there occurred a movement to form a new organization that hopefully would meet its perceived needs better than did the parent organization—an organization in which the participants should have had an active part, but one in which they perceived they could never play a meaningful role. The National Association of Emergency Medical Services Physicians (NAEMSP) came to be in this fashion. Prehospital emergency physicians who were (and most still are) members of the American College of Emergency Physicians (ACEP) believed that ACEP was not meeting the needs of the prehospital physicians and formed a new, separate organization with its own goals and structure. Of further note is the pervasive drive of many academicians to form groups separate and distinct from those of the clinicians. The formation of the University Academic Emergency Medical Services (now the Society for Academic Emergency Medicine) characterizes this type of development. The parent paid inadequate attention to its children and the family split. The kids ran away!

This story has been repeated again and again. But, the subgroups are subspecializing more and more, each with a smaller base of supporters, organized by specific narrow sets of interests rather than by the overall delivery of prehospital emergency medical care. Today, the EMS educators are forming a new organization because they perceive their needs are not being met by any of the existing EMS organizations. The flight physicians are organizing separately from other emergency and prehospital physicians. On and on it goes—more trees are cut down and new fences put up in the forest of EMS. This pattern has occurred in every other branch of medical care. Such factionalism characterizes each of the other disciplines of medicine and has led to difficulty identifying patient advo-

> We can preserve the independence of our vital components in a manner that shares what is common to us all: our victories, our problems, our ideals, and our dedication.

cates. Lack of advocacy is one reason underlying the uncomfortable position in which medicine in the United States finds itself today.

Common Needs

It is important to recognize that each strand of EMS has some needs that are specific to the group forming the new organization. For example, many problems encountered by the helicopter pilots are specific to piloting a medical helicopter; many problems encountered by helicopter crews seem distinct from those that occur in other parts of the prehospital EMS system. Yet, experiences and problems that seem specific to the air-medical component of the prehospital EMS system impact the other strands of the EMS system and must be shared with those groups. The same can be said of EMS educators, some of whose many needs are specific to the educational process. But EMS educators must train people to function within an EMS system.

Most problems are common to all EMS providers; each component is an integral part of the whole EMS system. To be effective, the entire profession must be aware of the problems others encounter because the solutions to individual problems affect the other components of the system. And, the strength of the EMS rope lies in the integrated processes provided by the system and the cooperation between the respective segments.

There is a potential danger if each component of the EMS system peels away from the rest of the EMS community and tries to mark its own territory: "Stay out—*it's mine,* and mine is too unique for you to understand." In the process, we increase the risk of falling prey to the divisive subspecialization that plagues the rest of the U.S. healthcare system. Our common interests, goals, and experiences make EMS a unique entity in the medical community. We provide universal access to optimal care at the lowest possible cost. Others should look to us as the example for delivery of accessible, cost-effective healthcare. The American colonies once made a choice and their rallying cry was "join or die." All of the components of EMS must come together now, or wither away in independence, divorced from their natural, professional, and historic allies. We can preserve the independence of our vital components in a manner that shares what is common to us all: our victories, our problems, our ideals, and our dedication.

Working Together

We need to meet together under a common banner and continue to learn from each other. The scope of the current organizations must and can widen to become more inclusive. The World Association for Emergency and Disaster Medicine (WAEDM) is pursuing this goal at the international level through the formation of the International Federation for Emergency and Disaster Medicine. Societies across the world with similar goals and interests should join this federation so they all can share and contribute to our combined experience and vision. The time is at hand to build a new union. The NAEMSP can work to splice together the many strands of the U.S. EMS profession to form a strong rope that can bind our individual needs to our common purposes. The leaders are at hand; let us join and thrive. Together we stand, divided we fall.

Source

Reprinted with permission from Prehospital and Disaster Medicine, *July-September 1992. Marvin Birnbaum, MD, PhD, is the editor of* Prehospital and Disaster Medicine *and director of the EMS program at the University of Wisconsin-Madison.*

The "E" in EMS Doesn't Stand for Emotion

Richard A. Keller

Far too often, emotions cloud the real issues when it comes to providing emergency services. Author Richard Keller suggests ways to remove the emotion from EMS.

THE BATTLE LINES HAVE BEEN DRAWN and the troops mobilized as the public and private sector armies prepare for their next skirmish in the ambulance wars.

Their weapons aren't missiles and guns, but emotions and appeals. The battlefields themselves are city council chambers, county commissions, and courtrooms. The battle cries are "home rule," "public safety," "no more profits," "the rights of small business people," "long-term member of the community," and "we can do it better."

EMS and Emotion

The "E" in EMS has come to stand for emotion. Emotional pleas arise from fire departments claiming that they should be the total provider for both fire and EMS. The arguments continue that the fire department should capture these "new" revenues to offset the costs of other operations, and that the community has the sole right to determine how emergency medical and ambulance services are to be provided.

Across the table, the private ambulance companies are crying foul, saying that it's unfair for municipalities to take away their livelihood. They describe their long-term roots in the community and their provision of ambulance services for decades. Discussions of capitalism and the American way are commingled in these conversations.

Each side attacks the other, confusion reigns, and the public suffers. The public/private competition in emergency medical services is marked by picketing and invasions of city council and county commission meetings by paramedics and EMTs from both sides. Strategies include press conferences, letters to the editor, and intense lobbying of local officials. Positions are supported by anecdotal evidence and the negative outcomes of isolated incidents.

The typical confrontation between a public department and a private company competing to provide ambulance services can best be described as ugly, nasty, and detrimental to the industry. It's time to retrench and redefine emergency medical systems. Even more important, it's time to refocus energies and efforts on providing the patients with the best possible service with the resources available.

Reviewing the Fundamentals

A few givens need to be restated. An emergency medical system requires the interaction, coordination, and integration of multiple organizations, including the dispatch center, public safety agencies (both fire and law enforcement), hospitals, trauma centers, state and local EMS oversight agencies, and private ambulance services. EMS is not the sole responsibility of, nor can it be provided by, a single agency. Any perception to the contrary cannot be allowed to continue.

Another fact is that out-of-hospital medical services are a healthcare issue. Services must be medically driven, and medical direction and control, quality improvement, and clinically proven treatment protocols are essential elements of an EMS system.

An often-ignored truism is that fragmentation of an EMS system damages patient care and the system's financial stability. In their turf wars, many system participants ignore the issue that creating many small emergency medical services causes far-reaching harm. Varying levels of care, inefficient operations, difficulties in providing oversight, and cost increases are some of the results of fragmentation.

Finally, the cost of providing the service *is* important. In arguments offered by both public and private sides of the issue, revenue—whether its gain or loss—is at the forefront, when realistically, the true and total costs of the system should be analyzed first. Only when the costs have been calculated should revenue sources be examined.

It's not appropriate to justify a medical transportation system's structure based on money that can be gained. Justification must first be accomplished in identifying the system that provides the desired level of service at the most reasonable cost.

The Important "Es"

It's time to take the emotion out of this controversy. There are three more important "Es" that the "E" in EMS should stand for: effectiveness, efficiency, and economy.

Effectiveness

Measuring effectiveness appropriately refocuses the system on the patient. Effectiveness measures, including dispatch, on-scene, and response times, and morbidity and mortality rates (patient outcomes), can gauge a system's performance. They can also be compared with community expectations as success indicators.

All of these factors outweigh any emotional pleas or discussions. An EMS system's effectiveness *can* be measured, and this should be the guiding factor in how the system is structured and who should deliver its various service components.

Efficiency

With the intense pressure in healthcare to reduce and stabilize costs, efficiency is essential for medical transportation organizations to survive. For an organization to provide out-of-hospital care efficiently, it has to meet a number of criteria.

It is important that the system's volume be adequate to support the

---

The Important "Es" of EMS:

• Effectiveness

• Efficiency

• Economy

Source

Reprinted with permission from Fire Chief, *May 1994. Richard A. Keller is a partner at Fitch & Associates, Inc. He is nationally known for his work in EMS system operations, reimbursement, and design. He is a principal author of the book* EMS Management: Beyond the Street, *2nd ed.*

infrastructure and capture some economies of scale. Small, geographically restricted organizations will not be able to deliver services at an efficient, low per-unit cost. Expansion of services through mergers and alliances of many types, therefore, will be necessary for successful out-of-hospital care providers.

Labor is the largest expense for out-of-hospital care organizations, so it's important that this valuable resource be used wisely. Efficiency will create situations where resources have to be allocated based on demand. Flexible deployment strategies and variable staffing patterns are crucial in accomplishing this, and public and private services are already incorporating these approaches into their out-of-hospital care delivery components.

Vertical and horizontal integration of emergency medical and medical transportation services is critical to lowering per-unit costs. Horizontal integration is expansion over a broader population base, while vertical integration includes the provision of multiple service lines. Potential examples include wheelchair, non-emergency, emergency, and air medical transportation services. Hospital medical transportation services have concentrated on vertical integration, while public and private services have addressed it in a more limited way.

Economy

Economy is achieved by capturing the greatest value for the money spent on personnel and non-personnel services and expenses. Though all organizations try to get the best value from their resources, external pressures will continue to make economy an important part of EMS.

Conclusion

EMS systems that survive long term will be those that incorporate these three "E's" into their operations and missions. Emotion is out. Effectiveness, efficiency, and economy are in.

EMS cannot be used to increase productivity or fill unused capacity, nor can it be viewed as a source of revenue to support other operations. Providing EMS and other medical transportation services is not an inalienable right of the incumbent.

Competition is high and likely to intensify between the various provider types, as well as between providers of the same type. The organizations that are going to successfully compete and survive are those that focus on providing the best possible service and out-of-hospital medical care at the lowest cost.

Health reform efforts are designed to encourage this, and the public and politicians are demanding it. The community should expect a high level of quality that is not anecdotal but documentable and is provided at a reasonable cost.

Creating Interagency Partnerships: When Collaboration Overcomes Competition

Jay Fitch, PhD

Collaboration has replaced competition in many ways, and many partnerships that were once thought unlikely have been formed. A number of collaborative approaches are detailed here that can change your competitors into partners.

CREATING INTERAGENCY PARTNERSHIPS is not just a new management phrase, but a creative way to work together that can improve the outcome for all involved. Throughout the world, across the country, around your town, and within the organization in which you work, new relationships are being created that are fundamentally different from those of 10 years ago. In those days, government and business were commonly conducted with competition as the main underlying theme. Today, more collaborative approaches are developing.

Recent world events are clear examples of these approaches and the new wave of leadership that has taken advantage of them. The collaborative manner in which the United States approached and consulted with other nations to support the Gulf War against Iraq, the new mutually supportive relationship between the United States and Russia, and the reunification of Germany all substantiate the premise that things are different today.

Throughout the nation, there are examples of entire industries acting differently to become more productive. If a group of United Auto Worker's Union members from the early 1970s were to visit an autonomous work group at Ford Motor Company in the 1990s, they wouldn't understand that every worker participates in decisions—nor would they understand that every worker is expected to shut down the production line if quality doesn't meet the agreed-upon standard. There is a significant difference between the authoritarian approach used in factories just 10 years ago and the team concept used today.

Healthcare and public safety organizations are being impacted by the transition from competition to collaboration. Hospitals that fiercely competed at every level five years ago are finding common ground to share services and reduce costs. Cities and public safety agencies, which would not even provide mutual aid for one another a few years ago, are now utilizing automatic aid and moving toward sharing specialized resources (such as haz-mat) on a regional basis.

Changes in leadership styles, which have been noted in the professional literature and are common in other industries, are beginning to be practiced by both EMS and fire agencies. Authoritarianism is slowly giving way to practices that share leadership responsibilities, power, and control. Leaders are learning to create partnerships with other stakeholders to improve outcomes. Changes between organizations and changes within organizations are happening. But what has caused this to occur?

There are two fundamental and intertwined reasons that more collaborative processes are being used: the increasing demand for quality and economic pressures experienced by public and private EMS organizations in the 1990s.

Motivational Factors Supporting Partnerships

There are two fundamental and intertwined reasons that more collaborative processes are being used: the increasing demand for quality and economic pressures experienced by public and private EMS organizations in the 1990s.

Quality

Consumers today demand quality in the products and services they buy. Individuals will pay a premium price for goods and services that they perceive to be of higher quality. Honda developed a reputation in the automobile industry for offering high-quality, low-maintenance automobiles. One could drive a Honda several years, and, because of its high resale value, it could be sold for almost as much as one paid for it.

The quality of the product made Honda a great value. One of Honda's secrets was using production methods that resulted in fewer errors and rejects. Honda's success and the success of others using these principles have set off a quality revolution that is touching every industry and profession.

The quality movement (or at least its acronyms) has taken the healthcare profession by storm. QA, QU, TQM, and CQI are all approaches designed to reduce errors and provide better value. To accomplish any well-defined quality program, managers must focus and measure outcomes, while at the same time paying particularly close attention to people and process issues.

To help hospitals focus on outcomes and improve both quality and cost effectiveness, the federal government now routinely publishes survival rates by hospital and procedure for major metropolitan areas. The thought was that those hospitals that do a large volume of kidney transplants, for example, are able to do them better and less expensively than a hospital that only does three or four kidney transplant procedures per year but feels they have to offer these services to be competitive in the market. The result of disseminating survival information was the closing of a number of marginal programs and the development of strategic alliances between the remaining healthcare facilities to provide the part of the continuum of care that they provide best.

Partnerships are being created within organizations, as well as with external, competing organizations. Individual leaders are recognizing that development of strategic alliances between management, employees, and other stakeholders is key to the organization's success. When you boil this down to the most simplistic level, it means helping others redefine their goal within the framework of the organization's goal.

A universal truth about quality is that doing the job right the first time is less expensive than doing it over to get it right. This is true whether building a car, transplanting a kidney, or immobilizing a patient before transportation to the hospital. The quality movement has largely been a mechanism of empowering individuals to become more responsible for the organization's desired outcomes. People involved and invested in the organization are more likely to do things right the first time.

Economics

Economics also play a major role in this paradigm shift toward strategic alliances inside and outside organizations. On a global level, the U.S. government sought others to share the cost of the Gulf War. In the auto industry, alliances between auto manufacturers and component suppliers have become commonplace. In healthcare, hospital linkages with physician practices are routine. In EMS, more alliances are being developed between organizations to share resources than ever before. These have taken many forms, including public-public alliances, public-private partnerships, and shared service relationships among private companies. The goal is to provide better value to their respective customers and constituency groups.

While some progress has been made, more is required. Improvements that have been made in EMS quality and efficiency to date could be likened to picking up the fruit off the ground beneath a fruit tree. The requirements of the future will necessitate shaking the tree trunk. The biggest "shake" will be reducing service duplication and fragmentation. Functions likely to be combined in creative partnerships include dispatch, medical control, training, maintenance, and supply functions. Agencies and firms will increasingly look at options to share services that will reduce costs and provide better value for the customer and taxpayer.

Examples of EMS Partnerships

Creative public-private partnership experiments are under way in many areas of the country. In suburban Chicago, for example, a number of fire departments have had a long-standing contract with Metro Paramedics to provide EMS service on behalf of the fire departments. Metro personnel and vehicles are housed in fire stations and are otherwise indistinguishable from sworn fire personnel.

In Arlington, Tex., a shared communications center, utilizing both public and private employees, dispatches all emergency resources, including the private ambulance service. In Bloomfield Hills, Mich., the private ambulance service provides initial and ongoing training under contract to public entities. In Richmond, Va., a unique arrangement has been organized to provide EMS services under the umbrella of the Richmond Ambulance Authority. In this system, fire department personnel provide first response and heavy rescue capabilities, while multiple volunteer organizations and a private company contract to provide transport and non-emergency services. A number of different approaches can be considered, but a key question must be answered: Does the arrangement create added value for constituents?

Partnerships between public sector agencies are also becoming more

The future of EMS lies in the cooperation of stakeholders in developing community-based partnerships that provide good value to their constituent groups.

common. Individual departments, which face expanding overhead without additional revenue, are considering consolidation as a mechanism to reduce overhead costs without negatively impacting services delivered. Examples range from automatic aid and sharing high-dollar specialized services to full consolidation of services.

A number of departments provide service to outlying areas through contractual agreements, but partnerships go further. The fire and life safety departments of Springfield and Eugene, Ore., are examples of two public agencies that have created an effective partnership. In those communities, Eugene provides haz-mat and neo-natal transport services for both cities, while Springfield manages the membership program and has the responsibility for billing and collection services for both departments.

Shared services and joint ventures are more formal partnership mechanisms that are being considered in many service sectors. Arrangements can involve public agencies, private agencies, or a combination of the two. These approaches involve setting up a separate organization with governance shared by the participating agencies. Jointly operated communications centers and air medical services are common examples of this type of approach. Hospitals are moving to jointly develop free-standing MRI units, specialty centers, and, in some cases, the community's ambulance service. For example, the hospitals in Peoria, Ill., jointly own and operate Advanced Medical Transport of Central Illinois. This ALS system provides service for the city of Peoria and surrounding areas and provides non-emergency service in the region.

Even professional associations recognize the importance of establishing partnerships. One of the most innovative partnerships was developed last year between the American Ambulance Association and the Congressional Fire Services Institute. Through this project, AAA funded an intern position with the institute to serve as a liaison and to educate members of Congress on fire and EMS issues. "It is a bit unusual," said David Nevins, executive vice president of AAA, "but we realized that the time had come for more direct communications between the public and private sectors. We saw this as an opportunity to develop a better relationship with the other associations and organizations involved in EMS."

Each of these examples illustrates a particular type of a partnership. Any number of creative combinations of resources can be developed. Don't be limited by those suggested here. In the complex economic and political times in which we live, creative thinking must become as natural as breathing.

Moving Toward Creating Partnerships

Healthcare and public safety organizations are in another important transition period. Clearly, the future of EMS lies in the cooperation of stakeholders in developing community-based partnerships that provide good value to their constituent groups. Instead of drawing lines in the sand, individuals and organizations must recognize the forces at work in our society and economy that are driving these changes. Some paradigm shifts are beginning to occur as individuals and organizations learn to "think outside the box" and discover new ways of working together, instead of competing against one another. Gerald McManis, who is well known for his work with competing hospitals, has suggested the following six steps.

Recognize everyone must give up some power to gain power. Compromises have to be made, and everyone has to approach the situation willing to give something up.

Reach agreement early on assumptions about the future. This step is time intensive, but without these fundamental agreements, goals and future directions can be difficult to achieve.

Make sure the process has integrity: Don't game it. There must be respect and trust at all levels within the respective organizations for this process to be successful. Consensus building doesn't just happen; it is the result of a deliberate process.

Establish a strong "case for cooperation." Identify the risks for each organization if they continue independently, as well as the benefits to each if they collaborate. But most important, focus on the benefits to the community.

Recognize each entity has its own culture and operating style. Regardless of the level of collaborative effort, potential gulfs caused by past history and differing philosophies must be bridged.

Create a compelling shared vision. Too many leaders dismiss this as unnecessary and have a failed joint planning effort to show for it. When people are faced with new paradigms, such as creating partnerships and collaboration, instead of competition, they need time to let go of the old ideas and embrace the new. The powerful force of a shared vision may be the only thing that keeps everyone on track when the going gets rough.

Conclusion

In the years ahead, producing higher-quality EMS and medical transportation services with fewer resources will simply be an economic fact of life. Creating partnerships that emphasize collaboration instead of competition is a creative way to work together that can improve the outcome for all involved.

Source
Original article.

A Primer on Politics: The Politics You Hate Today Were Created for a Reason 200 Years Ago

Stephen F. Dean, Jr.

Winston Churchill was fond of saying that politics were almost as exciting as war, and just as dangerous. In war, Churchill explained, you can only be killed once, but in politics you can be killed many times. Former County EMS Director Steve Dean provides an EMS "political IQ test" and outlines three decision models commonly used by politicians.

IF YOU ASK PARAMEDICS or EMTs what is wrong with their systems, you'll get a list of items that will vary depending on their locale. But if you ask why those problems can't be solved or have not been solved, invariably you will get a single answer: politics.

When people hear the word *politics*, they often think of dirty deals, corruption, and frustration. These images are in contrast to the principles of quality patient care and certainly the opposite of our ideals of American democracy and liberty.

Most paramedics and EMTs do not have a useful concept of politics or an understanding of why the political system works the way it does. Even if you do have an understanding of how the system works, it is difficult, at best, to make sense of the most complicated political goings on in any community—EMS politics.

One definition of politics is discussed below. The principles of self-rule, representative democracy, and separation of powers are examined, as well as how these principles affect the way local politics are conducted. Finally, three models or means of analyzing local political events are described. These models should enable EMTs and paramedics to make sense of some of the bewildering decisions that are generated by the political system.

Politics and Self-Government

Politics are defined by some political scientists as the pursuit of power. The pursuit of power in emergency medical services is the attempt to control the development and implementation of the policies governing the response to medical emergencies and the treatment of patients. The people who make those decisions control emergency medical services.

In the United States, the most influential emergency medical service policymakers are not physicians, administrators, or consumers. They are the mayors and council members who govern the thousands of political entities across the United States. Surprisingly, the most important EMS decisions take place on the local level, not the federal level.

Three general characteristics about the local political environment explain a great deal of the behavior and activity that occurs there. While most of us do not think of Civics 101 being relevant in our day-to-day lives, we live each day with the consequences of decisions made by the founding fathers more than 200 years ago. It was, in fact, February 21, 1787, that Congress endorsed the plan for delegates from all states to meet in Philadelphia for a constitutional convention.

Self-Rule

I used to wonder why EMS policy and EMS systems were different in every community. Part of the answer is that the constitution of the United States was based on the principle of self-government. The writers of the constitution felt that local groups of citizens (i.e., cities and counties) could best determine the rules and laws under which they would live. The federal government would only make laws and act in a very few specifically defined areas. Thus, each community is free to establish the type of system best suited to its own needs.

Representative Democracy

It was also determined that the manner in which these local governmental entities would make decisions would be by democratic rule; that is, people would vote when a decision was to be made. However, not everyone gets to vote on most issues. Instead, citizens elect representatives who conduct the affairs of government for them. Thus, EMTs and paramedics do not get to vote on issues of vital interest to themselves even if the issues do become the subject of governmental activity.

Separation of Powers

The third characteristic of government is separation of powers. Instead of establishing a single entity that would conduct all facets of government, three entities were established: a legislative branch for policy promulgation, an executive branch for policy administration, and a judicial branch to make sure the legislative branch, executive branch, and all the citizens followed the rules. Even on the local level, there is not a single entity or person who makes EMS decisions. There are several legislators (council members or commissioners) and possibly an executive (mayor or chairman) as well.

Effects of the Principles

How do these principles affect the day-to-day lives of EMTs and paramedics? Well, for one thing, it means that when there is a problem in EMS, paramedics who are concerned do not get together, get their guns, and go somewhere and solve the problem. There is no riot, no battle. If there is a government entity involved, a government process will be followed.

It also means that when there is a problem, it is usually solved by each of the thousands of local entities in their own way. Just because there is a solution that works in one locale does not mean that other locales will adopt the same solution.

Policy issues are not resolved by "quick thinking" or "fast action." The political process is designed to be slow and resistant to the passions of the moment. The premise is that, with the passing of time, people will have more opportunities to examine issues rationally and dispassionately. However, this is just the opposite of the orientation of prehospital per-

> The political process is designed to be slow and resistant to the passions of the moment. The premise is that, with the passing of time, people will have more opportunities to examine issues rationally and dispassionately.

sonnel who live in an environment where seconds count. For better or worse, there is no "lights and siren" approach to most issues.

The Political Decision Makers

The application of these principles in the local setting results in there being a council composed of several members, usually an odd number, who promulgate policy. There is also usually a mayor or administrator who is in charge of implementing the policy.

However, there are many variations of this basic structure. In some entities, the mayor is part of the council. In others, the administrator is not elected but is hired to work for the council or board of supervisors. When examining the local political scene, it is helpful to know how many legislators there are and whether the administrator is elected or hired, and also whether the administrator is really part of the council or independent.

Making Sense of Local EMS Politics

The great challenge to paramedics, EMTs, and politicians alike is trying to make sense of the bewildering events surrounding EMS in the local community. One night at a county board meeting at which I was in attendance, a particularly bright and informed commissioner stated that he could not begin to understand the politics of EMS and did not have any hope of ever understanding them. This is not uncommon.

As is usually the case, most people underestimate the complexity of EMS. The number of organizations having an interest in EMS policy usually makes agreement on any issue difficult. There may be two or more fire departments, ambulance companies, police agencies, and hospitals all involved in a single "system." The possibilities for conflict are mind-boggling. When you bring your problems to the local political forum before a group of elected officials who know little or nothing about EMS, you can readily see why the results are often bewildering.

Three Policy Models

Making sense of how decisions are made and why is difficult but not impossible. However, the means of interpreting all of this lies in a most unlikely place: the Cuban missile crisis. What does the Cuban missile crisis have to do with emergency medical services? At first glance, it would appear to be not much. However, if the words *crisis, showdown,* and *eyeball-to-eyeball* sound like familiar terms in your EMS system, then politics in your system may have a lot more in common with the Cuban missile crisis than one would expect.

Dr. Graham Allison, who was a policy adviser to President Reagan and a political scientist, wrote an analysis of the Cuban missile crisis titled "Essence of Decisions." The interesting thing about the analysis was that it used three different models to examine what occurred during the crisis.

Figure 5.1

Political IQ Test

*Answer the following questions in order to determine your awareness of,
and ability to influence, the local political scene.*

A. How Much Do You Know About Your Local Political Bodies?

1. Which political body in your community is authorized to regulate local emergency medical services (i.e., county or city commission)? (Score 5 points if you know.) _____

2. Do you know the names of the members of your local city or county commission? (Score 1 point for each name.) _____

3. Do any of the commissioners know your name? (Score 5 points for each.) _____

4. Are you a member of a union or a professional organization that actively lobbies and educates local officials about EMS? (Score 5 points for yes.) _____

B. Policy and Political Analysis *(Score 2 points for each correct answer. Circle the true or false answer.)*

T F 5. Individual personalities will not dramatically affect policy selections and political actions of organizations.

T F 6. Individual EMTs and paramedics cannot influence local political decisions.

T F 7. Organizations act in predictable ways.

T F 8. Organizational behavior cannot be predicted by examining the SOPs of an organization.

T F 9. Organizations always act in a rational manner.

T F 10. Organizations always act in their own self-interest.

T F 11. Politicians usually decide their votes on critical issues after carefully considering the testimony presented at public hearings.

T F 12. Politicians prefer not to meet with constituents or voters.

T F 13. Politicians generally do not listen to or consult with their staffs.

C. Political Tactics *(Score 2 points for each correct answer. Circle the correct answer.)*

14. Publicizing a fatal system error (one in which a patient dies) in the media will most often accomplish which of the following?
   a. Sell lots of newspapers
   b. Publicize the flaws in your system
   c. Result in those responsible for the error covering themselves in defending the system
   d. Provide elected officials a chance to posture on an issue
   e. Occasionally start the process of correcting the error
   f. All of the above

15. The use of surprise in politics
   a. Alienates the opposition and hampers meaningful negotiations

   b. Stops communication between parties
   c. May result in the embarrassment or temporary setback of the opposition
   d. Is effective
   e. a, b, and c above

16. The media in a political confrontation
   a. Usually do not understand EMS well enough to provide a very accurate description of the real issues
   b. Tend to portray the issue in terms of good versus evil
   c. Will direct attention to issues for only a short period of time and then go to another issue
   d. All three above

Answers:
14–f, 15–e, 16–d
5–13 are false,

Scoring:
0-20 points = politically unconscious
21-40 points = politically conscious
41-60 points = politically astute
61-80 points = run for mayor
81 or more = chief of a volunteer ambulance service

An "analytical model" is nothing more than a set of questions or equations that, when answered, provide key pieces of information about an event. The three models described below provide information about political events in much the same manner that a primary and secondary survey provide information to an EMT or paramedic about the condition of a patient. When the information from all three models is examined collectively, it provides a comprehensive explanation.

Model I—Action as a Result of Choice (Rational Actor Model)

The most common means of reviewing or analyzing decision making is the rational actor model. In this model, the problem, the alternatives, and the cost of those alternatives are identified, and then the decision is made by choosing the alternative that has the least cost and will most closely achieve the goal of the organization. If one has a general idea about the values and goals of an organization, one may use this model to predict its policy selections.

Most people use this model to analyze decisions and policy outcomes. However, the weakness of the model is that it assumes that both individuals and organizations act predictably on rational choices. The model fails when decisions are acted on by different groups of people who have competing interests. The next two models deal with this situation.

Model II—Action as a Consequence of Organizational Output

In Model II, government action is viewed as being largely determined by the standard operating procedures and programs of the various organizations within the government or involved in the decision-making process. In the long run, decisions are mainly influenced by the operating procedures of the organization.

Dr. Allison lists the following as the types of questions one would ask based on a Model II analysis:

- What organizations are involved in the decision?
- What organizations traditionally act on the problem and with what influence?
- What standard operating procedures (SOPs) or programs do these organizations have for making information about the problem available at various decision points?
- What SOPs do these organizations have for generating alternatives and for implementing alternative courses of action?

Model III—Action as a Result of Bargaining by Players

Perhaps the most interesting model described by Dr. Allison is Model III, which analyzes governmental action as the result of political bargaining among individuals. In this model, governmental action is viewed strictly as a result of bargaining. Given the tenor of local politics, this is often a very illuminating model. Questions posed by this model include

- What are the existing channels for producing action on this kind of problem?
- Which players and what positions are centrally involved?
- How do pressures of the job, past answers, and personality fit the central players on this issue?
- What deadlines will force the issue to resolution?
- What foul-ups are likely?

The thrust of these questions is to determine how organizations usually approach a problem and what individuals within the organization deal with the problem.

The Models at Work

Here's an example of how the models collectively provide insight into the workings of EMS politics.

During the 1970s, a five-county metropolitan region received a grant to establish a regional emergency communication system in which a seven-digit medical emergency telephone number would be established and calls would be routed to the appropriate EMS agency using computers. Theoretically, the company with the closest ambulance to the scene of the emergency would receive each call.

At the time the regional center received funding, there was no 9-1-1 telephone number, while there were more than 50 seven-digit emergency medical telephone numbers. A number of agencies could respond to calls, including county services, fire department services, a hospital ambulance service, and numerous funeral home and private ambulance services.

Based on Model I analysis, it appeared that the attempt to establish a single emergency telephone number and dispatch the closest ambulance to the emergency would be a great improvement over the current system. The equipment costs were to be paid by the grant, and a funding source had been established for the operating costs.

Reviewing the Model II questions, it became clear in this situation that the SOPs of the one particular county were biased toward internal information. The elected officials relied on their own fire and EMS officials for information.

This was the one county in the region that had established its own EMS service. The county was quite proud of its service and had traditionally operated independently of the other counties. The regional proposal would have resulted in some emergency calls originating within that county being diverted to at least one private ambulance company that had a substation in that county. The county service was bitterly opposed to this plan.

A Model III analysis showed that in addition to the organizational conflict, this situation was further complicated by the fact that the executive vice president of the regional communications organization had been previously employed by the private ambulance company with the substation in the county. As a result, the county EMS personnel were quite sus-

Source

Reprinted with permission from JEMS, *March 1987. At the time of original publication, Stephen F. Dean, Jr., was the director of Fire and EMS Administration for Pinellas County, Fla. He holds a bachelor's degree in political science and a master's degree in health administration.*

picious of the regional organization and particularly its vice president. The county EMS service successfully went over the heads of the regional organization to the grant agency to change the dispatch policy. As a result, all emergency calls received by the regional agency originating from that county went to the county EMS agency regardless of which unit was closer.

While a great deal of communications equipment was bought with grant funds, the regional concept failed. In the end, the communications center was established for one county only.

A Model I analysis of this entire episode would have resulted in one being puzzled about the outcome. However, most EMTs and paramedics instinctively realize that the Model I explanation is too shallow. The interaction of agencies and personalities as examined in Models II and III show the "real" situation and provide rational explanations for the failure of the regional concept.

Conclusion

In the preceding discussion, politics have been defined as the pursuit of power, and that pursuit of power was examined in the context of the local political scene. With this information, EMTs and paramedics may be better able to make sense of the complexities of local EMS politics and thereby relieve some of the frustration that all of us must feel as we look at a system that appears to be unresponsive and unmoving.

John Naisbitt in his book *Megatrends* and Alvin Toffler in *The Third Wave* both discuss the decentralization of political power in the United States and the movement of power away from the federal government to state and local governments. There will probably be more opportunities, not fewer, for EMTs and paramedics to participate in local government decisions concerning the provision of emergency medical services in their communities. Using the questions in each of the models will provide EMTs and paramedics a great deal of insight into the local political process. This will enable EMTs and paramedics to do themselves and their patients a great service by influencing the decisions made by local politicians, which will have a great impact on the quality of care that patients receive.

Evolving Systems and Standards

EMS SYSTEM CONFIGURATION varies widely in the 200 most populous United States cities. Some cities provide only basic life support (BLS) emergency care to their citizens. Others staff all vehicles with at least one advanced life support (ALS) provider (all-ALS system). Many systems use a combination of BLS and ALS units in a variety of tiered configurations (mixed BLS/ALS system). Non-transporting first responder units with or without defibrillation capability are becoming more frequent in all system configurations.

What should be the minimum acceptable level of care on every transporting ambulance in urban and suburban (non-rural) EMS systems? A recent survey of the systems in place today revealed that all but three of the 200 most populous cities include some degree of ALS ambulance coverage. Is it medically, economically, or morally defensible to accept less than all-ALS coverage (at least one ALS provider on each transporting ambulance unit)? We believe not.

Cardiac Arrest in BLS and ALS Systems

Eisenberg has recently shown that there is a "dose-effect" relationship between EMS system configuration and outcome from out-of-hospital cardiac arrest. This is one appropriate end point by which to judge an EMS system's effectiveness because cardiac arrest tests every component in the system. The problem occurs frequently; it has an easily measured outcome (life or death); and effective treatment is available, practical, and time dependent.

BLS-only systems result in approximately a five-percent survival from out-of-hospital cardiac arrest. Mixed BLS/ALS systems that provide either BLS or ALS treatment and transport based on presumptive patient needs are rapidly disappearing (82 percent of the top 200 cities respond with ALS to all emergencies, up from 63 percent the previous year). Having the

ALS in Urban and Suburban EMS Systems

Joseph P. Ornato, MD; Edward M. Racht, MD; Jay Fitch, PhD; and John F. Berry, MPA

Is there a significant difference between ALS and BLS systems in cost and manpower training? The authors explain why there should be all-ALS coverage for both urban and suburban systems.

9-1-1 center operator attempt to triage a BLS or ALS responder unit to a call based on the caller's description or having BLS units transport selected patients to the hospital is a potential "failure point" in any EMS system. This is analogous to a two-tiered police system in which one type of unit—armed or unarmed—is sent to each emergency call. It is just a matter of time until someone makes a wrong triage decision. In Kansas City, Mo. (an all-ALS system by the above definition), 11 percent of routine non-emergency transports that were thought to require BLS-only care at the time of dispatch actually received an ALS skill or procedure during the run.

Mixed BLS/ALS Versus All-ALS Systems

Braun and colleagues have recently suggested that the optimally efficient EMS system should provide a mixed BLS/ALS response. We believe that their conclusion is incorrect because it fails to take into account the nominal cost differential between mixed BLS/ALS and all-ALS systems. When the costs of emergency and non-emergency services are compared, the cost of upgrading from a mixed BLS/ALS response to an all-ALS system is minimal when spread among thousands of calls.

For example, in Richmond, Va., a city that has combined its emergency and non-emergency components into one system, the difference amounts to less than $2.88 per ambulance run over all system responses (Box 5.1). This is actually an overestimate of the true cost per run because an all-ALS system can always send the nearest vehicle (whether assigned to emergency or non-emergency duty) to an emergency call, resulting in a need for fewer ambulances to adequately cover a service territory compared with a mixed BLS/ALS system. Such a configuration never allows a "failure point" to occur in the 9-1-1 center because there is no triage of calls to a BLS or ALS response. Such errors not only jeopardize patient care, but may require dispatch of a second unit (the ALS response) to work a life-threatening call, tying up two units instead of one. Thus, there is no substantive economic justification for not upgrading to an all-ALS system.

A mixed BLS/ALS response also exposes the system to additional risk of litigation. In a recent study, the most frequent causes of litigation in an urban EMS system related to acts of omission, including not providing ALS care or not arriving in a timely manner. An all-ALS system reduces this risk by guaranteeing that the patient will be assessed and treated by an indi-

---

Box 5.1

Cost Comparisons for a BLS Versus ALS System

Personnel Cost

$3,000 per year differential between ALS and BLS provider

Each person works 2,496 hours/year (48 hours per week)

A 24-hour unit, 365 days = 8,736 hours per year

Number of ALS full-time equivalents (FTEs) per unit = 8,736/2,496 = 3.5 FTEs

Seven units x 3.5 = ALS FTEs = 24.5 total ALS FTEs

Total personnel cost differential = 24.5 x $3,000 = $73,500 per year

Non-Personnel Cost

ALS equipment/supplies, approximately $15,000 per unit

Average life expectancy of equipment = seven years

10 full sets of ALS equipment required for seven units (reserve + on line) = $15,000 x 10 = $150,000

Average life expectancy of equipment of seven years = $21,428 annual cost

Total Incremental Cost

Personnel	$73,500
Non-personnel	$21,428
	$94,928

Per-Transport Cost

$94,928 per year/33,000 transports = $2.88 per transport

vidual who has the highest level of skill in the profession. Examples of cities with all-ALS systems include Pinellas County, Fla.; Fort Wayne, Ind.; Kansas City, Mo.; Reno, Nev.; Tulsa, Okla.; Fort Worth, Tex.; and Richmond, Va.

The cardiac arrest patient is not the only beneficiary of an all-ALS system. In addition to airway management, IV line, and assessment skills, ALS providers can administer medication. The recent discovery that long-term disability from spinal cord trauma can be lessened in some patients by the early administration of methylprednisolone suggests that field ALS skills could become even more important in selected injuries.

A First Responding Tier

Adding a first responding, defibrillating tier to an efficient ALS system can yield 25 percent or more out-of-hospital cardiac arrest survival in mature EMS systems. From a medical standpoint, this is the most effective EMS configuration known. But is it cost-effective to add a first responding, defibrillating tier followed by an all-ALS response? We believe it is.

BLS ambulances or first responding units can be upgraded to automated defibrillation capability with minimal expense and training. Automated defibrillators cost approximately $3,000 to $8,000 and require only two to four hours of additional training for first responders or emergency medical technicians. This is a nominal expense compared with the cost of a typical ambulance ($50,000 to $100,000) or a fire truck ($250,000 to $500,000).

Conclusion

We believe that ALS with a first responding tier capable of rapid defibrillation is the minimum acceptable level of care in an urban or suburban EMS system. Just as police and fire protection is mandated by law, we believe the public has a right to prompt, trained, equipped ALS care and that such a level of emergency response can be provided by upgrading an existing BLS or mixed BLS/ALS system at a modest incremental expense. The only exception would be in rural areas where the population density and volume of EMS calls could not justify the expense of maintaining an all-ALS system. It is time for emergency physicians in all urban and suburban practice environments served by less optimally configured EMS systems to present these arguments to their local government officials and demand a system upgrade as soon as possible.

References

Bracken, M. B., M. J. Shepard, W. F. Collins, et al. "A Randomized, Controlled Trial of Methylprednisolone or Naloxone in the Treatment of Acute Spinal-Cord Injury: Results of the Second National Acute Spinal Cord Injury Study." *New England Journal of Medicine* 322 (1990): 1405-1411.

Braun, O., R. McCallion, and J. Fazackerley. "Characteristics of Midsized Urban EMS Systems." *Annals of Emergency Medicine* 19 (1990): 536-546.

Source

Reprinted with permission from Annals of Emergency Medicine, *December 1990. The authors include Joseph P. Ornato, MD; Edward M. Racht, MD; Jay Fitch, PhD; and John F. Berry, MPA. Sponsored by the Internal Medicine Section of Emergency Medical Services, Medical College of Virginia at Richmond.*

Eisenberg, M. S. "Quality Assurance: Is It Possible?" EMS Forum, ACEP Scientific Assembly, San Francisco, November 1987.

Eisenberg, M. S., A. P. Hallstrom, M. K. Copass, et al. "Treatment of Ventricular Fibrillation with Emergency Medical Technician Defibrillation." *Journal of the American Medical Association* 251 (1984): 1723-1726.

Eisenberg, M. S., B. T. Horwood, R. O. Cummins, et al. "Cardiac Arrest and Resuscitation: A Tale of 29 Cities." *Annals of Emergency Medicine* 19 (1990): 179-186.

Goldberg, R. J., J. L. Zautcke, M. D. Koenigsberg, et al. "A Review of Prehospital Care Litigation in a Large Metropolitan EMS System." *Annals of Emergency Medicine* 19 (1990): 557-561.

Keller, R. A., and M. Forinash. "EMS in the United States: A Survey of Providers in the 200 Most Populous Cities." *JEMS* 15 (1990): 79-100.

Ornato, J. P., E. J. Craren, E. R. Gonzalez, et al: "Cost-Effectiveness of Defibrillation by Emergency Medical Technicians." *American Journal of Emergency Medicine* 6 (1988): 108-112.

Overton, J. "The Use of Advanced Procedures on Presumptively Defined Basic Life Support Ambulance Responses." Presentation to Board of Trustees, Metropolitan Ambulance Services Trust, Kansas City, Mo., November 1989.

Weaver, W. D., L. A. Cobb, C. E. Fahrenbruch, et al. "Use of the Automatic External Defibrillator in the Management of Out-of-Hospital Cardiac Arrest." *New England Journal of Medicine* 319 (1988): 661-666.

Unexpected ALS Procedures: The Value of a Single-Tier System

Bryan Wilson, MD;
Matthew C. Gratton,
MD, FACEP; Jerry
Overton, MPA; and
William A. Watson,
PharmD, DABAT

Many viewpoints exist about how an EMS system should be structured. If the fundamental rule of medicine—"do no harm"—is applied to EMS, then systems must be designed to protect both patients and staff members. One of the compelling reasons to consider an all-ALS system design is presented in this article.

MOST EMS SYSTEMS IN THE UNITED STATES were developed along the historical and political perspectives of local and regional governments rather than as a result of careful scientific scrutiny. An important component of EMS system design is the type of service provided—either a single-tier system that utilizes advanced life support (ALS) response equipment and personnel, or a multi-tier system that utilizes both ALS and basic life support (BLS) response equipment and personnel. A recent review of 25 mid-size cities in the United States indicated that 60 percent used a single-tier EMS system and 40 percent used one of three basic designs of a two-tier system.

In a single-tier system, ALS personnel and vehicles are used for patient evaluation and transport regardless of the patient's condition or destination. While there are several variations of two-tier systems, generally there is an initial decision by a dispatcher to send a BLS unit, an ALS unit, or both in response to a patient call. When a BLS unit is dispatched, the patient is evaluated and BLS personnel determine the prehospital care requirements. If it is determined that the patient either requires or likely will require ALS care, a second unit with ALS capability may be requested and dispatched. This second triage potentially delays necessary patient care and transport until the ALS unit arrives at the scene. If the BLS personnel fail to recognize a condition that may require ALS care, no ALS unit is sent to the patient.

It is possible that an all-ALS system would provide better patient care by providing a universally higher level of care to all patients from the time of the first EMS unit's arrival to the patient. The proponents of single-tier, all-ALS systems cite better patient care, enhanced cost effectiveness, and elimination of the need for initial triage of ALS and BLS care as the advantages of a single-tier system. The supporters of a two-tier system also cite enhanced cost effectiveness by minimizing the ALS personnel and equipment required and using less expensive BLS units and personnel to respond to non-emergency calls not thought to require ALS-level care. In this system, ALS personnel can be trained more rigorously and monitored more closely, and can better maintain their ALS skills.

The frequency with which BLS units are dispatched to non-emergency patients who later require ALS intervention recently has been reported in a two-tier system. However, the frequency of such occurrences has not been reported in a single-tier system in which ALS personnel evaluate the patient and determine their prehospital healthcare needs. The purpose of this retrospective study was to determine the frequency of

ALS care provided on ambulance calls initially dispatched as "non-emergency" in a single-tier, all-ALS system.

Methods

A retrospective review of the records of all prehospital patient transports dispatched as non-emergency by the Metropolitan Ambulance Services Trust (MAST) in Kansas City, Mo., from January 1, 1989, to January 1, 1990, was performed. Non-emergency calls were those dispatched as Code-3 calls. Calls that were upgraded to Code-2 (non-life-threatening emergency) or Code-1 (life-threatening emergency) prior to the arrival of the EMS unit were excluded and reviewed separately to compare the frequency of ALS-required cases. Three interventions were defined as ALS care for the purpose of this study: treatment interventions, including administration of medication and endotracheal intubation; access interventions, including placement or attempted placement of an intravenous (IV) catheter; and diagnostic intervention, including electrocardiographic (ECG) monitoring.

The computer-managed MAST database, which included information on all MAST dispatches, was used to identify study cases. The MAST uses the Missouri Ambulance Report Form to document all transports and EMS care provided. The report forms for all transports during which medication was administered or endotracheal intubation was performed were reviewed by one investigator. A randomly selected sample (10 percent) of report forms documenting patient calls receiving either an IV or having an ECG performed also were reviewed. Report forms also were reviewed to identify documentation of the procedures performed, whether the required medical control contact was made, and whether, based on MAST protocols, the procedure was indicated. Information obtained from the report forms review was compared to the MAST database information to determine the accuracy of data input into the database management system.

The MAST system is a single-tier, all-ALS, public utility model, EMS system that provides emergency and non-emergency service for 475,000 citizens in a 400-square-mile area (Kansas City and the immediate surrounding area, 1980 census) with response time compliance standards set at 90 percent for all levels of response.

Dispatching is performed by a system status controller (SSC) using a fluid status management plan with computer-aided dispatch to achieve the required response time standards. Each SSC has a minimum of two years experience as a field paramedic, and has participated in 55 hours of classroom training and 60 to 80 hours of practical training required for Kansas City SSC certification. Dispatch priority is determined using a priority-based dispatch system developed by Dr. Jeff Clawson. These protocols have been modified locally by the Emergency Physicians Advisory Board and are more conservative than the original dispatch protocols.

The caller's complaint undergoes triage by the SSC as Code-1 (life-threatening emergency), Code-2 (non-life-threatening emergency), Code-3 (non-emergency), or Code-4 (scheduled transfer). All calls received via 9-1-1 or the seven-digit emergency telephone line are dispatched only as Code-1 or Code-2, regardless of the complaint. A separate, dedicated non-emergency telephone line also is available, and calls received on this line are prioritized as any one of the four codes. The prevalence of ALS care performed in the two groups, Code-3 and Code-3 upgraded during response, were compared using Chi Square analysis. Statistical significance was defined as $p < 0.05$.

Table 5.1

Advanced Life Support Interventions Used by the Metropolitan Ambulance Services Trust

	Medication	ET	IV	ECG
Code-3	24	3	296	545
n = 6.053	(0.7)	(0.05)	(4.9)	(9.0)
Upgrade calls	42	2	76	118
n = 309	(7.5)	(0.6)	(24.6%)	(38.2)

ET = endotracheal intubation; IV = intravenous catheter insertion attempted; ECG = electrocardiographic monitoring; cs = %

Prehospital and Disaster Medicine © 1992 Wilson et al.

Results

During the 12-month study period, a total of 42,064 responses and 33,933 transports (80.6 percent) were performed by MAST. Of these, 6,362 calls initially were prioritized as Code-3; 309 were upgraded en route based on additional information obtained from the caller by the SSC.

One or more ALS interventions were performed in 710 (11.7 percent) of the 6,053 calls in which paramedics arrived at the patient Code-3. Code-3 responses that were upgraded en route were more likely to require a procedure (144/309, 46.6 percent) than were those initially defined as Code-3 ($p < 0.0005$).

The type of interventions used are shown in Table 5.1. A statistically significant difference ($p < 0.0005$) between the groups was found for the prevalence of each intervention.

Report forms for 127 separate treatment or access interventions performed during each Code-3 call were reviewed. The accuracy of the database entry was determined by comparing all reviewed report forms to the database information for the Code-3 calls. There was a 97.6-percent agreement between the computer-managed MAST database information and report form documentation.

Discussion

Only one study has reported the frequency with which ALS care was provided to patients initially prioritized as non-emergency. Curka, et al., performed a three-month retrospective review of a two-tier EMS system and found that 1.8 percent of patients initially dispatched as BLS later required or involved ALS intervention. However, such a study of a two-tier system has limitations. It is unknown whether the BLS personnel assessing the patient always will recognize a situation requiring ALS and request ALS support. Secondly, if an ALS situation is recognized, other factors may preclude the BLS personnel from requesting ALS support, such as short transport time or the unavailability of a close ALS unit. A single-tier, all-ALS system with ALS personnel performing patient assessment should determine more accurately the number of patients in need of ALS intervention.

The results of this study demonstrate that 11.7 percent of calls dispatched by trained SSCs as non-emergency in a single-tier, all-ALS system received unpredicted ALS care. Several factors that can affect the frequency of unexpected ALS care include the dispatcher's ability to establish call priorities, the necessity of the care provided, and the accuracy of the database information.

The ability of the SSCs to perform a variety of functions was determined in a recent quality assurance report (unpublished). Audiotapes of 233 calls dispatched as chest pain were reviewed, and 1.7 percent of the calls were prioritized incorrectly from the information provided by the caller. The ability of MAST's SSCs to prioritize calls accurately also is supported by the comparison of Code-3 calls to those calls upgraded to Code-1 or Code-2 before arrival of the unit at the scene. Upgraded calls statistically required a significantly higher frequency of ALS care. This supports the ability of SSCs to use dispatch protocol to obtain additional information from callers and to identify patients who are likely to require ALS care, thus necessitating an upgrading of the code.

In other systems, the use of specific dispatch protocols to identify critically ill patients has been demonstrated. The use of dispatch protocols also has been shown to increase dispatch accuracy.

A second major issue that would affect the results of the study is whether the ALS procedures performed during prehospital patient care actually were necessary (i.e., followed established protocols). The MAST protocols developed by the Emergency Physicians Advisory Board define which interventions can be performed in certain medical situations. If the paramedic believes that an intervention is necessary but it is not indicated by protocol, the paramedic is required to contact a base station physician and request approval. Monitoring of the ECG is mandated by some protocols (i.e., chest pain, shortness of breath, etc.) but otherwise is left to the paramedic's judgment. Paramedics do not need protocol support or base contact to initiate ECG monitoring. Of the 127 treatment or access interventions reviewed, only three percent were performed without base station approval or without following the established protocol. When these cases were discarded from the evaluation, the frequency of unpredicted ALS procedures in the Code-3 cases was 11.4 percent. This does not change the interpretation of the study results.

It remains unknown whether the ALS treatment provided altered patient outcome; this was not a goal of the study. Other investigators have demonstrated improved patient outcome when ALS services are utilized.

With a 97.6-percent agreement between report form documentation and database entries, database accuracy should not have had a significant confounding effect on these data.

Conclusion

The results demonstrate that 11.7 percent of patients whose priority was established as non-emergency by dispatchers unexpectedly received ALS care after evaluation by ALS personnel. These results lend support to the use of a single-tier, all-ALS system when considering EMS system design implementation.

References

Braun, O., R. McCallion, and J. Fazackerley. "Characteristics of Midsized Urban EMS Systems." *Annals of Emergency Medicine* 19 (1991): 1469–1470.

Clawson, J. *The Medical Priority Dispatch System 1986 edition.* Salt Lake City: Medical Priority Consultants, Inc., 1986.

Curka, P. A., P. E. Pepe, V. F. Ginger, and R. C. Sherrard. "Computer-Aided EMS Priority Dispatch: Ability of a Computerized Triage System to Safely Spare Paramedics from Responses Not Requiring Advance Life Support." *Annals of Emergency Medicine* 20 (1991): 446.

Eisenberg, M. S., B. T. Horwood, R. O. Cummins, et al. "Cardiac Arrest and Resuscitation: A Tale of 29 Cities." *Annals of Emergency Medicine* 19 (1990): 179–186.

Kallsen, G., and M. Nabors. "The Use of Priority Medical Dispatch to Distinguish Between High and Low Risk Patients." *Annals of Emergency Medicine* 19 (1990): 458–459. Abstract.

Ornato, J., E. Racht, J. Fitch, and J. Berry. "The Need for ALS in Urban and Suburban EMS Systems." *Annals of Emergency Medicine* 19 (1990): 1469–1470. Editorial.

Slovis, C., T. B. Carruth, W. Seitz, et al. "A Priority Dispatch System for Emergency Medical Services." *Annals of Emergency Medicine* 14 (1985): 1055–1060.

Stout, J. "Ambulance System Designs." *JEMS* 11 (1986): 85–98.

Source

Reprinted with permission from Prehospital and Disaster Medicine, *October–December 1992. At the time of original publication, Bryan Wilson, MD; Matthew C. Gratton, MD, FACEP; and William A. Watson, PharmD, DABAT, were affiliated with the Department of Emergency Medicine, University of Missouri, Kansas City. Jerry Overton, MPA, was the executive director of Metropolitan Ambulance Services Trust, Kansas City.*

Accreditation Part 1: Why Accreditation?

Ellen Stewart

The following three short articles detail the impact accreditation has made in the ambulance service industry. The first article discusses why the process is important, the second article outlines how to submit the written application with the best chance for success, and the third article explains the expectations of the CAAS on-site reviewers.

YOU'VE LIVED IN YOUR HOUSE for years now, but the carpets still look clean, the landscaping is pleasant to the eye, and the roof is intact. All of those immediately visible things that show your home has been smoothly run are in place. Your house is ready for the market—until the appraiser comes. When was the last time you noticed the patterns in your heating bills so that you can demonstrate that your house is well insulated? Have your community codes changed, and if so, have you stayed within the code? Does that crack you filled in two years ago represent some structural damage that should actually have been repaired? You may have some work to do.

The scenario of putting your home on the market is analogous to what the CAAS accreditation process is all about. Sometimes we get so comfortable in our day-to-day operation, we neglect to look back at the structure on which it is built. And we forget the importance of keeping records that will prove our efficiency.

The Commission on Accreditation of Ambulance Services (CAAS) was established to set and assist providers in maintaining the highest standards of performance in their communities. Using the standards as a guide, agencies are now beginning to truly clean house, to evaluate in depth the way they do business—not only the delivery of patient care, but also relationships with other agencies and the community, administrative policies, operational procedures, record-keeping, compliance monitoring, and financial practices.

Over the past year, CAAS has been occupied with reviewing the 19 agencies that stepped forward early to subject themselves to this new process. But the primary questions at the recent AAA Conference and Trade Shows were not concerned as much with when the announcement would come, as with what those agencies had to go through to get there, and why.

The *why* of accreditation is in the learning experience, the self-evaluation it demands, and the promotion of excellence that is the result. It is as much a team-building experience as it is an examination of performance. And it is the only means by which the industry can monitor itself on a national basis. The accreditation process includes a comprehensive self-assessment and an independent, outside review of the EMS organization. This independent process provides verification to the applicant's board of directors, city council, medical community, and others that the service has met the most stringent ambulance industry standards.

Five Steps to Accreditation

Self-Assessment

Standards for the Accreditation of Ambulance Services is a publication of the standards adopted by the commission's board of directors in 1991. This booklet alone is an invaluable quality improvement tool as it enables the service to compare its current operation to national standards. If the service decides to pursue accreditation, the booklet serves as a checklist for preparation and implementation of any necessary changes.

Application

Once the service feels adequately prepared for the accreditation reviews, it will purchase and complete a comprehensive application package. The application package asks the agency to answer questions about its operation as well as provide documentation of compliance with the standards. Agencies completing the application package will find the team approach to its preparation essential, as well as of great professional benefit to those involved. Often, one individual will be assigned to coordinate the overall preparation. A team of key personnel can then be assembled to prepare the various components. When complete, the application package is submitted to the commission along with the appropriate application fee.

Evaluation

The commission's staff conducts an off-site review to ensure completeness of the submitted application before scheduling an on-site review. If any needed information is missing, the agency is notified and has an opportunity to submit the missing materials.

The on-site review consists of visitation, interviews, and observation by a team of three reviewers. The reviewers' role is to gather information needed to verify that the service meets (or exceeds) each of the standards established by the commission. Based on the information provided in the application package and information gathered during the on-site review, the reviewers prepare a comprehensive report of their findings.

Deliberation

The review team findings are presented to the independent, impartial panel of commissioners, which makes the actual determination of whether the service meets all requirements. If the review process identifies deficiencies, the service will have up to one year to correct the deficiencies. Depending on the type and number of deficiencies, a second on-site review may be required to verify compliance with the standards before accreditation can be approved.

Accreditation

If successful, the service will be recognized nationally for meeting the commission's high standards. Accreditation is granted for a one-year or five-year period. One-year accreditation signifies that the service sub-

Source

Reprinted with permission from the Ambulance Industry Journal, *November-December 1992. At the time of original publication, Ellen Stewart was the project director of CAAS, located in Dallas.*

stantially complies with all critical standards of the program, but that some deficiencies do exist. The agency will have one year to correct the remaining deficiencies, and if done, will be eligible for the remaining four years of accredited status. As an accredited ambulance service, the service can use the commission's logo on its ambulances and in its advertising. The commission also provides press releases and promotional materials to help publicize the service's accomplishment.

The Impact of Accreditation

Accreditation through CAAS assures local officials and the medical community that the service is operating in accordance with nationally recognized standards of excellence. Many local officials are expected to begin requiring ambulance accreditation as part of their franchise or contract bidding process. Services that have received accreditation may also experience a competitive advantage when marketing their services.

The commission has provided each state EMS office with a copy of its standards in hopes that the standards will lead to future improvements in local and state minimum standards. In time, states may accept ambulance accreditation in lieu of regulatory inspections, just as many states have accepted accreditation by the Joint Commission on Accreditation of Healthcare Organizations (JCAHO). Acceptance of accreditation may also lead to improvements in ambulance services claims processing and reimbursements by governmental and third-party payers.

The commission has already received hundreds of inquiries about accreditation. Applications are processed on a first-come first-served basis, and the applicant can anticipate a three-month period from the submission of the application to the scheduling of the on-site review.

For more information on the commission's activities, publications, and fee structures, contact the Commission on Accreditation of Ambulance Services, Ellen Stewart, project director, or Don Kerns, executive director, P.O. Box 619911, Dallas, Tex. 75261-9911, (214) 580-2829, fax (214) 580-2816.

CREDIBILITY AND FINANCIAL SUCCESS may soon require that ambulance services become accredited according to national standards. Many companies are using the accreditation process not only to perform a quality check on their operations, but also to gain the confidence of the public, government agencies, allied health professionals, and employees. Unfortunately, many small and medium-size services have neither the experience nor the resources necessary to complete the accreditation document. By following a few simple project management rules, these firms can successfully respond to the accreditation criteria established by the Commission on Accreditation of Ambulance Services (CAAS).

Producing an accreditation document can be simplified when the company follows standard project management process—much like building an aircraft carrier or constructing a house, though on a smaller scale. This process involves planning for and organizing the needs of the project, managing the project while the work is in process, and finally, packaging and submitting the document.

Accreditation Part 2: Preparing and Packaging Your Accreditation Document

Kyle R. Gorman

Planning

Planning and organizing are crucial to the successful project. Before the planning begins, however, the company should address two important factors. First, the project must have the unconditional support of company executives. Second, one person in the organization should have both the responsibility and authority to oversee the process from start to finish. Without corporate support, it may become more difficult to motivate personnel who have responsibilities on the project. Without a project manager, the project may succumb to lack of direction.

The first task of the project manager is to evaluate the organization. Specifically, the organization's mission, the personnel and management team, the personnel policies, the clinical quality assurance process, training programs, A/R management strategic and tactical planning, the management hierarchy, and many other facets of the organization must all be carefully considered. The project manager should note both formal and informal policies. For example, unwritten policies that are being followed by the management team should be addressed so that they may be formalized later in the project.

Once the strengths and weaknesses of the company are known, the project manager should evaluate the standards required by CAAS. Each requirement and each question should be carefully read and compared to the current practices of the organization. This will identify the work to be accomplished during the project. Although the disparities between the accreditation requirements and the current organizational standards may be substantial, few companies will meet or exceed all the standards without some adjustment in policies, procedures, or practices.

In addition, as part of the project start-up, the manager must identify the constraints within which the project must operate. Time deadlines, budget restrictions, quality and quantity of personnel on the project team, and restricted management hierarchies are some of the constraints that must be considered.

Once the manager has identified the work that needs to be done, a plan must be developed for accomplishing that work. This planning should be performed in four phases: dividing the work into manageable tasks; determining the order in which the tasks must be completed; matching those tasks with resources; and delegating the responsibility for those tasks. Although the first three are self-explanatory, managers frequently fail to delegate properly.

Most project managers will delegate writing tasks to other managers or employees; therefore, important points about delegation must be considered during the accreditation project. First, deadlines must be established for return of materials. Just as building a house requires that the foundation be laid before the walls are put up, the accreditation project requires that certain materials be produced before other phases of the project commence. Team members who are not aware of time constraints may not return materials on time, and this delay may slow production of other aspects of the project.

Second, team members must "buy into" the task and the time frames. An agreement should be reached with each person to whom work is delegated that specifies the task and the completion date of that task. This agreement ensures that the participant has ownership in the task and will thereby have an increased sense of responsibility not only in complying with deadlines but also in quality performance.

Third, the manager must remove internal barriers that might inhibit the individual's ability to accomplish the task. The people involved in this project must have access to information, equipment, and other assistance.

Managing the Work Flow

Once the planning phase of the project is completed, the managing phase begins. The three most important factors in the managing phase are monitor, monitor, and monitor. The manager must continually evaluate and review to ensure compliance with quality standards, deadlines, and appropriateness of information.

If work is unsatisfactory or late, the manager must prepare to either shift or add resources to the process in order to ensure that the production schedules are adhered to. There is danger in adding or shifting resources—these strategies usually add a substantially higher cost. The manager must consider how much these added resources will affect the budget constraints established during the planning process.

When preparing for accreditation, managers assigned to writing or gathering information will often delegate some of those tasks, but the project manager must ensure that team members continue to be responsible. Again, constant monitoring of the process will help to keep all members of the team on course.

As the work proceeds and the document begins to take shape, the manager must begin to prepare for its packaging by evaluating the packaging needs (i.e., the number of binders per document, number of pages, types of tabs, etc.).

Resources for printing need to be established at least four weeks before the submission date. Printing service firms and photocopying companies frequently need time to prepare any custom-made materials that the manager may want to attach to the document. Further, by scheduling printing and copying in advance, the manager enables copying services to plan for the time and materials they need. Some printers actually print additional amounts (sometimes at least 10 percent) so that last-minute defects can be quickly replaced.

The person managing the accreditation process may be required to write materials for submission to the CAAS and will often be asked to review and edit the materials submitted by others. Therefore, a clear, succinct writing style is important because short and to-the-point writing invites confidence. If a company lacks the information required by CAAS, no amount of quality writing will help it meet the standards, but if a company does have the substance to qualify for CAAS accreditation, poor writing can inhibit, delay, or even halt the process. In any case, regardless of the writing style, it is of primary importance to be honest about the company. Never, under any circumstances, should a writer lie or make false representations about the company.

Two of the most frequent errors made by business writers today are prolixity and turgidity. To be prolix is to go on and on without ever coming to the point. This writing style, of which most of us are guilty, is weary, tiresome, and distracting. Turgid writing is overblown, pompous, "fluffy," and overly boastful. Readers do not appreciate an author who waxes eloquent in praise of his company and who continually boasts without writing anything that supports his opinion. When writing or editing, remove every word or phrase that does not directly support your point. Continually search for ways to "boil down" the sentence to its simplest elements.

Another frequent mistake is that writers fail to answer the questions. Too often, complicated, wordy responses are submitted that never really answer the question being asked. Answer the question!

The document should be reviewed throughout for uniformity and continuity. Occasionally, especially when several people are participating in preparing the document, inconsistencies will arise. For example, a job title in one part of the document may be referred to as director of training

Source

Reprinted with permission from the Ambulance Industry Journal, *March-April 1992. At the time of original publication, Kyle R. Gorman was the total quality manager for Buck Medical Services in Portland, Ore.*

and in another part might be referred to as training officer. These and other inconsistencies are confusing for the reader and might reduce the document's positive impact.

Packaging and Submitting the Document

As with writing style, a document that is presented professionally will not help a weak company attain accreditation, but a poorly presented document may weaken a good firm. The best rule for submitting your document is "the simpler, the better." Avoid complicated and distracting binders, indexes, and tables of contents. Opt instead for a simple straight-forward document.

Because the CAAS requires three copies of each document, copying services are a critical part of the project. A good rule of thumb is to arrange for backup copying, because Murphy's Law dictates that the likelihood of copying machine failure is proportional to the importance of the documents being copied.

Dividing the document into logical components that fit easily into the binders without overstuffing helps the document reviewers. They can more easily turn the pages and cross-check references without fear of tearing the loose-leaf pages.

CAAS recommends that each section of the document contain all the necessary documentation within that section. Some providers have answered questions in one section and have provided the supporting documentation, such as policy manuals, in another. With this style of compiling the document, the reviewer's job is much more difficult; all sections of the document must then be made available to each reviewer, and cross-checking between sections, and at times between binders, is much more difficult.

As one final quality control measure, each copy of the document should be reviewed by the management team before the information is submitted to CAAS. This typically involves going through each document, page by page, to ensure that the copying firm has not omitted any pages, that any last-minute inserts are in place, and that any torn or damaged pages have been replaced. This final quality check helps to reassure all members of the team that the project is complete.

The accreditation process can be likened to peer review on the corporate level. Whether your company elects to pursue accreditation for competitive reasons or to gain the confidence and respect of employees or regulators, you can simplify the process by using a few simple project management techniques. These techniques will not help a poor company achieve accreditation, but they may help a good company prove that it deserves to accredited.

Accreditation Part 3: What to Expect from an On-Site Reviewer

Jimm Murray

THE ACCREDITATION PROCESS GOES SLOWER than you might expect in the beginning stages, and seems to go too quickly when the moment of truth comes and you open your front door to a team of three on-site reviewers. The beginning stages are time intensive for you, the applicant, in filling out all the detailed information called for in the accreditation application booklet and making copies of all appropriate information that will confirm your written statements.

The following are a few things you can expect, and some you should not expect, about the accreditation process and the site visit.

The Application

You can expect that your application will take on proportions best measured in pounds of weight, especially if you have detailed policy and procedure manuals for the various departments of your company. The CAAS staff, who will conduct the off-site review of your application materials, needs certain documentation to confirm your narrative explanations, and you will want to purposely submit additional material that spotlights some of the innovative or creative things you may be doing.

You can expect it will take you more time than you planned to complete the application packet and finally get it sent off to Dallas to start the formal review.

You should expect the off-site review to take more time than you imagined, for a couple of reasons. First, yours is probably not the only application that has been received by CAAS for a thorough review. Second, CAAS wants to be very methodical in ensuring they have not missed any of your required explanations.

The On-Site Review

You can expect to be assigned three reviewers to which you have no prior objections. You can expect to get reviewers that will have spent many hours poring over your written information to get a feel for your company and its operations. Lack of preparation will only make a reviewer look and feel dumb on site if he's looking for the wrong things or asking the wrong questions.

During the on-site review, expect the reviewers to ask questions of you or your staff members that you may have already answered in the original application material. The on-site review is to confirm to the CAAS commissioners that the practices you have documented in your application are verifiable and legitimate.

Source

Excerpted and reprinted with permission from the Ambulance Industry Journal, *January-February 1993. At the time of original publication, Jimm Murray was the director of the Office of Emergency Medical Services and Injury Control for the Wyoming Department of Health.*

Expect reviewers to talk to your division or department heads, but to also talk to billing clerks and field paramedics. The best business and medical practices are of no value if they are not carried out uniformly by everyone in the company.

Expect reviewers, in a methodical and unemotional way, to look for the correct answers and paperwork that will confirm your compliance rather than look for things to fail you on. The approach is similar to supervisors who walk into work each morning expecting good things out of their people rather than being surprised when they occur.

Don't expect the reviewers to have much time to fraternize with you or your people. First, there is no free time budgeted in the trip, and second, it is best to let your evaluation stand on its own worthy merits rather than on any appearance of impropriety. The reviewers use lunch and dinner to get away by themselves to review what they have covered and to plan for the next set of standards to verify. The smart reviewer will use the evening hours to start writing up individual reports of what has been seen and heard, rather than waiting until the final day in town to do it all.

If you have carefully lined up a tight schedule of substations for reviewers to visit and "screened" employees to meet them, expect a "what are you trying to hide" look from the reviewers. The more accommodating and open you are with the reviewers and their schedule, the quicker and smoother the review will go. By your actions, let the reviewers know you have nothing to hide, that all your people may be interviewed, that any ambulance may be viewed, that any substation may be visited, and that any file may be opened.

Don't expect the reviewers to indicate whether or not you have passed or failed. Each reviewer has his own assignments, and while some areas overlap, many don't. It would be unfair for a site review member to make a "guesstimate" as to what your overall ranking might look like. Your overall ranking is the responsibility of the three-member panel of commissioners. You will receive a copy of the tentative evaluation from the CAAS staff and will have an opportunity to rebut or disagree with anything before it goes to the commissioners.

Companies who apply will get an opportunity to compare their services to a "gold standard" and can identify areas on which to concentrate their improvement efforts. The accreditation process is a win-win situation.

System Design Considerations

EXACTLY WHAT IS AN EMS SYSTEM? It is commonly understood to be the resources used to deliver medical care to those with an unpredicted immediate need outside a hospital or other emergency medical facility.

This definition includes several diverse actions by many individuals, agencies, and providers.

Anatomy of an EMS System

A Call for Emergency Medical Assistance

Most requests for assistance come through a telephone call to an emergency number. Enhanced 9-1-1 systems can automatically identify the location of the call, even when a distraught person fails to provide an address.

Receipt of the Call

Once the call is made, it must be properly routed to police, fire, or ambulance. Most true EMS systems have established communication protocols through which the initial call-taker obtains all the information needed for any type of emergency (location, type of emergency, etc.) before routing the call to another organization so that the system can respond even if the caller should hang up or drop the phone.

Dispatch of a Service Provider

As soon as the basic information is received, the proper agency must be notified and the information obtained by the call-taker must be transferred to the proper dispatch location. This may be done by telephone, radio, computer lines, or a combination. The call-taker may transfer the information needed to dispatch the proper response and continue to talk to the caller to obtain additional information or to provide advice on how to handle the emergency until help arrives.

Improving Emergency Medical Services Systems

Carol S. Werner and Bruce A. Smith, PhD

This overview was initially published by the International City Manager's Association as a primer for local officials considering system changes. It provides a solid synopsis of the issues and a process to use when making changes.

In the dispatch protocol of a good EMS system, the type of response for any given emergency will be specified, with the responsibilities of all service providers established in advance.

The next step is the dispatch by one or more service organizations of appropriate personnel and equipment to the scene of an emergency. The service provider can be a uniformed officer with basic first-aid training or paramedics in an ambulance ready to provide advanced life support services. A fire engine might respond if its equipment is needed, for instance, to remove someone trapped in a car.

In the dispatch protocol of a good EMS system, the type of response for any given emergency will be specified, with the responsibilities of all service providers established in advance. This is particularly important when several providers must respond to a call. In many states, it has been established by law that the medical responder has the final say on any activity that may affect the medical condition of a victim. Clear definition of roles and responsibilities at the scene of the emergency will improve the chances for successful treatment.

Treatment on the Scene

The ability of responding personnel to stabilize patients at the scene varies with the level of system preparedness and provider training. It is widely recognized in medical circles and validated by several studies, that advanced life support (ALS) treatment has a dramatic effect on morbidity and mortality rates when compared to lower levels of care. In heart attack cases, for example, studies have shown that when a fire service first responder unit reaches a victim within four minutes of the attack and an ALS ambulance arrives within eight minutes, save rates are greatly increased over rates achieved with basic life support (BLS) response.

Whether or not ALS equipment is available, the training of EMS personnel plays a large part in determining the victim's potential for recovery, the length of hospital stay, and total rehabilitation time.

Transport to a Medical Facility

Failure to transport a patient to a medical facility is the single biggest reason for liability actions against EMS systems. Although a patient has the right to refuse transport (by signing a waiver), the responder should never advise against transport and should always make a serious effort to transport the patient.

Where the patient is to be taken may be an important issue. When there are several hospitals with trauma centers nearby, and especially when some of them are public and others are private, the issue must be addressed. In any case, the medical facility where the victim is taken should be considered part of the EMS system. It should have a trauma center staffed with trained emergency medical specialists certified by the American Board of Emergency Medicine.

Once the patient is in the medical facility and the initial treatment is completed in the emergency room, the EMS system's direct service delivery ends. However, the system still has two more activities to complete: billing and collecting for the services rendered, and monitoring of the services delivered.

Billing and Collection

If no charge is made for EMS, the local government is subsidizing the federal and state governments and the private insurance industry, since these parties offer substantial reimbursement for emergency medical treatment and transportation as part of their coverage. Over the past few years, more and more governments have adopted a fee-for-service approach to funding. Public policy may demand that the local government subsidize the EMS system in some areas, but the total costs need not be borne by local taxpayers.

What should you charge for services? A user-fee cost analysis will ensure that all of the costs associated with the service are recognized. Another measure is to look at the charges made by similar jurisdictions in the state for the same level of care. The Medicare reasonable charge profiles typically represent minimum rates.

Collection can be done by local government staff, but it is also a task easily contracted out.

Monitoring

Once all the pieces of an EMS system are in place, standards, procedures, and protocols for each area should be monitored routinely by independent parties to ensure compliance with changing EMS standards and local fiscal policy.

How much of this system must the local government manager manage? The answer varies by state, county, and locality. As a general rule, a local government or EMS authority probably will not be responsible for the medical issues but will be responsible for many, if not all, of the operational issues. But since the operational issues are related to the medical issues, it is important to involve all parties in the system design. State regulations will determine some aspects of the design. Additional guidance is available from the many organizations involved in various aspects of emergency care.

How can you determine what EMS your community needs? If there are unmet needs, how can you go about meeting them? The rest of this report discusses these questions.

Improving an EMS System

Organize for Success

The evaluation of an existing EMS system cannot be the responsibility of any one individual. It requires the input, effort, and dedication of several professionals representing a wide range of interests and expertise. One way of mobilizing this support is by forming an EMS task force or advisory board. A good EMS task force will include representatives of the following groups.

- Medical community. If EMS services are currently in place, there is probably also a medical control board that can

The EMS task force may be given the limited mission of evaluating existing systems and identifying needed improvements, or it may be established as a standing body to provide ongoing oversight.

work with the task force. Representatives from the medical community on this board will probably include an emergency room physician, a surgeon, an emergency room nurse, a general practitioner, and a hospital administrator. If there is no medical control board, it is important that physicians currently involved in medical control, including ambulance medical service directors, be represented on the EMS task force.

- Public sector. The public sector should be represented by an elected official from each government that will use the system.
- Private sector. Taxpayer associations and private ambulance companies may be represented, and other interested citizens may be included as well.
- Governmental staff. The EMS task force will usually require staffing, which can most easily be provided by staff members of the local government.

The EMS task force may be given the limited mission of evaluating existing systems and identifying needed improvements, or it may be established as a standing body to provide ongoing oversight. Either way, it will work with the local government, the medical control board, the EMS administrative agency or ambulance authority, and the contractors or providers, if any. Each of these parties is discussed below.

Local government. Whether it is a city, county, or regional authority created by a joint-powers agreement, the local government generally is responsible for deciding on the level of sophistication of the EMS system, adopting the rules that will govern the system, and establishing the operational, medical, and monitoring aspects of the system. Thus, it will decide what type of system to develop, what type of clinical standards are appropriate, who will establish and monitor these standards and medical protocols, and whether the system will be publicly or privately operated or a combination of the two. In addition, the local government will decide whether the system should be competitively bid, who will bill and collect, who will establish the rates, who will own the equipment, and what part the government will play in financing the equipment.

Medical control board. The EMS medical control board will generally include a properly qualified medical director, EMS physicians, and representatives of emergency facilities. The board is responsible for setting standards, medical protocols, pre-arrival instructions, and the qualifications of all personnel. It must have some funding and must have the authority and resources to maintain continuity of patient care. A key responsibility of the board is to conduct effective and timely system audits to ensure compliance with both clinical and operational standards.

EMS administrative agency or ambulance authority. In many areas, a multi-jurisdictional agency or authority is created to coordinate the EMS system. The agency's board of directors will represent the business, financial, healthcare, and legal professions, and its staff will be the primary liaison between the participating governments and the service providers. Often such an authority is established to address problems that arise when mini-systems in an incorporated city and unincorporated county are providing different levels of care.

Contractor or provider. The function of the contractor or provider is to manage and deliver services. The contractor may be a private operator with an exclusive franchise for both emergency and non-emergency transport, or a combination of a private operator and a local fire department or volunteer rescue organization that functions as a first response provider.

In some areas, the contractual provider is the fire department (usually for emergency services only), with private ambulance companies providing backup emergency services, while also serving the non-emergency transport market. Proponents of integrated EMS systems point out that this arrangement is inefficient because expensive care is funded by the taxpayers, often with high risk of liability to the local government. However, opponents of exclusive franchise-area arrangements argue that monopolizing non-emergency services as a way of subsidizing emergency services constitutes an unfair, if not illegal, method of putting primarily non-emergency ambulance services out of business. One solution is to allow the emergency contractor to compete with non-emergency services in the area.

Develop Standards

Once the general organizational structure of the EMS system has been determined, the next step is to develop the ideal standards for the system. This is a very important step because the decisions made now will be translated into the definitions of the EMS system later. Quantitative standards should be developed for as many of the areas as possible.

These standards are really goals that you would *like* to achieve—performance levels that the system could attain if there were not budgetary constraints. But of course there *are* budgetary constraints. Is it futile and superfluous, then, to set ideal standards? No, it's not, because the industry is changing so rapidly. Long-range goals enable the local government to make conscious tradeoffs among standards not only now but later on, and to quantify these tradeoffs. If resources change, the goals establish how the system should change.

There are at present no nationally accepted standards for the components of an EMS system. Many in the industry feel that EMS standards should be based on community standards of care even if national guidelines are established in the future. Guidance on the development of local standards is or will be provided by the American College of Emergency Physicians and the American Ambulance Association.

To set standards for an EMS system, start by separating the medical or clinical protocols from the operational standards.

> Many in the industry feel that EMS standards should be based on community standards of care even if national guidelines are established in the future.

The operational standards adopted by a jurisdiction will vary to some degree by the type of service, organizational unit, and provider or providers. Standards should be developed for each of the following.

The emergency telephone system. The standard 9-1-1 telephone system allows three-digit dialing, but does not identify the caller's location. The enhanced 9-1-1 system automatically identifies the location but requires an investment in computer hardware and software to provide this feature. The third choice is the use of one emergency number for all types of emergency services—police, fire, and ambulance. A seven-digit number that is easy to remember may be acceptable in some areas. If a seven-digit number is used, the exchange should be one that can be reached from all locations in the jurisdiction without incurring a long-distance charge.

Call-taking and dispatching. The call must be answered by someone who knows the EMS system and the agencies that respond to all the other types of emergencies handled by the emergency number. Call-takers must be trained to deal with people who are under a lot of stress and who may be irrational.

One call-taking and dispatch procedure that has proven to be very costly is call screening. Initially developed to minimize the costs due to "dry runs" (non-transports) and chronic system abusers, call screening has caused unnecessary deaths.

Dispatch and communication links. The receipt of a call and the taking of information helps no one unless the information can be passed on to the service provider. Computer transmission is the quickest way and may be the most cost effective. Information from all incoming calls is immediately entered into the computer. Telephone links are also effective, but they should utilize direct pickup lines that do not require dialing. Radio is also a viable alternative.

System status management. Call demand varies from hour to hour, from day to day, and from place to place. At certain times of day, there are more EMS calls from one location than from another—more from the freeway, for example, than from residences. Also, at certain times of day there are many times more calls than there are at other times. The formal or informal protocols and procedures that determine where and how many ambulances will be placed to handle these calls are known as system status management (SSM).

SSM is the process of matching supply and demand efficiently to optimize response time and reduce cost. One measure of SSM effectiveness is the unit hour utilization ratio. A unit hour is defined as a fully staffed, equipped, and available ambulance on the street for one hour. If a system operates one unit for 24 hours and transports 12 patients in that period, its unit hour utilization ratio is 0.50.

The art of SSM is predicting where the calls will occur in a geographic area and placing units strategically to respond to those calls. SSM requires ambulance movement because the pattern of calls shifts hourly, and it dictates where the available ambulances will be when the next call is received. It ensures that enough units are in service to meet demand and reduces unit hours when demand is low.

Many older EMS systems have not implemented SSM. They operate the same number of units 24 hours a day, seven days a week. Sometimes, therefore, all ambulances are busy when a call comes in, and sometimes many ambulances are idle. The old—and costly—solution for this problem was simply to add more units rather than to redeploy unit hours.

Urban EMS systems generally have higher unit hour utilization ratios than those in rural areas because of higher population density and call demand. Systems that operate on 24-hour shifts cannot expect the same employee performance as those that operate on shorter shifts. A utilization rate of 0.50 on a 24-hour shift would be considered very high by industry standards, whereas the same utilization rate would be considered low to normal on a 12-hour shift.

Response time. Response time is measured from the moment the call-taker obtains the address and complaint to the moment the ambulance actually arrives at the address of the call. Sophisticated systems measure this time in seconds.

Measuring response time by average criteria is misleading. Many systems now measure response time on a fractile basis, which is a much more consistent and difficult standard than averages. If an ambulance service measures response time on an average basis, it may locate all units close to areas of high call volume and sacrifice calls on the periphery. For example, seven out of 10 callers may be within three minutes or less, while it may take 15 minutes to reach three callers. The average response time would be 6.6 minutes, which sounds acceptable. For three callers, however, it is not acceptable.

But suppose the system measures response time on a fractile basis and has a requirement that 90 percent of all calls must be answered within eight minutes. In the above example, the system would be out of compliance by 20 percent.

It is more difficult to serve areas with a dispersed population and low call volume than to serve areas with a concentrated population and high call volume. For this reason, different standards may be necessary for different areas. In rural areas, the limit might be 25 or 30 minutes, and in remote wilderness areas, it might be an hour. To be a valid measure of performance, the standard for response time must be realistic and achievable.

Response options. Who should be dispatched to an emergency? How many units? When is a second unit required? These issues must be addressed in the standards. There are various possibilities that have worked in various locations. The final policy must consider the existing providers.

The simultaneous dispatch of the closest fire engine company and the closest advanced life support (ALS) ambulance is the state-of-the-art response to life-threatening emergencies. In many areas, fire department personnel have basic life support (BLS) training and can provide a high level of initial medical intervention. The personnel on the ambulance must be trained to BLS standards at a minimum, and optimally to ALS standards. When the ambulance is staffed with ALS personnel and the first responders are trained at the BLS level, the response can provide a very high quality of service and will have a dramatic effect on patient survival.

A second alternative is to dispatch an ALS-staffed ambulance as the sole responder, unless circumstances require additional resources. This response provides high-quality medical care, but in some cases additional manpower may be needed.

A third alternative is for the call-taker to ask enough questions to determine whether an ALS response is required or a BLS response is sufficient and then to dispatch the ambulance accordingly. This approach is typically used in systems that do not have the resources to provide an ALS unit for every emergency call. To avoid liability, it is very important to develop priority dispatch protocols in accordance with established medical protocols.

Equipment. Ambulances must meet the minimum standards adopted by the state or other cognizant agency for such vehicles. The ambulances should be inspected periodically and maintained on a regular basis. The equipment that should be on each ambulance will be determined by the medical control board or medical director.

Manpower and training. There are several levels of training for ambulance personnel, and the titles vary around the country. BLS training is the minimum standard recommended by the U.S. Department of Transportation for ambulance attendants. It consists of 80 to 120 hours of medical training in advanced first aid, oxygen therapy, splinting of fractures, cardiopulmonary resuscitation, and other skills that serve to stabilize a patient's condition in a prehospital setting. Upon successful completion of an approved BLS training program, the candidate is certified as an emergency medical technician (EMT). With the completion of an additional module for ambulance transport, the candidate is certified as an emergency medical technician-ambulance (EMT-A). The training required for an EMT-A is 110 to 150 hours, with annual recertification.

The emergency medical technician-defibrillator (EMT-D) level involves special training in the use of defibrillators for cardiac arrest cases. First responders and transport personnel trained at this level can be effective when ALS is not available or has not yet arrived at the scene. This is a particularly viable alternative to ALS in rural areas where ALS is either prohibitively expensive or not available.

The next level, emergency medical technician-intermediate (EMT-I), requires about 400 hours of training and is usually categorized as ALS because candidates receive training in IV therapy, the initial list of cardiac drugs, defibrillation, shock therapy, and other ALS techniques.

The final step is emergency medical technician-paramedic (EMT-P). This step requires 750 to 1,100 hours of training. The training completes the Department of Transportation modules for cardiac care (normally to the advanced cardiac life support level established by the American Heart Association), advanced airway management, and other advanced training in trauma and medical emergency invasive therapies. The National Association of Emergency Medical Technicians provides a national registry program for EMT-As and EMT-Ps.

The current practice in most states is to require that at least one person on each BLS ambulance be trained to at least the EMT-A level. To be considered an ALS ambulance, at least one person must be trained to the EMT-I level, and a second person must be an EMT-A. Some areas require EMT-P training for both individuals before an ambulance can be considered ALS.

Record-keeping and reporting. Records should be an integral part of the EMS system. While service delivery is the paramount concern, procedures to gather the information needed to bill must also be performed.

If possible, the third-party payer should be billed directly. The bill should provide all the information that the third-party payer requires, and should be on the proper forms. When a third-party payer does not exist or is unknown, the patient should be billed—even though full payment may seem unlikely—since most people can make at least a partial payment. Guidelines on collection can take into account the patient's ability to pay. In developing guidelines, consider not only policy issues on billing and subsidies but also characteristics of the accounts receivable system, provisions for transition between service providers, and policies for dealing with delinquent accounts.

Monitoring. The final component of the EMS system is monitoring. Periodic reports should be made to the local governments to inform them of the quality of services being provided. These reports should identify areas that need improvement and changes that must be made in response to problems that arise. Monitoring should be the responsibility of someone other than the service deliverers and should include independent medical control.

Evaluate the Existing System

After the EMS task force has assembled all the EMS system goals, existing EMS components can be measured against these goals. This evaluation will identify both the good points and the deficiencies of the current system. In addition to looking at the current system in relation to goals, the local government may also want to evaluate the service from the patients' point of view. Finally, an integral part of the evaluation will be a determination of the true costs of providing service, regardless of who pays the bill.

Who can undertake this task? How can it be carried out? Exactly what needs to be done? Although situations differ somewhat, the process is much the same in all places. Let's start with the question of who.

An evaluation of a complex system such as an EMS system requires the dedication of sufficient manpower to complete the project in a reasonable time. A larger jurisdiction may have an office that does management analysis, for instance, a budget office, a planning office, or a productivity office. In smaller jurisdictions, one person may do this job part time. In either case, management responsibility for the evaluation should be assigned to one individual to ensure accountability. This could be a governmental official or a local, independent emergency physician. Numerous private consultants are also available. The actual evaluation work will involve members of the task force (or their staff) and members from the provider community in addition to in-house staff.

Inventory Resources

If an EMS system needs improvement, it makes sense to take advantage of all the resources available in the community. However, they must first be identified and quantified.

Private ambulance providers are obviously an important resource. Identify the companies in the immediate area. Study their businesses and assess their capacity to serve an integrated EMS system. Interview the principals of each company, review its equipment, review its record in the state, and review the training and certification of its personnel.

If the search is extended to companies serving other markets, a key consideration is the quality and depth of their management. Expansion into a new market may dilute a provider's managerial talent. A good candidate's "bench strength" must be sufficient to provide the services required.

The information gathered on each potential public or private provider will be useful later in the development of the final system configuration and in the procurement process.

Make Initial Cost Estimates

The evaluation of the existing system in a previous step should give you a basis for cost estimation. Data on billing and collection, as well as other fiscal matters, should be gathered from all public and private providers in the area. It is important to include both direct and indirect costs.

The major categories of costs to be calculated are total costs of the system (by component), revenues to be generated (by source), and cost per capita to the taxpayers. When gathering cost data from the public sector, make sure that all costs are included—pensions, other benefits, and costs borne by other departments, such as equipment maintenance. If possible, use actual audited costs rather than budgets.

The direct costs to taxpayers for EMS in the United States range from zero to $25 per person per year. Some of the public sector services with good reputations, such as Johnson County, Kan., Dallas, and Houston, operate with good response times and performance but enjoy high taxpayer subsidies.

The usual cost of a fully loaded, paramedic-staffed ALS vehicle is approximately $500,000 per year.

The costs of a service are often subject to interpretation. The fire department EMS system in Monterey Park, Calif., apparently yields net revenues in the community, but some observers believe this is misleading. They point out that when the paramedic firefighters are staffing ambulances, they are not available to fight fires. Thus, a portion of their salaries and benefits should be counted as an EMS cost rather than as a fire department cost.

After the costs of the EMS system are calculated, review and analyze the system design and standards once again. The EMS task force may aspire to a level of service that cannot be provided efficiently by local providers, whether public or private. In this case, the local government can consider a regional or countywide system and regional or national procurement, or it can decide to change its design or standards.

Consider Procurement Alternatives

Deciding how services are to be provided is a critical step in the design of an EMS system. Communities that have depended on their fire department to provide EMS face the issue of privatization. Some of the hospitals or trauma centers to which patients are taken may be private sector organizations. But should the private sector also be involved in responding to calls, providing care at the scene of an emergency, and transporting patients?

The decision to privatize an EMS system can have a long-term effect on the community. Privatization is not the solution to all problems. However, EMS appears to be an ideal candidate for privatization for three reasons. First, there are many private companies in the industry, so competition exists. Second, private companies can expand beyond a single market to realize economies of scale, thus making it easier to afford state-of-the-art technology and to attract and retain highly trained and motivated management and field personnel. Third, private companies deal routinely with billing and collection, which the public sector is usually not well organized to handle.

Procurement alternatives available to any locality will be partly defined by the geographic and demographic characteristics of the area. The alternatives will also be defined, and perhaps narrowed, by the community's perception of its current EMS system. Procurement is generally complicated by subjective evaluations of quality, budgetary constraints, political pressures, and union demands. Yet another complicating factor is that the EMS standards and levels of service are continually evolving.

Some of the more common alternatives in type of vendor and type of solicitation process are described below.

Type of vendor. There are many kinds of EMS providers, both in the public sector, whether paid or volunteer, and in the private sector, where companies range in size from single-ambulance operators to large, multi-state networks.

Public sector. Government began to take an active role in address-

Procurement is generally complicated by subjective evaluations of quality, budgetary constraints, political pressures, and union demands. Yet another complicating factor is that the EMS standards and levels of service are continually evolving.

ing concerns over the quality of EMS in the mid-1960s. In 1966, the Division of Medical Services National Academy of Sciences-National Research Council (NAS-NRC) published a landmark white paper titled, "Accidental Death and Disability: The Neglected Disease of Modern Society," which implied that emergency ambulance services were a municipal responsibility. In the 1970s, the public image of the firefighter as the first to respond to a medical emergency was enlarged by a popular TV show called, appropriately, "Emergency." But in many parts of the country, EMS was *not* a public sector responsibility—and still isn't.

Private sector. Fifty years ago, emergency transport was largely provided by morticians because they had vehicles that could transport the seriously ill. While some might argue that this presented a conflict of interest, mortuary companies provided effective transport, and many of them trained their employees in the best life support care available at the time. As technology brought sweeping changes to communications, prehospital care techniques, equipment, and vehicles, the private sector took the lead in improving personnel training and setting quality standards. Today, the primary industry association of private sector ambulance service providers, the American Ambulance Association, has more than 500 members and supports a wide variety of programs, including a management training institute.

Hospital-based systems. In some places, hospital-based systems were developed because fire department-based systems did not seem to meet medical standards for prehospital care. In other areas, hospitals were motivated not only by their interest in providing high-quality medical care but also by a business need to expand their market.

Volunteer services. For a long time, America had strong volunteer EMS systems. But changing technology, increased liability exposure, ever-increasing regulatory and performance standards, and lifestyle changes have combined to cut back volunteer EMS services sharply.

Type of procurement. The decision to bid or renegotiate EMS in a community is rarely easy, and the procurement process is time consuming and expensive for both the community and the bidders. To attract an adequate number of qualified bidders, the services to be provided and the contract conditions must be carefully defined. The most typical procurement models are described here.

Negotiated contract. If citizens and officials are satisfied with existing services, a negotiated contract may be the most cost-effective arrangement. The recommended contract is based on performance and gives some assurance that the standards the community has established will be met, and monitored, within the subsidy or budget structure the EMS task force has agreed on.

Public convenience and necessity ordinance. Many cities regulate their emergency responders through ordinances that prohibit unbridled and destructive competition. Some of these ordinances are local, and some are statewide. Their purpose is to restrict access to the marketplace when the current providers are fulfilling their publicly defined responsibilities. As new system needs are identified, reimbursement can be negotiated to match the new costs before the improvements are implemented. This is usually the easiest system to modify because of the natural quid pro quo, with government desiring high-quality service and the provider being assured of marketplace protection as long as the community's needs are met.

Sole-provider franchise or franchise territories. There are no true franchises for ambulance services, because franchising is a property right, and ambulance services always operate within some level of revocable government authority. However, "franchise" is often the term applied to arrangements that grant a geographical territory to a company, often exclusively, in exchange for a stated level of service. Like the public convenience and necessity ordinance, the franchise creates a natural public-private partnership. It should be noted that the establishment of an exclusive service area requires state action to avoid antitrust litigation.

National or regional procurement. If local providers are not able to provide the quality of service desired, national or regional competitive procurement may be an option to consider. In deciding whether to launch what can be a time-consuming and expensive process, it is important for the local government to consider whether its population and demographics offer an attractive market for high-quality providers. If the opportunity to serve a large market for non-emergency transports exists, bidders will be more interested in providing emergency transport at a reasonable cost. In addressing this question, look at the dynamics of the service area—not just the size and type of population, but also its geographical dispersion and its proximity to major population centers and medical services. On average, there is one patient transport per day (either emergency or non-emergency) for every 7,000 people. Naturally, areas with a high concentration of elderly or convalescent people will have higher rates of non-emergency transport, and areas with more crime and poverty will have higher rates of emergency calls.

The local government will also need to decide whether it is necessary to create an exclusive service area for one provider to supply both emergency and non-emergency transport. While total exclusivity might be necessary in some systems to make providing high-quality service economically viable, in other systems it is better to let competition, rather than the government, level the playing field for non-emergency services. An exclusive emergency contractor who is performing well in both the emergency and non-emergency markets may be just as successful financially as if the government had put everyone else out of business. This issue is difficult, but it must be addressed squarely on the merits of patient care and system stability.

National or regional procurement will generally take one of the following forms:

- Two-phased request for credentials and request for proposals (RFC-RFP). This procedure has its fans and its foes. It is

Source

Reprinted with permission from ICMA *(International City Managers Association)* Management Information Service, *November 1988. Condensed for republication. At the time of original publication, Carol S. Werner was a senior consulting manager with Touche Ross. Bruce A. Smith, PhD, was a manager for Touche Ross.*

somewhat less expensive for the bidders to submit qualification or credential packages, but a certain amount of preproposal expense is required to understand the jurisdiction and its needs. Those who oppose this procedure maintain that it tends to decrease the number of bidders.

• Requests for proposals (RFP). This form of solicitation can have the disadvantage of bringing in too wide a variety of responses. Also, it is costly and time consuming both for the evaluators and for the bidders.

• Single-variable bid. If a jurisdiction can clearly articulate the services to be let, it may make sense to base the procurement on a single variable such as price, assuming that the competing vendors' abilities to meet the terms of a performance-based contract can be fairly evaluated.

Sample proposal contents. There are any number of public requests for proposals that can be used as guides in developing one for a local EMS system. The American Ambulance Association serves as a resource for sample RFPs.

Conclusion

The EMS industry in the United States has changed dramatically in recent years and is continuing to evolve rapidly. It is extremely complicated and involves a broad spectrum of professionals in both the public and private sectors. Poor systems can result in liability judgments for preventable loss of life. For these reasons, local governments must continually evaluate their EMS systems.

For a well-designed and effectively implemented EMS system, opportunities exist to align the profit motive with the public interest and minimize costs to the taxpayer.

E MERGENCY MEDICAL SERVICE SYSTEMS throughout the nation are faced with the inevitable prospect of change. Increasing demands for service, coupled with shrinking tax bases, are squeezing services as never before. Public policy questions regarding upgrading or changing an EMS system are frequently clouded by the emotions of providers, patients, and taxpayers.

Local decision makers often contemplate change without fully understanding the individual elements that contribute to an effective and efficient EMS system. Larger than a single service, the system must be viewed holistically. Is the current system functioning well? Could it be improved? Or must it be redesigned to better serve the community? Before major system upgrades or changes are contemplated, a number of fundamental system components should be reviewed. Community officials considering such a review are encouraged to use this guide.

The questions are organized to address issues related to the system's structure and organization, operational aspects, clinical components, and fiscal considerations. For each component, there is a single key question that needs to be answered. In addition, reviewer instructions are offered on some of the specific items that can be included in any internal or external analysis.

System Structure and Overview

A clear understanding of the system's legal and established mandates is necessary to provide a foundation from which the system can carry out its mission. The four key areas that provide a foundation for the system and its structure follow.

Enabling legislation. Does the system have the legal authority necessary to fully accomplish its mission?

An assessment of state and local legal and administrative authority for providing EMS services should be undertaken. Clear and concise legislative authority is necessary for an EMS system to function well. A detailed understanding of statutes, ordinances, and regulations is necessary before long-lasting change is contemplated. Legal authority to alter or implement a new system design may be necessary. Special consideration should be given to language that accommodates future growth or multiple jurisdictional participation.

Program description. Does a clear and accurate description of the system exist?

A clear, concise description of how the EMS program is organized

25 Crucial Questions When Upgrading an EMS System

Jay Fitch, PhD

Whenever local officials contemplate system design upgrades or other changes, it's important for them to first understand how components of the existing system are performing. Answers to the following 25 questions form a good starting point when considering an upgrade to EMS systems.

should be developed. This should include background information about the geographic area served, demographics, socioeconomic factors, relationships with other ground and air providers, and the general role of hospitals and trauma centers.

Current administration and leadership. Are the leadership roles and responsibilities clearly defined, and do these responsibilities support the system structure?

The review should describe the roles of the current EMS administrators, explaining those internal management systems established to provide clinical, operational, and fiscal monitoring of the EMS program.

Fiscal issues. Does the system have adequate funding to accomplish its mission?

The funding and budgetary structure for the EMS program, including a comprehensive analysis of how effective the billing and collection services are, should be described in detail.

Operating Conditions and Issues

This group of items determines how service is provided and the standards and benchmarks employed by the system. The performance levels should be compared to similar organizations.

Response time performance. Does the system set, monitor, and achieve appropriate response times?

Response times have been proven in clinical literature to be a key determinant of patient outcome. They are also often measured incorrectly, quoted out of context, and compared without due regard for statistical accuracy.

A determination of current response time standards, as well as the adequacy of the standards, should be undertaken. The review should address the data collection system and reporting methods used for response times. The communities may request that the review team make recommendations about establishing an optimal standard and an approach to ensure response time compliance. This should include a cost analysis for implementing any recommendations.

System utilization. Does the system use its operational resources wisely?

The current system utilization should be evaluated. This evaluation should employ appropriate utilization ratios and measure the system's performance compared to similar systems. The number of patient requests for service and transport should be compared to the routine availability of ambulance units. Run volumes and any significant variances should be quantified. Identify utilization problems and provide recommendations describing methods of improvement. A detailed explanation of the financial impact of these recommendations should be provided.

Levels of service. What level of service does the system provide?
Describe and differentiate the levels of service throughout the ser-

vice area. The review should include a comparative analysis of relationships between the fire department first responder BLS (or ALS) units and the transporting EMS service advanced life support response. Describe the role of the private providers in the non-emergency market.

Staff diversity and turnover. What is the gender and ethnic makeup of the staff? At what rate does turnover occur and for what reasons?

The workforce is changing in EMS. To understand this in relation to the current system, the review should determine the makeup and turnover rate of the providers. The reasons for any excessive turnover should be identified and compared to similar systems and communities. A detailed assessment of staff morale and overall job satisfaction should be a component of the review.

Relationship with the labor force. How receptive is the labor force to system development and change?

Existing union agreements should be reviewed. The level of cooperation between labor and management should be objectively assessed. Any system design changes should be evaluated with due regard for the continued stability of the labor force.

System management and services. What are the strengths and weaknesses of the existing agencies in the system?

The review process should describe the network of providers within the community and how they are managed, regulated, and controlled. Compare the system to acceptable standards and practices found in other communities. Indicate strengths and weaknesses in the management of the system and provide recommendations for improvement. Identify cost implications of these recommendations.

Performance reporting. Does the system objectively measure and report its performance?

The methods used to verify the level of performance of the EMS program should be identified. Recommendations for an effective management information system and performance reports should be made, identifying the fiscal impact of these systems.

First responder/medic assist performance. Does the system have effective early response capabilities?

How are first responder services currently provided? The review should describe the current training levels, response times, and routine availability of first response personnel. Strengths and weaknesses of the first responder service should be identified, and recommendations for improving the service to optimal levels should be provided. Any cost implications of these improvements should be profiled.

Utilization of public and/or private providers. What agencies currently provide services?

The review should address the use of public and private providers in the current system. Compare the benefits of using either type of provider, and make recommendations regarding the overall mix of providers needed to ensure an optimal service level.

Liability issues. Does the system manage its liability risks?

All potential liability issues, within the context of the level of care being delivered, should be identified in the review. The magnitude of any such issues requires evaluation. In addition, any potential liability issues involving the labor force and anticipated system upgrades must be determined. Liability issues may be mitigated through the design of a more optimal EMS system.

System dispatch. Does the system utilize nationally accepted processes for medical dispatch?

Current dispatch methods should be studied, including protocols, procedures, training certifications, and quality improvement components used in dispatching all medical resources of the system. Compare the methods with acceptable standards used in similar systems. Describe the strengths and weaknesses of the current dispatch system, and provide recommendations about improving these services with the associated costs.

Clinical Issues

These issues relate to the clinical efficacy and methods used to ensure high levels of clinical quality within the system. Systems that internally and externally review their clinical processes on a routine basis are generally more sophisticated than those that do not.

Medical protocols, procedures, review, and control. Do medical control processes reflect current standards of practice?

Medical protocols, procedures, controls, and standards used in the current system should be described and compared to those widely accepted standards found in the medical literature. Strengths and weaknesses in the current processes should be identified. The review should provide recommendations about an optimal system of medical control, as well as the cost and funding options for providing this service.

Quality improvement. How does the system monitor and improve quality?

The review should evaluate the EMS system's quality improvement processes and compare them to acceptable standards and programs of other jurisdictions. The strengths and weaknesses in the current QA/QI process should be identified. Recommendations about developing an optimal QA/QI program and the costs of such a program should be provided.

Interactive medical control system. Do system personnel have access to physicians when dealing with difficult cases?

A comprehensive review of the on-line medical control, including analysis of the service components rendered, levels of service and costs, and the performance of the medical control system, should be provided. Recommendations about improving medical control to optimal levels and any associated costs should be identified.

Physician involvement. Are experienced emergency physicians actively and routinely involved in the system and its oversight?

Physician involvement levels and authority should be assessed. Reviewers should provide recommendations about improving physician involvement to optimal levels and identify any associated costs.

Financial Issues

These issues deal with the fiscal viability and stability of the EMS system. Although systems are funded through a variety of mechanisms, developing sound fiscal processes is critical to the system's long-term success.

System resource requirements. Do the resources consumed by the system accomplish its mission compared with other high-performance systems?

The review should analyze resource consumption for all system participants. These costs should be objectively quantified using full cost methodologies. Some individual EMS department's costs include "off-budget" or other allocated expenditures from other departments' line items. Detailed review of line-item budgets and cost justifications must be used to verify assumptions regarding resource consumption requirements.

Capitalization of equipment and system infrastructure. Does the system depend on municipal budgetary limitations for capital resources?

The review should evaluate the impact of all budgetary cycles and the nature of capital equipment funding. The review should determine if critical equipment is scheduled for replacement at predefined intervals, and if these schedules are followed.

Subsidy and user fees. What is the current mix between subsidy and fees? What is the optimal subsidy/fee tradeoff?

An analysis determining what potential subsidy level may be required to provide optimal service should be completed. Recommendations should be made to demonstrate how the subsidy could be structured and used most effectively. The reviewer should use the most relevant ratios possible (e.g., per capita, per transport, etc.) to evaluate the level of subsidy required. The review should compare projected levels of subsidy to acceptable standards in other cities, as appropriate. The relationship between the level of subsidy and the level of revenues generated from fees charged should be compared. The review should provide recommendations about any subsidy or user fees necessary to provide optimal service levels. Financial impact projections of the recommendations should be provided.

Cost recovery. Does the system effectively recover its costs?

The project should review cost recovery methodologies. Statutory and regulatory requirements for EMS system billings and collections should be analyzed. User fees and alternative revenue sources should be evaluated. The review should analyze billing hardware, software, and procedures, and compare and contrast these to similarly sized systems. Specific methods and procedures that can enhance cost recovery within the bounds of generally accepted industry practices should be identified.

Source

*Copyright © 1991
Fitch & Associates, Inc.
Reprinted with
permission.*

Financial systems integrity. Are the financial systems both sound and externally reviewed?

The review should determine the adequacy of external controls to ensure the integrity of financial and operational systems that materially impact the financial performance of the system. Assessment procedures consistent with those used in an independent audit process should be used.

Other

Unique factors for consideration. Are there any other questions that must be asked to objectively evaluate this system due to the unique nature of the community or the situation?

Each community has unique factors that impact each of the other issues listed above. The review should seek to determine if there are any issues of significance, internally or externally, that would alter the analysis and, thus, impact the outcome of the review.

Conclusion

These 25 questions will stimulate discussion of the EMS system's components and their functionality. The process described, however, is difficult and time consuming. Its success depends on the use of standardized assessment criteria, detailed collection of both qualitative and quantitative data, and finally, an impartial analysis to objectively determine how the system is performing. From that foundation, conclusions can be drawn about the operational, clinical, and fiscal requirements of the EMS system and how the community can best be served in the future.

Procurements: Why Structured Is Better

Jay Fitch, PhD

Once a decision has been reached to competitively procure either a public or private ambulance service, local officials must use caution to ensure success. In this article, the author outlines elements for a successful procurement process and reviews a failed procurement to illustrate key points.

FOR A NUMBER OF REASONS, local governments consider the procurement process a means of providing their communities with high-quality emergency and medical transportation service. Communities may be seeking to increase the quality of their service, reduce costs, or answer the essential contracting question.

The essential question local governments need to ask when considering a procurement process is, "Should we focus our energies on making government a better buyer of EMS or a better producer?" A well-designed process can ensure that government meets its objectives by becoming an informed buyer, regardless of the method ultimately selected to provide service.

Four key factors often impact a community's willingness to consider a procurement process. They are system design considerations, political concerns, economic factors, and medical quality issues. Once the determination is made to conduct a procurement, communities need to promptly make public policy decisions, determine the form of competition, and decide on a bid structure to be utilized. A carefully structured process provides the best opportunity to achieve the desired outcomes.

System Design Considerations

Most EMS systems were born of necessity 20 to 25 year ago. Many no longer reflect their communities and current EMS needs. Frequently, EMS designs that initially worked well become dysfunctional over time. EMS systems are "entropic." That is, if left alone long enough, the systems will begin to disintegrate.

High-performance EMS systems are designed to achieve clinical excellence, response time reliability, customer satisfaction, and economic efficiency—simultaneously and consistently. There may be several reasons that a system no longer meets these objectives. Current first responders and providers may not be keeping up with the host of innovations flooding EMS. The system may no longer be as operationally efficient as it once was. Or there may not be enough revenue to support the expanding system and related expenses.

The term *system design* refers to the EMS system's underlying legal and organizational structure, financing strategy, business and medical oversight structure, and system safeguards. A myriad of system designs are in use today, each with particular strengths and weaknesses. These design features can be objectively profiled against the factors that distinguish the community as unique along each of the political, economic, and clinical quality dimensions. In professionally designed procurements, the unique community factors are given due regard in the planning process.

System design questions are confusing and require time-consuming objective analysis to assess the current and future issues that will impact the EMS system over time. Governments attempting to procure the best service possible from public or private sources will require an increasingly structured approach.

Political Considerations

When community leaders contemplate using a structured procurement process, there is usually political fallout from groups who would rather directly influence the provider selection decision. Politics are involved in every system. However, when local officials are guided to deal with public policy issues rather than emotional issues, the "back room" political nature of the process can be diminished.

Elected officials are often subjected to tremendous lobbying efforts by both public employee unions and private providers in an unstructured process. Sometimes, the process becomes so embroiled in politics that it cannot be successful.

Determining public policy issues early and focusing on *what* is to be accomplished by the system rather than on *who* is to accomplish it also improve the potential for a positive outcome. Otherwise, the process can become a "ready, fire, aim" situation.

Economic Considerations

In addition to design and political issues, there are a number of economic factors that must be considered. They include local socioeconomic trends, demographics, system revenue sources and mix, and the economies of scale the provider can achieve in the procurement.

Economies of scale are determined by market and medical trade area considerations and not just jurisdictional boundaries. Even studies conducted for the federal agency charged with funding EMS reimbursement have concluded that "the ambulance industry is a natural spatial monopoly." Inadequate economies of scale can result in the provider's reduced capability to deliver the desired clinical and financial performance.

Clinical Considerations

The medical oversight function in a structured procurement is a "system process" rather than determined solely by the provider's internal policies. The medical standard of care is defined by medical authorities before the process begins. The standard of care encompasses such things as response time standards, priority dispatch protocols, medical protocols for first responders, medical protocols for air and ground ambulance crews, transport or destination protocols, equipment standards, and minimum certification requirements for all persons involved.

The level of service to be provided by both transporting ambulances and first response units is another key clinical question that must be clearly determined prior to the procurement. Other decisions include issues such as who has the responsibility for both interactive and off-line medical direction. Clinical standards and the process to upgrade standards must be clearly articulated before the procurement to avoid providers requesting additional reimbursement as the system evolves.

Public Policy Issues

The American Ambulance Association has outlined 12 public policy issues that cover design, political, economic, and clinical dimensions. They are an outgrowth of the combined experiences of those who conducted successful structured procurements and those who participated as providers. The issues include service area definition, market and market rights, flexible versus specialized production method, system revenues, business and legal structure, forms of competition, duration of market rights, contractor's consideration, performance security, medical oversight, first responder services, and control center operations. Each of these is described in detail in the association's contracting guide for municipal officials.

Communities are well advised to determine the implications of potential public policy decisions prior to undertaking a procurement. Trying to "sort it out" during the procurement, or worse, after the fact, often degenerates into a series of symptom-driven policy crises. As rapidly as one policy issue is resolved, another develops.

Forms of Competition

While overly simplistic, there are several fundamental types of competition. They include no competition, benchmarking, competition within the market, and competition for the market.

In systems with no competition, a public or private provider is selected without any real competition or threat of competition. The problem with this approach is that organizations may stop innovating, grow inefficient, or stagnate because they have the "right" to that market.

Benchmarking is based on market comparison and is usually used in systems with well-defined contracts. The incumbent provider's performance is measured against the standards of the industry's highest quality and most efficient systems. Benchmarking provides a fair approach to competition but must be administered carefully.

Competition within the marketplace allows multiple providers to compete for business within the market. Retail competition is a dangerous form of competition for EMS systems.

Competition for the marketplace is the mechanism routinely used for the initial selection of providers in a structured procurement. In this approach, competition is held between organizations interested in and qualified to serve the market.

Bid Structure

Bids are typically structured in one of three ways: multiple bid variable, single bid variable in which service levels are established as constant and price is the variable, and single bid variable in which price is held constant and service levels are compared. Sophisticated procurements limit the bid variables.

Procurements with more than one bid variable force the bidder to guess the desired mix between service level and price. Infinite variations among the bids make rational (apples to apples) comparisons impossible. Either of the single variable bid methodologies can be used to determine a clear winner. The most common method of achieving an apples-to-apples comparison is to hold the price constant and objectively compare services. Finally, scoring bid documents and presentations must be accomplished in an impartial and objective manner.

In its contracting guide, the American Ambulance Association recommends that a community's procurement process be professionally managed. "In selecting an individual or firm to conduct the system evaluation, redesign the system, and manage the procurement process, the most important qualification is experience in successful high-performance EMS system design." In some cases a poorly managed procurement is worse than no procurement. A procurement attempt in Sacramento, Calif., is an excellent example of a process that went awry.

Sacramento's Failed Procurement

At stake in Sacramento was a five-year, countywide contract for nearly 70,000 9-1-1 transports, approximately $28 million in revenue per year. In January 1992, San Jose, Calif.-based PacMed (now AMR-West) received the unanimous endorsement of the county's selection committee, outscoring other bidders by a significant margin.

However, five months later, the county board of supervisors, after intense lobbying from local ambulance providers, set aside the bids and recommendations by both the county's selection committee and health director. This decision came after bitter political debate and legal wrangling. The *Sacramento Bee* newspaper called the move "a triumph of politics and parochialism over the public interest."

The combined cost of this exercise was a staggering $1 million. But there is much to be learned by both providers and county governments in this failed bid process. To gain a deeper understanding, a chronology of events and an analysis of why they happened must be reviewed.

In the late 1980s, Sacramento County had 23 response zones served by seven private providers and three municipal services. The newspapers began detailing system problems beginning in 1988. These included poor equipment, extended response times, and labor strife that plagued the system. Medical control, monitoring, and the level of care provided were also major issues. The General Accounting Office characterized the county's EMS communications system in one study as one of the most convoluted in the nation.

The board of supervisors removed Sacramento County from the seven-county EMS oversight agency and created a monitoring group that reported to the county health director. The county retained a local firm specializing in market research as its consultant, and a decision was made to seek competitive bids. Tension from the local providers mounted.

EMS Coordinator Bruce Wagner began assembling the request for proposal (RFP) in early 1990. "I threw in everything but the kitchen sink to see what would happen." Specifications were "borrowed" from 12 other communities, according to Wagner. A cut-and-paste approach was used in the hopes that potential bidders would tell them what would and would not work.

After reams of written comments, the county changed numerous provisions and released the final RFP in October 1991. Several firms refused to participate, as it was clear that the system and the procurement had been poorly designed. Five proposals were received from three outside firms and two local companies.

The county's 14-member selection committee reviewed the proposals. This committee included fire officials, EMS physicians, a paramedic, and an attorney. After scoring the proposals, a recommendation was prepared for the board of supervisors in January 1992.

The board delayed taking action and asked for a formal report from the county health director, Ron Usher. The scoring process was challenged, protests were reviewed, and the county deemed them to be without merit. In the meantime, the local paramedic union voted to endorse PacMed's selection.

The director's 30-page report was presented and workshops conducted. The board again delayed a decision and discussed rescoring the proposals. One supervisor was quoted as saying, "The problem is you didn't come up with the right answer." Another said, "It's awfully hard to ask elected officials to throw out companies with 52 years of service."

It is clear that the only winners were lawyers and lobbyists. "It became a lose-lose situation," said Paul Shirley, PacMed president. "We put our cards on the table face up. We will be at a disadvantage in any future procurement. In essence we've now run a training ground for local providers." Over $250,000 was reported to have been spent by PacMed alone on this procurement process.

The failed procurement process in Sacramento took three years. Outside providers would not be blamed for failing to become involved in a second procurement, regardless of how flawed. The *Sacramento Bee*

Source

Original article.

reported that the state attorney general was investigating possible anti-trust violations during the bid process.

"Just say no" is a popular phrase in fighting drugs in our society. The lure of success in bidding can be just as addictive as narcotics. Both are expensive habits. And although it's hard to "just say no" to a poorly structured procurement, it can be good advice.

Remember that there are a number of steps necessary for a successful procurement. They include adequately addressing system design, political, economic, and medical considerations, and developing an appropriately structured bid process. If these steps had been followed, the procurement nightmare suffered in Sacramento could have been avoided.

References

U.S. Department of Health and Human Services. *Project Hope Report*. Washington, D.C.: U.S. Department of Health and Human Services, October 1991, xii.

Contracting for Emergency Ambulance Services. Sacramento, Calif.: American Ambulance Association, 1994.

Innovative Methods for Providing EMS

Integrating Paid and Volunteer Staff

Jonathan Politis, REMT-P

Volunteer agencies are increasingly using fully or partially paid personnel for those times during the week when volunteers are not available. Accomplishing this task in a positive manner that supports volunteerism is the focus of this article.

VOLUNTEER SERVICES ACCOUNT for the majority of EMS delivery organizations in the United States, especially in the East where the tradition of volunteer fire and emergency services is deeply rooted in culture and political climate. Volunteer services date back to 1736, when Benjamin Franklin established the Union Volunteer Fire Company in Philadelphia. The provision of volunteer emergency medical services became a natural extension for many volunteer fire departments. Independent ambulance and rescue squads also began to develop in many communities.

While rural volunteer services are common nationwide, major population bases in the East are served by predominantly volunteer services. For example, Nassau County, New York, with a population of three million people, is served by all-volunteer fire and predominantly volunteer EMS. While this is one of the largest population bases served by volunteers, it is not unusual on the East Coast.

During the 1980s, many volunteer services became severely strained in their ability to provide service. A decline in the ability to staff units with an adequate number of competent volunteers can be traced to many factors. With increasing awareness of EMS and higher public expectations, a corresponding increase in the demand for EMS became evident. Many services began to notice their annual call volumes steadily increasing—especially during the daytime hours, which are typically hours of peak demand and the time when volunteer staffing is often least available. During this same period, the public began to expect immediate response and a high degree of clinical sophistication. Accordingly, increasing standards and organizational requirements meant a decreasing number of members and increased strain.

In addition, economic factors began to reduce the time available to pursue this volunteer avocation. Two wage-earner households became the norm as people struggled to make ends meet when faced with increased housing and other costs. On an administrative level, most volun-

Inconsistent leadership and the lack of a strategic long-term plan are common factors among volunteer organizations "in trouble." Many problems, such as recruiting, training, and staffing, cannot be solved in the short term.

teer organizations were led and managed by many of the same volunteers who were already overextended with training and duty-hour requirements. Constant regulatory mandates translated to more administrative and training time needed to bring their organizations into compliance. In addition, many of those same organizations depended on donations and annual fund drives to finance their operations.

These types of clinical, administrative, and financial demands have and will continue to be a major source of strain for all volunteer organizations. As we move further into the 1990s, this pressure will become more acute for volunteer organizations as they grapple with increasing regulatory mandates and the costs of financing their services.

Long-Term Problems, Short-Term Leadership

Most volunteer organizations elect leaders on an annual or biannual basis, which leads to constant leadership turnover. Along with turnover comes changing agendas and short-term planning. Inconsistent leadership and the lack of a strategic long-term plan are common factors among volunteer organizations "in trouble." Many problems, such as recruiting, training, and staffing, cannot be solved in the short term.

Once members are recruited, the training process to become an EMT often takes six months. After EMT training, at least another six months are frequently required to gain sufficient experience and confidence to act as a crew leader. Many groups typically wait until staffing problems are evident and then react by initiating a membership drive. By the time the drive is actually implemented, and new members are accepted for membership, another six months elapses. If they are accepted in the middle of a class semester, more time elapses before training begins. During this 18- to 24-month process, the staffing problems become worse and the new EMTs are forced to take calls without experienced partners. Then, retention of the new members becomes a problem and a whole new spiral of crisis begins. While this example may seem far-fetched, it is only one example of why many groups are in trouble.

The corporate structure of many volunteer groups requires that all leaders be elected and policy be voted on by the membership. This format virtually guarantees a short-term approach to organizational issues that plague emergency services. Unless they have a written, long-term plan and the staff to carry it out, crisis management prevails. While many hospitals are voluntary organizations, too, their corporate bylaws structure the organization with a board of directors that sets policy and a chief executive or operating officer who carries it out. While the workers are involved in problem solving and suggesting policy changes through a total quality management (TQM) process, they do not vote on every decision in the daily operation of the hospital. While voluntary EMS is not as complicated as hospital administration, the same issues of governance, finance, policy, and control exist.

Is Volunteerism Really Dead?

While changes in values, economics, and lifestyles have made recruiting and training volunteers more challenging, volunteerism is not dead and never will be. Many organizations continue to succeed and prosper in spite of new challenges. However, in the complex climate of emergency services, new approaches and a shift in the volunteer organization paradigm are necessary. The missing element in volunteer emergency services is a long-term approach to leadership and administration—a career chief operating or executive officer.

Some of the most highly successful volunteer organizations in the United States have career leadership, administrative, and support staff. The American Heart Association, American Red Cross, and Boy Scouts of America are good examples of volunteer organizations that have paid leadership and a mix of volunteer and paid staff to fulfill their missions. For volunteer emergency services to survive beyond the year 2000, they will need to change their organizational paradigms to more closely match that of a nonprofit volunteer hospital or service organization.

The Similarities Between Volunteer Nonprofit Hospitals and Volunteer EMS

In following the evolution of hospitals from just before World War I to today, there is a striking similarity to volunteer EMS. Private, nonprofit hospitals were viewed as charitable institutions that initially existed on donations and philanthropy by the wealthy. Staffing consisted of significant numbers of volunteer personnel, and the hospital board was, of course, volunteer. Eventually, the hospitals sought public subsidies. Parochialism and poor transportation often spawned a small institution in nearly every community, each receiving donations and tax subsidies.

Eventually, taxpayers began to question these subsidies and push for hospital consolidations and fewer subsidies. Accordingly, hospitals began charging for their services. Over the next 50 years, hospitals evolved, physical plants improved, and consolidations and networks developed—all in an effort to improve market share and regional viability.

Hospitals have evolved over the last century through many of the same crises that voluntary EMS is just now facing: the need for career administration, integration of paid staffing, charging for services, consolidations to improve service, and so on. Unlike hospitals, where professional licensure has all but relegated volunteers to the coffee shop, volunteers can continue to be a viable part of EMS for many years to come.

But, volunteer services will need to redefine and reshape themselves to remain viable in the future.

Uni-Dimensional Thinking

Many individuals tend to be uni-dimensional in their thinking, considering organizations to be completely paid or completely volunteer. However, another alternative exists: integration of paid and volunteer staff in the same organization. While implementing this type of program is not easy, the advantages outweigh the disadvantages for many organizations. For all-volunteer services, adding paid staff can relieve administrative burdens and improve staffing levels and clinical sophistication. It also allows an organization to bring a consistent long-term approach to planning, policy development, training, and support services. If handled properly, paid staffing results in more consistent operations and allows better service and long-term organizational survival. However, adding paid staffing in a haphazard manner can quickly cause a volunteer organization's demise.

For all-paid services, volunteers can add to organizational depth and provide tremendous reserve capacity. Volunteers bring many talents to the organization. In most cases, the range of talents being volunteered would be costly to pay for or couldn't be hired at all. But people will volunteer their time to help the community, especially through high-profile emergency work. They also bring a sense of community involvement. In short, they bring additional staffing, depth, and a brain trust to be tapped when needed. However, volunteers are not free. There are costs associated with the training and development of every staff person. Management must carefully survey their organizational climate and be willing to spend the time necessary to recruit, train, and retain volunteer resources.

Volunteer Organizational Governance—Who's Driving the Bus?

While organizational governance may seem like an odd subject to review, it must be evaluated prior to employing anyone. Governance is the organizational design that determines who sets and implements policy, makes decisions, sets parameters of power among officers, and establishes the chain of command. The most common mistake made by volunteer groups is to begin hiring staff before fundamental issues of governance have been identified and changed. A common formula for failure is for a group structured as a membership corporation (membership meetings to elect operations officers, voting to pay bills, voting members in or out, etc.) to begin hiring paid field staff. The volunteer leadership is not available when they are working, and policies are inconsistent and change with the whims of the membership. The problem quickly develops into "nobody's driving the bus," and friction and segregation develop among the groups. While these problems create organizational dysfunction, the underlying issues that created the need for paid staffing go unsolved.

The Hospital Paradigm

The first major issue for the volunteer group to tackle is changing the organizational design to more closely resemble other nonprofit organizations. Most are structured with a board of directors that sets policy, and a CEO or COO who carries out policy and manages the organization on a daily basis. The staff (both paid and volunteer) answer to the CEO/ COO, who in turn answers to the board. This is a painful change in groups that decide at monthly meetings what type of Band-Aids to buy and who will be the next chief. Obviously, the membership (staff) loses power to vote on every issue. However, any volunteer organization contemplating hiring paid field staff has problems complex enough to need full-time leadership with excellent management skills.

Therefore, step number two is to hire a full-time executive or operations officer. His role is to work closely with the board to identify issues, plan, organize, and implement solutions. After these two major changes are made, the board and CEO may be able to rectify staffing issues without hiring staff. If paid personnel are needed, they will have a leader to direct their activities and set a tone in concert with the board.

Groups that decide to omit these steps end up with poorly supervised paid staff, conflicting personal agendas, friction, and turmoil—all of which are very damaging. Everyone (paid and volunteer staff) must answer to the CEO for true integration to occur. If volunteer and paid staff answer to different chains of command, segregation and an "us versus them" organizational tone often result.

Not every volunteer group needs a CEO and hospital-type governance, but voluntary EMS organizations large and complex enough to consider hiring paid staff need to be governed and managed differently to survive. When considering the integration of paid and volunteer staff, changes in organizational structure/governance are the most painful, but are also the most important changes to be made.

Short-term leadership, elected by a popularity contest, manages for the short term. Today's increasingly complex volunteer EMS organizations need long-term solutions. Failure to implement these changes leaves an unsupervised paid staff developing its own agendas, and nobody "driving the organizational bus."

Hiring the Right People

The Leader

The leader sets the tone for the entire organization. Therefore, hiring the right person for the job is a high priority for any new board. Integrating paid and volunteer staff is very challenging, and the leader must be absolutely committed to such a combined effort. There will be many critical moments along the way where the leader will be subtly tested, and many eyes will be watching to see if the leader "walks his talk." Any leader with a disguised contempt for either paid or volunteer staff will soon be discovered at some critical moment. Finding a person with the maturity and the management and people skills to make this marriage succeed is of paramount importance.

> Today's increasingly complex volunteer EMS organizations need long-term solutions.

The leader also must be able to work cooperatively with the board. Autocratic personalities and people with inflated egos will inevitably have difficulty with cooperation. The ability to work cooperatively with the board, volunteers, and paid staff will make the difference between success and failure. Many of these qualities are difficult to determine from reading a resume and interviewing someone. As the old saying goes, people are as perfect as they will ever get on their resumes. Two of the best ways to "smoke out" a potential leader's best and worst qualities are by carefully checking references, talking with former employers, and utilizing an "assessment center" to evaluate candidates. The following are some key traits to look for in a leader.

Listening skills. Listening is an essential skill needed for problem solving and negotiation. Look out for people who finish your sentences, interrupt, and formulate their responses before they have heard the whole message.

Win-win. People who have a poor life script (I'm OK and you're not) usually attempt to win every discussion or issue. An honest desire to satisfy needs is key to win-win negotiation.

Communications skills. Excellent verbal and written communications skills as well as teaching skills are important. The leader needs to be able to constantly communicate and have everyone understand his vision of where the organization is going.

Follow-through. Many people have great ideas and can communicate well, but what translates ideas into reality is the ability to follow through and execute them. What type of track record does the leader have in making things happen?

Situational leadership style. Can the new leader adapt his leadership style as the organization and situations evolve? Knowing when and how to be directive rather than supportive or vice versa is essential to leading.

In short, a great resume and a nice suit won't make a paid/volunteer integration work. Take the time to determine what qualities are needed in a leader, assess the candidates, and check their backgrounds.

Paid Staff

While good players may grow on trees, good player-coaches do not. Hiring a group of "hot-shot" medics fresh out of school with a pocket full of the latest EMS merit badge cards is a formula for failure. The paid clinical staff should play the role of player-coaches—providing unit staffing and patient care and being coaches, mentors, and role models in the grooming of new people. As a part of a new experiment, they, too, will be under intense scrutiny to see if they "walk their talk." Just as great care is taken in hiring the leader, the same care must be exercised in hiring clinical staff. Some important traits to look for follow.

Look out for "pups." Generally speaking, "pups," "rookies," or freshly trained people want to do everything until they are more seasoned and settle down. Rookies are not usually pulled off the bench to be coaches. Rookies want to run with the ball all the time. Avoid hiring "pups." What are needed are experienced people who don't have to prove to themselves they are competent practitioners.

Leadership. Paid staff also need the leadership and teaching experience to know when to be supportive and when to be directive. In terms of experience, hire the most mentally mature, medically experienced people available.

People skills. Again, staff need to like people and have a proven ability to work with and get along with others. Don't be afraid to call previous employers, as well as references. The background information revealed is sometimes amazing. They will be acting as the role models for current and future members, intended or not. They need to set the best possible example and be part of the organization's solution, not a new set of problems.

Role perception. Paid staff need to clearly understand their role as player-coaches and as key elements in solving the organization's problems. Their role is to assist with training and support functions, and to treat patients. They exist to help build the organization and make it strong. Anyone not mature enough to work cooperatively with the leadership to strengthen the organization will quickly become a liability.

Flexibility. Just as the leader will need to be flexible in leadership style, the staff need to be flexible as well. The organization will be evolving, and new challenges will constantly require their attention. They need to be flexible enough to solve new problems.

Once the very best people are hired, time needs to be spent training them in exactly what their roles and specific responsibilities are.

The Volunteer Staff

Just as paid staff must understand their roles, the volunteer staff must, too. With paid staff suddenly arriving, many volunteers will assume the "paid scum" are there to be the maids and butlers of the organization—with all cleanup and maintenance dumped on *them*. While they may play an important role in support functions, the presence of paid staff cannot be an excuse for volunteers to shirk their responsibilities. The majority of support functions will naturally shift to the paid staff, but volunteers must continue to be accountable for their responsibilities. If either group starts dumping on the other and the problem isn't resolved quickly, they will begin to polarize and segregate rather than integrate.

Volunteers who won't work with paid staff are just as destructive as paid staff who won't work with volunteers—it works both ways. While paid and volunteer staff responsibilities will differ, both must be expected to fulfill their work responsibilities. Often there are volunteers who see themselves as "gold card" members who can put themselves above everyone else. This is very destructive and must be dealt with swiftly for the good of the entire organization.

> While paid and volunteer staff responsibilities will differ, both must be expected to fulfill their work responsibilities.

A recruiting program must be aimed at bringing new people in all the time, not just when a staffing crisis exists. Volunteers must be an integral part of the emergency response organization and not treated as reserves, auxiliaries, or window dressing.

Playing Well Together: Those Critical Moments

Amazingly small issues have the potential to become major issues because of the perception of discrimination. The leadership must set the tone. It's a careful balancing act to "feed the hungry beaks" of both groups. It takes attentive listening, a keen sense of fairness, and good conflict resolution skills to make paid/volunteer integration work.

An immediate perception of many volunteers when paid staff are added is that they are being phased out and the organization will soon be all paid. Constant communication and troubleshooting is important to dispel these types of destructive rumors. Otherwise they can destroy morale, cause turnover, and become a self-fulfilling prophecy.

When paid staff are added, some volunteers will decide to "vote with their feet." In most cases, the people lost are those who were looking for an excuse to exit. If you start losing large numbers of your very best people, quickly take stock of what you are doing.

Everybody from the board to the field staff needs to understand why people volunteer, and work to keep the flow of new volunteer members constant. A recruiting program must be aimed at bringing new people in all the time, not just when a staffing crisis exists. Volunteers must be an integral part of the emergency response organization and not treated as reserves, auxiliaries, or window dressing. They must continue to be treated as peers by the paid staff and vice versa. Mutual respect is something that must be continually earned. Organizational "dead wood" and people not fulfilling responsibilities erode the mutual respect that is essential among the staff.

Among the paid staff, a destructive perception is that they will work themselves out of a job by grooming new volunteers. To prevent that perception, determine a minimum level of paid staffing and stick to it—even if extra volunteers are available and overtime will be incurred. The wrong message to send the key support staff is that doing their job will result in their demise.

Professionalism

Remember that professionalism has little to do with pay status and everything to do with a member's attitude, conduct, appearance, and performance. Don't make the mistake of referring to the paid staff as the "professional" staff. Your paid staff should be called paid or career staff. Everyone, paid or volunteer, is expected to be a professional and should be treated that way.

If there is a training or qualification process that is required by the organization, everybody, paid and volunteer, must be required to do it. From an operational and clinical performance point of view, staff is staff. The public has a right to expect excellence regardless of membership type. The only responsibilities that should differ are the administrative and support duties that paid staff are expected to do.

Everybody is expected to complete training and vehicle inspections and perform competently.

By the same token, everybody must be issued the same basic uniform. Issuing different types of uniforms to paid staff and volunteers only enhances the perception of "gold card membership" in the organization. This creates controversy. Consider setting up some type of an annual uniform allowance program, which allows members to add and maintain uniforms based on work or duty hours.

You're Not in Kansas Anymore

There are naturally differences between paid and volunteer staff. Frankly, the paid staff will be there for 40 hours each week, while most volunteers will be there less than half that time. Paid staff will naturally have different needs than most of the volunteers.

Then there is the federal Fair Labor Standards Act. If a volunteer would like to become a member of the paid staff, they are no longer a volunteer. A common mistake is allowing a paid staff member to continue to volunteer in the same capacity, or requiring paid staff to volunteer for a certain number of hours to help maintain a volunteer perspective. Both of these practices are illegal. Any organization hiring paid staffing must become familiar with the FLSA or risk major fines. One of the biggest dilemmas is when volunteers apply for employment. If they are good enough to volunteer, are they automatically "player-coach" material? Not necessarily. Be sure that everyone understands the expectations of paid staff and how there are administrative differences. However, if you have people who are qualified for a job and are desirable, they should be hired. Otherwise, a very bad message is sent to the membership, and morale suffers. Remember, once hired, a person is no longer a volunteer, and a hole must now be filled on the volunteer duty schedule with a new volunteer.

There will always be administrative differences between staff; just remember to keep the operational differences, real or perceived, as few as possible!

Listen, Listen, Listen

The total quality management process, where employees (paid and volunteer) are involved in addressing quality and operational issues, is vital. With the change in organizational governance, volunteers no longer vote on all issues. The TQM process uses quality circles of employees to address issues, find solutions, and keep people involved in the organization. One dilemma to be faced is the obvious difference in proficiency among staff members. A 40-hour-per-week employee works in the field on "auto pilot"; a 12-hour-per-week volunteer does not, even though both could be competent care providers.

Quality circles must be properly charged with the organization's

> The TQM process uses quality circles of employees to address issues, find solutions, and keep people involved in the organization.

Source

Original article. Jonathan Politis, REMT-P, is the chief of the Colonie EMS Department in upstate New York, a combination career-volunteer department. He has been an active EMT since 1971, as well as a paid firefighter, a state EMS training coordinator, and a paramedic training program coordinator.

parameters so that a small group of zealots does not develop unrealistic expectations for the total organization.

When paid staffing is implemented, leadership must be absolutely committed to making this integration work. It takes listening, conflict resolution, fine-tuning, and patience.

The New Paradigm

Over the last decade, controversy over whether municipal or private concerns can provide the best EMS has been plentiful. Because of the old volunteer EMS paradigm, most volunteer organizations have been functioning at anything but state-of-the-art levels. With a new organizational paradigm, nonprofit volunteer EMS systems could become as effective as their hospital counterparts in the delivery of high-quality, low-cost emergency medical care.

Both governmental and for-profit services have significant drawbacks. Government services are typically very expensive and often provide low performance. For-profit services, while less expensive, have the profit motive that can hinder many decisions. Accordingly, in some states "for profit" hospitals are against the law. Could it be that EMS should be provided by neither government nor private enterprise?

Could the new EMS paradigm be a regional nonprofit volunteer organization run like a volunteer hospital? Given that over half of the EMS organizations in most states are voluntary nonprofit groups, it is definitely possible. But to do so will require a reinvention of the volunteer service, reshaped to accept the challenges as we move toward and beyond the year 2000. There are no secrets to this new paradigm. It involves reorganization, long-term planning, leadership, and the ability to integrate both paid and volunteer staff. While the new paradigm is technically possible and administratively feasible, it will require hard work to gain political acceptance in many groups. Are you ready for the new volunteer paradigm?

IMAGINE AN EMS SYSTEM in which providers can move easily across jurisdictional lines, communications are possible from any ambulance to any hospital, all ambulances have the same equipment, and all hospitals participate fully and accept and transfer patients as needed to provide proper care. Imagine a system where funding is equally distributed to all jurisdictions. Sound like an EMS utopia? Theoretically, this is how a state-provided EMS system should work. But do such systems really work? Do they even exist?

During the early development of EMS, the idea of a regional approach to the delivery of EMS was advocated. In 1966, the National Academy of Sciences, National Research Council (NAS/NRC) published *Accidental Death and Disability—The Neglected Disease of Modern Society.* In this premier document, the NAS/NRC called for the adoption—at the state level—of general policies and regulations pertaining to ambulance services, as well as the provision of ambulance service at local levels. In 1972, the then Department of Health, Education, and Welfare funded five EMS demonstration projects. Each of these projects explored a different approach to regionalization. It was concluded that a regional approach to EMS was feasible, provided there was a recognized and accepted lead organization responsible for the implementation and continuation of the system.

The EMSS Act of 1973 (P.L. 93-154) provided the legitimacy and funding necessary for the development of EMS systems. The "1200" series of funding, as it came to be known, led to the development of EMS systems on a statewide and regional basis. An "eligible entity" under the law was defined as

- A state
- A unit of local government
- A public entity administering a compact or other regional arrangement or consortium
- Any other public entity or nonprofit private agency

In addition, the law required that priority be given to applications submitted by states, local governments, or public regional entities. Thus, funding was now available for developing and providing statewide EMS systems. This was especially attractive to those states that did not have established public regional organizations. The law also required that 25 percent of the annual appropriation would go to rural EMS, precluding large metropolitan jurisdictions from receiving all of the funding.

Given the provisions of the EMSS Act of 1973, the development of state-provided EMS systems would seem to be a logical approach. And indeed it was for a number of states. However, with the demise of federal

Statewide EMS Provider Systems: Do They Work?

Bruce J. Walz, PhD, NREMT-P

Several states have developed statewide approaches to responding to EMS situations. Geography, financing, historical system development, and politics are major factors in creating such systems. This article discusses the pros and cons of providing EMS on a statewide basis. In the companion article, Idaho's state EMS director outlines the roles and functions of the state EMS office.

A statewide system provides a means for these resources to be shared.

funding for EMS in 1981, many statewide systems collapsed into little more than a central office struggling to meet statutory requirements. In other cases, state or other funding replaced federal dollars, allowing some state-provided EMS systems to continue and even expand. Given these extremes, it is no wonder that the effectiveness of statewide EMS systems would be questioned.

Advantages of a Comprehensive State-Provided EMS System

Given the many components necessary for the development of an EMS system, it would not be feasible for each locality or jurisdiction to form its own. Indeed, the term *system* carries the connotation of some degree of integration, making a regional or statewide approach seem logical. Perhaps the most important advantage of this approach is the ability to have a single focus for all EMS activities. Providers, hospitals, consumers, and government agencies need only turn to an identified official or organization. Additionally, such a central focus provides a continuity of vision, which can serve as a common thread to hold an otherwise fragmented state-provided EMS system together. The central organization can also mediate jurisdictional disputes, including political jurisdictions, clinical services, and professional practice concerns.

Integration of resources is another important advantage of a statewide system. Not every community has the clinical expertise needed to care for all patients. Rather than duplicate such services, a statewide system provides a means for these resources to be shared. Suppose a young woman is injured in a car crash. Paramedics on the scene determine that she has life-threatening, multi-system trauma. A helicopter is requested and she is flown to a state-designated level one trauma center. After stabilization and initial recovery, she is transferred to a rehabilitation facility near her home. Following a significant stay, she returns home and eventually resumes her pre-crash lifestyle. The resources involved in the young woman's recovery included trained paramedics, helicopter evacuation, a trauma center, and a rehabilitation facility. All of these are necessary for a total response to a trauma incident, but they are also very expensive. Facilities such as trauma centers and rehabilitation hospitals cannot be supported by a single community. It would also not be cost effective to duplicate such specialized centers in every jurisdiction or region. By categorizing resources and establishing echelons of care, patients can be directed to the facility most appropriate to meet their needs without regard for political or system boundaries.

One of the original 15 components identified in the EMSS Act of 1973 is communications. As with any system, communications are what hold it all together. Most of the daily EMS activities depend on communications, whether for medical control, arranging for an interhospital transfer, or disaster response. By having a central focus, existing systems can be integrated and new systems developed that will respond to the needs of all EMS system providers and users. One need only look at the expansion of a universal access number, 9-1-1, across states and the nation and its effect on medical response. As the demand for frequencies becomes more acute in urban areas, a consolidated, statewide communications system provides for more efficient use of the limited radio spectrum currently available for the emergency services. We must learn from the military and from disaster response literature about how essential a coordinated communications network is. A sound communications system provides for the delivery of prompt, efficient, and proper emergency medical care, both in the prehospital setting and at the interhospital level. In addition, a well-established central communications system provides a means to coordinate disaster and mutual-aid response.

In addition to communications, a standardized approach to patient record-keeping is needed. Such standardization is advantageous at a number of levels, but most importantly for system review and evaluation. All facets of the system can be evaluated because the same information is available at all levels, or at least linked by some common identifying criteria. Once a patient enters the EMS system, it is necessary to track that patient through to discharge, even if the patient is transferred to other facilities.

Of all the advantages of a statewide system, the most complex is funding. In a statewide approach, funding can be coordinated across the various jurisdictions. A united front can be presented when approaching state legislatures for support. If necessary, and politically possible, funds can be moved from more affluent parts of the state to impoverished areas. Such an approach is currently being used by some states to reduce inequity in local school systems. The entire resource and tax base of the state can be used to fund programs and activities that no one jurisdiction or region alone could afford. Montgomery County, Md., for example (located within the Washington metropolitan area), is one of the richest counties in the nation. In contrast, some counties on Maryland's eastern shore are among the poorest. By initiating a statewide approach to EMS funding—using eight dollars from every biannual vehicle registration—Maryland has been able to support a statewide EMS system that equally benefits all areas of the state.

Closely related to funding at the state level is the advantage of consolidated procurement. Imagine the increase in purchasing power when a whole state joins together to buy supplies and equipment. In one state, a cardiac monitor manufacturer tried to introduce its product to EMS providers. The state had negotiated a contract with another manufacturer and the "state price" was so low that the other manufacturer could not match it. Combined procurement also leads indirectly to standardization.

One more advantage of providing EMS on a statewide basis is brought about by geography. The location, size, or shape of a state may lend itself to the establishment of a statewide EMS system. As an ex-

In a statewide approach, funding can be coordinated across the various jurisdictions.

ample, Delaware, with only three counties, uses a statewide system approach to EMS.

Disadvantages of a Statewide EMS System

Those aspects of a statewide system that make it appealing may also be the aspects that present the most difficulty. Trying to be all things to all people has never led to great success, only mediocrity. And that is how many state-provided EMS systems are viewed—as mediocre systems

State EMS Offices
Dia Gainor

In state government, the public expects certain programs to exist. For example, the state department of transportation is responsible for all of the bridges in the state, and the state department of education should manage teacher and curriculum standards. Most citizens will recognize the purpose of these programs. But a state office of emergency medical services does not have the same level of public recognition or expectations about what that office does and what its mission is. Often, EMS providers do not understand all the responsibilities of their state EMS office.

Each state has an office of emergency medical services, although the name varies. Each has a lead manager, most commonly called a director. Most often the EMS office is within the state department of health, public health, human resources, or public safety. In a few states, EMS offices are self-governing agencies guided by a commission. Staff size ranges from four to 86.

Funding for State EMS Programs

Revenue for state offices varies considerably. State EMS offices either weave a patchwork quilt of funding sources or have dedicated funds independent of the state general funds. In a few states, federal funds are the sole means of support. Federal funds are usually channeled through another state office to EMS in the form of block grants, like the U.S. Department of Transportation 402 funds and the Centers for Disease Control's Preventative Health and Health Services block grants. Other grants, like the EMS for Children and Trauma Systems Planning

and Development programs are competitive, and often available on a time-limited basis.

Dedicated funding sources are derived from assessed fees or "piggy-backed charges" on existing fines, protecting the EMS dollars. Dedicated funds can be moving violation fines, vehicle registration fees, driver's license fees, and DWI convictions, for example. Without dedicated funds, state EMS offices depend on general funds. Economic shortfalls may reduce budgets in a given year.

State EMS Activities

State EMS offices have mandated programs often set forth in state laws. Some of those laws may have been written in the early 1970s, during the EMS Systems Act of 1973, with subsequent block grant funding. Typical state EMS responsibilities include systems planning, eligibility determination/certification of prehospital care personnel, data collection and analysis of prehospital response documentation, standard setting and provision of EMS training, inspection and licensure of EMS vehicles or services, public information programs, EMS communications systems development and management, patient care standards and protocol development, legislative issues, and grants to regional and local EMS organizations. These activities vary among states. Some states may be responsible for even more programs.

Many states have an EMS advisory committee. Some committee roles may be purely cosmetic, built on compromise. One need only look at the political diversity present in any state to see that a statewide approach to EMS systems is fraught with difficulty. Add this to the individual needs of local hospitals, the egos of providers, and the traditions of the local delivery system, and the opportunity for success is minimal.

The major advantage of a single statewide EMS system is that it provides one central focus of leadership. This may appear to be a simple concept, but not necessarily in the realm of EMS. There are various components and levels of providers in the typical EMS system, each with its

while other committees may be intimately involved in planning and program development. Either extreme can result in damage to the overall EMS system through neglect or the emergence of a political beast that slows and strangles even the best ideas.

The advisory committee, at the state or local level, is a valuable source of advice, input, strategic planning, and problem identification. Other groups outside of the government can provide the state EMS director with insight about that EMS system. Provider or instructor associations and human interest groups, such as trauma victim coalitions, or state chapters of clinical specialists, such as emergency physicians or surgeons, can act in this capacity. Consultants can help when addressing a specific problem. An interdisciplinary team approach was introduced by the National Highway Traffic Safety Administration to conduct technical assessments of state EMS systems and has been used by the majority of states. The team concludes its review of the current status of the state system by writing an incisive report that includes recommendations for system improvement based on the expertise of the team members.

A state EMS program has the most influence in state government itself. The state EMS director is in a position to educate the governor, legislators, and other state agencies, and can offset negative impact to the system. A cause in dire need of a solution can be effectively introduced to these players, especially when the state EMS office can supply the appropriate statistics, problem statements, or issue analyses.

State EMS offices regularly communicate with their fellow EMS offices across the country. Sometimes this interaction can be as simple as confirming that a reciprocity candidate's certification

is current, or it can be as complex as a few state EMS directors collaborating on a major project or document. The National Association of State EMS Directors is an active, productive organization that augments the individual states' capabilities through information sharing, expertise, and formal participation in other national organizations.

Federal agencies influence state EMS offices through funding or introducing standards and guidelines. Very few federal agencies have had a consistent level of participation in EMS system development. The U.S. Department of Transportation National Highway Traffic Safety Administration has probably the most notable history in EMS involvement, having set the standard for prehospital care curriculum, the registered "star-of-life" insignia, and demonstration project initiatives throughout the country. Other agencies are newly emerging forces that have already proven to be valuable assets to state EMS systems, like the U.S. Department of Health and Human Services, Division of Trauma and EMS. Although rarely regulatory in nature, federal agency activities often set the standard and indicate the trends occurring in EMS.

The state EMS office performs important roles in setting and enforcing standards, coordinating federal mandates, providing grants and other funding to local and regional systems, and a host of data gathering and public information programs designed to improve the provision of patient care.

Source
Original article. Dia Gainor is the Idaho State EMS director in Boise, Idaho.

own identified leadership. To bring together such diverse and powerful groups as hospitals, nurses, and physicians, each with a traditional power base, is a difficult task. Even if a leader is mandated by law, many of these groups possess sufficient power to control or influence the leader's position. In addition, traditional politics may also be a factor. For example, the state EMS director may be a political appointee and change with administrations. Or the director may only come from a particular area of the state or from a particular group (e.g., nursing).

As in any dynamic group, certain group members may exert more control than others. This can easily occur in a statewide EMS system. For example, a major jurisdiction may not have the resources to train its EMS personnel to a particular level. Because of the jurisdiction's influence, the whole state could be trained at a lower level.

The same situation can occur with funding. Areas of the state that contribute the most will naturally have the most influence. Therefore, poorer sections of the state may not be able to share equally in the decision-making process. Likewise, more affluent areas may provide a higher level of EMS response than other areas.

Political and funding concerns can easily lead to a policy of "the lowest common denominator." In this situation, statewide decision making is based not on what a jurisdiction or region of the state is capable of, but on what the least funded or supportive area of the state can bear.

For example, the 1993 American Heart Association ALS guidelines placed new emphasis on the use of transcutaneous external cardiac pacing (TECP). As EMS systems update their protocols based on these new guidelines, a decision will have to be made on allowing TECP as a field skill for ALS providers. From a clinical and training point-of-view, TECP use by field personnel is straightforward. However, a cardiac monitor with pacing may cost over $10,000. In a state-provided EMS system, where such equipment is purchased or subsidized by the state, the expense of upgrading all ALS units may override the clinical advantages of TECP. In addition, to maintain standardization and "political correctness," jurisdictions or regions of the state that could support such equipment with local funds are prohibited from doing so. The desire to maintain a system of equality that does not offend areas or jurisdictions that cannot compete stymies initiatives and advancement in all areas of the state.

Although statewide systems may provide a central focus for the delivery of EMS, medical control is often a local responsibility. The state medical director may establish medical control guidelines and protocols, but in many states, the ultimate responsibility for prehospital providers rests with the local medical director. Because of this, field providers who are certified or licensed by the state may not be able to function statewide. In Maryland, for example, paramedics are certified by the state but "practice" in the field under the license of a local medical director. This system works well for paramedics who only function in one jurisdiction; however, many providers function in multiple jurisdictions. A career paramedic may work in county A, volunteer in county B, and work part-time in county C. The paramedic is now responsible to three medical directors, must participate in continuing education in each jurisdiction, and usually takes a biannual recertification exam for each county. In addition, the National Registry recertification requirements must be met to maintain state certification. Yet, this is a "state-certified" paramedic.

Administration of an EMS system that serves an entire state inevitably leads to the development of some form of bureaucratic structure. In large states, this structure may have many levels. Individual EMS organizations, such as rescue squads, may be organized within counties. A group of counties will form a region, and the region will interact with "the state." Each of these levels has the potential to have its own administrative structure and political process. The "grass roots" provider can easily become isolated from the decision-making process of the central EMS office.

Feeling disenfranchised from the EMS system may lead to poor morale, substandard care, and lack of initiative on the part of field providers and local components of the EMS system, such as the community hospital and local medical director. All too often, this creates an "us versus them" attitude among field providers. Such an attitude undermines both the support for the statewide EMS system and the public's and political leaders' impression of the EMS community.

Source

Original article. Bruce Walz, PhD, NREMT-P, is the director of continuing education programs for JEMS *magazine.*

Conclusion

Given these advantages and disadvantages, can EMS provided on a statewide basis really work? The answer is yes and no. In some respects, a statewide system presents many advantages, most notably in the development of echelons of care and the integration of a statewide communications system. The mere existence of a statewide approach will ensure at least a central focus for EMS delivery. However, a statewide system also has the potential to foster conflicts and inequity within the system. This can lead to poor morale and inferior care.

What is the answer then? Perhaps there is no *one* answer. EMS systems are dynamic entities forced to exist in a political realm while trying to meet the out-of-hospital medical needs of all citizens. Because of this, no one system will ever be perfect. However, by understanding the limitations of the various approaches and the historical development of these systems, healthcare planners and EMS managers can make a more informed judgment on how best to meet the needs of their service areas.

References

Division of Medical Sciences. *Accidental Death and Disability: The Neglected Disease of Modern Society.* Washington, D.C.: National Academy of Sciences-National Research Council, 1966.

Emergency Medical Services Systems Act of 1973. Public Law 93-154. 93rd Cong., 1973.

Hanlon, J. J. "Emergency Medical Services: New Program for Old Problem." *Health Services Reports* 88 (1973): 205.

The Drought in Rural EMS

Lee Reeder

Rural hospitals continue to close at an alarming rate. As a result, the importance of and demand for EMS in these communities increases. This article reviews the issues that face rural EMS systems in the areas of finance, personnel, communications, and system development.

RURAL EMS IN THE UNITED STATES needs help, and its people know better than to expect a handout. Services, government agencies, and thousands of individuals will have to combine hard work, pioneering spirit, and a sense of community to ensure quality emergency medical care in rural America.

So concludes a report drawn from the National Rural EMS Needs Workshop, conducted in March 1989 at the EMS Today Conference in San Diego and sponsored by the National Rural Health Association. The invitational workshop combined the knowledge and experience of 42 rural EMS administrators and managers from 22 states with national rural EMS studies and surveys in an attempt to identify problems and offer solutions. Also present were two members of the federal Office of Technology Assessment (OTA), an advisory arm of Congress.

The findings of the San Diego workshop were then used in a workshop on rural EMS held in May 1989 by OTA. The OTA workshop was conducted as part of a larger study by that organization on rural health. OTA will merge the results of the San Diego workshop with six reports it has commissioned to form a background paper on rural EMS for Congress.

Janet Reich, chairwoman of the NRHA's Rural EMS Task Force, said the NRHA-sponsored report could be a useful tool. "Hopefully, individual states will use this as a guideline to look at programs they can implement to address their problems," she said.

The following is a summary of draft reports made by the five workshop groups. The areas of training, communications, systems, finance, and personnel were covered.

Training

The group report on training identified research and quality assurance as "two focal and overriding needs."

Group members agreed that valuable information could be gained by an in-depth study of rural training programs. Their report stated, "If we could identify eight to 10 training programs from varying environments and have them showcased in a seminar to share the secrets of their success, we would probably discover some inconsistencies in what makes training programs work well."

Asked to relate training problems to the U.S. Department of Transportation standard curricula, the group consensus was that redevelopment of national standard curricula needed to be preceded by serious research. To form a baseline, according to the group, researchers must first determine the knowledge required to carry out both the actual and ideal duties of EMS field personnel. This research should be conducted in consultation with EMTs of all levels, training and service administrators, educational psychologists, nurses, and physicians. From there, the group recommended that researchers study curriculum design and "how people learn and remember practical skills."

The gradual inclusion of specialty courses into the standard curriculum—on subjects ranging from farm rescue to hazardous materials to high-angle rescue—was also listed as a concern. These courses, the group concluded, would best be taught on an as-needed basis.

Some solutions and models related to quality assurance (QA) in training were offered by the group. These included

- Developing a strategy or campaign to make QA a priority for personnel at all levels
- Organizing a conference to showcase model QA systems
- Conducting research in rural areas rather than extrapolating data from urban studies
- Establishing a multidisciplinary committee to evaluate and suggest implementation models after research

The report added that medical director involvement was critical throughout the training process and that state and federal governments should be responsible for technical and financial research assistance in addition to planning and implementation.

Instructor training and sophistication were cited as concerns because of the limited student pool in rural areas. The group report stated, "Due to low population density, aging population, perceived need for physically fit, young individuals, and lack of access to training resources (financial, human, materials, and equipment), the pool of EMS provider trainees is grossly decreased in rural communities."

The lack of prospective trainees due to low population in many areas is often compounded by the overall perception of the "typical" EMS responder. The training group report stated that instructors "need to be skilled at adapting curricular requirements/materials to atypical students." These students include the reading and learning disabled, high school students, and culturally different, handicapped, or elderly people.

The importance of not overlooking the young and old in the available student pool was also stressed. "Training personnel and service directors can learn to take advantage of the strengths of the individual or group and work within their limitations," the report stated. "For example, while retired people may have some physical limitations, their overall judgment and stability may far outweigh their limitations. High school students are frequently enthusiastic and have fresher learning skills; their limitations generally are in the areas of life experience, judgment, and empathy."

Other training problems cited by the group included a lack of "quality clinical interaction both for initial training and continuing education" and a lack of leadership and management training.

The public access problem goes deeper in many rural areas, especially along highways where there are often no telephones for many miles. Response times become much longer when people are forced to travel great distances to reach telephones.

Communications

The report by the communications group drew a picture of an EMS system still plagued by "dead spots" in emergency radio coverage and public access to EMS.

Local and regional levels of government were identified as primarily responsible for developing 9-1-1 central access/dispatch wherever possible to ease the problems of public access to EMS in rural areas. The group report stated: "According to a survey by the National Association of State EMS Directors, only two states, Connecticut and Maryland, reported that 100 percent of the population can access emergency services by dialing 9-1-1. Twenty states and territories reported less than 50-percent 9-1-1 coverage, and four states did not respond. Many rural areas are not covered by 9-1-1 central access/dispatch systems."

The public access problem goes deeper in many rural areas, especially along highways where there are often no telephones for many miles. Response times become much longer when people are forced to travel great distances to reach telephones.

Recommendations from the communications group included the suggestion that local, regional, and state agencies work together to install emergency call boxes along major rural highways.

Educating the public was recognized as key to the goal of improved public access to EMS. Local, regional, and state agencies were identified as having responsibility for such educational programs.

Coping with equipment deficiencies was also listed as a priority by the group.

Members felt that more emphasis should be placed on new equipment to cover radio dead spots, citing a recent NASEMSD survey in which 31 states reported a lack of EMS radio system coverage in rural areas. The group recognized that rural areas will need some help in reaching this goal. Its report stated: "Covering these radio dead spots will require capital equipment investments beyond the capabilities of most rural ambulance services."

Those necessary capital investments include VHF and UHF relays, radio-telephone switching systems, microwave relay, cellular telephones and—possibly in the future—mobile satellite.

The solutions, which include standards for frequencies, dispatch centers, and equipment, would require funding and technical assistance from state and federal governments.

Communications planning, coordination, and training were also addressed as major problems. Solutions to planning and coordination problems included standards for medical control and dispatch communications; coordination with local hospitals; frequency coordination in cooperation with FCC-designated frequency coordination; disaster response (including mutual-aid frequencies and interagency participation); air-to-ground radio frequencies; local and regional EMS planning participation; coordination with other public safety agencies; and interstate coordination.

Communications training was specifically cited as a pressing need. The training level of rural dispatchers was termed "especially important" in rural areas because of long response times. Solutions to training shortcomings included establishing standardized EMS communications protocols; conducting standardized training for all EMS dispatchers (including police and fire departments); training in-hospital medical personnel to communicate with EMS responders; conducting QA reviews for communications operations; and providing continuing education for EMS communicators.

Systems

In the draft summary of the systems work group, NASEMSD President Barak Wolff defined the two greatest systems problems as "lack of effective medical control and inconsistent and poorly defined EMS systems in many rural areas."

Wolff's summary stated, "Historically, there has been a lack of consensus standards for the roles, responsibilities, and training required by physicians serving as EMS medical directors in an 'off-line' capacity. Coupled with this is the problem that, in many states, there is no legal requirement for 'off-line' medical direction, particularly for transporting or first response basic life support (BLS) level services. Further, where medical direction is available, there is often a lack of clear authority and liability protection to support local physicians in implementing the desired standards."

Some of the training deficiencies cited were in emergency medical techniques and procedures (including ACLS and ATLS) and experience in organization, management, and evaluation of EMS systems. The problem, according to the summary, is especially acute in smaller rural emergency departments, where medical directors are "expected to provide this service for no compensation, like the volunteers they are to supervise."

Because many rural medical directors are not trained specialists in EMS, group members agreed that consensus standards and clear guidance on medical control should be more widely distributed and shared.

The group identified several areas of responsibility for states, including providing emergency medical training and continuing education to rural nurses and physicians. The state programs, which would involve the assistance of medical schools, professional associations, hospitals, EMS regional offices, and local systems, should—according to the summary—include ACLS, ATLS, base-hospital courses, and EMS systems and medical control topics.

Other solutions on the state level to systems problems included the "need to adopt standards and/or issue guidelines that require EMS medical directors for all prehospital providers and identify the roles, expectations, and authority for the position." The summary added that states should

"The lack of a clear and consistent definition of an 'EMS system' contributes to public and professional confusion, makes it difficult to make comparisons between geographic areas, and inhibits smooth jurisdictional transitions."

work to ensure there are "no liability impediments to the provision of medical control."

One of the biggest problems of rural EMS systems is public perception. The report stated, "The lack of a clear and consistent definition of an 'EMS system' contributes to public and professional confusion, makes it difficult to make comparisons between geographic areas, and inhibits smooth jurisdictional transitions."

Other recognized system problems were a lack of consistency between states for EMS authority and responsibility; a frequent lack of professional and expert EMS management in smaller and more rural services; uninformed public expectations of rural EMS that lead to a lack of regard and support for rural services; and extreme distances from many rural communities to tertiary care facilities.

Suggested solutions to some of these problems included using a national consensus group, such as ASTM, to formally define an EMS system; having all states "define the authority, responsibility, and minimum standards for the development and implementation of EMS systems"; developing model federal laws "to encourage states to implement comprehensive EMS acts"; having post-secondary schools and professional associations create training programs and curricula that are accessible to rural EMS managers; having universal support and participation in public awareness campaigns; and promoting overall cooperation that would lead to better EMS access and rapid transportation.

Finance

The finance workshop group presented a picture of rural providers battling for revenues against declining economies and a lack of state and federal support.

The four major problems identified by the group were "poor availability of local financing resources, poor local financial management practices, restricted market share for rural agencies, and inequitable Health Care Finance Administration (HCFA) reimbursements for ambulance services."

The financing resource problem was blamed on declining economies in many rural areas, the high tax burden on rural property owners, and a lack of discretionary income available in the rural population to support charitable contributions.

Group members recommended a revision of the HCFA formula for determining Medicare reimbursements for ambulance services under Part B, saying, "The current formulae, based on prevailing local rates, do not accurately reflect the true costs of providing service, yet, in many rural areas with an aging population, these reimbursements reflect a large percentage of the agency's revenue." Correcting the problem, according to the group, is the responsibility of the federal government.

Responsibility for solving other funding problems was placed, for the most part, on EMS officials at the local level. The report stated, "We feel that rural administrators must take a lead in billing for, and collecting, EMS service fees that are based on the cost of providing the service." Subscription plans were also presented as a solution. In addition, the finance group urged that rural EMS administrators "take an active role in seeking out and applying for grant funds, and for charitable contributions to their local service agencies."

Other solutions presented by the group included forming special ambulance taxation districts in some areas and broadening the range of billable services, such as providing physical examination services to health insurance companies and performing some home healthcare services.

The group felt that direct funding and financial incentives could, in effect, be used to make local rural services more self-reliant. The report stated, "Our recommendations . . . are to reinforce the concept of using grant monies for building stronger statewide infrastructures for EMS systems and networks, and providing grant money to local agencies and for the development of special projects that can be reasonably expected to be self-sustaining with little or no additional federal or state funding."

Such funds could, according to the group, be well spent educating rural administrators. "Poor management practices in rural EMS agencies are often the result of ignorance on the part of rural EMS administrators and managers," the report stated. "Many management-level people in the rural areas are volunteers or poorly paid part-time employees with little or no management education or experience."

Research and information systems were seen by the finance group as possible solutions to management problems. The group recommended that research be undertaken to identify effective rural financing practices and that a clearinghouse be established for compiling and disseminating such information to rural EMS administrators and managers.

The federal and state roles in solving management problems, the group felt, should come in the forms of financial, technical, and consultative assistance for management-level educational and training programs.

Again, research was cited as a partial solution to the problem of a small market share caused by service areas that have a small population base. The report stated, "We felt additional research was needed to determine the relationship of market share to the marketability of rural EMS agencies, to determine the impact of larger systems in the local delivery of prehospital care, and to determine what relationship hospital closures have on the market share of rural EMS agencies."

Mergers and acquisitions to form larger services were recommended as solutions to the market share problem. The group also recommended that services realize some of the benefits of a larger market share by consolidating such things as equipment and supply inventories, personnel, education and training programs, and maintenance and repair facilities.

The group was not optimistic about the prospect of federal funding for rural EMS agencies. "Our group noted a serious lack of confidence in the ability of the federal government to provide operating revenues for

Support from employers—allowing employees time for training and response—is considered vital to enlarging the pool.

the direct provision of prehospital care. The removal of federal funding in 1981 is considered by many to be a primary cause of the current financial crisis in rural EMS agencies, and we are hesitant to recommend reliance on the federal government to fund local prehospital care systems."

Personnel

As one might expect, recruitment and retention rated highest on the personnel work group's list of problems in rural EMS. Group members stressed a need for social and psychological research to determine why some communities can retain adequate personnel levels while others have recruitment and retention problems.

The group, through discussion, realized the reasons for poor retention are varied and that a combination of many solutions is needed to address the problem. Among the group's recommendations were that the following be provided:

- Compensation and allowance for training, including supplies
- Readily available recertification training and continuing education and the reduction or elimination of associated fees
- Medical insurance coverage and adequate wage-replacement insurance for on-the-job incidents
- Malpractice/liability insurance
- Retirement benefits for paid and volunteer EMTs
- Psychological support, such as critical incident stress debriefings and for other conditions such as burnout
- Nominal pay for volunteers and increased compensation and benefits for paid EMTs
- Income tax credits for active volunteers
- Public information and education programs to promote the recognition and status of EMTs
- Employer support for employee volunteer efforts
- Assurance on the part of local government of the availability of EMS in the community
- Management and leadership training

Another problem rural areas face that relates directly to the recruitment and retention problems is the deficient pool of available EMS personnel.

Support from employers—allowing employees time for training and response—was considered vital to enlarging the pool. Providing employers with incentives was seen as a solution to the lack of such support. Offering incentives to prospective EMS personnel was also listed as an effective solution for increasing the workforce.

Other solutions to this problem included consolidation of small services; developing tiered response systems to increase the availability of advanced services; opening systems to equal opportunity utilization of the available pool; developing auxiliary components to help provide nonresponse services to the organization; expanding public relations efforts; and increasing exposure of EMS systems to high school students.

The group gave equal weight to the importance of occupational health and felt that educational programs, proper equipment, and health examination and maintenance were vital in rural EMS.

Some recommendations of the group included provisions for health and stress education programs; improved equipment and techniques for their use; regular medical exams, immunizations, and health maintenance programs; critical incident stress debriefings; driver training; and exposure reporting and follow-up.

Lack of adequate risk management was also seen as a shortcoming of rural EMS as a whole. "It is suggested that line-of-duty insurance programs—including medical, workers' compensation, liability, employment disability, legal defense funding, death benefits, and professional malpractice—would serve to reduce the perceived problem. It is further suggested that establishing liability limits would tend to reduce expenses for rural services."

Finally, ineffective interrelationships were seen as a serious problem in rural EMS. The report stated, "To increase the effectiveness of rural EMS systems, we must foster positive, mutually supportive interrelationships among the various agencies and personnel who make up the system." Those agencies and personnel include dispatch, law enforcement, fire service, hospital/medical care facilities, medical personnel, and local governments.

"In many areas, these interrelationships are strained and do not promote effective operation," the report continued. "In fact, in some areas negative interrelationships discourage recruitment and retention of EMS personnel."

Solutions to the problem, for which state and local levels are responsible, include

- Establishing programs to ensure coordination of all EMS services
- Improving management through training and technical assistance
- Establishing that local governments are responsible for interagency coordination
- Defusing interagency conflicts
- Working to eliminate competition between the various levels of EMS care
- Increasing positive recognition and support provided to local EMS units by hospitals and physicians providing joint training programs for all emergency service providers
- Encouraging medical community involvement with other public safety agencies when medical issues are involved

The group also recommended that the federal, state, and local levels be responsible for the encouragement and support of joint disaster planning programs.

Source

Reprinted with permission from JEMS, June 1989. Lee Reeder is the special projects coordinator for Jems Communications. He has planned the educational programs for four Emergency Vehicle and Fleet Management Conferences and has published fleet management articles in JEMS and Ambulance World, an Australian EMS publication.

The responsibility for most of the personnel group's solutions was placed on the state and local levels. The federal government's responsibility, according to the group, is primarily one of support for volunteer efforts, public relations activities, tax credits, and other incentives.

Conclusion

The San Diego workshop served to identify many of the problems that confront rural EMS and to offer solutions. The predominant question many have—according to frustrations expressed by rural EMS personnel in a recent *JEMS* survey—is whether serious consideration is being given to these problems on a national level.

Some of those who attended the San Diego workshop expressed reserved optimism. Michael French, state EMS director for Wisconsin, citing recent work by the Office of Technology Assessment and interest in Congress, said, "There hasn't been a time I can recall when there has been so much interest in the problems of rural EMS, so I have to think that something will come out of this."

Marvin Hayes, a regional EMS coordinator in Oklahoma, attended the workshop and said the effectiveness of the information will depend largely on the initiative of individuals. He said the information should be used by state, regional, and local EMS personnel to make representatives at all levels of government aware of the problems of rural EMS and of the need for legislation.

Integrating Medical Helicopters Into EMS

Christine M. Zalar, RN, MA

Air medical programs have played an integral role in the development of EMS systems but are often taken for granted. This article stresses the significant contribution made by the air component, and how using these programs wisely can enhance patient care in the future.

THE DEVELOPING ROLE OF AIR MEDICAL transportation services has been to support EMS system expansion into a larger geographic region. Since the inception of the first hospital-based flight program at St. Anthony Hospital in Denver in 1972, air medical transport has gradually found a contributing role within the horizontally integrating EMS system that has since evolved. Medical helicopters and airplanes are being used as a complementary adjunct to the ground ambulance services that are the core of EMS system response. Further, air medical transport has brought the critical care and emergency experiences and skills of nurses and physicians to scene and interfacility transports.

The process of integrating air medical services into the ground system has not been without conflict, turmoil, and competition. The maturation of both industries—and external pressures such as healthcare reform—has created an environment for survival, resulting in consolidation within each of the separate industries, as well as a need for intensified collaboration between the two industries. The resulting movement toward horizontal integration has become a synergistic alignment of the complementary services that the ground and air providers offer. In medical transportation services, the fully integrated system will focus on developing relationships that match the most efficient emergency, non-emergency, and critical care ground providers with efficient medical helicopter and medical airplane services. Each of these industry "service segments" overlap to a small degree, with each contributing to the overall EMS delivery system in its own unique manner. This article is an analysis of the role and contributions of the medical helicopter.

Effective Utilization of Medical Helicopter Resources

In 1990, the Association of Air Medical Services (AAMS) published a position paper on the appropriate use of emergency air medical services. The general criteria outlined by AAMS for dispatching emergency air medical units addressed both patient transports from hospital facilities and scene responses. Generally, the AAMS criteria include the following:

- The patient requires critical care life support at a clinical level that is unavailable from local ground ambulances.
- The patient's clinical condition dictates minimal out-of-hospital transport times.
- The potential exists for delays via ground transport, which may include route obstacles and traffic that may worsen the patient's clinical status.

- The patient cannot be accessed by ground units.
- The patient's medical needs require specific treatment not available at the local referring facility, and/or the patient has been receiving specialized care from a non-local hospital.
- Transport of the patient by ground would deplete the local community of its EMS coverage.

The AAMS position paper further details specific medical and surgical conditions that are appropriate for air medical transport.

The overlap of the capabilities of ground ambulances, mobile intensive care units, and air medical resources was further addressed by Boyko in the development of the Patient Transfer Pyramid. The Pyramid addresses three tiers of clinical services—basic life support, advanced life support, and critical care—and their corresponding modes of transport. By assessing the patient's medical condition, a proper match can be made for the appropriate clinical capabilities and transport vehicle that most effectively meet the patient's need.

The AAMS position paper and the Transfer Pyramid are broad guidelines that EMS systems can apply to their local and regional transport protocol and destination policies.

Helicopters Enhance Patient Access to Tertiary Services

Turmoil in the healthcare system of the United States has centered on providing universal access, which means that healthcare services are provided to everyone, regardless of financial or health reasons. There is a whole other side to the access issue that medical transportation services are well positioned to address—the area where "access" encompasses how patients are transported to the healthcare services that they need. Specifically, this area is the transport of emergent, critically ill, or injured individuals to the appropriate facilities that have the services needed for their medical condition. Air medical transport coupled with an effective ground transport system significantly improve patient access to healthcare services.

Patients in rural areas have limited access to specialized healthcare services, resulting in documented increases in patient morbidity and mortality. Obstacles such as time and geographic terrain can be minimized with appropriate use of a medical helicopter. In the regionalization process, the geographic location of healthcare services is less important than the presence of rapid, efficient transport and clinical care capabilities. Expensive, but medically necessary, tertiary services can be centralized when medical helicopters are able to provide the "access" within a 100- to 150-mile radius of rural constituents. In essence, the medical helicopter expands the scope of service that local EMS providers can offer their patients.

Many rural community hospitals cannot maintain specialized services and facilities for more critically ill and injured patients. Centralization of special and tertiary healthcare services is inevitable. Physician specialists, expensive technology, and related support services can be centrally located within a 100-mile radius. Patients requiring these services can be effectively transported by air medical transportation.

Medical helicopters provide critical means of access to the closest open facilities. Data from the American Hospital Association reflect that 84 hospitals permanently closed their emergency departments in 1991. In 1992, 39 community hospitals closed, down slightly from the 45 community hospitals that closed in 1991. However, the trend that has reduced the number of local healthcare facilities continues. During a 10-year period (1982 to 1992), a total of 509 community hospitals closed. In that same 10-year period, the total number of community hospitals fell 8.8 percent, the number of urban hospitals declined by 1.1 percent, and the number of rural hospitals fell 17.2 percent. However, the number of emergency department visits increased by 2.5 percent, totaling over 2.3 million additional patients.

Centralized tertiary and specialty services create economies of scale, with effective access provided by medical helicopters. These helicopters are able to transport clinical services and equipment to the patient in order to initiate sophisticated clinical care prior to the patient arriving at the destination hospital. In this manner, patients directly benefit from the advanced clinical capabilities and equipment brought to a hospital or an accident scene as part of the medical helicopter response.

The effective transport time to definitive care is drastically reduced through the use of air medical transport. The "golden hour" for trauma and cardiac patients, both of which are time-sensitive medical conditions, has been significantly enhanced through air medical transport. Through medical helicopters, the clinical capabilities of rural and community hospital personnel is often complemented, and at times exceeded. In some rural areas of the United States, medical helicopters are often the only available advanced clinical care response.

Research by Smith, et al., defined formulas for evaluating air versus ground transport times. The mathematical formulas in the research were designed to provide triage criteria for appropriate utilization of air medical services. The formulas lead to appropriate utilization of helicopter transport based on distance, extrication time, and rendezvous with predetermined landing zones. The basis of the research was that time is a critical factor for the transport of patients by helicopter. Findings concluded that ground transportation can effectively be used within a 66-kilometer distance as long as the patient is not entrapped, there are no obstacles such as road blocks or tortuous routes, and the patient's medical needs do not exceed the clinical capabilities of the ground transportation system.

The operational range of a helicopter or fixed-wing air ambulance is greater than that of ground ambulances, resulting in greater efficiency of operation. Ground ambulances operate effectively for emergency response within confined geographic areas. In addition, ground ambulances can effectively provide interfacility transports within a 30- to 50-mile ra-

Medical helicopters provide critical means of access to the closest open facilities.

The expertise of the medical flight crew enhances the care provided by rural and community hospitals and ambulance services.

dius. However, ground ambulances are traditionally staffed with two paramedics as a maximum level of care. In some instances, ground critical care units may include specialty teams such as neonate or pediatric transport specialists (RNs, respiratory therapists), or a critical care nurse.

Helicopters effectively serve up to 150 miles and are staffed with a registered nurse and paramedic team or a physician and nurse team. The experience level generally required for flight nurses is a minimum of three years of critical care or emergency nursing. For paramedics, the required experience level is traditionally at least three years of advanced life support in emergency rescue experience. The physician medical crew member may be a senior resident in emergency medicine or a staff emergency medicine physician. The result is that air medical transport provides rapid access to medical care and a higher level of patient care en route, with a decreased transport time to the receiving facility.

Lutz reported in *Modern Healthcare* that sparsely populated areas have long been underserved by even basic-level emergency ambulance support. In these areas, the adjunctive role of the medical helicopter may actually represent the primary transport means for patients to access advanced life support care in the out-of-hospital environment.

The expertise of the medical flight crew enhances the care provided by rural and community hospitals and ambulance services. This is a result of the level of experience of the medical flight crew and the number of experiences resulting in higher clinical proficiencies with the types of patients that a rural community hospital may see only a few times in a given year.

Research Supports Appropriate Use of Medical Helicopters

In those instances in which medical crew capabilities were comparable to those of ground ambulance personnel, and therefore time was the key factor, research conducted by Reddick reported that 33 percent of the patients were found to benefit from rapid air medical transport. In the sparsely populated areas of rural communities—where time is of the essence—the length and duration of EMS transports give a significant advantage to air- versus ground-transported patients. Rural EMS ground ambulance systems have undergone significant deterioration due to a lack of funding, a decrease in the number of volunteers able to provide service to the community-based ambulance, the loss of skill proficiency due to the low number of patient encounters, and an increasing difficulty to maintain certification due to requirements for continuing education.

Research conducted by Boyd indicated that patients transported by ground had the same mortality as was predicted by trauma scoring methodologies. However, patients transported by medical helicopter had a 25-percent reduction in predicted mortality. Further, Boyd's research indicated that the reduction in mortality for the airborne patients demonstrated the most impact with the subsection of patients who had a probability of dying of greater than 10 percent.

Moylan compared survival rates of patients with multi-system injuries. The research indicated that overall survival was 89 percent for helicopter patients, compared with 61 percent for ground ambulance patients. The significant survival advantages were attributed to the more aggressive therapeutic interventions that were performed during air transport compared with those of ground transport.

Further research by Baxt and Moody compared trauma patients transported by standard ground prehospital ambulance and those transported by medical helicopter staffed by a physician and a nurse. The study demonstrated a significant reduction—52 percent—in predicted mortality for the group transported by medical helicopter. This study was repeated by numerous others, and other trauma centers in different geographic locations conducted similar comparisons with the same results.

More recently, American Hospital Association statistics indicated that, in 1991, the average length of stay by a patient who had been brought to that hospital's intensive care unit by air was reduced by more than 50 percent compared with traditional ground services. Further, the actual costs incurred by such airborne patients were similarly reduced by more than 50 percent. In 1991, research reported in the *New England Journal of Medicine* (November 1991) illustrated that the rate of mortality decreased by 48 percent for those patients transported by helicopter intensive care units versus conventional ground vehicles. Research justifying the use of medical helicopters was conducted by the state of Connecticut in 1989. It concluded that over a three-year period, during which 1,798 patients were transported by critical care helicopter, only five percent of the flights were judged to be unjustified.

Conclusion

Research conducted by Bruhn, et al., comparing the true costs of air medical versus ground ambulance systems, found that helicopter emergency transport services are not costly when compared to similar services by ground. In the research model, staffing, response times, cost comparisons, and benefits of air versus ground were examined. The research, however, did not yield a result that air should replace ground. It further supported the need for integrating both air and ground service and coverage to optimize the limitations and expenses of each transport segment.

Access to care must also include the means by which patients who are not proximal to primary, tertiary, or specialty services are able to be transported and cared for en route should the need arise. Providing optimal levels of clinical and transportation services should be the goal of an integrated EMS system. Achievement of this goal, and providing patients the access to healthcare services, mandates continuous collaboration between ground and air providers.

> Patients transported by medical helicopter had a 25-percent reduction in predicted mortality.

Source

Original article. Christine Zalar is a partner at Fitch & Associates, Inc. She is widely recognized as one of the nation's leading experts on air medical and hospital-based EMS/medical transportation systems. She is also a principal author of the book EMS Management: Beyond the Street*, 2nd ed.*

References

AHA Hospital Statistics, 93/94. Chicago: The American Hospital Association, 1993.

Association of Air Medical Services. "Position Paper on the Appropriate use of Emergency Air Medical Services." *Journal of Air Medical Transport* 9, no. 9 (1990): 29-33.

Baxt, W. G., and P. Moody. "The Impact of a Rotor Craft Aeromedical Emergency Care Service on Trauma Mortality." *Journal of the American Medical Association* 249 (1983): 3047-3061.

Boyd, C. R., K. M. Corse, and R. C. Campell. "Interhospital Transport: Air vs. Ground." Presented at the second annual Eastern Association for the Surgery of Trauma Scientific Meeting, Longboat Key, Fla., January 1989.

Boyko, S. M. "The Transfer Pyramid: An Educational and Marketing Tool." *Journal of Air Medical Transport* 9, no. 11, 12 (1992): 9, 11.

Critical Care System of Connecticut: Three-Year Report, 1985-1988. Hartford, Conn.: Department of EMS/Trauma, Hartford Hospital.

Lutz, S. "Hospitals Move to Hub of Rural Emergency Care." *Modern Healthcare* 23, no. 16 (1993): 31-42.

Moylan, J. A., K. T. Fitzpatrick, A. J. Beyer, et al. "Factors Improving Survival in Multi-System Trauma Patients." *Annals of Surgery,* 207 (1988): 679-685.

Reddick, E. J. "Evaluation of the Helicopter in Aeromedical Transfers." *Aviations Space Environment Medicine* 50 (1979): 168-170.

Smith, J. S., B. J. Smith, S. E. Pletcher, et al. "When Is Air Medical Service Faster Than Ground Transportation?" *Air Medical Journal* 12, no. 8 (1993): 258-261.

A Community-Based Ambulance Model

Dale J. Berry

Hospitals and hospital-affiliated services provide EMS in a large number of small to medium communities throughout America. Many of these services have changed from hospital-based to community-based services. This article describes that evolutionary process in one midwestern community.

THE CRISIS THAT OCCURRED in Washtenaw County in 1981 was not unique. The county, with 268,000 residents, would be without ambulance service within 48 hours, and officials were trying to figure out a solution to the problem. How did things get so bad?

Washtenaw County is located 30 miles west of Detroit in southeastern Michigan. After the funeral homes left the ambulance business in the late 1960s, the county depended on private ambulance service to provide emergency medical care and transport.

Ambulance services bid and received two- to three-year contracts to serve the community—including the urban areas of Ann Arbor and Ypsilanti, and the vast rural area containing many small cities and towns. Eighty percent of the county's 720 square miles was rural, which was the primary reason why the county wanted to bid out ambulance service. Providing ambulance service to the 214,000 residents of the urban area was easy. Serving the remaining population in the rural areas was the challenge.

During the 1970s, a number of small private ambulance providers were under county contract, one after another after another. A cycle occurred that is still very familiar to some EMS markets. The successful ambulance company would gain the county contract and concentrate on providing emergency ambulance service. When emergencies overloaded the contractor, non-emergency transports waited. Often, the provider wouldn't take the non-emergency customers seriously.

A second ambulance company—sometimes the loser in the bid process—would concentrate on the non-emergency customers. This "cream skimming" would reduce the revenue to the first provider in a market too small to support more than one service at the quality levels the community expected.

In the summer of 1981, the cycle began to change again—but it happened much more quickly than ever before. In the midst of a five-year agreement, the primary provider appeared before the county board of commissioners and explained that an additional $180,000 cash infusion was needed immediately, or it would be forced to close its doors within 48 hours. The commissioners, who were dissatisfied with the level of ambulance service they were receiving, refused to pay, forcing the crisis reported on the front page of the local newspaper the next day.

County emergency management leaders scrambled to make backup arrangements, in case the provider followed through with its threat to close. Unfortunately, the other local "cream skimming" provider was too small to offer adequate countywide coverage. Services in adjacent counties could provide only limited assistance.

The county did not want to enter the ambulance business itself. Although it had always wanted excellent ambulance service, it felt that private organizations could do a higher-quality job at lower costs. It was about this time that the area hospitals stepped in.

Washtenaw County has five general hospitals. St. Joseph Mercy Hospital, the second largest with 558 beds, stepped in first. St. Joe's approached Washtenaw County and offered to enter into negotiations to purchase the primary ambulance company.

The University of Michigan Medical Center, the largest area hospital with over 900 beds, immediately became concerned, fearing that its market share would quickly erode. It began exploring the start-up of a competing ambulance company.

In the next 48 hours, discussions at the highest levels of all five hospitals set a course of action that was designed to stabilize the crisis and provide a long-term solution. A four-phase plan was devised.

The hospital chief executive officers agreed that they would form only one ambulance service, and that hospital ownership would not be a permanent solution. They reasoned that even one high-quality ambulance service probably could not survive on its own. The burden of subsidizing operations would fall on the hospitals if they remained the owners.

However, the hospital CEOs did agree that hospital ownership, for a period of time, was necessary. In 1981, only the hospitals had the financial resources, the expertise, and the interest to fix the situation.

Phase One—Financial Management

Phase One began in August 1981 and included getting the existing ambulance service and the community through the crisis period. Not all of the hospitals could react quickly. Formal involvement by the University of Michigan Hospital required action by the board of regents, a process which could take six months or more.

A third hospital, Beyer Memorial, was owned by the People's Community Hospital Authority. With only 48 hours to consider the situation, the hospital was not even sure that its enabling legislation would allow it to contribute funding jointly with other hospitals for this purpose.

The remaining two hospitals, Saline Community Hospital and Chelsea Community Hospital were eager to assist. Both with less than 100 beds, they were located in the rural areas of the county, which would be affected most by the lack of a countywide ambulance provider. All five hospital CEOs agreed that St. Joseph Mercy Hospital would act as the lead hospital in the initial stages of the venture because of its size and corporate structure.

St. Joe's immediately entered into an option agreement to purchase the primary ambulance company, pending successful resolution of the company's liabilities. The hospital arranged for emergency financing through a local bank, in exchange for financial control of the company. An option was also negotiated to purchase the assets of the second, "cream skimming" ambulance company.

During the five-month financial management period, outstanding debt with banks and suppliers was successfully negotiated and reduced. New equipment was ordered, and employees were laid off. Most were rehired after being scrutinized through a new hiring process. A $2 million credit line was authorized by the St. Joseph Mercy Hospital board of trustees, following consultation with the other four hospitals.

Phase Two—Single Hospital Ownership

On December 15, 1981, Phase Two began as the hospital exercised its options and purchased the primary ambulance company, as well as the assets of the second company. Huron Valley Ambulance, Inc., (HVA) was formed—named after a prominent river valley that runs through the community.

Phase Two included several important tasks. The first involved completing negotiations with the federal government regarding the IRS debt and putting new equipment on line.

The company also began offering paramedic advanced life support service. This upgrade in quality had been on the drawing board for at least four years but was never implemented by the former companies due to financial limitations.

The company was converted to a nonprofit corporation, and an IRS 401 (c) (3) tax exemption was obtained. The company also began consolidating operations and cutting costs.

A new county contract was negotiated. A premise to this contract was the trust that the county placed in the hospitals. In prior ambulance contracts, the county had defined a number of operational configurations that had become outdated. As one example, the old contract specified station placement when a system status management deployment plan was badly needed.

The county believed that the hospitals would operate the ambulance service in the best interest of the community, particularly after the planned conversion to a community-based structure. As a result, most performance benchmarks were left up to the hospitals and the ambulance service itself.

An Ambulance Service Advisory Council was also created by the five hospitals to monitor the operational performance of the company. The council concentrated on monitoring patient flow to ensure that hospital market shares remained steady. Three years of transport data were obtained from the former ambulance companies and compared to the patterns of the new ambulance entity. No changes in patient flow were found with the new company now under single hospital ownership.

Phase Three—Joint Hospital Ownership

Phase Three began in July 1983, when all five hospitals bought into the ownership of HVA. A percentage formula was used that generally equated to the ambulance transport market share of their emergency departments. St. Joe's and the University of Michigan Medical Center each owned 37.5 percent of the company, Beyer Hospital owned 15 percent, and Saline and Chelsea Hospitals each owned five percent. The $2 million dollar credit line was continued and shared by the five owners.

During joint hospital ownership, the company continued to make improvements. The HVA board of trustees was made up of the five hospital CEOs, who attended monthly meetings faithfully with great interest. On April 30, 1984, a day etched in everyone's memories, the ambulance service became profitable.

As the hospital CEOs began the transition to community ownership, they started recruiting new members for the board of trustees. This was an extremely difficult task, given the history of previous ambulance companies, the negative publicity, and the unlikely plan that the company could remain self-sufficient. Recruitment was also more difficult because the hospital CEOs realized that the company could only survive if the best and brightest community leaders were selected.

Four outside trustees were initially recruited, including an emergency physician, a marketing executive and former chamber of commerce president, a construction company owner, and a prominent volunteer community leader. A banker and an attorney were added shortly thereafter.

By December 1984, the company was regularly operating in the black and improving quality. As the hospitals prepared for final transition to community ownership, they pondered what to do about the debt. The ambulance company had drawn down $1.6 million of the $2 million hospital credit line to subsidize early operations.

The hospitals never expected the ambulance company to repay the debt. In fact, the debt was structured in a way that would trigger principal payments only if certain healthy financial performance was achieved. The debt was also provided interest free.

The hospitals were now receiving other requests to collaborate on projects that were of interest to the community. Although they were not opposed to helping some of these groups, they were concerned about the precedent they might set if HVA didn't repay the debt. They also felt that burdening the ambulance company with significant debt in the community ownership phase would hamstring the company and make future financing much more difficult.

To resolve this problem, the hospital CEOs decided to "pay back" the hospitals prior to converting to community ownership. Because the debt was interest free, the board voted to draw down an additional $200,000 from the hospital line of credit. With these funds, the ambulance company purchased zero coupon bonds payable with interest to the hospitals in the amount of $2 million dollars in 1995. These were then accepted by the hospitals as payment in full and the debt was erased.

The hospital CEOs also drew down the remaining $200,000, which they gave to the company to use as a "rainy day" fund. This money, which has been invested, remains in the company nine years later.

Phase Four—Community Ownership

On January 1, 1985, the company became "community owned." Technically, HVA is a private, nonprofit corporation, and there are no owners as such. The company operates in the public interest. Should the company ever be dissolved, IRS regulations require that the assets be distributed only to other tax-exempt, nonprofit organizations or to the government.

HVA is governed by a volunteer board of trustees made up of nine community leaders. A trustee can serve two three-year terms and then must step down for a minimum of one year. The present board is designed so that three trustees "turn over" each year. The remaining six trustees vote to fill the vacant positions. The executive director of HVA, who is also the president and CEO of the company, serves on the board as well.

There are no formal eligibility criteria for becoming a trustee. The board is concerned about changing political interests and generally prefers not to have trustees who are officials of county or local government. They feel that it is important that HVA be shielded from any change in the political climate. The board also makes every attempt to attract top community leaders with a variety of expertise and interest. The board meets approximately eight times per year. It has one standing committee that advises management on investment strategy. Other special committees are periodically created for special purposes, such as nominations or board composition.

12 Years After Start-Up

Today, Huron Valley Ambulance is very successful—well beyond the original expectations of the five hospitals and the county. The primary 9-1-1 service area has grown to 1,000 square miles and 400,000 residents, in all or part of six counties.

The service has grown from 12,000 annual transports in 1982 to 30,000 transports in 1992. The annual operating budget is in excess of $7 million. A four-percent operating profit is budgeted each year, and this goal has been met or exceeded every year since 1985. Although the service is nonprofit, this surplus is necessary to keep up with growth and technology. It is far less than what would be considered a reasonable return on investment in the for-profit sector.

All operating surpluses in excess of five percent are shared with HVA employees through a performance-based compensation program. The program, which is based on team performance, depends on the entire organization achieving five predetermined quality indicators.

HVA has also grown from a fleet of nine original ambulances to 28 units. Ninety-two percent of all deployed unit hours are ALS, and only paramedic units are used in the system status plan. HVA operates two neonatal intensive care units and one adult mobile intensive care unit. System status management and priority call handling/medical self-help have been used since 1982.

In 1993, HVA became one of only 20 ambulance services in the country to be accredited by the national Commission on Accreditation of Ambulance Services.

The communications center is fully computerized with AVL. HVA also was the first private ambulance service in Michigan to utilize ANI/ALI direct transfer of 9-1-1 emergency calls to paramedic dispatchers. In addition, eight local fire departments are dispatched from the dispatch center.

HVA also operates one of Michigan's largest EMS education programs, employing five full-time instructor-coordinators who teach external programs.

What Makes this Model Successful

A number of significant events in the history of HVA have made the company one of the most successful ambulance services in the country using the community-ownership model.

First, without a doubt, was the vision and cooperation of all community hospitals. In most communities, this would have never occurred because hospitals often look out for themselves instead of collaborating to do what is right. In Washtenaw County, the hospitals put aside their competitive interests to form HVA, rather than form expensive, individual, competing ambulance services.

These hospitals also realized that the company would be more successful under a community-based model. Even though many hospitals are struggling today, the public has a perception that there is unlimited financial depth for projects like this. Changing to community ownership has fostered a greater sense of "pride of ownership" in the community.

As one example of this support, $400,000 was raised in contributions from the community in 1987 to build a new headquarters building in what was one of the largest ambulance fundraising projects in the history of the country. This included over $100,000 in donations from community physicians.

A second significant historical event was when the hospitals freed HVA from debt before putting community ownership in place. This, combined with a credit line from a consortium of community banks, made HVA a financially strong organization from the beginning.

The third significant point is the quality of community leadership. When new community leaders are asked to serve as trustees, the sights are set very high. Each community leader who has volunteered to govern HVA has a unique perspective and provides expert guidance. The leaders also have the foresight to limit themselves to policy decisions and let company managers implement those policy decisions without unreasonable scrutiny.

The fourth strength of the organization is its focus on entrepreneurial leadership. Operating HVA in an entrepreneurial way is paramount to every HVA manager.

Finally, the focus is on quality. Everything HVA does, from top to bottom, revolves around continuous quality improvement. "If it ain't broke," HVA looks for ways to make it even better.

The community ownership ambulance model works. Typically, this model is common in small towns using volunteer staffing. But it can also be successful on a larger scale. Huron Valley Ambulance is an excellent example of the community-owned model in a service area of 400,000 people.

Source

Original article. Dale J. Berry is the executive director of the Huron Valley Ambulance, Inc., community-based ambulance service in southwestern Michigan.

EMS Visions of the Future

Public Sector EMS

James O. Page

Veteran Fire Chief and JEMS Publisher Jim Page analyzes the trends in EMS delivery and outlines his perspective on the challenges and possibilities for public sector services in the years ahead.

THE MAYOR OF AN IMPORTANT California city was faced with a political, practical, and philosophical problem. His fire chief had recommended that the city fire department take over emergency ambulance transportation from a private ambulance company. The city manager endorsed the plan and the city attorney declared it legal. But the local newspaper and the chamber of commerce opposed the move. Two members of the city council were outspoken in their opposition to it, and the mayor knew that the private ambulance company probably had contributed to the campaigns of one or more council members.

Adding to the weight of the issue was the mayor's experience in both government and business. He knew that, except in some special situations, government is not as nimble, efficient, or economical as small business. He also knew that the trend in local government was to downsize, not to add employees, as the fire chief had proposed. At the end of a long city council meeting, where the full spectrum of opinions was put forth, it was the mayor's task to bring the matter to some resolution. He looked uncomfortable.

Finally, after summarizing the various and divergent opinions that had been offered, and after hearing each of the council members give an obligatory speech on the matter, the mayor revealed how he would vote. He started by saying that he believed there were many traditional government functions that could be performed more efficiently and economically by private enterprise. But, he said, there are some unique functions of government that are extremely time sensitive and have life-or-death consequences for people.

As an example, the mayor pointed to national defense. There is no doubt that the private sector could manage the functions of the U.S. Department of Defense with greater efficiency and economy. However, the mayor commented that he did not want to see the commander in chief in the position of having to call a low-bid defense contractor to protect our nation against attack by a foreign power. National defense is very time sensitive, and it can have life-or-death consequences, he pointed out.

Next, the mayor turned to police and fire protection. He advised that if he were to awaken to the sounds of a burglar forcing entry into his house, he wanted to be able to dial 9-1-1 with the knowledge that his call would cause a prompt response by well-trained career law enforcement officers who were directly accountable to and through public officials in a chain of command that included the city council. As with fire protection, he pointed out, police protection is time sensitive and can have life-or-death consequences.

Finally, he arrived at the point of his speech. Ambulance services are also time sensitive and can have life-or-death consequences for people. The mayor may have been jaded by many years of mediocre ambulance service in his community, underscored by the failure of county government to cure the problems. However, he was sincere and persuasive in advocating that ambulance service be viewed in the same light as national defense and public safety. When he called for a vote, a majority of the members of his city council opted in favor of a fire department ambulance service.

That anecdote more or less frames the issue of public sector ambulance service, although the larger topic of public sector provision of or participation in EMS services tends to be less of an either-or proposition. Whether it's the smaller or larger version of the issue, however, there are few topics that arouse such intense interest, feelings, and debate at the local government level.

Popular Methods of EMS Delivery

There has never been a complete national census of EMS in the United States. Therefore, it is impossible to precisely measure many factors, including the ratio of public and private sector participation in delivery of prehospital emergency medical services in every community and county throughout the nation.

Since the early 1980s, the only reliable source of this type of information has been the annual survey conducted by *JEMS (Journal of Emergency Medical Services)*. That survey and report covers the 200 most populous cities in the United States, from New York City to Brownsville, Tex. (pop. 98,962). The 200-City Survey is commonly relied on as an indicator of trends in EMS.

The 1994 version of the 200-City Survey revealed that private ambulance services were considered primary providers of prehospital EMS in 48 cities (24 percent), while various cooperative arrangements between fire departments and private ambulance companies were used in 32 additional cities (16 percent).

The 1994 survey revealed that in 70 (35 percent) of the 200 most populous cities, fire departments were considered the primary provider of prehospital EMS. Another 32 (16 percent) cities used third-service public agencies as their primary providers. An additional 14 (seven percent) of the 200 cities used hospital ambulance systems as their primary providers, and the four remaining cities used alternative designs, which make up only two percent of the total (Table 5.2).

So, depending on how you view the cooperative arrangements that exist between fire departments and private providers in 32 cities, fire departments and third-service EMS agencies currently are the primary providers in 51 percent to 67 percent of the nation's 200 most populous cities. Unfortunately, due to the absence of reliable data, there is no way of knowing whether these percentages and ratios apply in smaller communities and rural areas of the nation.

Trends and Potential for Growth

As illustrated in Table 5.2, between 1992 and 1993, there was a small percentage increase in the number of fire departments and third-service agencies defined as primary EMS providers, while there was a small decrease in the number of private ambulance companies serving in that role. Is this a trend, or is it a statistical anomaly?

A review of survey results from 1989 through 1993 reveals no net changes greater than two percent over that five-year period, except in the category of alternative delivery methods (from nine cities in 1989 to four cities in 1993). However, a close look at the data reveals some important turbulence within the categories. For example, some private providers were replaced by fire department ambulance services. Some fire department ambulance services were replaced by private companies, and at least one third-service program was converted to a fire department ambulance system. So, the totals fail to reveal shifts in categories on a city-to-city basis.

Also not yet apparent is the ultimate effect of some important national developments. Not necessarily in order of importance, they are the rapid consolidation of the private ambulance industry, the fire services' need for non-tax-based sources of revenue

---

Table 5.2

Comparison of Provider Mix from 1992 to 1993*

Provider Type	1992		1993	
	Percent	Number of Cities	Percent	Number of Cities
Fire Department (CT/DR and SS)	34	68	35	70
Private (Including PUM)	25	50	24	48
Fire Department and Private Provider	17	34	16	32
Third Service (Co, Muni, and PT)	15	30	16	32
Hospital Systems	6.5	13	7	14
Alternative Delivery Method (PD, Nonprofit Pri, and Vol)	2.5	5	2	4

* Data collected in 1992 and 1993 but reported in 1993 and 1994 200-City Survey results.

(and recognition of ambulance transportation as a revenue source), financial shortfalls at all levels of local government, and the anticipated reform of healthcare delivery and finance.

Consolidation of the Private Ambulance Industry

Since August 1992, when a new private ambulance company called American Medical Response (AMR) launched a public offering of its stock on the New York Stock Exchange, AMR and at least four other companies have been raising capital and buying smaller ambulance companies from coast to coast. The effect of this consolidation has been to change the "mom and pop" traditions of private ambulance companies to the realm of big business. Presumably, those in charge of these new or expanded corporations are savvy business people with hefty credit lines, political acumen, and the need to build market share. Presumably, they will do all in their power to prevent public agencies from depleting the market share of their companies. Presumably, they will actively try to convince elected officials to privatize ambulance services in those locales where fire departments or third-service agencies now provide medical transportation.

Fire Service Need for Non-Tax Revenues

Competing with this trend is the recognition by public fire protection agencies that they need increased revenues from non-tax sources. Traditionally, fire departments have been financed by local property tax revenues. However, in the aftermath of California's Proposition 13 property tax roll-back in 1978, many states have enacted laws that have reduced this form of finance for local government operations. During the same period, federal revenue sharing has dried up, creating ever-greater pressure on local governments to provide basic services with less resources.

Although the reduction in frequency and severity of structure fires throughout the United States has been widely reported, the impact of this success on fire service productivity and staffing is not recognized to the same degree. A public fire department is labor intensive and expensive, and all public expenditures must be justified in the current economic environment. However, fire protection is an emotional issue with citizens and their elected leaders, and the size and expense of the fire protection force cannot be reduced in proportion to the reduced frequency and severity of fire incidents.

In many places, the productivity issue has been partially resolved by coincidence, as most public fire departments have increasingly provided first responder services on emergency medical incidents. In fact, in a majority of public fire departments in the United States, first responder services on emergency medical incidents represent two-thirds or more of all emergency activity. This partial solution to one problem, however, compounds another.

In the 200 most populous U.S. cities, for example, more than 90 percent of fire departments are responding to all or most reported out-of-hospital medical emergencies as first responders, thus expending personnel and physical resources, and—in most cases—receiving no compensation for those services. The commitment of personnel to this activity, plus wear and operational costs for fire apparatus, represents a large expenditure of public funds.

Aside from the benefits of having trained first-aid or emergency care personnel arrive on scene within four to five minutes (in most cases), there is other value in fire department first responder services, which generally is not compensated or accounted for. For example, the prompt arrival of first responder fire companies allows ambulance service providers (public or private) to operate with longer response times (e.g., eight minutes or less in 90 percent of all responses). When the first responder units are able to provide advanced life support (ALS), they "stop the clock" for the ambulance service—meaning that the physiological deterioration of the patient or victim can be stopped or reversed even though the ambulance may be three or more minutes distant.

Other value is to be found in the labor expended by fire company personnel, such as lifting or moving the patient to a location where emergency care can be administered. Even after the ambulance has arrived on scene, fetching equipment and the gurney from the ambulance often is a task handled by fire company first responders, in addition to assisting in emergency care procedures. Carrying the patient to the ambulance, loading gurney and patient into the ambulance, and retrieving equipment, supplies, and debris often is another task performed by firefighters. In some cases, where both members of the ambulance crew are required in the patient compartment, a firefighter may drive the ambulance to the hospital.

As mentioned, although these services represent value and cost to public fire protection agencies, there has been no compensation for them in most systems. Generally, the reimbursement policies of third-party sources limit payment to the agency or organization that provides medical transportation. In the severe cost-recovery environment of local government, it is not surprising that fire departments have begun to look with interest at medical transportation as an extension of their first responder services, and as a potential revenue stream.

Local Government Financial Shortfalls

Financial shortfalls at the local government level not only have fed the increased interest in fire department emergency ambulance services, but they have caused serious budget problems for most of the so-called "third-service" ambulance organizations and "separate service" fire department ambulance organizations (Box 5.2).

In these provider types, EMS personnel usually are "single role" (as opposed to "dual role, cross trained"), meaning that all labor costs and all or most administrative costs must be borne by the EMS function. In systems using dual-role personnel, labor costs and administrative overhead are generally shared with the fire protection function, resulting in significant economies. The net effect is that third-service and separate service EMS operations tend to be the most expensive provider types on a per-capita or per-patient basis.

These provider types usually were designed on the rationale that EMS is a specialty, requiring the complete dedication and attention of personnel. However, experience in many systems has demonstrated that the rigors of the job—without diversion or transfer to other less stressful and demanding roles—causes a high degree of attrition and job-connected disability. These human factors, plus relative costs of operation, place these provider types at some degree of risk in the current economic environment.

Healthcare Reform

The national dialogue over healthcare reform began to produce revolutionary change in the healthcare industry long before a plan was put forth by the Clinton Administration in 1993. Apparently convinced that change was inevitable, hospitals in many areas began to merge into networks and negotiated with insurers and employers to secure group healthcare arrangements. Insurers and employers began to negotiate with physician groups to serve as "preferred providers." After more than two decades of struggling for acceptance, the concept of the health maintenance organization (HMO) came into its own.

These changes, most of which occurred before Congress even began to debate the Clinton plan, effectively made the independent hospital and the private practice physician almost obsolete. Eventually, once the structural rearrangement of hospital organizations and physician practice is nearly universal, peripheral services, such as ambulance service, will be forced to accommodate the new order.

Among the new realities of this managed healthcare concept is the insignificance of city, town, or county boundaries. Previously, ambulance service providers could operate within a defined geographic area and transport emergency patients to the nearest appropriate facility. In some cases, secondary transport of the patient to a more distant facility has been necessary. However, the economic incentives of the new order will compel providers to transport to facilities that are contracted with the patient's insurer when it's safe to do so. That may require an ambulance to travel many miles from its assigned service area.

Anticipated for the future is a system of capitation, wherein an HMO or other insurer will seek to contract for ambulance service to all of its members at a capitated rate. That is, if an HMO has 10,000 members, and if it's expected that five percent

---

Box 5.2

Glossary of Provider Types

Fire Department—
Cross trained/dual role: Fire department-based responders trained as both firefighters and EMTs (basic, intermediate, or advanced). The same personnel may be used to perform both fire protection and EMS.
Separate service: Fire department-based EMS responders who may be sworn or uniformed personnel (and who may be classed as civilians) but who have no direct fire-suppression responsibilities.

Hospital Based—A hospital-owned and operated ambulance service.

Private—A privately owned, for-profit company or corporation engaged in the provision of medical transportation or EMS.

Public Utility Model (PUM)—A regulated-monopoly ambulance system that selects the exclusive provider based on a competitive procurement process. These systems are usually single tiered, providing emergency and non-emergency service with an all-ALS fleet. Commonly, a quasi-governmental entity supervises the contract and performs billing/collection services.

Third Service—
Municipal: Funded and operated by municipal government using local government employees. Not administered by the police or fire departments.
County: Funded and operated by county government using county government employees. Not administered by the police or fire departments.

of those members will require emergency ambulance transport in a given year, it may offer a contract to one or more ambulance providers to serve all of its members during that year for the total amount of $150,000. That would be an average of $300 per transport.

In this example, which is purely hypothetical, if the ambulance provider (or group of providers) who contracts with the HMO can profitably transport 500 patients—in accordance with the HMO's response time and clinical care standards for an up-front payment of $150,000—all parties should be satisfied. However, if more than 500 members require transport during the year, or if unexpected costs alter the ambulance provider's break-even point, it could suffer financial peril. On the other hand, if only 4.5 percent of the HMO's members require transport during the year, an extra $15,000 in profit could be realized.

Depending on the progress in healthcare reform, medical service areas (which could encompass numerous communities and portions of two or more counties) could be served by multiple HMOs, each of which would negotiate a capitated rate for its members. Or there may be a regional federal agency to control costs and serve as a single payer. In either event, traditional methods of billing and collecting for ambulance services may be changed radically. In the previous example of a capitated system, one check would be issued, in advance, for serving an estimated 500 people. The costs of billing those customers would be eliminated, as would the uncollectibles.

That's a simplistic example of how capitation could affect emergency ambulance service. For public ambulance services, the biggest question is whether the organization and its elected city or county officials can be flexible enough to accommodate this concept. In most areas, it would be necessary to form ambulance service cooperatives consisting of multiple providers. Numerous contracts between public agencies, and between public agencies and private ambulance companies, will be necessary to meet the demands of a capitated system.

The alternative is for an entire medical service area to be served by a single private ambulance service. That is probably the goal of the large companies that are consolidating the private ambulance industry. While the numbers of players and related agreements in a cooperative system may seem ominous, spreading the risks among numerous providers may be preferable to concentrating the potential for financial loss on one provider.

Conclusion

Growth of fire department ambulance services using dual-role, cross-trained personnel is likely, but not without competition from the private ambulance industry. Other public sector provider types, such as third-service and separate service fire department systems (using single-role personnel), are not likely to grow for economical reasons if nothing more, and may even lose ground in the foreseeable future. Regardless of provider type, however, the challenge to the public sector will be quickly understanding and adapting to the new order of healthcare reform.

Returning to the logic of the mayor who voted to replace a private ambulance company with a fire department emergency ambulance system, there are some responsibilities of government that are time sensitive and have life-or-death consequences. In the face of complex and confusing times and issues, such as healthcare reform, people tend to seek familiar and comfortable methods for meeting their basic needs. In the vast majority of communities where public agencies provide ambulance service, public opinion polls have rated those services at or near the top of the rankings.

Whether or not public agencies can find their place as ambulance service providers in the new order of healthcare delivery and finance, the role of first responder fire companies is not likely to change. One question remaining—the answer to which could hold the solution to public-private conflict over the delivery of ambulance service—is whether the value inherent in fire department first responder services will be compensated appropriately.

Source

Original article. James O. Page is an attorney and the publisher and editor-in-chief of JEMS. *He served as the executive director of the ACT (Advanced Coronary Treatment) Foundation and was appointed in 1973 by the governor of North Carolina to create and lead that state's EMS agency.*

The Future of Private EMS

Ron Myers

Ron Myers, former president of the American Ambulance Association and an entrepreneur, makes predictions for the future of private ambulance services.

PEOPLE MAY DISAGREE ABOUT THE BEST way to provide emergency medical services—public or private, third service or hospital based—but everyone agrees that EMS has changed radically in the last 20 years. Standards for training, technology, and performance are steadily rising. The public's expectation of rapid, quality emergency medical care has also risen as a result of convincing proof that quality EMS saves lives.

Most of today's EMS systems were designed nearly two decades ago. They were based on shifting assumptions of EMS demand patterns, funding resources, and production methods. Many of the systems structured during this period have not responded well to the new realities shaping the future of EMS: increasing public expectations of service, new OSHA regulations, dwindling federal tax support for local services, uncertainties surrounding the national debt, possible capitated payment plans, integrated delivery services, healthcare reform packages, and in all likelihood, a continuing taxpayer revolution.

My predictions for the future are based on experiences spanning over 25 years in the private ambulance sector, delivering emergency and non-emergency medical services. But anyone who tries to peer into the crystal ball risks offending certain segments of the community. My opinions are admittedly biased. However, I have had the privilege of working with the public sector for many years and have listened carefully to the concerns of all providers.

The private ambulance sector is just beginning to bud, and its growth within the next decade will be faster than in its previous 30 years. Two big reasons for this growth are the graying of America and the newly formed, publicly held companies now entering the EMS field. Multinational companies and venture capitalists are also entering the picture. This was unheard of only a few years ago.

These new players have been lured by predictions of explosive growth, but they will approach the EMS delivery methodology much differently than others have in the last two decades. With healthcare reform developing, a higher level of service will be expected with the same or fewer resources. It sounds like a recipe for failure, unless the industry is approached in a "non-traditional" manner.

The private sector can make this transformation in a number of ways. But let's first acknowledge that the public sector does an outstanding job in many communities; some services have diversified from the typical fire suppression staffing patterns into more modern EMS staffing patterns. Second, let's recognize that there are quality private ambulance services as well as services with poor standards. This discussion will focus on quality providers. Poor examples hurt the industry, and most will fall by the wayside as the industry experiences its own "global warming."

Many U.S. cities are experiencing serious financial difficulties and are challenged by their taxpayers to become more efficient at all levels— federal, state, and local. Local tax dollars in stagnant systems can no longer carry the EMS expense load. The public sector, volunteer systems, and even some community hospital-based services are being forced to bill for their services on top of what is already being paid through taxes. The demand for higher levels of customer service and accountability increases when the public believes it is paying twice. In addition to justifying charges and collections received, the public sector is no longer able to hide behind the shield of sovereign immunities and protections against malpractice or shortcomings of system performances.

When communities decide to go to bid or when their service delivery costs become excessive, opportunities will be created. Dissatisfied taxpayers will look towards privatization. The private sector couldn't be in a better position—and the investors know it!

Corporations with revenues of literally hundreds of millions of dollars, led by seasoned senior executives, will have greater vision, superb strategic planning, corporate positioning, and, above all, a proven philosophy toward internal and external customer service. These key elements will enable the private sector to position itself as the logical alternative choice for EMS.

These corporations bring numerous advantages that will help them offer superior service and maximize resources, strategic development, and creativity. Historically, these advantages have been rare within our industry. Sophisticated inventory control systems and huge group purchasing capabilities will help drive down the cost of service delivery and maximize results for the larger corporate players. The drive for marketplace consolidation, including acquisitions and mergers, has already begun and looms even larger in the future.

> The drive for marketplace consolidation, including acquisitions and mergers, has already begun and looms even larger in the future.

The Public/Private Partnership

I believe the future belongs to the public/private partnership, where public agencies contract with private services. The taxpayers and customers will win in this progressive style of EMS delivery.

In a true public/private partnership, an independent body that fully understands how to construct and administer an objective bid process prequalifies the bidding parties. Expectations shift toward heavier accountability and a clearer understanding of productivity and cost requirements. Additionally, all of these quality systems need an external oversight review process. Political motivations must be replaced by performance evaluations. Communities that have contracted with private sector services have held providers more accountable than their public counterparts. The providers, in turn, have worked well within the system design and achieved the expected performance standards.

The ambulance treatment and transport providers must collectively achieve clinical excellence and state-of-the-art response time reliability.

Public policymakers must evaluate their EMS systems to see if the taxpayer and end users are getting the most service for the lowest cost. These comparisons must be determined against a system's true cost. Both the fees charged to the user and the subsidized or contracted tax dollars must be included. Opportunities for contract bids and procurement will become an even bigger reality with taxpayer pressure.

The contract bid process does not need to be a battle, but rather an understanding of the true meaning of free enterprise: "The one who does the job best wins." The well-educated community will make the complex decisions. Each community should structure its request for proposal (RFP) with a solid system design that includes appropriate medical and financial oversight and offers a level playing field for all sectors. Once these things have been realized, consistent, quality performance and long-term financial stability are the community's rewards.

The American Ambulance Association developed a Needs Assessment Workshop in 1982, facilitated by Jim Page. In the years since then, the creation of a level playing field has occurred. There is now an accreditation model and process available for ambulance services. The Commission on Accreditation of Ambulance Services (CAAS) has evaluated at least 100 services as of this writing. Accreditation is not limited to the private sector, but open to all providers. The process is similar to that of the Joint Commission on Accreditation of Hospital Organizations (JCAHO). I predict that within five years the federal government will require that all services be nationally accredited in order to receive federal funds for service delivery (similar to hospital requirements).

The CAAS process has raised respect for providers who have met the standards. By simply going through the application process, providers have also improved their operation's quality of service. In all probability, CAAS accreditation will be a prerequisite for bidding on a municipal contract. With these factors in mind, and healthcare reform imminent, if you are not accredited or not preparing for accreditation, you will be sealing your own tomb.

An important component in any community's success is a partnership with a quality first responder program. Historically, the fire department has delivered this vital service, and I believe they should be reimbursed for their efforts.

The ambulance treatment and transport providers must collectively achieve clinical excellence and state-of-the-art response time reliability. This is not merely averaging response times, but making fractile percentage measurements that achieve a set minimum response time reliability. To accomplish this goal, the transport provider must use the industry's most advanced communications technology and equipment, and encourage working partnerships among local agencies. Financial penalties should be assessed for poor response times.

Private providers have a long history of working with both government and privately operated EMS systems throughout the United States.

These proven designs deliver the industry's highest level of EMS performance and efficiencies in cities like Kansas City, Mo., Richmond, Va., Tulsa and Oklahoma City, Okla., Las Vegas, Syracuse, N.Y., Fort Wayne, Ind., Little Rock, Ark, Fort Worth, Tex., and many other cities. They are managed by leaders with proven ability in both the public and private sectors. In these systems, the ambulance contractors charge for their services, but they receive little or no tax subsidies. In many cases, these were troubled systems before the public/private partnership took the reins and accomplished immediate and dramatic improvements. Thus, taxpayers benefited, employees benefited, and most importantly, patients benefited.

Some of these systems function without a union, while several have unions. Both the public and the private sectors will see an increase in unionization of field personnel. In many cases, and especially in larger systems, operations are facilitated by the presence of a union. However, it is extremely important that labor leaders understand the emerging changes within the industry. Unions must also avoid work rules that can entangle the service, making it inefficient. They must refrain from creating any "featherbedding" jobs that are not productive.

Traditional Versus Non-Traditional Performance

The private ambulance sector has, for the most part, focused on one thing—ambulance service. This has generally set the sector apart from multi-service providers. The single focus has played a large role in the success private providers have enjoyed over the past 10 years. Non-traditional methodologies have been developed for improved performance.

Communities have shouldered the public sector with many responsibilities, including fire suppression, fire inspections, general public safety, evacuation and extrication services, EMS, first responder services, disaster coordination, hazardous materials, incident command, and many other services. Increased technology has reduced the need for fire suppression services, resulting in a shift toward EMS. However, EMS is being used to justify many fire department budgets. Unfortunately, in many cases, tradition has remained where changes are needed. For those guilty of becoming too expensive, underutilized, and overstaffed, the day of reconciliation will arrive.

Medium to high EMS call volume does not require traditional fire suppression scheduling—24-hour shifts. In a moderate to high demand system, 24-hour shifts are inefficient and often dangerous for the patients and personnel. They create increased fatigue, diminished clinical care efficiency, driving hazards, and lowered customer service standards. The public sector, in some systems, has adjusted its approach and started the process of change. If public sector providers continue to address the issues of efficiency and break away from tradition, they will continue to control the treatment and transportation methodologies of patients in their communities.

Primary healthcare services will become a major issue in value-added services when communities contract for EMS over the next decade.

The private sector's approach to EMS offers somewhat of a philosophical difference. The private sector believes that providing the service is not an issue of control or ownership, but a privilege and an earned right to serve the community. The private provider wants the opportunity to earn *the right* to serve communities that wish to contract their EMS systems. The EMS community knows that a single provider group or agency does not make the system work all by itself. Everyone, public and private sector, volunteers, hospital-based services, physicians, nurses, and even the National Guard and police officers, have a role and a responsibility to do the right thing for the community. All must operate effectively and efficiently for improved patient care. These are the major elements that will keep EMS an appreciating asset to our communities.

The Challenge for Excellence

Hands-on providers must meet the challenge of creating a clinical difference. Go for alphabet soup: Obtain all the extra certifications you possibly can, in addition to paramedic certification. Additional certifications and training, such as a specialization in pediatric advanced life support, basic cardiac life support, advanced cardiac life support, and so forth, will stretch the minimum standards.

A move toward advanced primary healthcare services will become a reality and a key issue in the healthcare reform packages within the next several years. Discussions about the pros and cons of physician extenders in the field have already begun. Primary healthcare services will become a major issue in value-added services when communities contract for EMS over the next decade.

Concepts never even imagined 10 years ago are just around the corner: mobile minor treatment services, including portable X-rays and the suturing of minor wounds on scene; follow-up doctor visits scheduled by computer; and more. These advances will help solve overcrowding in emergency departments and will speed up patient care services for minor illnesses and injuries. Additional training and certification through accredited colleges and teaching facilities will be explored for hands-on providers. The pressure to excel is on, and only time will tell how many communities will take the lead.

Dawn of Opportunity

I believe that the dawn of opportunity for private sector EMS is before us. Companies that run a professional, well-organized service will advance in many communities. It will be extremely important that they spend sizable dollar amounts and resources on educating their management teams and personnel. Communications will be a key survival issue for internal operational competency and meeting customer needs.

The goal is to become progressive and non-traditional. A vigorous approach toward hard work and appreciation for services delivered will make the difference in the next 10 years. Years ago, former EMS consultant Jack Stout predicted, "There eventually will be an 'oligopoly.'" In other words, a few providers will be serving most of the industry. There won't be just one provider type; however, major corporations will control a large part of the market share with only a small number of providers, similar to how the airline industry is structured today. With competent and reasonable regulation, and minimal government interference, public policymakers will create a level playing field and design excellence for EMS in their communities.

I believe the public and private sectors will eventually realize that the public/private partnership is the best model available for the benefit of our communities. The public's interests are best served when EMS systems are designed to deliver maximum performance at the lowest possible cost. In the midst of public pressures from both financial issues and various special interest groups, community leaders must remain committed to ensuring optimum quality and efficiency in EMS. I believe this is the new reality facing public policymakers. Predicting the future, however, is like nailing Jell-O to a post; it's tough to do.

Source

Original article. Ron Myers has been involved in private ambulance service since 1967. He is the immediate past president of the American Ambulance Association and the Ohio Ambulance Association.

Hospital-Based EMS Systems Evolve

Janet Blum

Hospital-based EMS system program director Janet Blum provides a vision for medical transportation services that supports hospital-based programs of the future.

NATIONAL HEALTHCARE REFORM IS CREATING an unprecedented restructuring of the healthcare system in the United States. Just as hospitals must change to achieve the goals of universal access, cost containment, and delivery of a quality product, medical transportation services must begin to transition into models that support healthcare network formation.

The manner in which transportation services will be provided in the future may differ depending on the geographic area and available resources. Rural and urban areas may develop dramatically different medical transportation delivery systems based on the transport needs of each region. What is certain, however, is that medical transportation systems must begin to view themselves as a part of larger healthcare systems, aligning transport service with hospital networks and regional health alliances. This network formation goes hand-in-hand with the concept of managed competition now being implemented in regions and states.

Managed Competition

To understand why medical transportation systems must begin to be integrated into hospital networks, one must first understand how healthcare reform is shaping healthcare delivery. Although individual states will have considerable flexibility in the implementation of healthcare plans, the basic benefit package and the method of financing premiums will be set at the national level.

Managed competition is the core concept behind federal healthcare reform. Under managed competition, large consumer purchasing cooperatives will be formed to negotiate for packages of healthcare services at fixed prices. All individuals within the purchasing cooperatives will be guaranteed healthcare coverage regardless of employment, personal resources, or pre-existing medical conditions. The purchasing cooperatives will negotiate with healthcare providers or networks for the most comprehensive healthcare package at the best price.

Although a basic benefit package for everyone will be mandated, healthcare networks will be motivated to provide additional and augmented services to receive and retain the purchasing cooperative contracts. These healthcare packages will include hospitalization, physicians services, prescription drugs, and some mental health and substance abuse coverage. Preventive services, such as routine medical exams and health education programs, will be the cornerstone of healthcare cost containment.

Although medical transportation services have not been specifically addressed, it is reasonable to assume that some level of medical transportation will be included as part of the basic healthcare benefit package. Consumer purchasing cooperatives seeking to acquire the most comprehensive benefit package for members would be wise to include medical transportation services in the bidding process. Hospital networks that can offer comprehensive medical transportation services to purchasing cooperative members will have a distinct advantage over those systems that do not.

Network Formation

Hospitals anticipating the formation of consumer purchasing cooperatives are considering ways to provide comprehensive health services within fixed budgets, while ensuring the high quality of services to patients. Clearly, hospitals that can achieve these goals will be the survivors of the reform era. Prudent hospital administrators are positioning their institutions to adapt to healthcare reform legislation through the formation of healthcare networks. Network relationships are taking a variety of forms. Hospital systems comprising tertiary and community hospitals are affiliated to pool resources. Hospital and physician partnerships are occurring. Payers are also examining new relationships with hospitals and physicians, creating new organizations able to bid hospital and physician services to the purchasing cooperatives.

Hospital networks are forming in an effort to control costs through the consolidation of services. Combining these hospital networks with associated services will encourage the centralization of advanced technologies and specialized services within tertiary institutions. The proliferation of sophisticated and expensive technologies will be contained by the mandate to operate efficiently within the fixed budgets created through the competition for purchasing cooperative contracts. The end result will be a need for medical transportation systems that can access technology centers from community hospitals with referral relationships within the network. Comprehensive medical transportation systems will become a critical component of hospital network formation. Centralization of technology and specialty medical services cannot occur without patient access.

Medical Transportation Services Within Hospital Networks

Healthcare reform is occurring, and hospital networks will be the driving force in the provision of services. What is changing for hospitals is the scope of services that will be mandated by the purchasing cooperatives. The preferred provider will be the hospital network that can offer comprehensive health services ranging from routine eye exams through open heart surgery. Medical transportation will become another service that individual hospitals or hospital networks will have to offer when bidding for purchasing cooperative contracts.

As hospitals establish regional networks of tertiary and community

> Hospital networks that can offer comprehensive medical transportation services to purchasing cooperative members will have a distinct advantage over those systems that do not.

Existing medical transportation systems should be positioning themselves, much as hospital networks are doing, to provide a full range of medical transportation services that support regional healthcare systems.

hospitals, the existence of quality medical transportation systems becomes critical. A key element of reform is ensuring the quality of healthcare within the framework of cost containment and universal access. As tertiary medical institutions become the focus of advanced technology that supports primary care community hospitals, quality medical transportation services must be available to transport emergency and non-emergency patients. The concept of quality transportation implies that the needs of the patients are matched by the appropriate transport modality and staff within a time frame that ensures optimal patient outcome. These key quality indicators require an integrated level of medical transportation that is not currently available in most systems.

Many hospitals currently support fragmented portions of an integrated medical transportation system. Most tertiary medical centers operate or support helicopter air ambulance or mobile intensive care unit services. Community hospitals are typically involved in supporting local volunteer or private ambulance services, either through direct funding or in-kind services. Rarely, however, does any integration of services between ground and air EMS systems operating within a region occur, resulting in duplication of services, inconsistent standards of quality, and fragmented access to the medically appropriate transportation service. Unfortunately, medical transportation services are often placed in a competitive role with each other rather than in a collaborative arrangement that focuses on making decisions appropriate to patient condition and available resources. An integrated system, which incorporates ground and air transport, ensures that the competitive issues are removed from patient decision making since there is a singular organization ensuring consistent quality medical transportation. Medically appropriate transport decisions can be made based on patient condition and availability of resources within the regional network.

Given that medical transportation will be required to support hospital network formation, two options exist for progressive hospital networks that wish to provide transport services. Networks will either develop internal medical transportation systems or will contract with existing independent providers offering comprehensive transport services. Existing medical transportation systems should be positioning themselves, much as hospital networks are doing, to provide a full range of medical transportation services that support regional healthcare systems.

Components of an Integrated Medical Transportation System

The components of an integrated medical transportation system include helicopters, fixed-wing air ambulances, and ground ambulances. Helicopters can transport those critically ill or injured patients who benefit from rapid transport or are inaccessible to ground ambulances. Fixed-wing air ambulance is capable of patient access and egress over long distances where extended ground transportation would negatively impact the patient's condition. Ground ambulances encompass both interhospital and prehospital services. Mobile intensive care ground ambulances offer hospital-equivalent intensive care en route, with the appropriate medical and nursing staff. Prehospital services are tiered to provide emergency access to services required by ill or injured patients and include advanced and basic life support units. All transportation modalities should be available within a hospital subsidiary transportation division or through a contract with an independent provider.

Another key component of an integrated medical transportation system is the communication center. A centralized communication center that triages, dispatches, and tracks location of ground and air ambulances becomes the focal point for interhospital transport within the network. Referring hospitals benefit from integrated, full-service transportation systems where one telephone call results in the patient being appropriately transported.

Additional components of an integrated medical transportation system include support services such as centralized billing and collections, management, and dispatch. The goal of an integrated system should be to achieve appropriate utilization of resources, control costs, and avoid resource duplication.

Source

Original article. Janet Blum is the program director for NorthFlight in Traverse City, Mich. The Traverse City program is a regional, integrated air and ground medical transportation system.

Benefits of Integrated Medical Transportation Systems to Hospital Networks

Integrated medical transportation systems are an implied component of healthcare reform that enables the centralization of technology by providing for the movement of patients between network hospitals. Hospital networks that support these full-service transportation systems will have an advantage in securing purchasing cooperative contracts. Patients will benefit from the care delivered by qualified staff working with appropriate equipment during transport between community hospitals and referral centers. The emphasis of healthcare reform on the prevention of illness or injury is supported by integrated transport networks, which improve patient outcome through the provision of appropriate care during transport, ultimately saving healthcare dollars.

A regionally integrated medical transportation system is expensive. To support this sophisticated transport system, cost containment and collaboration on a regional basis are required to sustain the spectrum of services, ranging from helicopter through basic life support transport. This level of cost containment is achieved through consolidation of existing services, such as competing helicopter systems, and reallocation of resources based on a regional needs assessment. Cost savings are achieved through centralization of such services as communication centers, management, billing, and purchasing. The end results are comprehensive medical transportation systems that support the establishment of hospital networks and facilitate excellence in patient transport in a cost-effective method.

What Does the Future Hold?

Jay Fitch, PhD

EMS systems have evolved rapidly and the pace of change is steadily increasing. In this original article, Dr. Jay Fitch describes why he believes EMS is dancing with destiny. He outlines 10 paradigm shifts that EMS will experience before the twenty-first century.

WE ARE LIVING IN ONE OF THOSE RARE times when divergent forces come together, offering exciting possibilities. What was the sense of purpose that propelled EMS forward in its developmental stages? Are those forces still present? If so, how can they be maximized? If not, how can they be reclaimed? Is EMS prone to go the way of the dinosaur in the impending evolution of society and healthcare? Or will EMS systems resemble chameleons, those adaptable animals who alter their color to blend with the changing environment?

Like the Dinosaurs, EMS Is Dancing With Destiny

EMS systems that have lost the excitement of discovery and lack an action orientation at every organizational level have much in common with dinosaurs. Both have a long and proud tradition. Both consumed large amounts of the resources and food around them. Both have had a long-lasting impact on the world. And both became endangered species. Will many of our EMS systems also become extinct?

No one knows scientifically why dinosaurs became extinct. One theory is that they simply could not adapt to their changing environment. It may be that even though food was plentiful, the dinosaur became nearsighted and couldn't see it, or got lazy and wouldn't reach for the food.

Many EMS systems today have the same problem. Like the dinosaurs, they have voracious appetites. So much time and energy is spent foraging for fiscal and political resources that fundamental service responsibilities are forgotten. Many systems are unaware that the world is radically changing. They are unwilling to look for resources in different locations or use what they have more wisely. Either foolish pride or nearsightedness keeps leaders from changing the ways in which they lead their organizations. And like the dinosaurs, EMS systems are dancing with their destiny.

Unfortunately, a number of EMS systems today are waiting for someone else to ensure their survival. In the 1960s, there were pioneering physicians, firefighters, and ambulance owners who were farsighted enough to dream of what was possible. Like small creeks that flow into mighty rivers, the dreams of leaders eventually shape the course of history. What dreams can you share today that may shape the course of history for the future of EMS?

My wish for the future is that "EMS Leaders—the Next Generation" will remember the prime directive, that is, to develop and sustain sophisticated, future-oriented EMS systems that are clinically effective, operationally efficient, and—at the same time—cost effective. I believe that we can retool traditional and dying EMS systems to dance with our destiny. The dance will not be easy, and it will require smashing more than just a few paradigms.

EMS Paradigms

A paradigm is an assumption, belief, idea, value, or expectation that forms a filter through which we make meaning out of life, create structure and process, view information, and make value judgments. This filter contains the rules and regulations by which we see reality. A paradigm sets the boundaries within which we are willing to process information and helps us solve problems. Our paradigms are what allow us to accept or cause us to reject new ideas, or keep us from seeing information in a new way. Our paradigms must change if we are to understand what is happening today and help shape the future.

Ten basic assumptions form the filter through which I see the future of EMS. I do not share them in order to lift them up as the only way to filter reality. By the time you read this, the list will have expanded and contracted several times based on my new learnings and the expansion of my paradigm boundaries.

- There is no one "best" system design.
- Patients will be seen as customers rather than victims.
- EMS will be more closely allied with the integrated healthcare system of the future.
- New internal partnerships will be forged between leaders and co-workers.
- The EMS workforce will be more diverse.
- Medical tasks and skills for EMS will be different.
- Reimbursement methods will shift significantly.
- If systems only improve what they are doing, they will fail.
- Bureaucracies and traditional practices that have stagnated EMS will be reshaped.
- EMS systems that will survive in the twenty-first century will initiate radical changes before the year 2001.

If these 10 assumptions are the filter through which you approach EMS leadership, what changes would you consider making in the style or tasks of your leadership? For a moment, set aside traditional practices and the personal assumptions that you have built your career on, and take a fresh, objective look at *new* paradigms for EMS leadership. Making a few adjustments here and there will not help. If we simply continue to do what we have done in the past, we will become increasingly irrelevant, and over time, extinct.

Making the Paradigm Shifts

The "best" system design. So often we get locked into the thought pattern that "our way" of providing EMS is the best way or the only way.

The best system is the one that is planned based on the unique needs of a community.

It simply isn't so. We must break that paradigm and realize there is no one right system design or method of providing EMS.

The best system is the one that is planned based on the unique needs of a community. Objective consideration must be given to the socioeconomic, demographic, geographic, and political dynamics of the community. In addition, existing services, service history, system oversight and safeguards, resource availability, and a multitude of other factors must be expertly blended to create a well-designed system.

Patients will be seen as customers rather than victims. The "S" in EMS stands for service. Service must be first. When patients are viewed as something less than valued customers, we devalue the patient and, ultimately, ourselves. Over time, we can become hardened, eventually treating customers as victims. Soon after, the system becomes a victim of its own callousness and insensitivity.

The system serves many customers. Co-workers are often the forgotten customer. The new paradigm requires that the service value all members of the team for the potential contribution they can make.

EMS will be more closely allied with the integrated healthcare system of the future. Crystal ball gazing may be futile in an unpredictable world. But many predict that healthcare will become significantly more integrated in the next decade. Hospitals are closing and merging at a record pace. Physician practices and other support services are being acquired. Major tertiary care centers are establishing networks, reaching out hundreds of miles in some cases. The entire healthcare system is being horizontally and vertically integrated to achieve cost savings.

Both public and private agencies must recognize that the deep-seated commitment to independence and autonomy may be their Achilles' heel in dealing with the integrated health networks of the future.

New internal partnerships will be forged between leaders and co-workers. Staff members will be treated neither as consumable items nor have their development constrained by dysfunctional labor agreements or past experiences. Instead they will be considered professionals and colleagues.

Some EMS services have rightfully earned the reputation as places where workers are stressed out, suffer from brown-out or burnout, or are otherwise professionally consumed. Other services have been likened to dysfunctional families, scarred by past abusive relationships and never able to break free to experience a fulfilling life. Neither is a place where you would choose to work.

Stress-related brown-out, rust-out, and burnout are all symptoms of arrested professional development in both the public and private sectors. They are common responses to non-stimulating environments. Brown-out refers to the intellectual "lights" being dimmed over time. Rust-out involves an organization's failure to appropriately involve or use the workers' energy. As a result, interest wanes. Often, rusted-out employees stay on the job but seek outside interests or employment. Burnout refers to the end-stage process in which an EMS employee can no longer be functional within the organization due to increasing levels of frustration or mental stress.

Vibrant EMS systems and their people are constantly learning, growing, and changing. As we move toward the twenty-first century, the distinction between worker and leader will be reduced. More workers will lead and more leaders will work in ways more visible to other workers. Leadership will become an increasingly shared responsibility among all members of the team.

The EMS workforce will be more diverse, and both minorities and women will be welcome. By the year 2001, one in four people in the United States will be non-white, making the emerging society the most diverse ever, according to *American Demographics* magazine. Currently, non-whites represent less than five percent of the nation's EMS workforce. This must change if EMS is to meet the challenge of recruitment needs. Minorities will be the largest growing segment of the EMS workforce.

The male-dominated world is disappearing outside our profession, and the "glass ceiling" that has kept women out of top fire department and EMS jobs is being broken. John Naisbitt, author of the book *Megatrends 2000*, indicates that women are increasingly taking their rightful leadership positions and have established themselves in future-oriented industries.

Inclusiveness will replace racism and sexism in EMS systems of the future.

Medical tasks and skills required for EMS will be different. As ALS skills are further compressed into the basic EMT's role, there are persistent questions about the clinical efficacy of full paramedic systems. Some believe that these changes will ultimately lead to a lower level of care that is more technical than professional. In contrast, skill expansion for paramedics has historically not been viewed as a priority. In the healthcare system of the future, paramedics with expanded skills may offer an entirely new dimension of service.

Rural EMS systems may become the best laboratory for expanded skills. Poor access to primary care offers an opportunity to develop radically different classifications of EMS/primary care workers. Urban, suburban, or rural, the EMS system must shift paradigms about its appropriate clinical roles and responsibilities if it does not want to become extinct.

Reimbursement methods will shift significantly. Most EMS systems are compensated through a mix of local tax dollars and user fees. That may radically change in the next decade. At a minimum, leaders can expect that the mix of tax support and user fees will continue to fluctuate.

Currently, EMS is paid for its services only when patient transport service is provided. There are no financial incentives to reduce transports. But under managed care, the key goal is to keep group members healthy and reduce utilization. As reimbursement incentives change to accomplish this goal, the EMS profession will be reshaped.

According to Laidlaw Medical Transportation Executive Don Jones,

> Vibrant EMS systems and their people are constantly learning, growing, and changing.

managed care organizations will become the largest payer for EMS services. The financial and operational results of that change could be profound. In 1994, there were over 300 multi-facility healthcare systems and 45 million Americans in some form of managed care.

In the future, EMS may be paid on a capitated prospective payment plan instead of on a fee-for-service basis. Simply defined, capitated payment means receiving a flat rate per enrollee, regardless of how much service they require.

If systems only improve what they are doing, they will fail. Many public and private EMS systems have become dysfunctional organizations, unable to cope with the increasing pace of change. Leaders of the organizations believe they are making progress and will eventually reach their goal. Unfortunately, by the time they reach the destination, the next leg of the journey is already underway. They will never catch up.

Incremental change, in which slow, steady progress is made, will not keep the organization viable in the future. Change is occurring at a much more rapid pace than ever before—clinically, operationally, and financially. EMS programs must not only improve what they have been doing, they must seek out new service opportunities, methods, and mechanisms.

Bureaucracies and traditional practices that have stagnated EMS will be reshaped. In other service industries, red tape is being reduced drastically. Organizations are streamlining everything to be more responsive. Institutions that cling to their bureaucracies are beginning to vanish.

The days of managing by rule making and other bureaucratic practices are as out of step with today's employees as a kitchen is without a microwave. And, although there has been movement toward meaningfully involving people in decisions that affect their future, this single area is resisted most by managers. Many older managers see this as a reduction in their organizational power. Unfortunately, failing to effectively energize workers impacts (and stagnates) almost every other aspect of the EMS organization.

In short, leading tomorrow's EMS organization requires recognizing and developing healthy responses to the changing needs within the workplace.

EMS systems that will survive in the twenty-first century will initiate radical changes before the year 2001. The transmission and reception of both knowledge and information are experiencing a series of quantum leaps. Change is a difficult and complex task that also occurs in quantum leaps. To be able to meet the demands of the future, start early.

When flying, for example, it is not uncommon to experience rough air or bad weather. The pilot proactively reviews weather forecasts, listens to the experience of other pilots ahead on the route, and tries to avoid the storm by anticipating the need to change altitude or direction. The most comfortable flights are those in which the pilot correctly anticipates the need for a change in altitude and executes that change before getting into the middle of the storm.

Likewise, EMS leaders will find it valuable to begin the change process early. Anticipate what will be required to survive and thrive, and seek the correct altitude early. Once in the middle of the storm, the risk of a crash for the system or the leader's career increases exponentially.

Breaking Through

Thinking about new paradigms and what the future holds can provide a pulse-quickening "high." It may be the stimulus needed to reconnect with the original reasons you became involved with EMS or provide the courage to leave if you no longer feel connected.

I have found both passion and energy in exploring and renewing my understanding that the "S" in EMS stands for a seven- rather than a four-letter word. For me, the "S" stands for finding new ways to be of service to other human beings in their time of need.

On a broader level, increasing individual commitment—coupled with energized leadership—can make a dramatic difference for the EMS profession. It may be the stimulus required to make the clinical, operational, and fiscal changes necessary for EMS to avoid extinction.

In any time of transition, such as EMS is now experiencing, there is an opportunity for those willing to accept, embrace, and lead the change process. While some individuals' careers and EMS systems may become extinct, most can—like chameleons—adapt to the challenges and thrive in the new EMS paradigm. Indeed, like dinosaurs, we are dancing with our destiny.

Source

Original article.

Case 5

The Richmond System Transformation

City officials knew that things were not going well in EMS. The public safety director determined that a full review of the system, including the city's contract with a private ambulance firm, was in order.

In the meantime, the Richmond, Va., EMS system teetered on the brink of collapse. Several years before, a number of private firms bid on and accepted a poorly structured city contract that split the city into response zones. Several zones were served by private firms, and others were served by volunteer rescue squads. Another private firm's contract was canceled after its owner was convicted of Medicaid fraud. The city asked Central Virginia Ambulance Service to assume that zone. The pressure on the company increased. The city underfunded the system and failed to provide adequate oversight and support. Medics were overworked, medical equipment was not available, ambulances were being repossessed, and the list went on. The outlook was grim.

When the consulting team arrived for the first meeting, city officials were discussing the option of calling in the National Guard to provide emergency coverage if the service abruptly ceased operations. It was quickly surmised that the National Guard's resources were not suited for such an operation. The fire department was not well positioned to support an emergency takeover, as there were only a handful of EMTs working there. Volunteer services from outside the area were willing to provide temporary assistance, but officials knew that this limited coverage would only last three or four days.

Crisis Contingency Plan

A crisis contingency plan was quietly prepared. Officials did not want their planning actions to further weaken the system. The private service was approaching insolvency. Failure to make payroll would trigger a media feeding frenzy and further undermine the fragile condition of the company. It was critical to extend the planning time so that officials could adequately complete emergency plans and evaluate options for the future. The city's monthly subsidy payments were changed to be paid biweekly to ensure that there were funds available to cover payroll. Ultimately, the company defaulted on its contract and a negotiated early termination was effected to coincide with the city's readiness to provide service.

City officials wanted to preserve their future system configuration options during the initial transition period. An interim system was created to manage operations and obtain the operational and financial data necessary for decisions related to long-term development of a stable system.

The Transition

During the transition, hundreds of decisions were made and then acted upon. The city invested $3.2 million in capital equipment and an additional million to fund the negative working capital required. A headquarters building was acquired and renovated, a medical control board was established, and the volunteer squads were assisted in upgrading to ALS status and becoming full members of the system.

System design constraints were reviewed and a variety of design options were objectively laid out. Difficult public policy decisions had to be made. Should the system continue to be private, be operated by the fire department or some other public agency, or become a regulated public utility?

Ultimately, the council requested that the consultants implement a modified public utility model system. The decision was based on the city's desire to ensure high-quality care at a reasonable price without day-to-day management responsibilities. In this approach, the hardware and other "system" components were kept in the public sector, while the responsi-

Chronology of Events

1985	"Zone system" with two private providers and four volunteer squads.
1987	One private provider convicted of Medicaid fraud; Central Virginia Ambulance Service assumes all private zones with no additional subsidy.
October 1989	City awards consultant RFP to review system.
November 1989	Consultant assessment begins as provider instability increases.
December 1989	Seriousness of situation communicated to city; provider ability to meet payroll questionable; city manager orders emergency plan development.
January 1990	Negotiations with provider to avoid insolvency and system failure.
February 1990	City council briefings; direction given to stabilize system; consultants negotiate with lien holders to avoid repossession of ambulances and equipment; preliminary agreement reached with provider to terminate agreement and take over system; city request that consultants manage interim system for 12- to 18-month development period.
March 1990	City creates nonprofit corporation to manage regional EMS system with council appointing the board of directors; system transition occurs smoothly.
July 1990	New vehicles and equipment begin arriving; ongoing discussion with volunteers about upgrading to ALS; medical control board appointed and begins meeting.
August 1990	System design specifications (RFP) process under way; first responder program plan developed.
December 1990	Pre-bid conference held; install and train on new CAD; response times improved.
January 1991	Search for executive director underway.
February 1991	Move to renovated headquarters building.
March 1991	Contractor selected; contract negotiated; council approval.
May 1991	State legislation introduced converting nonprofit corporation to government authorized ambulance authority.
July 1991	Contractor begins service; new authority director assumes responsibilities.

bility for managing the quality and operational aspects of the system were handled by a private company.

The Procurement Process

Implementing this option required a national competitive procurement process to select an operations contractor. As this process began, the system was "tuned" to demonstrate its ability to perform clinically, operationally, and financially.

The procurement process was both complex and comprehensive. Specifications for the contract ran several hundred pages. Potential bidders submitted qualifications statements. Although a number of firms expressed interest in bidding, many were not qualified. Following an objective review of their credentials, qualified firms submitted final proposals. The final step in the selection process was an oral presentation before the selection committee. The selection committee independently scored the proposals and presentations and selected Mercy Services of Grand Rapids, Mich., as the contractor.

According to city officials, the Richmond EMS system has been successful beyond what they initially thought possible. It continues to grow and evolve.

Case Questions

1. What were some of the underlying system design factors that may have contributed to the downfall of Central Virginia Ambulance Service?
2. What other actions could the city have taken to avoid a system collapse?
3. What other system design solutions could Richmond have used?
4. What was the reason given that the city implemented a modified public utility model?
5. Why is the procurement process with this type of system more complex?

Appendix: Case Study Summaries

CASES BASED ON THE EDITOR'S experiences and published media accounts have been used to illustrate the key points found in each section of *Prehospital Care Administration: Issues, Readings, Cases.* As is common with leadership issues, there are no definitively right or wrong answers to the questions presented at the end of each case. The cases all contain general EMS leadership concepts and practices that readers should be able to assimilate and articulate.

The following summarizes each case's issues and dimensions.

Case 1: What's a Supervisor to Do?

This case presents several issues related to managing human resources in an emergency medical services organization. It asks readers to evaluate their services' written policies and determine how those policies would guide them in deciding whether to terminate or rehabilitate an impaired employee.

Another dimension of the case relates to management information systems. The point made is that it is easier to recognize and deal with a performance problem in its early stages if systems are in place to ensure the supervisor is aware of the problem.

Also illustrated is the importance of planning how to investigate the matter, of understanding due process issues, and of preparing for both administrative and media review of actions taken.

Case 2: When Turf Wars Prevail

This case illustrates a number of operational components required for effective EMS systems. Readers are to use their own experiences to reflect on decisions made and potential opportunities for improving patient care and service.

The case highlights the negative clinical implications of a call screening system and asks the reader to identify key decision points and actions that could be taken by various participants to improve the system. It makes the point that the entire system could be improved significantly if individual provider agencies focused on developing the system rather than on protecting their own turf.

Case 3: Medicare Mistakes Can Be Costly

Case 3 presents two examples of how the Medicare program adjudicated compliance errors associated with Health Care Finance Administration regulations.

Readers are asked to outline the similarities and differences of the two examples. Other dimensions of the case include an analysis of the Medicare violations committed, processes that services should use to avoid violations, and steps that should be taken when administrators are notified of a pending Medicare investigation.

Case 4: How Much Is a Life Worth, Anyway?

In this case, two services that fail to adequately monitor clinical systems are mired in litigation and negative publicity. Addressed is the administrators' responsibility in preventing, investigating, and mitigating these situations.

The case makes the point that there are strong financial penalties for failing to manage services in a manner that reduces potential exposures.

Case 5: The Richmond System Transformation

This case describes a major system redesign. Underlying factors that may have contributed to the original system's failure are discussed. The case then asks readers to identify alternative actions and system designs.

The case also illustrates that the process of changing an EMS system in a major city is complex and time-consuming. Readers are asked to draw upon several of the readings from the section to identify system design and procurement issues.

Index

This subject index is designed to complement the size of this book and better enable the reader to find pertinent topics. The topics below are discussed within the specific pages listed.

About the Editor

DR. JAY FITCH IS PRESIDENT of Fitch & Associates, Inc., and has served as a firefighter, volunteer, EMT, paramedic, director, consultant, and author. He has been at the forefront of EMS for 20 years.

Over the past 10 years, Fitch & Associates has become the most widely utilized consulting firm in EMS, serving clients in 45 states and numerous foreign countries. Dr. Fitch has worked extensively in the areas of EMS system design, procurement, and operations management, and is known for shaping organizational thinking with a low-key, hands-on approach.

Dr. Fitch holds a doctorate in psychology, as well as degrees in public administration and adult education. He also holds the professional designation "Certified Healthcare Consultant" conferred by the American Association of Healthcare Consultants. His previously published books include *EMS Management: Beyond the Street* and the *Service First* quality improvement series.